Traumatic Brain Injury

Jack W. Tsao
Editor

Traumatic Brain Injury

A Clinician's Guide to Diagnosis, Management, and Rehabilitation

Springer

Editor
Jack W. Tsao, MD, DPhil, FAAN
Traumatic Brain Injury Programs (M96)
Wounded, Ill, & Injured Directorate
US Navy Bureau of Medicine and Surgery
Washington, DC, USA

Department of Neurology
Uniformed Services University of the Health Sciences
Bethesda, MD, USA

ISBN 978-1-4939-3968-8 ISBN 978-0-387-87887-4 (eBook)
DOI 10.1007/978-0-387-87887-4
Springer New York Heidelberg Dordrecht London

Softcover re-print of the Hardcover 1st edition 2012

Printed on acid-free paper

Springer is part of Springer Science+Business Media (www.springer.com)

For Emmanuel and Veronica

Preface

Traumatic Brain Injury: A Clinician's Guide to Diagnosis, Management, and Rehabilitation was written to enable medical professionals to quickly learn about the latest issues and treatments in this evolving clinical field. Traumatic brain injury (TBI) has been labeled one of the "signature injuries" of the military conflicts in Iraq and Afghanistan and in the USA, and the rise in public awareness of combat-related brain injuries has coincided with awareness of the potential long-term consequences of sports concussions. This book was developed as a result of a course on TBI which I directed for the American Academy of Neurology (one of the professional associations of neurologists in the United States) in 2008.

The term "TBI" describes a spectrum of injury ranging from mild (typically called "concussion") to moderate and severe (including penetrating brain injuries). Most TBI cases are of the mild variety, so the book focuses on this particular area. Readers will note that chapters discuss the most common clinical sequelae following TBI. The chapter authors were asked to summarize the key findings, issues, and treatments in their areas of expertise to enable this book to serve as a guide for busy clinicians managing patients with head injuries. To address a wide readership, initial chapters focus on acute clinical management including intensive care, imaging, neurocognitive testing, and sports and battlefield concussions. Later chapters discuss treatment of sleep disturbance, vestibular symptoms, headaches, seizures, and mental health consequences which might be seen after TBI. Finally, the book concludes with chapters on rehabilitation, including cognitive therapy, and gaps in knowledge with future research directions. As an aide to the clinician, an appendix reviewing ICD coding for TBI is also included.

I would like to thank my family for their support in the writing and editing process and Brian Belval, who was my initial publishing editor and who convinced me to take on the role of book editor.

Finally, as many of the authors of this book are United States military officers or government employees, it remains for me to issue a blanket disclaimer:

The opinions or assertions contained herein are the private views of the authors and are not to be construed as official or as reflecting the views of the Departments of the Navy or Army, the Department of Defense, or the Department of Veterans Affairs.

Bethesda, MD, USA Jack W. Tsao

Contents

Contributors

Aimee L. Alphonso, B.S. Department of Orthopedics and Rehabilitation, Walter Reed National Military Medical Center, Bethesda, MD, USA

Rocco A. Armonda, M.D. Department of Surgery (Neurosurgery), Uniformed Services University of the Health Sciences, Bethesda, MD, USA

Randy Bell, M.D. Department of Surgery (Neurosurgery), Uniformed Services University of the Health Sciences, Bethesda, MD, USA

John Betjemann, M.D. Department of Clinical Neurology, University of California at San Francisco, San Francisco, CA, USA

Justin S. Campbell, Ph.D. U.S. Navy Space and Naval Warfare Systems Pacific, San Diego, CA, USA

Anthony J.-W. Chen, M.D. Department of Neurology, VA Northern California Health Care System and University of California at San Francisco, San Francisco, CA, USA

Robert L. Collins, Ph.D., A.B.P.P. Neurology Care Line, Michael E. DeBakey VA Medical Center, Houston, TX, USA,

Department of Neurology, Baylor College of Medicine, Houston, TX, USA

Jay C. Erickson, M.D. Neurology Service, Madigan Army Medical Center, Tacoma, WA, USA

Alisa D. Gean, M.D. Department of Radiology, San Francisco General Hospital, University of California, San Francisco, San Francisco, CA, USA

Department of Neurological Surgery, San Francisco General Hospital, University of California, San Francisco, San Francisco, CA, USA

Brain and Spinal Injury Center (BASIC), San Francisco General Hospital, San Francisco, CA, USA

Division of Neuroradiology, 1X55, San Francisco General Hospital, San Francisco, CA, USA

Mel B. Glenn, M.D. Department of Physical Medicine and Rehabilitation, Harvard Medical School, Boston, MA, USA

Outpatient and Community Brain Injury Rehabilitation, Spaulding Rehabilitation Hospital, Boston, MA, USA

NeuroRestorative Massachusetts, Braintree, MA, USA

Community Rehab Care, Newton, MA, USA

Kim Gottshall, Ph.D. Physical Therapy Department, Naval Medical Center San Diego, San Diego, CA, USA

Department of Neurosciences, School of Medicine, University of California-San Diego, San Diego, CA, USA

Jeffrey H. Greenberg, Ph.D. Altarum Institute, Washington, DC, USA

Arthur Guerrero, M.D. Endocrinology and Metabolism Service, Department of Medicine, Tripler Army Medical Center, Honolulu, HI, USA

Michael E. Hoffer, M.D., F.A.C.S Department of Otolaryngology, Naval Medical Center, San Diego, CA, USA

Michael S. Jaffee, M.D., U.S.A.F. Department of Neurology, Uniformed Services University of the Health Sciences, Bethesda, MD, USA

Department of Neurology, University of Virginia, Charlottesville, VA, USA

Department of Neurology, University of Texas Health Sciences Center at San Antonio, San Antonio, TX, USA

Thomas A. Kent, M.D. Neurology Care Line, Michael E. DeBakey VA Medical Center, Houston, TX, USA

Department of Neurology, Baylor College of Medicine, Houston, TX, USA

Department of Psychiatry and Behavioral Sciences, Baylor College of Medicine, Houston, TX, USA

Theresa B. Lattimore, M.S.N., N.P-C. Traumatic Brain Injury Programs (M96), Wounded, Ill, & Injured Directorate, US Navy Bureau of Medicine and Surgery, Washington, DC, USA

Carson Lawall, M.D. Naval Medical Center San Diego, San Diego, CA, USA

Tuong H. Le, M.D., Ph.D. Department of Radiology, San Francisco General Hospital, University of California, San Francisco, San Francisco, CA, USA

Geoffrey S.F. Ling, M.D., Ph.D., F.A.A.N. Neurology and Critical Care, San Antonio Military Medical Center, Brooke Army Medical Center, Fort Sam Houston, TX, USA

Department of Neurology, Uniformed Services University of the Health Sciences, Bethesda, MD, USA

Department of Surgery (Neurosurgery), Uniformed Services University of the Health Sciences, Bethesda, MD, USA

Critical Care Medicine for Neurology, Anesthesiology, and Surgery, Uniformed Services University of the Health Sciences, Bethesda, MD, USA

Donald W. Marion, M.D. The Defense and Veterans Brain Injury Center, Henry M. Jackson Foundation for the Advancement of Military Medicine, Rockville, MD, USA

Scott A. Marshall, M.D. Neurology and Critical Care, San Antonio Military Medical Center, Brooke Army Medical Center, Fort Sam Houston, TX, USA

Department of Neurology, Uniformed Services University of the Health Sciences, Bethesda, MD, USA

David F. Moore, M.D., Ph.D., F.A.A.N. Department of Neurology, Tulane University, New Orleans, LA, USA

Ian C. Murphy, B.A. Department of Orthopedics & Rehabilitation, Walter Reed National Military Medical Center, Bethesda, MD, USA

Tatjana Novakovic-Agopian, Ph.D. Department of Neurology, University of California at San Francisco and Martinez VAMC, San Francisco, CA, USA

Karen Parko, M.D. Department of Clinical Neurology, University of California at San Francisco, San Francisco, CA, USA

VA Epilepsy Centers of Excellence, San Francisco VA Medical Center, San Francisco, CA, USA

Nicholas J. Pastorek, Ph.D., A.B.P.P. Rehabilitation Care Line, Michael E. DeBakey VA Medical Center, Houston, TX, USA

Department of Psychiatry and Behavioral Sciences, Baylor College of Medicine, Houston, TX, USA

Seb Potter, D.Clin.Psych. Lishman Brain Injury Unit, South London & Maudsley NHS Foundation Trust, London, UK

Adam Reuben, M.B.B.S. Emergency Medicine, Royal Devon and Exeter Hospital, Exeter, UK

Michael Russo, M.D. Department of Neurology, Uniformed Services University of the Health Sciences, Bethesda, MD, USA

Helen J. Ryland School of Psychology, University of Exeter, Exeter, UK

Shirley I. Stiver, M.D., Ph.D. Department of Neurological Surgery, San Francisco General Hospital, University of California San Francisco, San Francisco, CA, USA

Brain and Spinal Injury Center (BASIC), San Francisco General Hospital, San Francisco, CA, USA

Victoria Tepe, Ph.D. Defense Centers of Excellence for Psychological Health and Traumatic Brain Injury, Arlington, VA, USA

Survivability/Vulnerability Information Analysis Center, Booz Allen Hamilton, Dayton, OH, USA

Andra T. Tharp, Ph.D. Department of Psychiatry and Behavioral Sciences, Baylor College of Medicine, Houston, TX, USA

Brett J. Theeler, Ph.D. 187th Medical Battalion, Fort Sam Houston, TX, USA

James Tonks, Ph.D., D.Clin.Psych. School of Psychology, University of Exeter, Exeter, UK

Jack W. Tsao, M.D., D.Phil., F.A.A.N. Traumatic Brain Injury Programs (M96), Wounded, Ill, & Injured Directorate, US Navy Bureau of Medicine and Surgery, Washington, DC, USA

Department of Neurology, Uniformed Services University of the Health Sciences, Bethesda, MD, USA

Erik S. Viirre, M.D., Ph.D. Department of Neurosciences, School of Medicine, University of California-San Diego, San Diego, CA, USA

Naval Health Research Center, San Diego, CA, USA

Sharon R. Weeks, B.A. Department of Orthopedics and Rehabilitation, Walter Reed Army Medical Center, Washington, DC, USA

Jennifer M. Weil, Ph.D. Deployment Health Clinical Center, Defense Centers of Excellence for Psychological Health and Traumatic Brain Injury, Arlington, VA, USA

W. Huw Williams, Ph.D. School of Psychology, University of Exeter, Exeter, UK

Philip J. Yates, D.Clin.Psych., C.Psychol School of Psychology, University of Exeter, Exeter, UK

Department of Psychological Medicine, Devon Partnership NHS Trust, Exeter, UK

Overview of TBI

1

David F. Moore, Michael S. Jaffee,
and Geoffrey S.F. Ling

Abstract

The continued significant societal challenge of both civilian and military traumatic brain injury (TBI) makes the development of preventive strategies ranging from primary to secondary to tertiary pressing. The invisible and visible loss of societal productivity further underscores this urgency. The clinical complexity of traumatic brain has resulted in controversy, especially in the appreciation of concussion and its sequelae with the need to clearly define terms such as mild TBI and the persistent post-concussive syndrome or symptom complex. The following overview highlights some of the key areas of the required interdisciplinary approach to TBI.

Keywords

Traumatic brain injury • Concussion • Persistent post-concussive symptoms • Strain-rate continuum • Material properties • Pore viscoelasticity

Wartime Traumatic Cerebral Vasospasm: Recent Review of Combat Casualties

Accounts of neurological trauma are present in the *Iliad* and *Odyssey* of Homer from Greek antiquity, where concepts consistent with interpretation loss of consciousness, penetrating brain injury, spinal cord injury, and brachial plexus and nerve injury are present. These injuries concepts of the nervous system are well summarized with direct translation from ancient Greek in two review articles by Walshe (1997) and Sablas (2001). One important aspect of these oral tradition epics to the ancient Greeks may have been to preserve warrior knowledge about injury vulnerability allowing more formalized military training. It is clear that even in antiquity, traumatic brain injury (TBI) was described both in the military and civilian contexts.

The historical account of concussion is well summarized and described in the paper by McCory and Berkovic (2001). Initial use of the term "concussion" in the modern sense of an alteration or

D.F. Moore, M.D., Ph.D., F.A.A.N. (✉)
Department of Neurology, Tulane University,
New Orleans, LA, USA
e-mail: dmoore14@tulane.edu

M.S. Jaffee, M.D., U.S.A.F.
• G.S.F. Ling, M.D., Ph.D., F.A.A.N.
Department of Neurology, Uniformed Services
University of the Health Sciences, Bethesda, MD, USA

J.W. Tsao (ed.), *Traumatic Brain Injury: A Clinician's Guide to Diagnosis, Management, and Rehabilitation*,
DOI 10.1007/978-0-387-87887-4_1, © Springer Science+Business Media, LLC 2012

temporary loss of adaptive brain function or an abnormal brain physiological state as opposed to distinct brain injury was used by medieval Persian physician Rhazes (Muhammad ibn Zakariyā Rāzī, 826–925 A.D.). Subsequent to this and with Chauliac (1300–1368 A.D.), the concept of a brain concussion or "commotio cerebri" with a relatively benign outcome from "contusio cerebri" or brain injury such as a skull fracture with a poor outcome became accepted in Western medicine with some variation. In more recent discussion, the consideration of a structural versus a functional cause of concussion has been considered in light of modern medical advances and technologies but still contains significant indeterminacies depending on the length and time scale of the approach. For example, in acute concussion, neuroimaging is typically negative yet with more extended techniques such as diffusion tensor imaging (DTI) and susceptibility-weighted imaging; previously unrecognized lesions are becoming increasingly appreciated indicating sustainment of structural abnormalities (Niogi et al. 2008; Bazarian et al. 2007). The conception of the length and time scale of injury is fundamental to the subsequent discussion of TBI since at a molecular level membrane disruption may result in alteration in membrane channel physiology or mechanoporation with resultant abnormal ionic fluxes and altered cellular and axonal function. Distinct examples of pathological sensitivity to brain trauma are present in abnormalities of calcium channel subunits *CACNA1A* and CACH (Childhood Ataxia and CNS Hypomyelination) (Kors et al. 2001; Schiffmann and Elroy-Stein 2006).

Complexity of Intracranial Anatomy

The brain is a uniquely anisotropic organ with the gyrencephalic cortical gray matter (GM), broadly orthogonal white matter (WM) fascicles, and subcortical gray matter nuclei together with multiple solid fluid interfaces between the brain parenchyma and the cerebrospinal fluid (CSF) both internally as represented by the ventricles and externally by the subarachnoid space. The entire brain is tethered by the dura together with the bridging veins and other vascular structures surrounded by the CSF cushion of the subarachnoid space. The skull represents a further protective layer of similar complexity with the diploic bone structure, numerous air sinus cavities together with foramina for exit and entrance of various neuro-vascular bundles. The complexity of the intracranial contents is well illustrated in Fig. 1.1, an axial section of the brain from the Visible Human Project (http://www.nlm.nih.gov/research/visible/visible_human.html).

Definition of Traumatic Head Injury

The current definition of TBI is phenomenological. Often, there is confusion in the nosology of TBI especially in relation to mild TBI (mTBI), a term that implicitly refers to the TBI event consistent with acute concussion. TBI is categorized according to the clinical pillars of post-traumatic amnesia (PTA) and/or a disturbance of consciousness [either alteration of consciousness (AOC) or loss of consciousness (LOC)]. Both of these clinical features, although correlated, allow for independent diagnosis of TBI severity. The overall TBI diagnosis is due to the severity of *Primary Traumatic Brain Damage* that is brain injury that results from mechanical forces producing tissue deformation at the moment of injury with direct damage to blood vessels, axons, neurons, and glia. The Glasgow Coma Scale (GCS) is also used as a TBI severity and diagnostic scale with mTBI being a GCS of 13–15, moderate TBI having a GCS range of 9–12, and severe TBI having a GCS of 3–8. *Secondary Traumatic Brain Damage*, on the other hand, is by definition due to the complications of primary damage including brain tissue hypoxia, ischemia, hydrocephalus, raised ICP, and CNS infection. The TBI spectrum definitions for closed head are summarized in Table 1.1. TBI is dichotomized into penetrating (pTBI) and closed head injury (cTBI) with the subclassification of cTBI into mild, moderate, and severe TBI. Although there is variation between epidemiological studies and it is a truism that all epidemiological studies are, in some degree, biased due to a trade-off between the veracity of ascertainment and the extent of the population sampled, rough

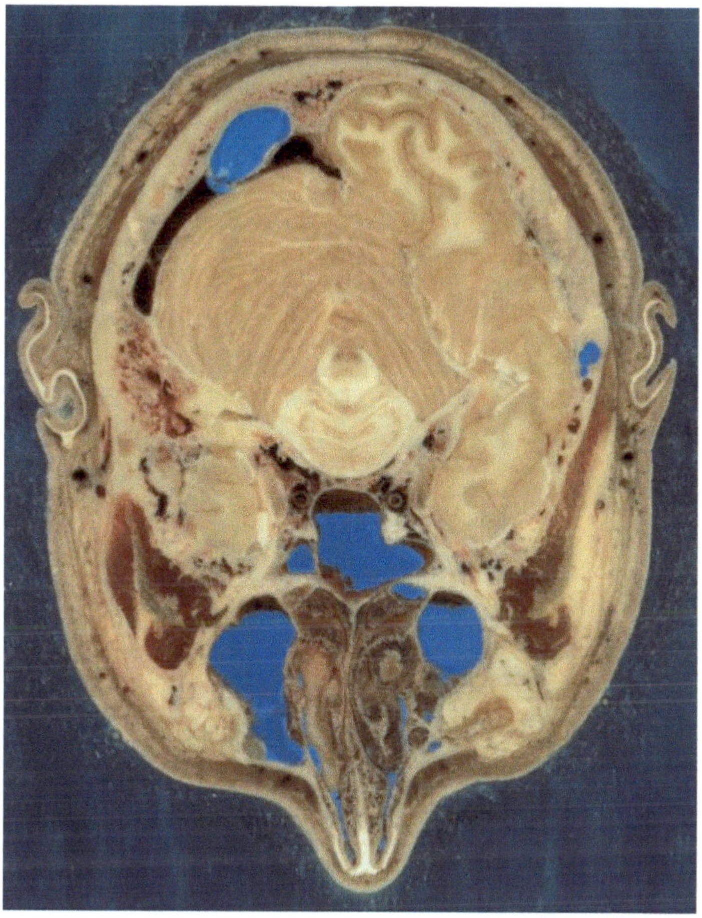

Fig. 1.1 Illustrating the intracranial contents illustrating the diploic nature of the skull bone, the numerous air sinus spaces together with the venous sinuses and dural sheathing. The gyrencephalic quality of the cortical ribbon is well seen in the occipital–temporal region. The complexity of brain anatomy has significant implications for the transmission of mechanical forces that may injure brain tissue. In particular, this is seen in the military context across impact to penetrating to blast brain injury

Table 1.1 Ascertainment of TBI according to the accepted severity scales

Definitions of TBI spectrum			
GCS	LOC	PTA	TBI
13–15	<1 h	<24 h	Mild or mTBI
9–12	>1 h and <24 h	>24 h and <7 days	Moderate
3–8	>24 h	>7 days	Severe

categorization suggests ~17% of cTBI being severe with ~13% being moderate and ~70% being mTBI (Zasler et al. 2007).

The above classification of TBI is inherently clinical and dependent on either direct observation or self-report. The current clinical trend is to attempt to redefine categorization of TBI in a patho-anatomic framework (Saatman et al. 2008). This is motivated, in part, by the recurrent failure of randomized clinical trials (RCTs) in TBI (except initially promising results with progesterone in moderate TBI), but also by a drive for standardization of common data elements (CDEs) to facilitate ongoing and new RCTs (Wright et al. 2007; Beauchamp et al. 2008; Xiao et al. 2008). CDE will also be particularly important in cross-sectional and longitudinal epidemiology studies allowing for "core" datasets to be acquired in studies with undoubted comparative value between study populations. A key epidemiological fact concerning TBI is that ~1.7 million civilian TBIs occur annually in the USA, with a cost to society estimated at 60 billion dollars both in direct medical costs and indirect costs due to lost productivity (Finkelstein et al. 2006; Xu et al. 2010) (http://www.cdc.gov/TraumaticBrainInjury/index.html).

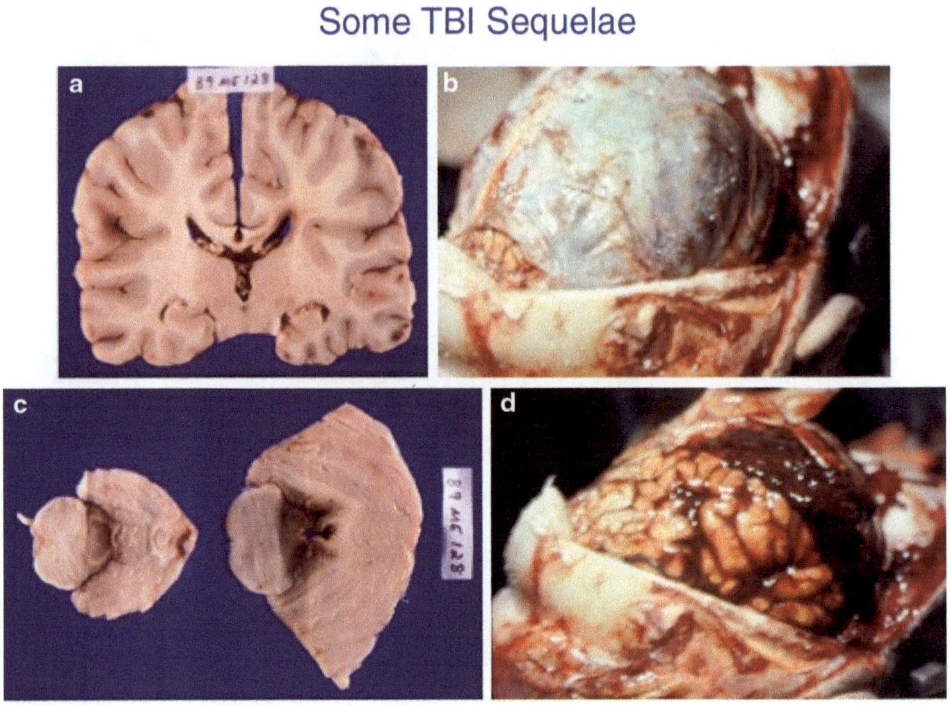

Fig. 1.2 Illustration of the neuropathology of traumatic brain injury. (**a**) and (**c**) illustrate the gross neuropathology of diffuse axonal injury with white matter hemorrhage in the corpus callosum (**a**) in the pontine white matter (**c**). (**b**) and (**d**) illustrate the subdural hematoma with (**b**) showing the dura intact and (**d**) the underlying hematoma with the dura reflected. (**e**) demonstrates cerebral contusion with bifrontal and bitemporal contusions; (**f**) the *left-hand side* of the image shows a coronal section that clearly shows the edematous and swollen brain compared to the normal brain tissue on the *right-hand side* aspect of the image. (**g**) shows a swollen optic nerve head in sagittal section due to chronically raised intracranial pressure. (**h**) illustrates delayed apoptosis of neuronal cells following TBI

TBI Spectrum: Neuropathology, Acute, Subacute, and Chronic Effects

In primary TBI, the spectrum of injury may range from diffuse or multifocal resulting in diffuse axonal injury (DAI) and diffuse vascular injury (DVI) to focal with intracerebral hemorrhage, subdural hemorrhage, epidural hemorrhage, and subarachnoid hemorrhage (Zasler et al. 2007). Other injuries include direct axonal injury, direct brain laceration, and contusion. Injuries from secondary TBI may also be diffuse or focal in the setting hypoxic-ischemic damage and brain swelling. While acute moderate and severe TBI may often require neurosurgical intervention, mTBI or concussion typically requires limited observation and intervention with recuperation occurring over several days to weeks. The prolonged sequelae of TBI are an opportunity for extensive rehabilitation care and therapeutic intervention. Of particular interest is the potential for metabolic abnormalities after concussion that if not adequately resolved may predispose the brain to more extensive damage if a further concussion occurs during the period of vulnerability—the second impact syndrome (Shaw 2002; Henry et al. 2010) (Fig. 1.2).

Concussion Biology and Mechanism

The neurobiology of concussion is incompletely understood and this has resulted in several theories ranging from interference with the reticular activating system or the cholinergic reticular inhibitory system to a paroxysmal depolarization shift of neurons resulting in "kindling" and a potential convulsive episode resulting in concussion

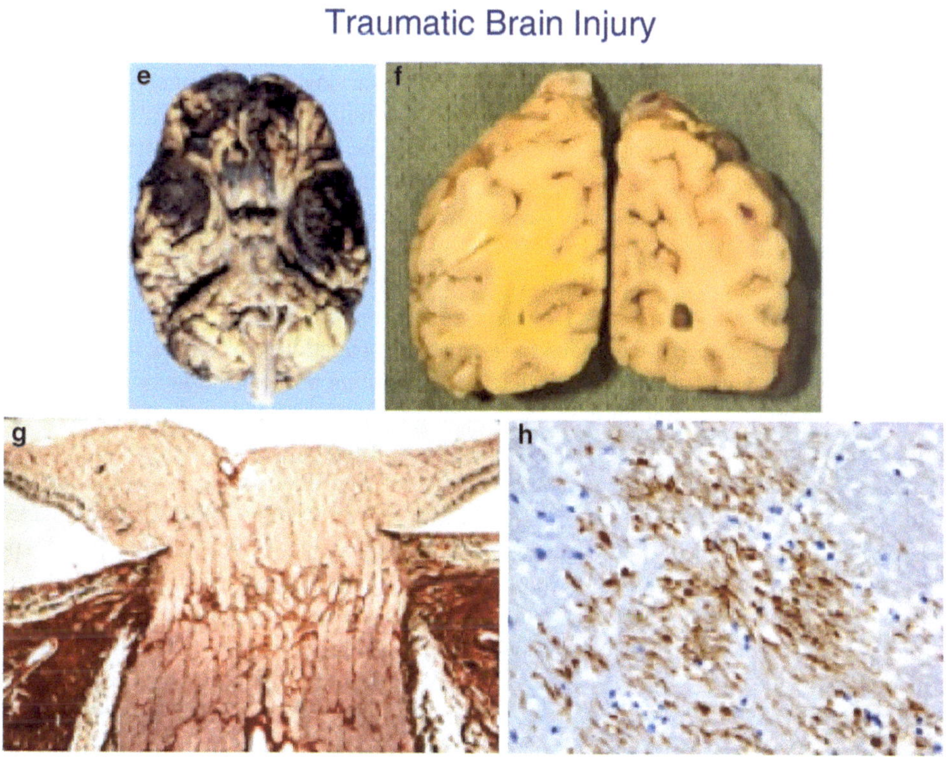

Fig. 1.2 (continued)

(Walker's Convulsive Theory) (Shaw 2002; Casson et al. 2008). From clinical neurology, it is a maxim that an alteration in consciousness results from either a bi-hemispheric process or a process in the posterior fossa. In relation to AOC and LOC, it is probable that most concussive processes result from a bilateral process suggesting more of a convulsive process secondary to a paroxysmal depolarization shift, although this cannot be stated with certainty. Similar reasoning is applicable to PTA with a resulting failure to lay down memory engrams bilaterally—the memory consolidation hypothesis (Shaw 2002).

The mechanical events precipitating concussion have been the subject of debate since the 1940s. Denny-Brown and Ritchie Russell (1940) demonstrated that injury in ketamine-anesthetized cats that were subjected to a concussive blow required that the head was able to undergo acceleration with associated translation and rotational effects. The blow was able to induce death without any rise in intracranial pressure but failed to result in concussion if the head was restrained and did not undergo acceleration. The cause of death appeared to be respiratory depression, but all brainstem reflexes were depressed with the respiratory centers being the most sensitive. Denny-Brown commented that "momentary deformity of the skull and stimulation of superficial structures, therefore appear to play no part" and finishes with "the nervous effect of a blow is thus considered to be due to the physical acceleration directly transmitted to each and every centre" (Denny-Brown and Ritchie Russell 1940). A threshold of 23'/s (angular minutes per second) was found for the cat with a higher value for the Macaque monkey. Subsequent to this, Holbourn in 1943 suggested that due to the incompressible nature of the brain linear acceleration would be unable to result in brain tissue injury; however, angular acceleration would result in shear strain and subsequent brain injury (Holbourn 1943). This was countered by Gurdjian and Lissner (1944) at Wayne State who suggested that concussion resulted from the pressure differential and the induced shearing strain on the brainstem with little reference to rotational injury.

More advanced interpretations of TBI using Newton–Euler equations describing combined translational and rotational dynamics indicate that movement may occur in all six degrees of freedom (along three translational orthogonal axes and three rotational axes, pitch, yaw, and roll), where the coordinate frame does not correspond to the center of mass of the rigid body. The equations clearly indicate that the translational and angular accelerations are coupled, resulting in both force and torque components on the brain. The exact components of torque and force will depend on the site and directionality of skull impact together with the duration of the mechanical jolt (Ivancevic 2009). The mobility of the skull on the neck probably also contributes considerably to the variation in the forces and, thereby, acceleration components experienced by the brain.

Constitutive Properties

The constitutive property of a material or a tissue is the equation and parameter relationship specific for the tissue between the applied stress field (σ) and strain deformation (ε). Typically, this may have a higher order tensor representation and involve varying elements of elasticity and viscosity. The unique nature of the brain compared to more typical engineering material is that it is soft and, further, biphasic in that it consists of a water-like component with an embedded matrix resulting in a pore-elastic tissue properties. Pore-elastic materials have different properties from more conventional materials, especially in terms of wave propagation (e.g., sound, blast). Pore-elastic mediums support both dilational and transverse waves but also include a further dilational wave that is of lower propagation velocity and termed by Biot as a dilational wave of the second kind (Biot 1992; Coussy 2004). This consideration and analysis were derived from propagation of elastic waves with the direction of propagation of the wave being longitudinal as opposed to rotational or transverse, where the direction of wave motion is normal to the direction of propagation resulting in a shear wave within the tissue. It is not at all obvious how a pore-elastic medium interacts with blast or shock wave propagation through a tissue. In Fig. 1.3, a lumped isotropic model of brain tissue is presented with varying mechanical elements that account for tissue viscoelasticity, shear thickening, pore elasticity, and

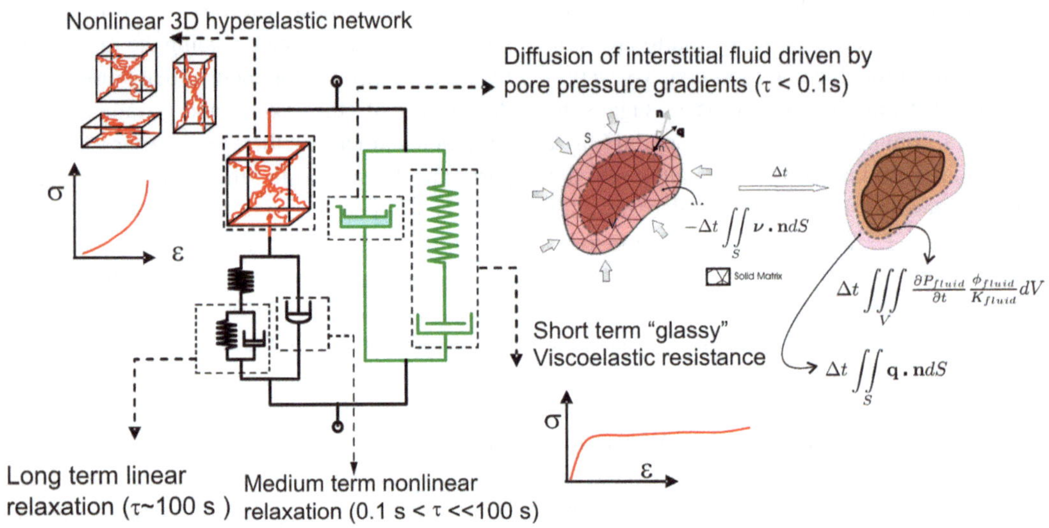

Fig. 1.3 Constitutive model of brain tissue illustrating viscoelasticity, shear thickening to increasing strain rate, tissue pore elasticity, and nonlinear relaxation effects to mechanical stress (courtesy Dr. Simona Socrates, MIT, and The Institute of Soldier Nanotechnology)

nonlinear tissue relaxation to stress. The brain is highly anisotropic with the potential for material properties to alter in a directional and regional manner so that the constitutive property of white matter is likely to differ from gray matter. The correct characterization of the material and constitutive properties of tissue is an essential prerequisite to the accurate validation of complex finite element models used to enhance understanding of mechanical and blast-related TBI.

Woodpecker Analogy

The woodpecker is a particularly instructive "experiment of nature" in relation to concussion. It is possible that further understanding of the biological and physical characterization of the woodpecker in relation to head impact may define those biological features that are adaptive and protective against concussion (Fig. 1.4). In a paper by Oda et al., the authors use finite element models (FEMs) of the woodpecker skull and examined the properties of the woodpecker that resulted in concussive stress wave dissipation. The analysis found that the unique shape of the head and neck tended to channel the stress wave away from the skull into the neck while the brain is tightly tethered by the dura and the small CSF space. Further, an adaptive hyoid bone anatomy together with the cancellous nature of the skull bone results in further stress dissipation from the concussion wave due to woodpecker impact (Oda et al. 2006).

The ability of the woodpecker to sustain repeated concussive impacts without biological effects is of significance and bears further study. The potential to inform preventive strategies to minimize concussion should not be underestimated. For example, consideration of head and neck posture during an impending concussion with increased neck rigidity may prevent extensive rotational acceleration and the incipient development of concussion.

Persistent Post-concussive Symptoms

A number of patients after a concussion fail to resolve clinically but develop persistent post-concussive symptoms (Cicerone and Kalmar 1995). This constellation of symptoms usually involves headaches, imbalance or postural disequilibrium, and memory difficulties that persist for several months from the concussive event (*International Classification of Diseases, 10th Revision*, Criteria for Postconcussion Syndrome, Code 310.2). The symptoms are often refractory to treatment but generally abate over months to years (Ropper and Gorson 2007). Up to about 15% of patients can be affected in civilian injury and concussion, but the statistics are study and

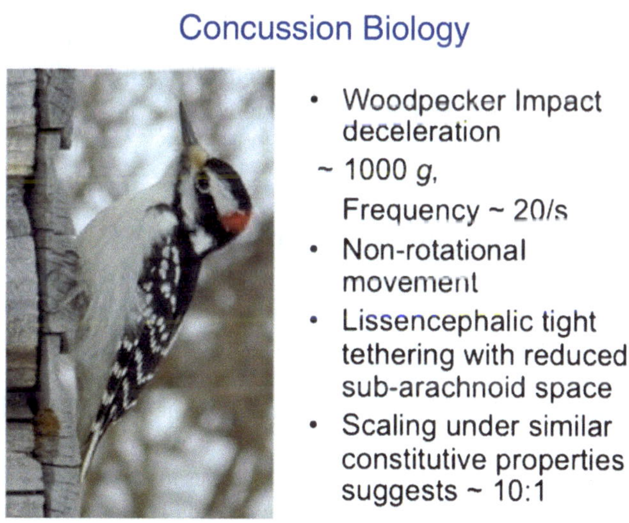

Fig. 1.4 The woodpecker species is uniquely adapted to high impact loading on the beak and head with unique biological adaptations to prevent concussion

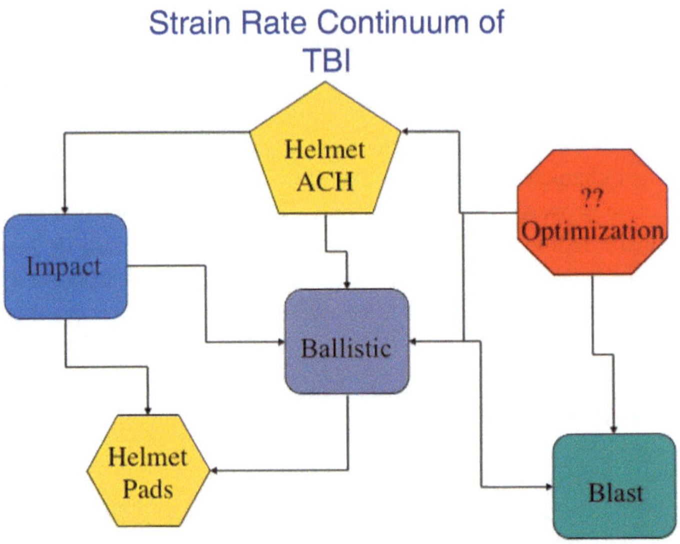

Fig. 1.5 Strain-rate continuum for traumatic brain injury, where the optimization of personal protective equipment (PPE) against impact injury may be enhanced by optimization of helmet pads placed between the helmet shell and the head. The ballistic protection is provided by the material composition of the helmet shell while mitigation of blast injury may require further head and facial coverage by appropriate protective materials. The simultaneous optimization and characterization of these diverse material properties capable of preventing head injury across the strain-rate domain are formidable

population dependent. Using an Illness Perception Model, Whittaker et al. (2007) were able to predict persistence of post-concussive symptoms in 80% of diagnosed patients in their population. The work suggests that patients may incorrectly attribute commonly prevalent symptoms to the concussive injury and become more at risk of development of persistent post-concussive symptoms (Whittaker et al. 2007). In a follow-on editorial, Wood (2007) comments on the efficacy of cognitive-behavioral therapeutic approaches in persistent post-concussive symptoms using brief early interventions (Wood 2007). Such studies may point to efficient mechanisms of preventing this important comorbidity of concussion in the civilian head injury population; however, the possibility of true structural and organic changes still must be considered, especially due to the known plasticity of the CNS (Niogi et al. 2008).

Strain-Rate Continuum of TBI

Stress is the force per unit area within the tissue with the resulting strain deformation field depending on the applied stress and the constitutive properties of the tissue. These measurements are often performed in a quasi-static fashion, where this may allow reversible mechanical changes in the tissue during application of the stress fields both in compression or tension. For TBI, traumatic events occur in a variety of ways, such as during motor vehicle crashes or following penetrating head injury from a bullet wound to blast-associated traumatic head injury. The rate at which stress is applied to the head or brain differs under these differing conditions but is related by the strain rate with vehicular head injury occurring at a strain rate <500 s^{-1}, while that of penetrating injury occurs at ~2,000 s^{-1}. With blast-associated head injury, the rate of strain can be in the range of ~2,000–10,000 s^{-1}. It is, therefore, possible to consider TBI from these diverse etiologies across a strain-rate continuum with the constitutive tissue properties often responding in a strain-rate-dependent manner (Saraf et al. 2007). This is particularly important where the requirement is to design helmets for prevention of head injury and to obtain full characterization of possible tissue injury parameters. For personal protective equipment (PPE) such as the advanced combat helmet (ACH), it is an exceptionally difficult engineering optimization problem to account for mitigation across all the strain-rate domains. This is illustrated in Fig. 1.5.

Neuroimaging of TBI

In recent years, the rapid advances of both structural and functional neuroimaging have allowed extensive clinical characterization of TBI for

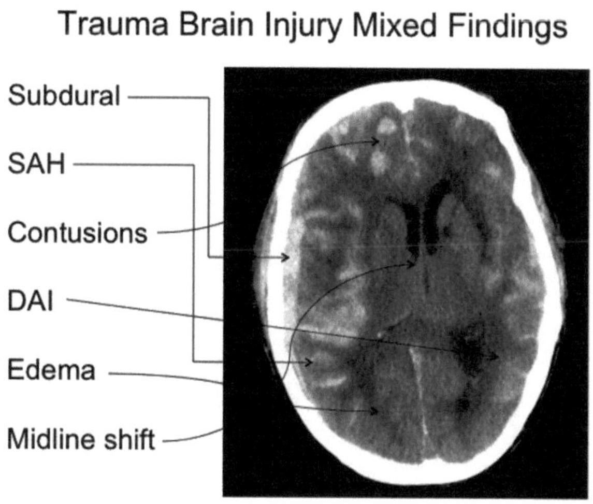

Fig. 1.6 Computer Tomograph (CT) axial image illustrating multiple simultaneous pathologies from subdural hematoma to subarachnoid hemorrhage (SAH), to cerebral contusions, to diffuse axonal injury (DAI), and to cerebral edema and herniation syndromes with midline shifts

immediate clinical patient care and for clinical investigation and research. It is now possible to understand various subcategories of TBI such as DAI with more investigative techniques such as DTI with such imaging metrics as fractional anisotropy (FA), mean diffusivity (MD), and radial and axial diffusivity (Gennarelli et al. 1998; Beaulieu 2002; Lee et al. 2006; Bazarian et al. 2007; Budde et al. 2007, 2009; Kraus et al. 2007; MacDonald et al. 2007; Mori 2007; Neil 2008; Niogi et al. 2008; Rutgers et al. 2008a, b; Wilde et al. 2008). The DTI studies performed in general concussion indicated reduction in FA with increases in isotropic DTI metrics such as MD. Injury severity is less in concussion or mTBI with some resolution appearing to occur across time, although there are currently only a limited number of longitudinal DTI studies in TBI (Bendlin et al. 2008). It can be anticipated that greater use of Positron Emission Tomography (PET) and Single-Photon Emission Tomography (SPECT) together with functional Magnetic Resonance Imaging (fMRI) will more fully allow the exploration of the metabolic, neurochemical, and functional neuronal aggregate changes in both resting connectivity and task-related connectivity in TBI. A particularly significant area, where noninvasive neuroimaging is likely to contribute substantial clinical insights, is in disorders of conscious states such as in persistent vegetative states and emerging levels of consciousness through the minimal conscious state to normal conscious cognitive states. The complexity of TBI as highlighted is well illustrated in Fig. 1.6, where multiple pathological processes are seen at a simultaneous play in a single patient.

Military Medicine Perspective on Brain Injury

The effect of blast in relation to TBI has been well described since World War I, with shell shock and concussion, in particular, described by the clinical descriptions of Gordon Holmes (1876–1965) (Lord SouthBorough 1922). The current military operations in Iraq (Operation Iraqi Freedom, OIF) and Afghanistan (Operation Enduring Freedom, OEF) have led to a resurgence of interest on the effects of blast and blast-associated polytrauma due to the extensive use of improvised explosive devices (IEDs). Part of the spectrum of blast-associated polytrauma includes the full range of TBI and, in particular, blast-associated concussion or mTBI. Current estimates for blast-associated TBI are ~130,000 service members since 2003 with ~4.5% of service members having persistent post-concussional symptoms (http://www.dvbic.org/TBI-Numbers.aspx). Blast may be defined as an "in-the-atmosphere" explosion characterized by the release of energy in such a short period of time and within such a small volume resulting in the creation of a nonlinear shock and pressure wave of finite amplitude,

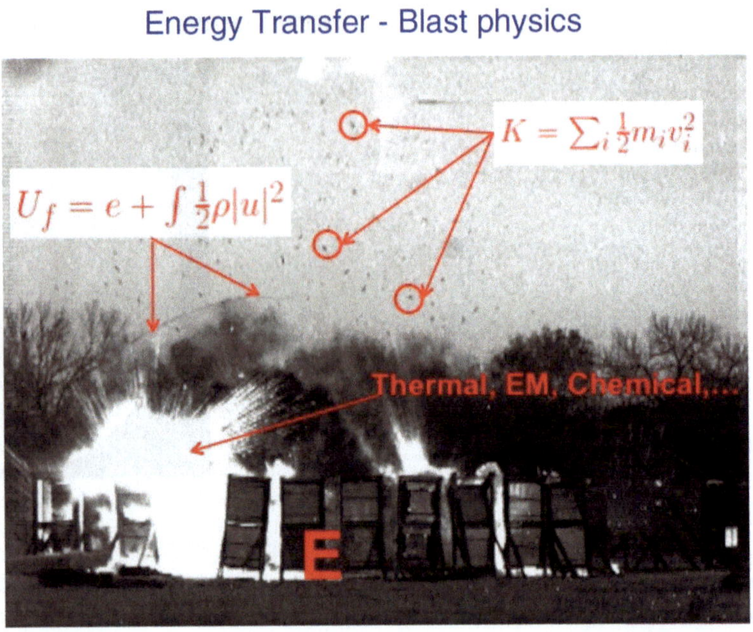

Fig. 1.7 Energy conversion (E) associated with a blast wave illustrating the shock wave front together with fragment kinetic energy. Other energy components are the blast-associated electromagnetic pulse, thermal energy, and chemical conversion

spreading from the source of the explosion (Moore et al. 2008). The energy conversion from a conventional blast can be chemical, electrical, thermal, and kinetic or pressure energy (Fig. 1.7). The kinetic energy of the blast is associated with fragments and results in their expulsion in advance of the shock wave front.

The "ideal case" of a blast pressure wave is the Friedlander waveform with a rapid rise-time to the peak positive pressure above atmospheric, the overpressure followed by an exponential pressure falloff together with a relatively prolonged subatmospheric underpressure. Typically, the timescale of the total explosive pressure event is tens of milliseconds. The prolonged underpressure component of the pressure waveform may exceed the critical tensile strength of the fluid component of a tissue allowing the development of cavitation.

Blast injury is defined as primary, where injury is related to the shock-wave overpressure and underpressure propagation through the tissue; secondary blast injury occurs from blast-associated fragments or shrapnel tissue injury; tertiary injury is secondary to falling debris or throwing of the dismounted service member or vehicle with subsequent tissue injury; quaternary injury develops from a variety of physical processes associated with explosive detonation, such as thermal, toxic detonation products while quinary injuries refer to the environmental hazard remaining after an explosive detonation (Mayorga 2007; Guy et al. 1998, 2000; DePalma et al. 2005).

The effect of primary blast on the CNS is still unclear but in military concussion it is unusual to be exposed solely to primary blast; rather such exposure is associated most commonly with tertiary blast injury (Warden et al. 2009). For this reason, blast-associated CNS injury is better considered as a constellation of blast component exposure resulting in a blast(+) syndrome of CNS injury. This results in the brain being exposed to mechanical events across the strain-rate continuum as previously discussed. The relationship of particular aspects of the blast wave exposure (that may be very complex due to reflection and augmentation) to clinical CNS injury is also unclear while ongoing efforts are well developed to computationally model all aspects of blast-associated phenomenon in virtual test facilities with bio-fidelic head models (Moore et al. 2009). One clinical aspect that has been noted in relation to blast-associated CNS injury is the increase in traumatic cerebral vasospasm, particularly in penetrating head injury (Armonda et al. 2006).

The peak overpressure is most simply dependent on the distance from the blast source but approximately scales according to the standoff distance divided by the cube root of the explosive weight (Hopkinson Rule) (Moore et al. 2008). The coupling of the nonlinear blast wave into biological tissue results in increased energy deposition at high strain rates in fractions of microseconds. The biological effect will depend on the constitutive tissue properties together with the largely unknown high-strain-rate tissue material properties for brain. Ongoing work is establishing brain material properties across the strain-rate domain from low strain rates seen in impact injury to intermediate and higher strain rates seen in ballistic and blast injury. The above concepts lead to a frame of reference debate in relation to blast-induced military concussion or mTBI, where it should be possible to rapidly approximate the potential exposure from any particular event to first-order accuracy.

Explosives' detonation results in the formation of a detonation wave of altering chemical composition with the rapid formation of a propagated, nonlinear shock wave representing a large discontinuous increase in pressure, temperature, and density in the gas flow. The propagation of the shock wave develops a 3D complex fluid flow field that is altered by ambient conditions and environmental boundaries. This may result in multiple wave reflections and potentially pressure field intensification up to eightfold.

The blast waveform can be regarded as a combination of compressive and tensile components that impose a stress on the tissue in a manner that is dependent on the strain rate together with the constitutive properties of the tissue. This, combined with the potential for CNS injury from ballistic fragment, acceleration–deceleration impact injury, as well as chemical, thermal, and electromagnetic radiation, results in a highly complex problem where dominating effects become very difficult to parse in terms of their biological effects on the CNS.

Overlap of Wartime TBI and Acute Stress Disorders

The effect of military concussion on the development of persistent post-concussion symptoms together with other co-morbidities such as post-traumatic stress disorder (PTSD) (Fig. 1.8) and depression is an area of active research (Hoge et al. 2008a, b). Current studies are cross-sectional in design and may not have accounted accurately for statistical use of structural equation type of models.

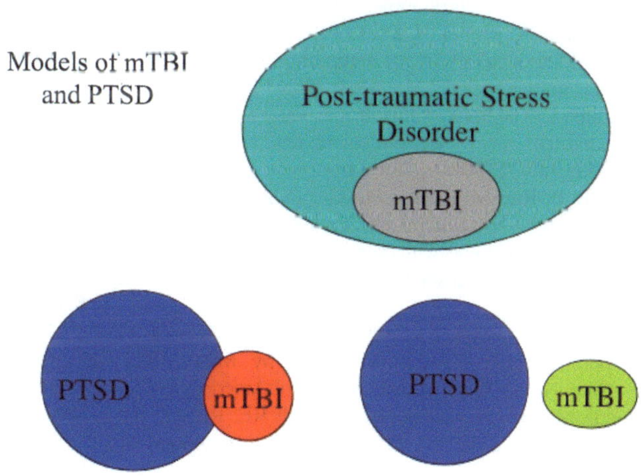

Fig. 1.8 Overlap of military concussion models and PTSD. The Venn diagrams represent various disease models of military mTBI and PTSD, where military mTBI/concussion is regarded as a subset of PTSD to where the two disorders are regarded as independent (*separated circles*). Clinical perceptions suggest that the two disorders overlap to a greater and lesser degree within any clinical evaluation

Further preliminary data from DTI suggests differences in blast(+)-exposed service members compared to non-blast-exposed service members in relation to such metrics as the FA, MD, and radial diffusivity.

Conflict of Interest Statement

The authors have no conflicts of interest to disclose. The views expressed in this chapter are those of the authors and do not reflect the official policy of the Department of the Army, the Defense Advanced Research Agency, the United Sates Department of Defense, or the US Government.

Acknowledgments This work was supported in full by financial aid from the Joint Improvised Explosive Device Defeat Organization (JIEDDO) and the Army Research Office. The authors appreciate the permission of Dr. James Smirniotopoulos, Radiology, USUHS, and Dr. Gerard Riedy, Radiology, WRAMC, for the use of the neuroimaging slide in Fig. 1.6. We also thank Dr. Simona Socrates for the use of Fig. 1.3 and Dr. Raul Radovitzky for permission to use Fig. 1.7.

References

Armonda R, Bell RS, Vo AH, Ling G, DeGraba TJ, Crandall B, Ecklund J, Campbell WW. Wartime traumatic cerebral vasospasm: recent review of combat casualties. Neurosurgery. 2006;59(6).

Bazarian J, Zhong J, Blyth B, Zhu T, Kavcic V, Peterson D. Diffusion tensor imaging detects clinically important axonal damage after mild traumatic brain injury: a pilot study. J Neurotrauma. 2007;24:1447–59.

Beauchamp K, Mutlak H, Smith WR, Shohami E, Stahel PF. Pharmacology of traumatic brain injury: where is the “golden bullet”? Mol Med. 2008;14:731–40.

Beaulieu C. The basis of anisotropic water diffusion in the nervous system - a technical review. NMR Biomed. 2002;15:435–55.

Bendlin B, Ries ML, Lazar M, Alexander AL, Dempsey RJ, Rowley HA, Sherman JE, Johnson SC. Longitudinal changes in patients with traumatic brain injury assessed with diffusion tensor inaging. Neuroimage. 2008;42: 503–14.

Biot M. Accoustics, elasticity, and thermodynamics of porous media - twent-one papers by M. A. Biot. Woodbury, NY: Accoustical Society of America; 1992.

Budde M, Kim JH, Liang HF, Schmidt RE, Russell JH, Cross AH, Song SK. Toward accurate diagnosis of white matter pathology using diffusion tensor imaging. Magn Reson Med. 2007;57:686–95.

Budde M, Xie M, Cross AH, Song SK. Axial diffusivity is the primary correlate of axonal injury in experimental autoimmune encephalomyelitis spinal cord: a quantitative pixelwise analysis. J Neurosci. 2009;29:2805–13.

Casson I, Pellman EJ, Viano DC. Concussion in the national football league: an overview for neurologists. Neurol Clin. 2008;26:217–41.

Cicerone K, Kalmar K. Persistent postconcussion syndrome: the structure of subjective complaints after mild traumatic brain injury. J Head Trauma Rehabil. 1995;10:1–7.

Coussy O. PoroMechanics. Chichester, UK: Wiley & Sons; 2004.

Denny-Brown D, Ritchie Russell W. Experimental cerebral concussion. J Physiol. 1940;99:153.

DePalma R, Burris DG, Champion HR, Hodgson MJ. Blast injury. N Eng J Med. 2005;353:1335–42.

Finkelstein E, Corso P, Miller T. The incidence and economic burden of injuries in the United States. New York: Oxford University Press; 2006.

Gennarelli T, Thibault L, Graham D. Diffuse axonal injury: a important form of traumatic brain damage. Neuroscientist. 1998;4:202–15.

Gurdjian ES, Lissner HR. Mechanism of head injury as studied by the cathode ray oscilloscope, preliminary report. J Neurosurg 1944;1:393–399.

Guy R, Glover MA, Cripps NP. Primary blast injury: pathophysiology and implications for treatment. Part III: injury to the central nervous system and the limbs. J R Nav Med Serv. 2000;86:27–31.

Guy R, Kirkman E, Watkins PE, Cooper GJ. Physiologic responses to primary blast. J Trauma. 1998;45:983–7.

Henry L, Tremblay S, Boulanger Y, Ellenberg D, Lassonde M. Neurometabolic changes in the acute phase after sports concussion correlate with symptom severity. J Neurotrauma. 2010;27:65–75.

Hoge C, Goldberg HM, Castro CA. Care of war veterans with mild traumatic brain injury -flawed perspectives. N Eng J Med. 2008a;360:1588–91.

Hoge C, McGurk D, Thomas JL, Cox AL, Engel CC, Castro CA. Mild traumatic brain injury in U.S. soldiers returning from Iraq. N Eng J Med. 2008b;358:453–63.

Holbourn A. Mechanics of head injury. Lancet. 1943;2: 438–41.

Ivancevic V. New mechanics of traumatic brain injury. Cogn Neurodyn. 2009;3:281–93.

Kors E, Terwindt G, Vermeulen F, Fitzsimons R, Jardine P, Heywood P, et al. Delayed cerebral edema and fatal coma after minor head trauma: role of the CACNA1A calcium channel subunit gene and relationship with familial hemiplegic migraine. Ann Neurol. 2001;49: 753–60.

Kraus M, Susmaras T, Caughlin BP, Walker CJ, Sweeney JA, Little DM. White matter integrity and cognition in chronic tarumatic brain injury: a diffusion tensor imaging study. Brain. 2007;130:2508–19.

Lee J, Choi CG, Chun MH. Usefullness of diffusion tensor imaging for evaluation of motor function in patients with traumatic brain injury. J Head Trauma Rehabil. 2006;21:272 8.

Lord SouthBorough, a., Committee. Report of the War Office Committee of Enquiry into “Shell-shock”. Military Handbook Series. Crawley, UK: Imperial War Museum; 1922.

MacDonald C, Dikranian K, Bayly P, Holtzman D, Brody D. Diffusion tensor imaging reliably detects experimental traumatic axonal injury and indicate approximate time of injury. J Neurosci. 2007;51:11869–76.

Mayorga M. The pathology of primary blast overpressure injury. Toxicology. 2007;121:17–28.

McCory P, Berkovic SF. Concussion: the history of clinical and pathophysiological concepts and misconceptions. Neurology. 2001;57:2283–9.

Moore D, Jérusalem A, Nyein M, Noels L, Jaffee MS, Radovitzky RA. Computational biology - modeling of primary blast effects on the central nervous system. Neuroimage. 2009;47:T10–20.

Moore D, Radovitzky RA, Shupenko L, Klinoff A, Jaffee MS, Rosen JM. Blast physics and central nervous system injury. Future Neurol. 2008;3:243–50.

Mori S. Introduction to diffusion tensor imaging. Amsterdam: Elsevier; 2007.

Neil J. Diffusion imaging concepts for clinicians. J Magn Reson Imaging. 2008;27:1–7.

Niogi S, Mukerjee P, Ghajar J, Johnson C, Kolster RA, Sarkar R, Lee H, Meeker M, Zimmerman RD, Manley GT, McCandliss BD. Extent of microstructural white matter injury in postconcussive syndrome correlates with impaired cognitive reaction time: a 3 T diffusion tensor imaging study of mild traumatic brain injury. Am J Neuroradiol. 2008;29:967–73.

Oda J, Sakamoto J, Sakano K. Mechanical evaluation of the skeletal structure and tissue of the woodpecker and its shock absorbing system. JSME Int J. 2006;40(3):390–6.

Ropper A, Gorson KC. Concussion. New Engl J Med. 2007;356(2):166–72.

Rutgers D, Filliard P, Paradot G, Tadie M, Lasjaunais P, Ducreux D. Diffusion tensor imaging characteristics of the corpus callosum in mild moderate and severe traumatic brain injury. Am J Neuroradiol. 2008a;29:1730–5.

Rutgers D, Toulgoat F, Cazejust J, Filliard P, Lasjaunais P, Ducreux D. White matter abnormalities in mild traumatic brain injury: a diffusion tensor imaging study. Am J Neuroradiol. 2008b;29:514–9.

Saatman K, Duhaime AC, Bullock R, Maas AI, Valadka A, Manley GT, Workshop Scientific Team and Advisory Panel Members, Collaborators (31), Brody D, Contant C, Dash P, Diaz-Arrastia R, Fertig S, Gean A, Goodman C, Gordon W, Hayes R, Hicks R, Langloi J, Marmarou A, Moore D, Murray G, Okonkwo D, Papa L, Phillips L, Plesnila N, Robertson C, Robertson C, Sahuquillo J, Silbergleit R, Steyerberg E, Stocchetti N, Teasdale E, Teasdale G, Temkin N, Thompson H, Tong K, Wilson L, Wright D. Classification of traumatic brain injury for targeted therapies. J Neurotrauma. 2008;25(7):719–38.

Sablas D. Functional neuroanatomy in the pre-hippocratic era: observations from the iliad of homer. Neurosurgery. 2001;48(6):1352–7.

Saraf H, Ramesh KT, Lennon AM, Merkle AC, Roberts IC. Mechanical properties of soft human tissues under dynamic loading. J Biomech. 2007;40:1960–7.

Schiffmann R, Elroy-Stein O. Childhood ataxia with CNS hypomyelination/vanishing white matter disease—a common leukodystrophy caused by abnormal control of protein synthesis. Mol Genet Metab. 2006;88:7–15.

Shaw N. The neurophysiology of concussion. Prog Neurobiol. 2002;67:281–344.

Walshe T. Neurological concepts in archaic Greece: what did homer know. J Hist Neurosci. 1997;6(1):72–81.

Warden D, French LM, Shupenko L, Fargus J, Riedy G, Erickson ME, Jaffee MS, Moore DF. Case report of a soldier with primary blast brain injury. Neuroimage. 2009;47:T152–3.

Whittaker R, Kemp S, House A. Illness perceptions and outcome in mild head injury: a longitudinal study. J Neurol Neurosurg Psychiatry. 2007;78:644–6.

Wilde E, McCauley SR, Hunter JN, Bigler ED, Chu Z, Wang ZJ, Hanten GR, Troyanskaya M, Yaltampalli R, Li X, Chia J, Levin HS. Diffusion tensor imaging of acute mild traumatic brain injury in adolescents. Neurology. 2008;70:948–55.

Wood R. Post concussional syndrome: all in the minds eye! J Neurol Neurosurg Psychiatry. 2007;78:552.

Wright D, Kellermann AL, Hertzberg VS, Clark PL, Frankel M, Goldstein FC, Salomone JP, Dent LL, Harris OA, Ander DS, Lowery DW, Patel MM, Denson DD, Gordon AB, Wald MM, Gupta S, Hoffman SW, Stein DG. ProTect: a randomized clinical trial of progesterone for acute traumatic brain injury. Ann Emerg Med. 2007;49:391–402.

Xiao G, Wei J, Yan W, Wang W, Lu Z. Improved outcomes from the administration of progesterone for patients with acute severe traumatic brain injury: a randomized controlled trial. Crit Care. 2008;12:R61.

Xu L, Wald MM, Coronado VG. Traumatic brain injury in the United States: emergency department visits, hospitalizations, and deaths. Atlanta, GA: Centers for Disease Control and Prevention, National Center for Injury Prevention and Control; 2010.

Zasler N, Katz DI, Zafonte RD. Brain injury medicine. New York: Demos Medical Publishing; 2007.

Imaging Diagnosis of TBI

2

Tuong H. Le, Shirley I. Stiver, and Alisa D. Gean

Abstract

Fundamentals and recent advances in imaging techniques and selection paradigms for the diagnosis of traumatic brain injury (TBI) will be discussed. Characteristic imaging findings for common TBI lesions will be described. Computed tomography (CT) is the modality of choice for the initial assessment of acute TBI. Magnetic resonance imaging (MRI) is recommended for patients with acute TBI when the neurological findings are unexplained by CT. MRI is the modality of choice for the evaluation of subacute and chronic TBI. Advanced MR techniques, such as diffusion weighted imaging, can improve the identification of otherwise occult lesions, especially with mild TBI.

Keywords

Imaging • Traumatic brain injury • Blast-induced injury • CT • MRI

T.H. Le, M.D., Ph.D.
Department of Radiology, San Francisco General Hospital, University of California, San Francisco, San Francisco, CA 94110, USA

S.I. Stiver, M.D., Ph.D.
Department of Neurological Surgery, San Francisco General Hospital, University of California, San Francisco, San Francisco, CA 94110, USA

Brain and Spinal Injury Center (BASIC), San Francisco General Hospital, San Francisco, CA 94110, USA

A.D. Gean, M.D. (✉)
Department of Radiology, San Francisco General Hospital, University of California, San Francisco, San Francisco, CA 94110, USA

Department of Neurological Surgery, San Francisco General Hospital, University of California, San Francisco, San Francisco, CA 94110, USA

Brain and Spinal Injury Center (BASIC), San Francisco General Hospital, San Francisco, CA 94110, USA

Division of Neuroradiology, 1X55, San Francisco General Hospital, 1001 Potrero Avenue, San Francisco, CA 94110, USA
e-mail: alisa.gean@radiology.ucsf.edu

J.W. Tsao (ed.), *Traumatic Brain Injury: A Clinician's Guide to Diagnosis, Management, and Rehabilitation*,
DOI 10.1007/978-0-387-87887-4_2, © Springer Science+Business Media, LLC 2012

Introduction

Traumatic brain injury (TBI) refers to injury to the intracranial structures following physical trauma to the head. TBI can be classified into *primary* and *secondary* injuries. Primary injuries are the result of direct trauma to the head and occur at the moment of impact. Secondary injuries arise as sequelae due to activation of excitatoxic, oxidative, inflammatory and other signaling cascades following the primary injury. Secondary injuries are potentially preventable and treatable, whereas primary injuries, by definition, have already occurred by the time the patient first presents for medical attention. TBI can be further divided according to *location* (intra-axial or extra-axial) and also by the nature of the *mechanism* of injury (penetrating/open or blunt/closed). The severity of TBI is classified clinically according to the universally accepted Glasgow Coma Scale (GCS). Patients presenting with GCS<=8 are designated as having a severe TBI, those with GCS between 9 and 12 are categorized as moderate injuries, and mild TBI (mTBI) encompasses patients with a GCS 13–15 (Teasdale and Jennett 1974). From the moment of impact, TBI is a dynamic process with varying therapeutic windows, and early diagnosis and intervention are imperative for favorable outcomes.

Diagnosis and management of TBI requires a multi-disciplinary approach, starting with a detailed history and physical examination, followed by appropriate diagnostic imaging, and subsequent medical and/or surgical intervention as deemed necessary. The goals of imaging include identification of treatable injuries, recognition of sources of potential secondary damage, and analyses of factors that may provide useful prognostic information for long-term outcome. Advances in medical imaging technology have resulted in an explosion of novel imaging modalities that have improved the sensitivity and specificity for early detection of TBI and added a host of valuable prognostic indicators and signs to help guide patient management. Consequently, clinicians are faced with the difficult task of selecting the most appropriate diagnostic test from an array of available imaging techniques. These decisions are of vital importance for optimal management, especially for injuries that require aggressive and timely intervention. In this chapter, recent advances in imaging techniques and selection paradigms for the diagnosis of TBI will be discussed. Characteristic imaging findings for individual lesions observed in TBI will be described in detail, including a discussion of the unique imaging features of blast-induced brain injury.

Imaging Selections

Conventional Radiography

Skull fracture, with or without signs of neurological injury, is an independent risk factor for a neurosurgically relevant intracranial lesion (Munoz-Sanchez et al. 2009). Therefore, in the setting of clinically occult TBI, the diagnosis of skull fracture serves to alert the clinician to the possibility of an immediate or delayed neurologically relevant intracranial lesion. Conventional radiography itself (film or digital) is not sensitive for detection of intracranial pathology and should not be performed to evaluate parenchymal damage in TBI (Bell and Loop 1971; Hackney 1991; Masters 1980). In mTBI, skull films rarely demonstrate significant findings; and in severe TBI, the lack of abnormality on skull films does not exclude major intracranial injury (Adams 1991). Patients who are at risk for acute intracranial injury, even without clinical evidence of a skull fracture, should be imaged by computed tomography (CT).

Computed Tomography

In the setting of acute head trauma, a non-contrast CT is recommended for patients with moderate and severe TBI (GCS ≤ 12) and in any patient with evidence of a penetrating injury. CT is not indicated for mTBI (GCS > 12) unless the patient meets one of the following criteria, that also

Table 2.1 New Orleans Criteria for mTBI—A non-contrast CT of the head is indicated if the patient meets one or more of the following criteria

Headache
Vomiting
Age > 60 years
Drug or alcohol intoxication
Persistent ante-grade amnesia (short term memory deficits)
Visible trauma above the clavicle
Seizure

Table 2.2 Canadian CT Head Rule for mTBI—A non-contrast CT of the head is indicated if the patient meets one or more of the following criteria

GCS < 15 two hours after injury
Suspected open or depressed skull fracture
Any sign of basal skull fracture
Two or more episodes of vomiting
Age ≥65 years
Amnesia before impact of 30 min or more
Dangerous mechanism (i.e., pedestrian struck by motor vehicle, occupant ejected from motor vehicle, or a fall from a height of at least 3 ft or five stairs)

include those recommended by the New Orleans Criteria (Table 2.1) and the Canadian CT Head Rule (Table 2.2), which consist of age > 60 years, persistent neurologic deficit(s), headache or vomiting, amnesia, loss of conciousness ≥ 5 min, depressed skull fracture, bleeding diathesis or anticoagulation therapy (Haydel et al. 2000; Jagoda et al. 2002; Stiell et al. 2001a, b, c). CT is the primary modality of choice because it is fast, widely accessible, and there are few contraindications to a non-contrast CT scan. Pregnancy, especially in the first trimester, is a relative contraindication for a CT scan. In the setting of TBI, one needs to balance the risks of the CT against how the information from the scan might alter the patient's management. Unlike Magnetic resonance imaging (MRI), CT can easily accommodate life-support and monitoring equipment. In addition, CT is superior to MRI for the dectection of skull fractures and radio-opaque foreign bodies. In fact, MRI is contraindicated in the presence of certain foreign bodies. Non-contrast CT scans provide rapid and accurate detection of space-occupying hematomas and associated mass effect, together with signs that reliably flag impending complications of herniation that would require immediate medical and/or surgical intervention. Intravenous contrast administration should not be performed without a baseline non-contrast exam because the contrast can both mask and mimic underlying hemorrhage. Addition of contrast, after the non-contrast scan, can, however, detect active extravasation and alert the clinician to a highly unstable lesion that has the risk for rapid enlargement.

CT angiography (CTA) utilizes iodinated intravenous contrast to delineate the vascular structures at high (sub-millimeter) resolution. CTA is best performed with multi-detector CT (MDCT) and rapid bolus contrast injection using vessel tracking technique. Typical imaging parameters include a slice thickness of 1.25 mm, with a 0.625 mm overlap, and a bolus injection rate between 3 and 4 mL/s. In suspected vascular injury, such as in the setting of a fracture traversing the carotid canal or venous sinus, CTA can serve as a useful screening method for vascular injuries such as carotid dissections, fistulas, and venous stenoses or occlusions (Enterline and Kapoor 2006).

Dynamic perfusion CT measures brain hemodynamics by tracking transient attenuation changes in the blood vessels and brain parenchyma during the first-pass of an intravenously-injected contrast bolus. Perfusion CT involves continuous cine scanning with a scan interval of 1 s and a total scanning duration of 40–45 s (Wintermark et al. 2005). Maps of cerebral blood volume (CBV), mean transit time (MTT), and cerebral blood flow (CBF) are generated from a voxel-by-voxel analysis of the change in attenuation over time. In severe trauma, CT perfusion has been shown to provide independent prognostic information regarding functional outcome with normal brain perfusion or hyperemia correlating with favorable outcome, and oligemia associated with unfavorable outcome (Wintermark et al. 2004). One potential limitation of dynamic perfusion CT is limited anatomic coverage, because only a few slices of the brain can be imaged on some CT scanners during the 1-s time acquisition window. Wider coverage can be achieved using a 40-mm-wide detector and toggling table technique or by the more recent availability of scanners with more multislice detectors (Siebert et al. 2009; Youn et al. 2008). Another limitation of CT perfusion is the additional radiation exposure that accompanies cine imaging.

Magnetic Resonance Imaging

Conventional MRI

MRI may be indicated in patients with acute TBI if the neurologic findings are unexplained by the CT imaging. Routine MR imaging typically includes T1- and T2-weighted spin-echo, gradient-echo, and inversion recovery MR sequences. MRI is preferred over CT for subacute and chronic TBI because of its superior sensitivity to older blood products. MR also demonstrates increased dectection of grey and white matter injury as well as lesions, especially shear injury, in the brainstem. MRI is comparable to CT in the detection of acute epidural and subdural hematomas (Gentry et al. 1988; Orrison et al. 1994). Compared to CT, MRI is more sensitive for detection of subtle extra-axial "smear" (i.e., very thin layer) collections, non-hemorrhagic lesions, and brainstem injuries. Fluid attenuated inversion recovery (FLAIR) MRI can also be more sensitive to subarachnoid hemorrhage (Noguchi et al. 1997; Woodcock et al. 2001).

Fluid Attenuated Inversion Recovery (FLAIR) imaging suppresses the bright cerebrospinal fluid (CSF) signal typically seen on conventional T2-weighted images, thereby improving the conspicuity of focal cortical injuries, white matter shearing injuries, and subarachnoid hemorrhages. Sagittal and coronal FLAIR images are particularly helpful in the detection of diffuse axonal injury (DAI) involving the corpus callosum and the fornix, two areas that can be difficult to evaluate on routine T2-weighted images (Ashikaga et al. 1997). Abnormal high signal in the sulci and cisterns of ventilated patients receiving a high inspired oxygen fraction greater than 0.60 (inspired oxygen fraction = [flow rate$_{air}$ × 0.21 + flow rate$_{oxygen}$]/[flow rate$_{air}$ + flow rate$_{oxygen}$ + flow rate$_{nitrous\ oxide}$]) can be observed on FLAIR sequences in normal, uninjured patients and should not be mistaken for subarachnoid hemorrhage (Frigon et al. 2002).

Gradient-Recalled-Echo (GRE) T2-weighted* imaging is highly sensitive to the susceptibility changes among tissues. The presence of blood breakdown products from brain injury, such as methemoglobin, ferritin and hemosiderin, alters the local magnetic susceptibility of tissue, resulting in areas of signal loss on GRE T2*-weighted images. Because hemosiderin can persist indefinitely, its detection on GRE T2*-weighted images is especially useful for the evaluation of remote TBI. Small foci of hemosiderin can, however, sometimes be resorbed; therefore, the lack of hemosiderin on GRE T2*-weighted images does not rigorously exclude old hemorrhage (Messori et al. 2003).

Advanced MRI Methods

Susceptibility-Weighted Imaging (SWI) further amplifies the susceptibility changes among tissues and blood products by combining magnitude and phase information from a high-resolution, velocity-compensated 3D T2*-weighted gradient echo sequence (Haacke et al. 2004). Conventional GRE T2*-weighted MRI relies only on the magnitude images and ignores the phase images, the latter of which contain valuable information regarding tissue susceptibility differences. In SWI, phase images are unwrapped and high-pass filtered to highlight phase changes. These are then converted to "*mask*" images that are multiplied with information from the corresponding magnitude images. The increase in tissue magnetic susceptibility contrast afforded by SWI is significantly more sensitive to small hemorrhages. SWI is 3–6 times more sensitive than GRE T2*-weighted imaging for detection of hemorrhagic DAI (Babikian et al. 2005; Tong et al. 2003, 2004).

Diffusion-Weighted Imaging (DWI) measures the random microscopic motion of water molecules in brain tissue. DWI is very sensitive to alterations in the pattern of water molecule movement that occurs following acute shear injury, and, thus, DWI has been particularly useful for the detection of DAI (Arfanakis et al. 2002; Huisman et al. 2003; Le et al. 2005; Liu et al. 1999; Niogi et al. 2008). DWI identifies more acute DAI lesions than fast spin-echo T2-weighted and/or GRE T2*-weighted images. Acute DAI lesions typically also show a reduced apparent diffusion coefficient (ADC), which measures the magnitude of water diffusion averaged over a 3-dimensional (3D) space. By comparison, chronic DAI lesions frequently demonstrate reduced fractional anisotropy (FA), which measures the preferential motion of water molecules along the white matter axons. The integrity of the white matter tracts can be further assessed with diffusion tensor imaging (DTI) with 3D tractography (Conturo et al. 1999; Mori and van Zijl 2002). Images of the white matter fiber tracts are generated based on the direction of fastest diffusion of water molecules, which is assumed to correspond to the longitudinal axis of the fiber tract. Unfortunately, there is still considerable variability in techniques used to prepare images of the fiber tracts using DTI tractography. Abnormalities identified within the white matter tracts created with DTI need to be carefully assessed for the parameters, technical expertise, and reproducibility of the image processing to distinguish true lesions from artifacts.

MR Spectroscopy (MRS) allows for in vivo measurement of the relative amount of metabolites in brain tissue. Common brain metabolites that are measured with proton (^{1}H) MRS include *N* acetylaspartate (NAA), creatine (Cr), choline (Cho), glutamate, lactate, and myoinositol. NAA is a cellular amino acid and is a marker of neuronal health. Creatine is a marker of energy metabolism and cellular density. Creatine is especially abundant in glial cells, and can serve as a marker for post-traumatic gliosis. Cho is a marker for membrane disruption, synthesis or repair. An increase in Cho is observed in myelin injury. MRS can detect abnormalities that may not be visible on conventional MRI (Garnett et al. 2000a, b). A reduction of NAA and an elevation of Cho have been shown to correlate with the severity of TBI, as measured by the GCS and duration of post-traumatic amnesia (Garnett et al. 2000a). A reduction in the NAA:Cr ratio also correlates with a worse prognosis following TBI (Sinson et al. 2001).

Magnetization Transfer Imaging (MTI) exploits the longitudinal (T1) relaxation coupling between bound (hydration) protons and free water (bulk) protons. Protons that bind to macromolecules are selectively saturated using an off-resonance saturation (radiofrequency) pulse. These bound protons subsequently exchange longitudinal magnetization with free water protons. The magnetization transfer ratio (MTR), a relative measure of the reduction in signal intensity due to the magnetization transfer (MT) effect, provides a quantitative measure of the structural integrity of tissue. In TBI, a reduction of the MTR correlates with a worse clinical outcome (Sinson et al. 2001).

Perfusion MRI employs either dynamic susceptibility contrast (DSC) or arterial spin labeling (ASL) imaging. In DSC-MRI, following intravenous injection of gadolinium contrast, continuous cine imaging of fast (echo-planar) T2*-weighted images is performed. As the contrast passes through the tissues, it causes susceptibility changes and associated reduction of signal intensity on T2*-weighted images. Maps of CBF, CBV, and MTT can be generated using pixel-by-pixel analysis of the signal changes. ASL-MRI is an alternative, safe, convenient noninvasive method to measure CBF by using the water molecules in arterial blood as a natural diffusible tracer. With ASL-MRI water molecules in inflowing arteries are "*labeled*" using radiofrequency (inversion or saturation) pulses proximal to the tissue of interest. Images of the tissue of interest are acquired after a short delay (usually 1 s) that allows the labeled blood water to flow into the imaging slices. The perfusion parameters are calculated by pair-wise comparison with baseline control images acquired without spin labeling. Based on the tracer half-life of blood T1, absolute CBF can be quantified. ASL scans can be repeated as often as necessary during the same scanning session without any added risks or cumulative effects.

Magnetic Source Imaging

Magnetic source imaging (MSI) utilizes magnetoencephalography (MEG) to localize weak magnetic signal generated by neuronal electrical activity. Electrical currents flowing within dendrites give rise to a surrounding magnetic field that can be measured by superconducting quantum interfering devices (SQUID). MEG provides a selective reflection of activity in dendrites oriented parallel to the skull surface. MSI integrates anatomic data obtained with conventional MRI and electrophysiological data obtained with MEG. So far, only two MSI studies have been published (Lewine et al. 1999, 2007). These MSI studies showed excessive abnormal low-frequency magnetic activity in mTBI patients with post-concussive syndrome. Additional research is warranted before MSI can be adopted in the clinical setting.

Positron Emission Tomography

Positron emission tomography (PET) utilizes positron-emitting isotopes, commonly 15-oxygen (^{15}O) to measure cerebral perfusion and oxygen metabolism, and 2-fluoro-2-deoxy-D-glucose (^{18}F-FDG) to measure cerebral glucose metabolism. ^{15}O-PET can define potential ischemic areas after brain injury, which is associated with poor outcome (Coles et al. 2004a, b; Menon 2006). ^{18}F-FDG can evaluate glucose metabolism in vivo. Acutely injured brain cells show increased glucose metabolism following severe TBI due to intracellular ionic perturbation (Bergsneider et al. 2001). Following the initial hyperglycolysis state, injured brain cells show a prolonged period of regional hypometabolism. Since glucose metabolism reflects neuronal activity, regional hypometabolism implies neuronal dysfunction. For that reason, ^{18}F-FDG has the potential to reveal cerebral dysfunction in regions that would appear otherwise "normal" on CT or MRI (Kato et al. 2007; Nakashima et al. 2007). Although ^{18}F-FDG PET imaging has made great progress in the field of oncology, it is relatively expensive and is not widely available for the evaluation of TBI.

Single Photon Emission Tomography

Single photon emission tomography (SPECT) uses gamma-emitting isotopes, e.g., ^{133}Xe and technetium-99-m-hexamethyl-propylamine-oxime (^{99}Tc-HMPAO), to measure CBF. It can potentially provide a better long-term prognostic predictor in comparison to CT or conventional MRI (Newton et al. 1992). For example, a worse prognosis has been associated with multiple CBF abnormalities, larger CBF defects, and CBF defects within the brainstem, basal ganglia, temporal and parietal lobes. SPECT can also show areas of perfusion abnormality following head trauma that are "normal" on conventional CT and MRI (Kinuya et al. 2004). However, due to its low spatial resolution, SPECT is less sensitive in detecting small lesions that are visible on MRI.

Imaging Findings

Missile and Penetrating Injury

In the United States, the majority of penetrating injuries are due to assaults and suicide attempts (Gean et al. 1995). More than 80% of gunshot wounds to the head penetrate the scalp and skull, and 80% of these patients die (Awasthi 1992). Missile injuries result in various forms of brain damage, depending on the mass, velocity and shape of the missile (Lindenberg and Freytag 1960). Missile injury is classified as superficial, depressed, penetrating, or perforating. In *superficial missile injury*, the weapon remains extracranial and the skull is intact, but brain damage can still occur as a result of the initial impact force (Fig. 2.1). High velocity, small shotgun fragments can cause intracranial injury even if they are superficial because the applied energy depends not only on the mass (m) but also on the

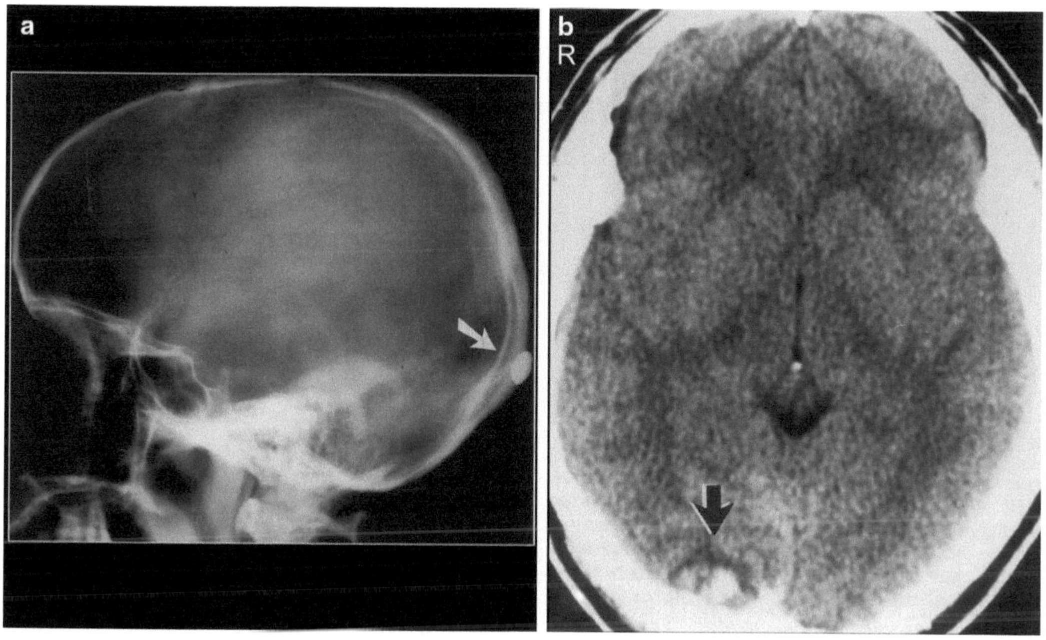

Fig. 2.1 Superficial missile injury. (**a**) Lateral skull film shows a bullet lodged within the soft tissue overlying the occiput. (**b**) Non-contrast axial CT, performed after removal of the bullet, demonstrates a subjacent left occipital lobe contusion (*arrow*). No fracture is identified on the "bone window" images (not shown). (Reprinted with permission from Gean AD. Imaging of head trauma. Philadelphia, PA: Williams & Wilkins-Lippincott; 1994, p. 191)

square of the velocity (v) (i.e., kinetic energy = $\frac{1}{2}mv^2$). With increases in velocity, an extracranial missile may have enough impact to cause a depressed skull fracture and subjacent parenchymal injury, resulting in a *depressed missile injury* (Fig. 2.2). However, the majority of ballistics penetrate skull, meninges, and brain, causing a *penetrating missile injury* (Awasthi 1992). The brain laceration caused by the missile is characteristically canalicular, with decreasing diameter from the entry site to the exit site. A high-velocity missile can generate enough shock wave damage to cause a contusion at a distance from the missile trajectory or even result in diffuse cerebral edema (Fig. 2.3). With even greater velocity, a missile can exit the contralateral side of the skull, resulting in a *perforating missile injury*. The exit site is usually larger than the entry site (Purvis 1966). Another distinguishing feature is that the inner table of the skull is beveled at the entry site while the outer table of the skull is beveled at the exit site (Fig. 2.4).

Blunt Injury

Primary Extra-Axial Injury

Pneumocephalus

Pneumocephalus (intracranial air) indicates a communication between the intracranial and extracranial compartments. Pneumocephalus can occur in the epidural (Fig. 2.6), subdural, intraventricular space or the brain parenchyma (pneumatocele). The most frequent cause of traumatic pneumocephalus is from a fracture of the posterior wall of the frontal sinus. With a calvarial-dural defect, rapid increases in pressure within the paranasal sinuses (e.g., from sneezing or coughing) may force air into the intracranial cavity. With a CSF leak, the decrease in intracanial pressure (ICP) also leads to a compensatory influx of air, resulting in pneumocephalus. Most cases of pneumocephalus resolve spontaneously. In rare instances, expanding tension pneumocephalus can cause mass effect, headache, stiff neck, stupor, and papilledema (Briggs 1974).

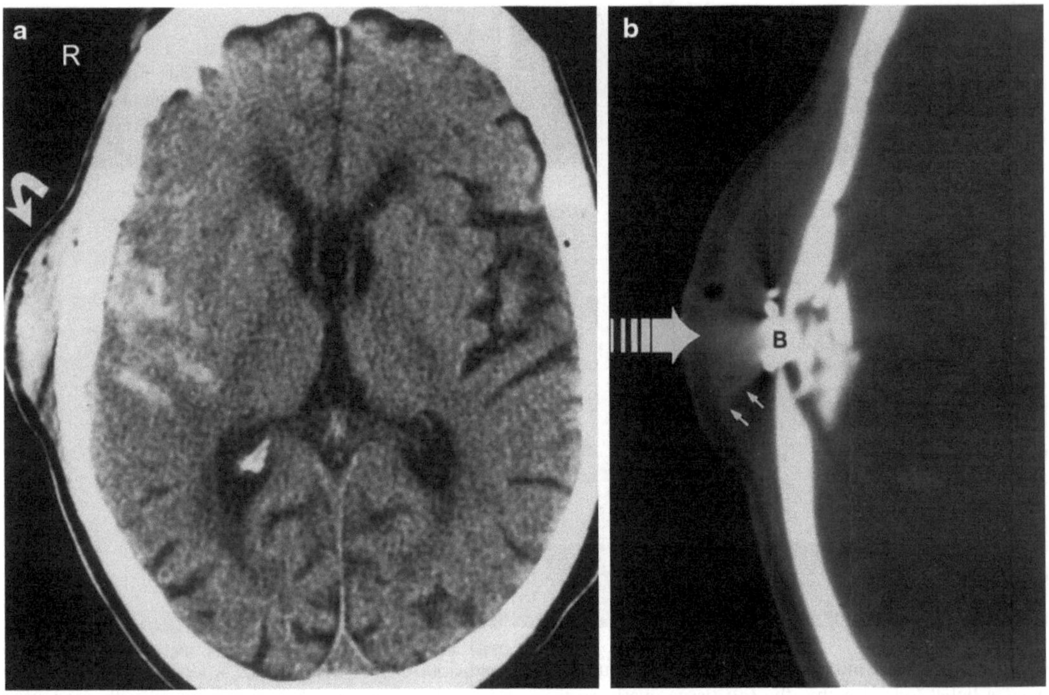

Fig. 2.2 Depressed missile injury. (**a**) Non-contrast axial CT image demonstrates posterior right temporal scalp soft tissue swelling (*curved arrow*) and a subjacent temporal contusion, subarachnoid hemorrhage, and effacement of the frontotemporal sulci. (**b**) CT image displayed in bone window reveals a bullet fragment (B) lodged within the outer table of the skull. Multiple bone fragments from the inner table of the skull are noted. (Reprinted with permission from Gean AD. Imaging of head trauma. Philadelphia, PA: Williams & Wilkins-Lippincott; 1994, p. 192)

Tension pneumocephalus requires immediate intervention. On imaging, the air usually collects ventrally since most patients are scanned in the supine position.

Epidural Hematoma

A hematoma that develops within the potential space located between the dura and the inner table of the skull is called an *epidural hematoma* (EDH). The EDH splits the dura from the inner table of the skull, forming an oval collection that can cause focal compression of the underlying brain. Because the EDH is subperiosteal, it rarely crosses cranial sutures, where the outer periosteal layer of the dura is firmly attached at sutural margins (Fig. 2.5) (Gean et al. 1995). At the vertex, however, where the periosteum is not tightly attached to the sagittal suture, the EDH can cross the midline.

EDHs are usually arterial in origin. Most EDHs occur at the coup site (i.e., the site of impact) and are usually associated with a skull fracture, commonly involving the temporal squamosa region where the fracture disrupts the partially embedded middle meningeal artery (Zee and Go 1998; Zimmerman et al. 1978). In children, EDHs may occur from stretching or tearing of meningeal arteries without an associated fracture. EDHs are less common in young children because the overall incidence of head trauma is lower the pediatric skull is more compliant, and the meningeal groove is more shallow. EDHs are also less common in the elderly because the dura in the elderly is more adherent to the inner table of the skull and is, therefore, not easily displaced.

On CT, an acute EDH appears as a well-defined biconvex hyperdense collection, with attenuation between 50 to 70 Hounsfield units (HU) (Fig. 2.6). On MRI, a thin dark line is observed at the inner margin of the EDH (Fig. 2.7). This line represents the two layers of displaced dura and confirms

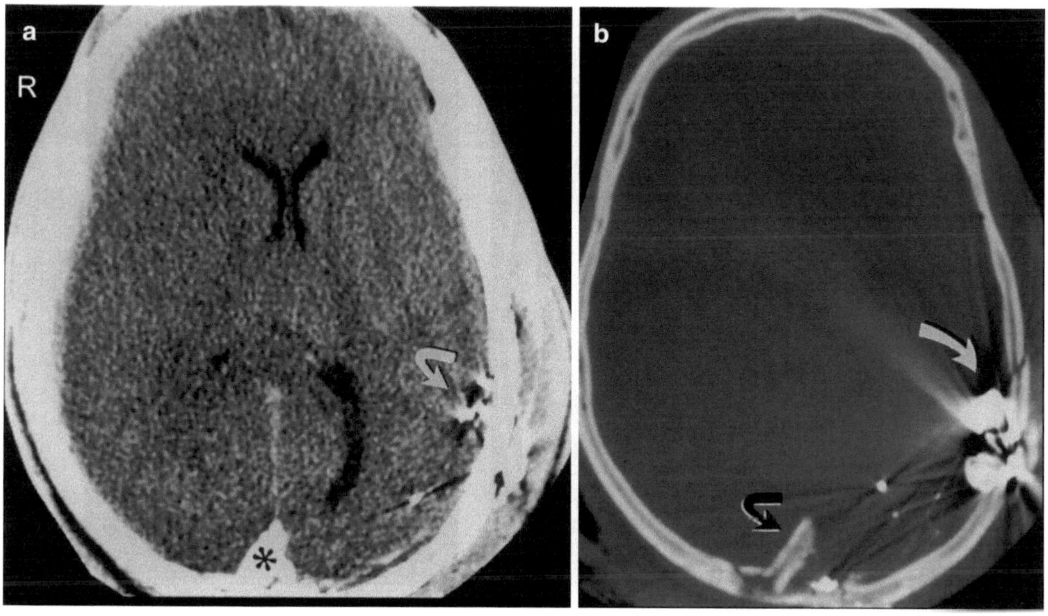

Fig. 2.3 Penetrating missile injury. (**a**) Non-contrast axial CT image reveals several metallic fragments within the left parietal lobe (*arrow*) with associated overlying scalp soft-tissue swelling. There is effacement of the right occipital horn and complete loss of gray-white matter differentiation due to cerebral edema. A bone fragment projects into the superior sagittal sinus (*asterisk*). (**b**) The corresponding bone-window image demonstrates a displaced fracture fragment projecting into the superior sagittal sinus (*black arrow*). Note how the donor site for the fracture fragment is the inner table of the skull—a finding consistent with the clinical history that the patient was shot in the occiput. Multiple metallic fragments and a comminuted skull fracture are seen in the left parietal region (*white arrow*). The patient died several hours later. (Reprinted with permission from Gean AD. Imaging of head trauma. Philadelphia, PA: Williams & Wilkins-Lippincott; 1994, p. 193)

the epidural location of the hematoma. Inward displacement of the venous sinuses also serves as a clue that the hematoma is located within the epidural space. As is the case with hematomas elsewhere, the MR signal characteristics of the EDH correlate with the age of the blood products (Gomori et al. 1985; Fobben et al. 1989).

An important imaging finding of the EDH that correlates with a worse prognosis is the presence of low-density areas within the hyperdense hematoma (the "swirl sign"), thought to represent active bleeding (Fig. 2.8) (Al-Nakshabandi 2001; Greenberg et al. 1985). It forewarns expansion of an arterial EDH. Patients with an expanding EDH tend to present early, with a poorer GCS, and a higher mortality rate (Pruthi et al. 2009). Contrast extravasation within the low density areas of the EDH due to active hemorrhage from an underlying dural vessel laceration has also been reported (Kumbhani et al. 2009). Thus, active extravasation on CT may be another potential biomarker for EDH expansion, and may warrant more aggressive clinical management. Midline shift > 1 cm and brainstem distortion are additional imaging findings that often require aggressive management.

Venous EDHs are less common than arterial EDHs, and they occur due to bleeding from meningeal and diploic veins or from the dural sinuses. They tend to occur in three classic locations: (1) the posterior fossa from rupture of the torcula Herophili or transverse sinus (Fig. 2.9), (2) middle cranial fossa from disruption of the sphenoparietal sinus (Fig. 2.9), (Le and Gean 2009) and (3) vertex due to injury to the superior sagittal sinus or cortical veins (Gean et al. 1995). Unlike the arterial EDH, the venous EDH rarely expands beyond its initial size because of the lower pressure imposed by venous extravasation. The venous EDH is less frequently associated with a skull fracture than is the arterial EDH.

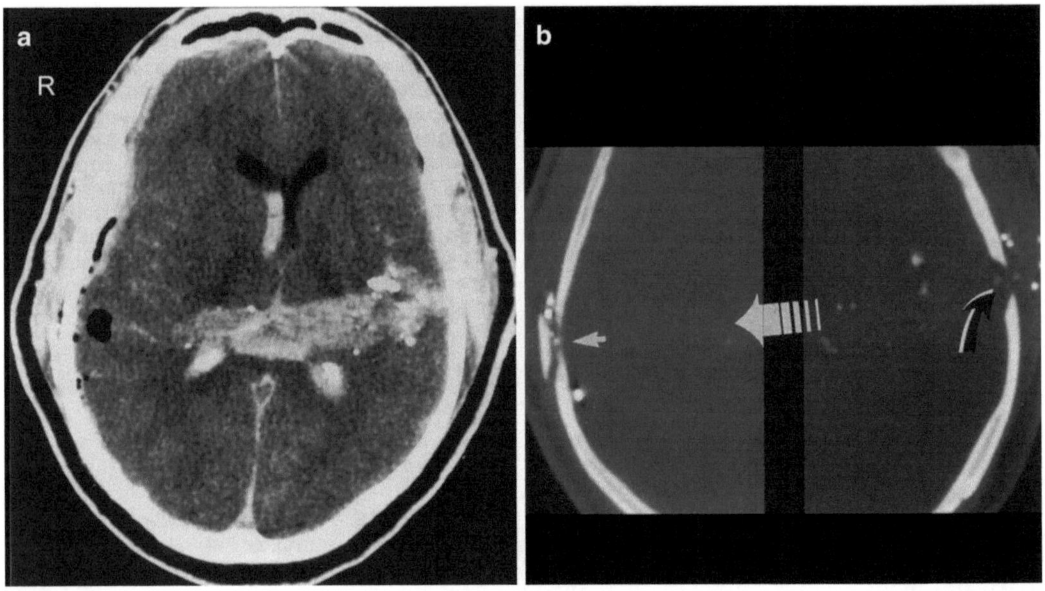

Fig. 2.4 Perforating missile injury. (**a**) Non-contrast axial CT image demonstrates a left temporal gunshot wound that crosses the midline and ultimately exits the right temporal skull on a higher section. Note how the brain injury typically has a canalicular shape with a diameter that decreases from the site of entry to its exit. There is intraventricular hemorrhage, a small right subdural hematoma, and a small amount of pneumocephalus. (**b**) Corresponding bone-window images are spliced together to illustrate how the entry and exit sites can be distinguished by the location of the calvarial beveling. At the entry site (*black arrow*), the inner table of the skull is beveled. At the exit site, the outer table of the skull is beveled (*small white arrow*). In this example, only a few bullet fragments actually perforate the skull at the exit site. A wedge-shaped bone fragment from the outer table appears to have been lifted off the calvarial surface. (Reprinted with permission from Gean AD. Imaging of head trauma. Philadelphia, PA: Williams & Wilkins-Lippincott; 1994; p. 193)

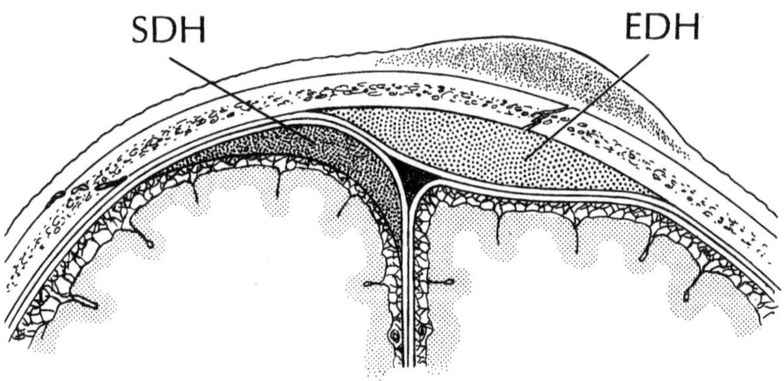

Fig. 2.5 Coronal diagram of the EDH and SDH. The EDH is located above the outer dural layer (i.e., the periosteum), and the SDH is located beneath the inner (meningeal) dural layer. The EDH does not cross sutures. The SDH does not directly cross the falx or the tentorium. (Reprinted with permission from Gean AD. Imaging of head trauma. Philadelphia, PA: Williams & Wilkins-Lippincott; 1994, p. 76)

Subdural Hematoma

The *subdural hematoma* (SDH) occurs above the arachnoid and beneath the inner meningeal layer of the dura (Fig. 2.5). Because the dura and arachnoid are not firmly attached, the SDH is frequently seen layering along the entire hemispheric convexity from the anterior falx to the posterior falx. The SDH usually develops from

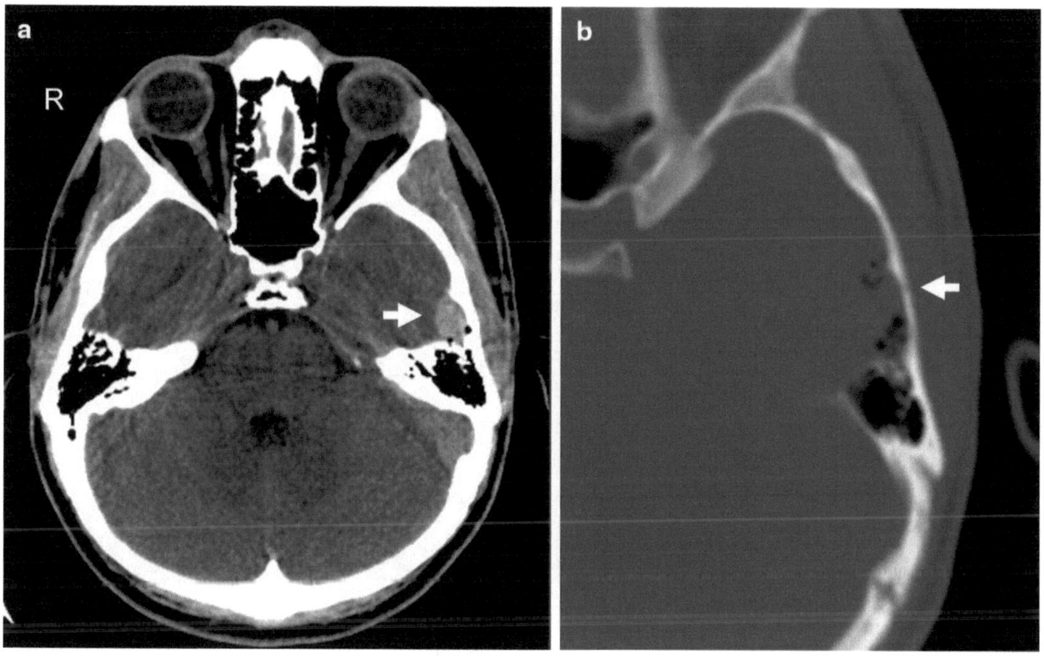

Fig. 2.6 Acute EDH. (**a**) Non-contrast axial CT shows a characteristic hyperdense, homogeneous, biconvex left temporal extra-axial collection (*arrow*). (**b**) An adjacent axial CT slice, displayed in bone window, reveals associated pneumocephalus and a linear non-displaced fracture of the left temporal bone (*arrow*)

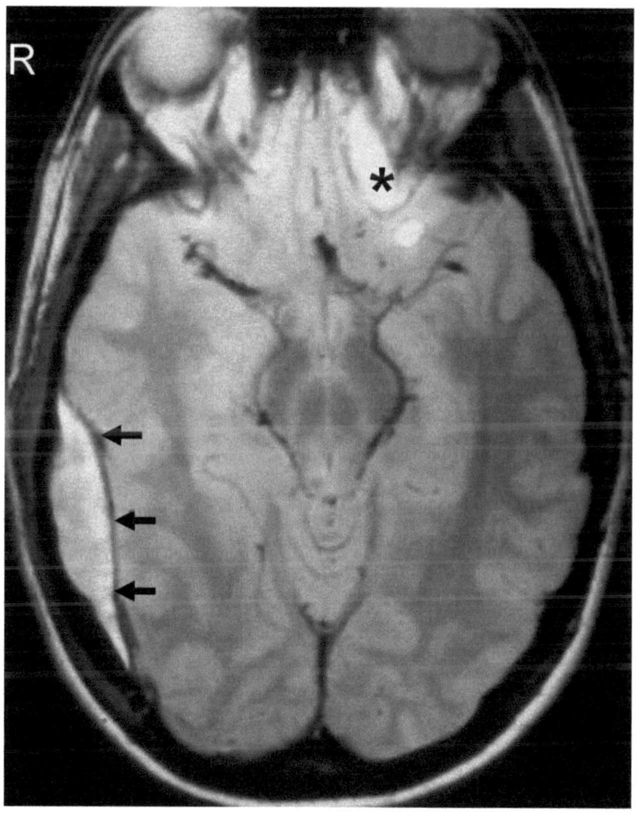

Fig. 2.7 Subacute EDH on MRI. Proton density-weighted axial MR image shows a thin dark line (*horizontal arrows*) displaced by the extra-axial collection, indicating the epidural location of the hematoma. A contrecoup left orbitofrontal contusion is also evident (*asterisk*). (Reprinted with permission from Gean AD. Imaging of head trauma. Philadelphia, PA: Williams & Wilkins-Lippincott; 1994, p. 119)

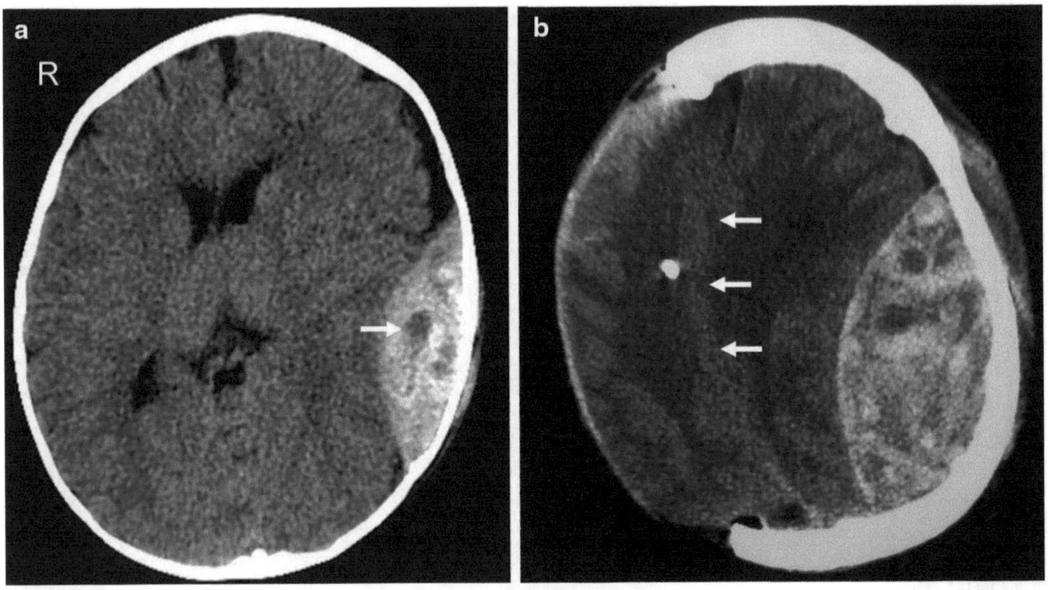

Fig. 2.8 EDH "swirl sign". (**a**) Axial CT image shows low attenuation areas (*arrow*) within a left frontotemporal heterogenous acute EDH. The heterogeneous density within this EDH is secondary to mixing of hyperacute (low attenuation) with acute (high attenuation) blood. (**b**) Axial CT image from another patient, performed following decompressive craniectomy, demonstrates right external herniation, left-to-right subfalcine herniation (*arrows*), and formation of a contralateral, heterogenous EDH

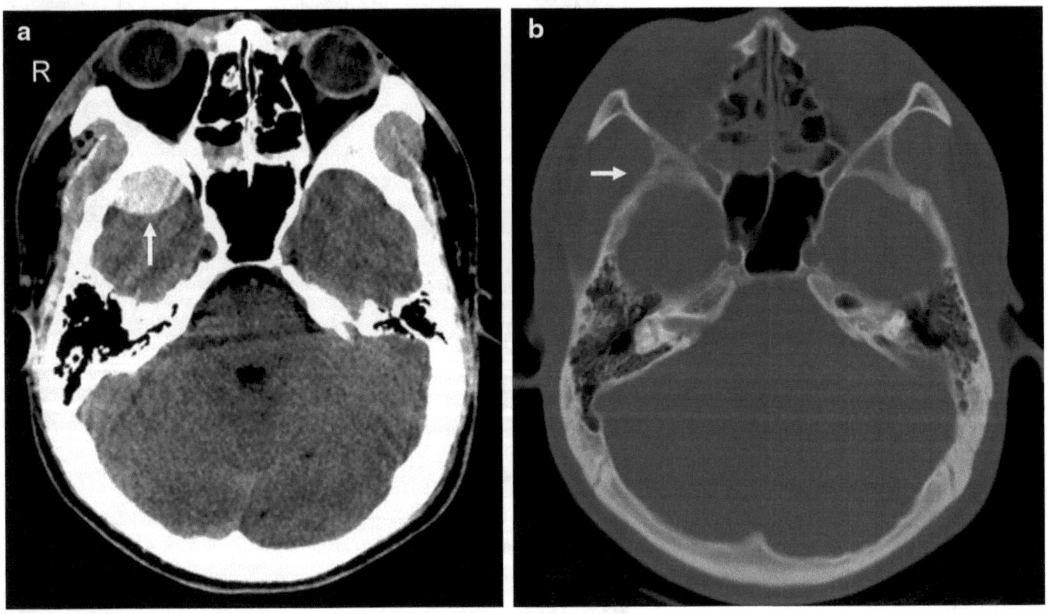

Fig. 2.9 Venous EDH. (**a**) Axial CT image shows a biconvex, homogeneous, high attenuation extra-axial collection within the right middle cranial fossa (*vertical arrow*). (**b**) CT image displayed in "bone window" reveals a fracture of the right greater sphenoid wing (*horizontal arrow*). The location suggests that the hematoma is due to disruption of the sphenoparietal sinus. (Reprinted with permission from Le TH and Gean AD. Neuroimaging of traumatic brain injury. Mt Sinai J Med. 2009;76:145–162)

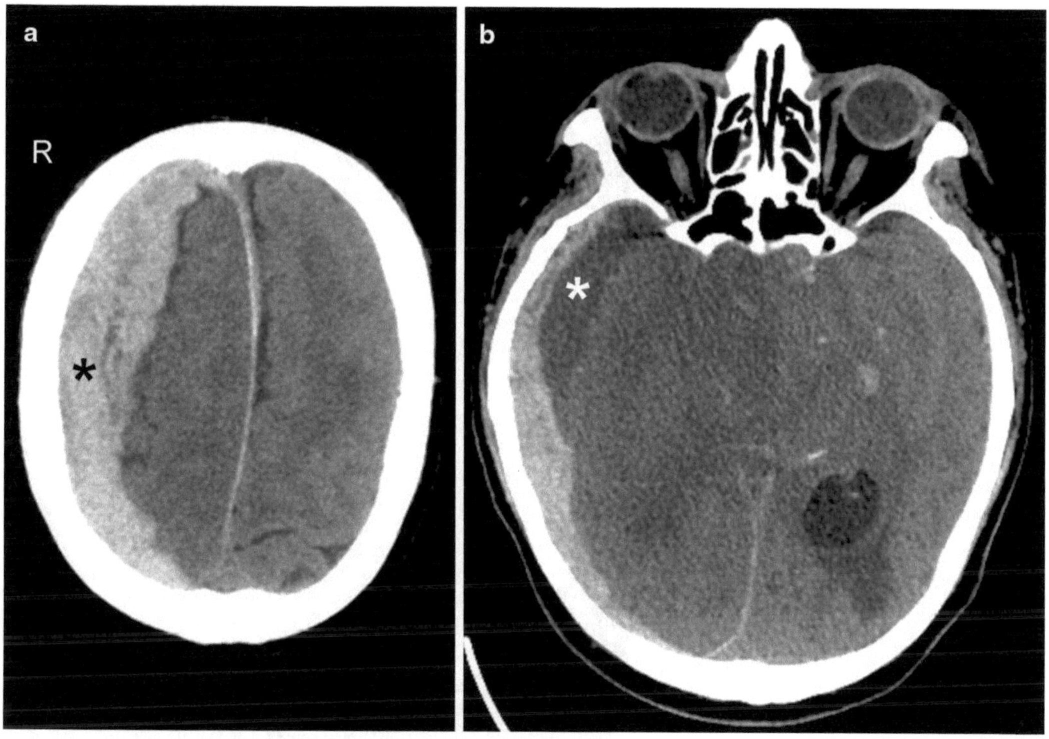

Fig. 2.10 SDH. (**a**) Non-contrast axial CT image demonstrates a right hyperdense, holohemispheric extra-axial collection (*asterisk*), causing mass effect and sulcal effacement of the right cerebral hemisphere. There is also mild right-to-left subfacine herniation. (**b**) Non-contrast axial CT image shows a low-density area (*asterisk*) corresponding to a chronic SDH component within an acute right temporal SDH. There is associated loss of gray-white matter differentiation and diffuse decrease in attenuation of the right temporal lobe and midbrain due to cerebral edema and ischemia. There is effacement of the cisterns. Multiple foci of small hemorrhages within the left temporal lobe indicate axonal injuries. There is also dilatation of the occipital horn of the left ventricle

laceration or disruption of bridging cortical veins, especially during sudden head deceleration. Disruption of bridging cortical veins can also occur with rapid decompression of obstructive hydrocephalus, when the brain surface recedes from the dura quicker than the brain parenchyma can re-expand after being compressed by the distended ventricles. SDH can also arise from injury to pial vessels, pacchionian granulations, or penetrating branches of superficial cerebral arteries. The incidence of SDH is higher in the elderly because the increase in extra-axial space from cerebral atrophy allows for increased motion between the brain parenchyma and the calvarium.

Most SDHs are supratentorial and located over the convexity, especially the parietal region. They are frequently seen along the falx and tentorium. Unlike EDHs, SDHs frequently occur at the contrecoup site. Because the SDH is often associated with parenchymal injury, the degree of mass effect may appear more extensive than the size of the SDH blood collection.

On CT, the acute SDH appears as a hyperdense, homogeneous, and crescent-shaped collection (Fig. 2.10a). Compared to normal brain (20–30 HU), the density (attenuation) of an acute SDH (50–60 HU) is higher because of clot retraction. The density of the SDH will progressively decrease as protein degradation occurs. Rebleeding during evolution of a SDH appears as a heterogeneous mixture of fresh blood and partially liquefied hematoma (Fig. 2.10b). A sediment level or "*hematocrit effect*" may be seen from either rebleeding or in patients with clotting disorders.

Between 1 and 3 weeks following injury, an isodense SDH phase occurs. The timing depends

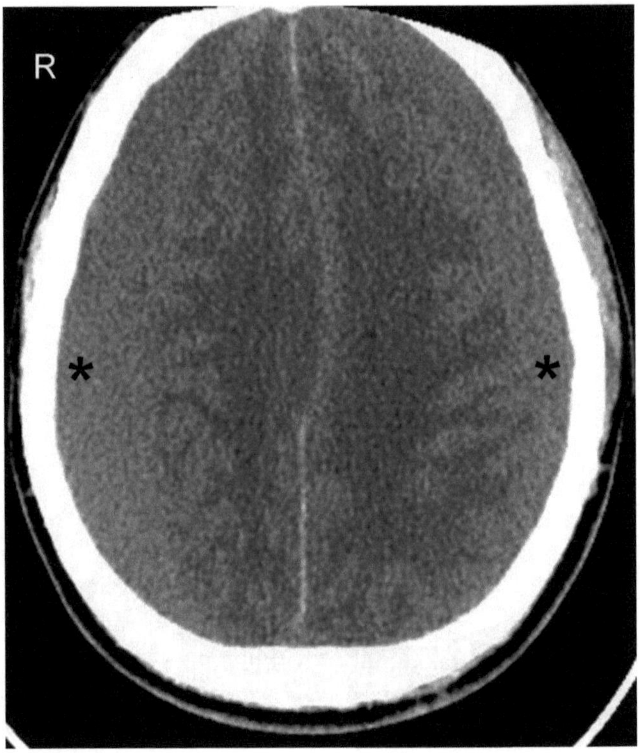

Fig. 2.11 Isodense subacute SDH. Non-contrast axial CT image shows bilateral isodense SDHs. During the transition from acute to chronic SDH, an isodense phase occurs. At this stage, the SDH (*asterisk*) can be difficult to differentiate from the adjacent brain parenchyma. Note displacement of the gray-white matter junction from the inner table of the skull (the "*thick gray matter mantle*" sign)

on the patient's hematocrit level, clotting capability, and presence or absence of re-bleeding. During this subacute period, a small thin convexity isodense SDH can be difficult to identify on CT (Fig. 2.11). Imaging findings such as sulcal effacement, effacement or distortion of the white matter (white matter "*buckling*"), abnormal separation of the gray-white matter junction from the inner table of the skull ("*thick gray matter mantle*"), distortion of the venticles, and midline shift are indirect signs that can improve detection of isodense SDHs.

The chronic SDH has density similar to, but slightly higher than, cerebrospinal fluid on CT (Fig. 2.12). It may be difficult to distinguish from prominent subarachnoid space in patients with cerebral atrophy. In these patients, a contrast-enchanced CT can improve detection of the chronic SDH by demonstrating an enhancing capsule or displaced cortical veins. Over time, activated fibroblasts and blood vessels from the dura organize within the SDH. The fragile penetrating vessels are prone to bleeding, which can lead to the dreaded "*chronic recurrent*" SDH. The chronic recurrent SDH may not be crescentic in shape because of dural adhesions, and it is typically heterogeneous with multiple internal septations, loculations, and fluid levels (Fig. 2.13f).

The MRI signal characteristics of the SDH vary depending on the age of the blood products (Gomori et al. 1985; Fobben et al. 1989). The acute SDH is isointense to brain on T1-weighted images and hypointense on T2-weighted images. During the subacute phase, when the SDH is isodense on non-contrast CT images, the SDH has a high signal intensity on T1-weighted images due to the presence of methemoglobin (Fig. 2.13a). The chronic SDH appears hypointense on T1-weighted and hyperintense on T2-weighted images relative to normal brain. The signal intensity of the chronic SDH is typically slightly higher than CSF signal intensity on T1- and T2-weighted and FLAIR images (Fig. 2.13b). The lack of beam-hardening artifact and the capability of multiplanar imaging make MRI particularly useful in identifying small convexity and vertex hematomas that may not be readily recognized on axial CT.

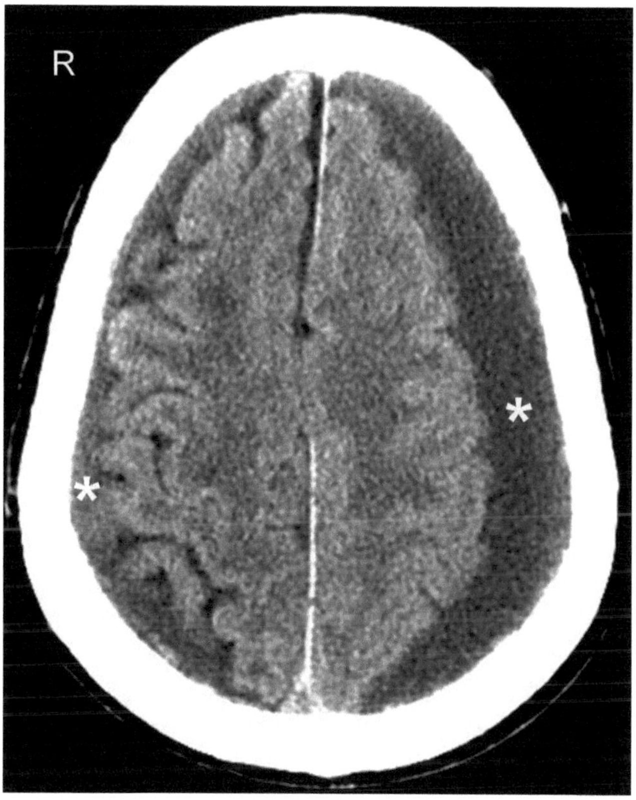

Fig. 2.12 Chronic SDH. Non-contrast axial CT image demonstrates bilateral low-density collections (*asterisk*) due to chronic SDHs. The chronic SDH has attenuation slightly higher than CSF

Subarchnoid Hemorrhage

Traumatic *subarachnoid hemorrhage* (SAH) can develop from disruption of small pial vessels due to skull fracture or brain motion, from contiguous extension into the subarachnoid space by a contusion or a hematoma, or from spread of intraventricular hemorrhage via the fourth ventricular outlet foramina. Common sites for traumatic SAH include the sylvian fissure, the interpeduncular cistern, and the high convexity. The greatest accumulation of SAH tends to occur on the con trecoup side.

On CT, acute SAH appears as areas of high density that conform to the morphology of the cerebral sulci and cisterns (Fig. 2.14). SAH along the convexity or tentorium can be difficult to differentiate from a SDH. A useful distinguishing clue is the extension of the SAH into adjacent sulci. Occasionally, "effacement" of the sulci due to the presence of intra-sulcal SAH is the only imaging clue of the presence of SAH.

Acute SAH is more difficult to detect on conventional T1- and T2-weighted MRI than on CT because intracellular oxyhemoglobin and/or deoxyhemoglobin is isointense to brain parenchyma. However, FLAIR is potentially more sensitive than CT, especially when at a volume of at least 1–2 mL is present (Woodcock et al. 2001). Subacute SAH, when the blood is isointense to CSF on CT, is better recognized on MRI because of the high signal intensity of extracellular methemoglobin. SAH more than 1-week old would be difficult, if not impossible, to detect on CT. Chronic SAH is better detected on MRI and is invisible on CT. Old blood products, such as hemosiderin in the subarachnoid space ("superficial hemosiderosis"), are best detected on SWI and GRE T2*-weighted images (Fig. 2.15) and appear as areas of decreased signal intensity

Intraventricular Hemorrhage

Traumatic *intraventricular hemorrhage* (IVH) can result from rotationally-induced tearing of subependymal veins along the surface of the ventricles, from contiguous extension of a parenchymal

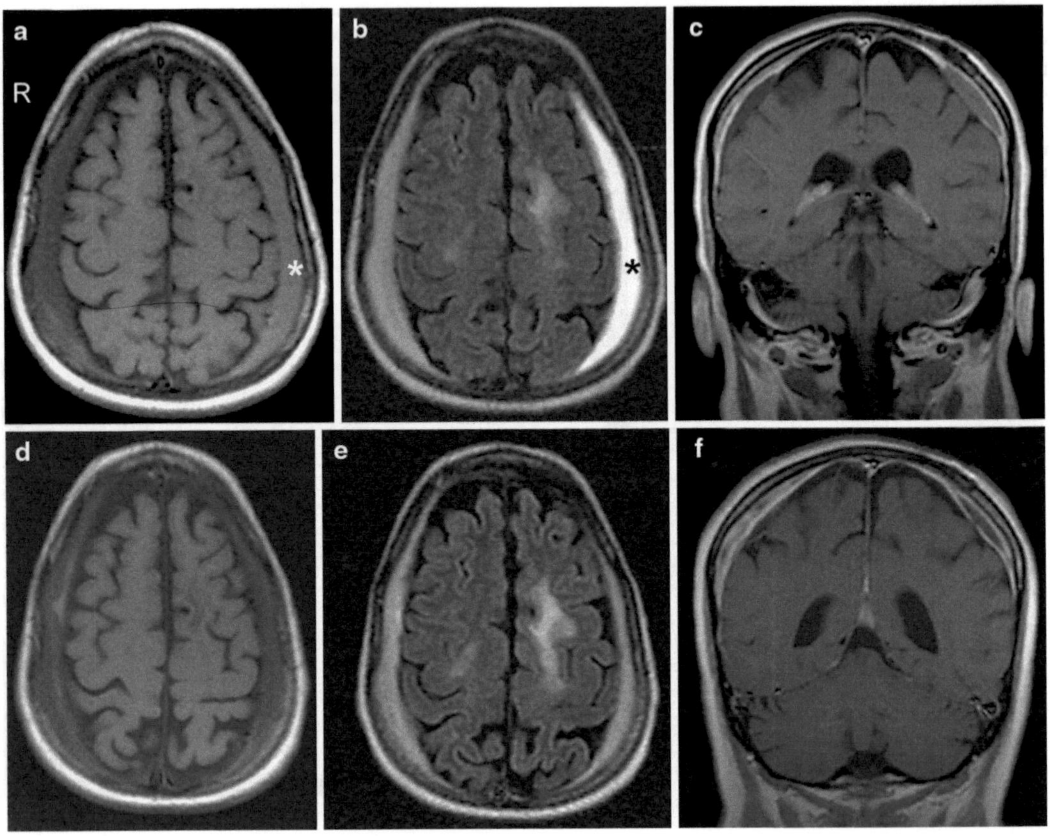

Fig. 2.13 MRI of SDH. (**a**) Axial T1-weighted MR image, performed on a 0.7 T open MRI, reveals bilateral holohemispheric SDHs. The subacute left SDH has signal intensity relatively higher than adjacent parenchyma due to the presence of methemoglobin. (**b**) The corresponding FLAIR image shows that the subacute left SDH is quite intense. The chronic right SDH has signal intensity higher than the suppressed CSF signal. (**c**) The SDHs also have enhancing capsules, as seen on the coronal T1-weighted post-contrast image. (**d**) Axial T1-weighted image, performed 2 months later, shows evolution of the left SDH, which is now low in intensity. (**e**) Both SDHs are now of similar intensity on FLAIR. (**f**) Coronal T1-weighted post-contrast image shows heterogenous enhancement within the right SDH due to the presence of activated fibroblasts and blood vessels from the dura organized within the SDH

hematoma into the ventricular system, or from retrograde flow of SAH into the ventricles (Fig. 2.14). Direct penetrating wounds can also cause IVH. Patients with IVH are at risk for developing non-communicating hydrocephalus from obstruction of the aqueduct due to ependymal proliferation ("ependymitis") and/or communicating hydrocephalus from obstructive scarring of the arachnoid villi.

On CT, acute IVH typically appears as a hyperdense collection layering dependently within the ventricular system, forming a CSF-blood fluid level (Fig. 2.14). Sometimes, a tiny collection of increased density layering posteriorly in one occipital horn may be the only clue to IVH. Occasionally, the IVH appears "tumefactive" or "mass-like" as a cast within the ventricle.

Primary Intra-Axial Injury

Diffuse Axonal Injury

Traumatic *axonal injury* refers to white matter damage arising from shear-strain deformation of brain tissue following rotational acceleration and deceleration injury. When the skull is rapidly rotated, axial stretching, separation, and disruption of the white matter fibers occur because the non-rigid brain and brainstem lag behind. *Diffuse axonal injury* (DAI) indicates extensive injury to

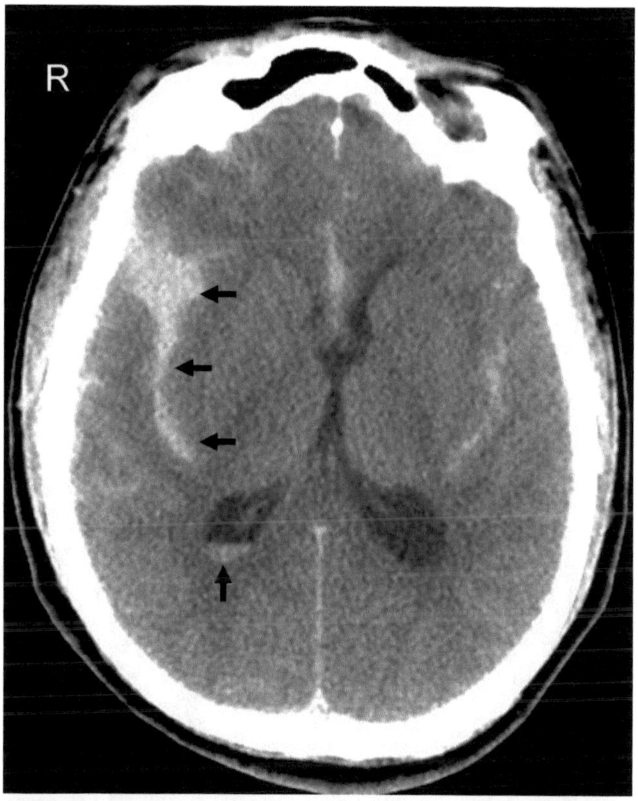

Fig. 2.14 SAH and IVH. Non-contrast axial CT image demonstrates bilateral high attenuation collections conforming to the sylvian sulci due to acute SAH. The greatest collection of SAH is within the right sylvian sulcus (*horizontal arrows*). Small high-density collection layering within the occipital horn of the right lateral ventricle is compatible with acute IVH (*vertical arrow*)

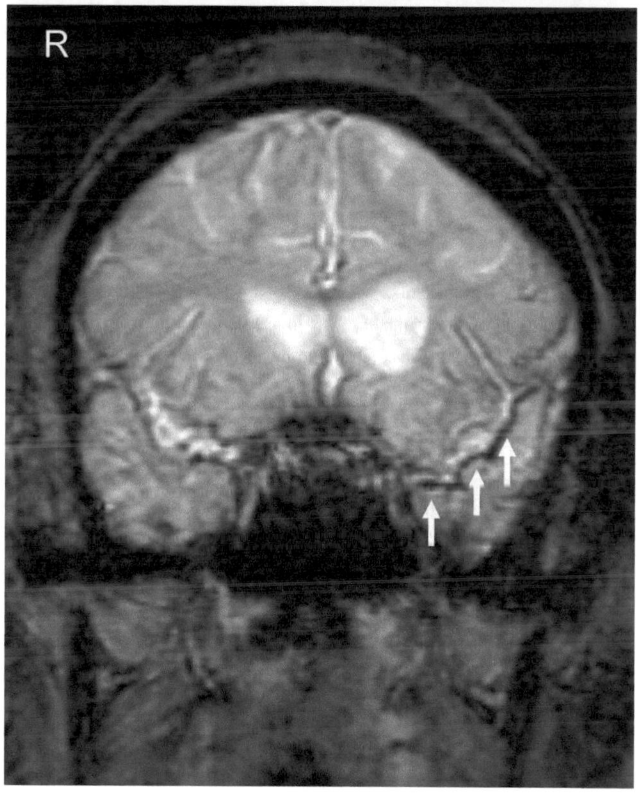

Fig. 2.15 Chronic SAH on GRE MRI. Coronal GRE T2*-weighted image demonstrates bilateral decrease in signal within the temporal sulci, with the greatest accumulation within the left sylvian sulcus (*arrow*) due to hemosiderin deposits (superficial siderosis)

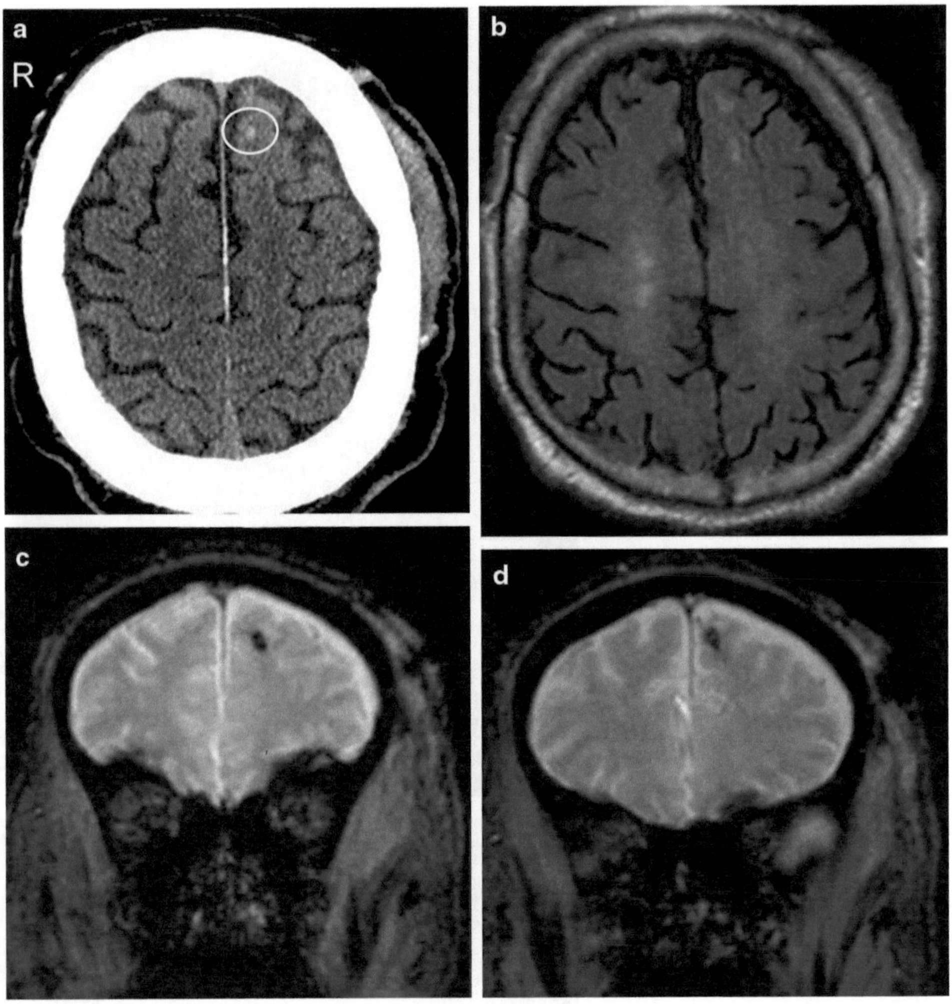

Fig. 2.16 Grade I DAI. (**a**) Non-contrast axial CT image reveals a small high-density focus within the subcortical white matter of the left frontal lobe, compatible with hemorrhagic shear injury. (**b**) Follow-up axial FLAIR image demonstrates a corroborated subcortical focus of T2 hyperintensity. There is an additional left frontal subcortical focus of FLAIR hyperintensity that is not visible on the CT image. Nonspecific T2 signal abnormality within the bilateral centrum semiovale is also noted. (**c** and **d**) Coronal GRE T2*-weighted images show corresponding foci of hemorrhagic shear injury within the left frontal lobe

the white matter and occurs in up to 50% of severe head trauma cases (Jennett et al. 2001). DAI is of special interest because it is believed to be responsible for the majority of unexplained cognitive deficits following head trauma. DAI is under diagnosed by conventional imaging techniques (Inglese et al. 2005; Mittl et al. 1994).

DAI tends to occur in three classic regions ("*shearing injury triad*"): the lobar white matter, the corpus callosum, and the dorsolateral quadrant of the rostal brainstem adjacent to the superior cerebellar peduncle. The location of DAI generally correlates with the severity of the trauma (Gennarelli et al. 1982). Mild (Grade I) DAI typically involves only the peripheral gray–white junction of the lobar white matter, commonly the parasagittal regions of the frontal lobes and the temporal stem (Fig. 2.16). With moderate (Grade II) DAI, the corpus callosum, particularly the posterior body and splenium, in addition to the lobar white matter, is involved (Fig. 2.17). In severe (Grade III) DAI, the dorsolateral midbrain, in addition to the lobar white matter and corpus callosum, is affected.

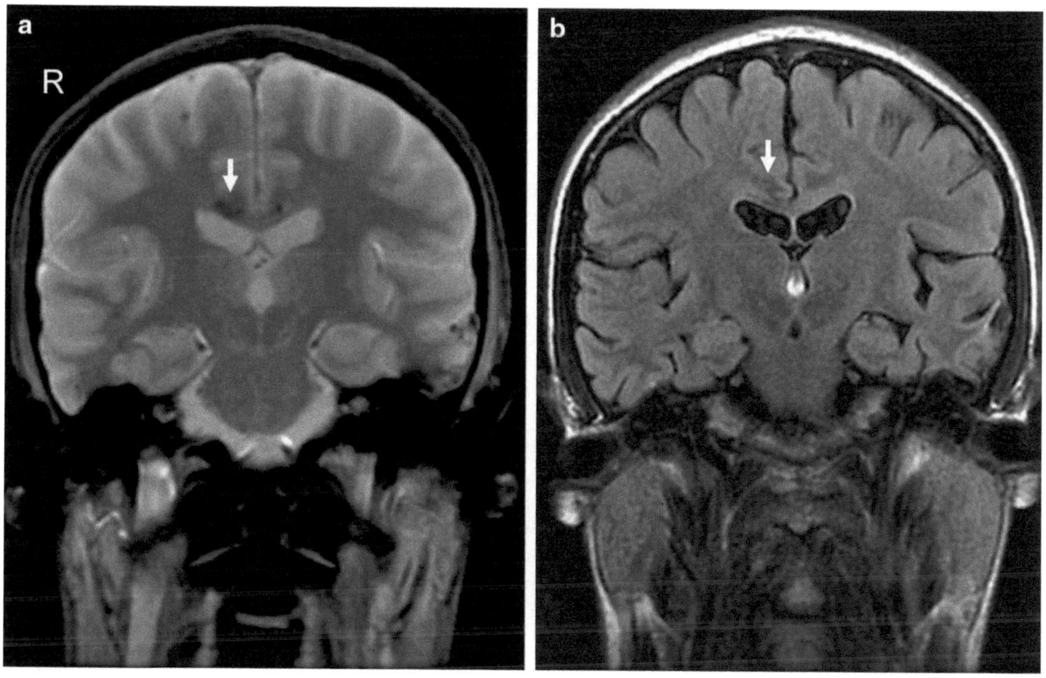

Fig. 2.17 Grade II DAI. (**a**) Coronal GRE T2*-weighted image demonstrates multiple foci of low signal (hemorrhages) within the peripheral gray-white junction of the bilateral temporal and right frontal lobes. Abnormal foci of low signal are also seen within the corpus callosum (*arrow*). (**b**) The callosal injury is low in signal intensity on FLAIR (*arrow*) and is not as easily detectable

On CT, DAI lesions appear as small high attenuation foci (shear hemorrhages) at the gray–white junction of the cerebral hemispheres (Fig. 2.16a), corpus callosum, and the dorsolateral midbrain, depending on the severity of the trauma. Because of its higher sensitivity to blood products, GRE T2*-weighted MRI reveals more hemorrhagic DAI lesions than CT (Mittl et al. 1994). Even so, detection of hemorrhagic shear alone does not fully describe the extent of DAI (Adams et al. 1991). FLAIR MRI can identify additional non-hemorrhagic foci of DAI but still underestimates the true extent of the diffuse white matter damage (Ashikaga et al. 1997). Non-hemorrhagic acute DAI lesions appear as multiple small foci of increased signal on T2-weighted images and decreased signal on T1-weighted images. On DWI, acute DAI can show reduced ADC (Fig. 2.18) and reduced FA. In subacute DAI, intracellular methemoglobin from petechial hemorrhage appears as an area of central hypointensity on T2-weighted images and hyperintensity on T1-weighted images. The conspicuity of DAI on MRI eventually diminishes as the damaged axons degenerate and the edema resolves. Chronic DAI imaging findings include nonspecific atrophy, gliosis, wallerian degeneration, and hemosiderin staining. The FA is generally reduced in chronic DAI.

MRI is superior to CT in detecting axonal injuries, especially when susceptibility-weighted sequences and higher field strength magnets (3T) are used (Lee et al. 2008). Yet even with MRI, the incidence of DAI is still thought to be underestimated. Advanced MR imaging methods, such as DTI with 3D tractography (Fig. 2.18), have shown potential in improving the detection of white matter injury in both acute and chronic DAI (Arfanakis et al. 2002; Huisman et al. 2003; Le et al. 2005). MRS and MTI can also offer additional prognostic value in DAI (Sinson et al. 2001).

Cortical Contusion

The *cortical contusion* is a hemorrhagic parenchymal injury ("brain bruise") involving predominantly the superficial gray matter with relative

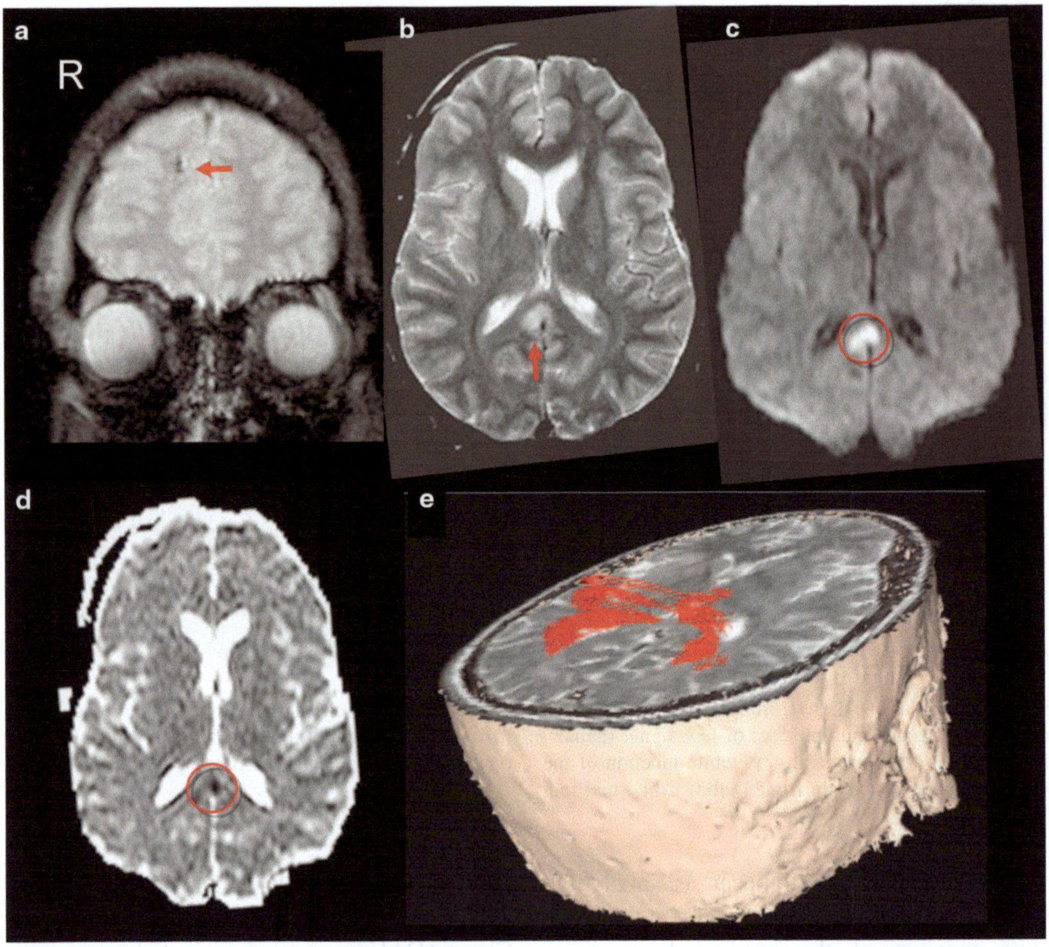

Fig. 2.18 Grade II DAI (Acute) on DWI. (**a**) Coronal GRE T2*-weighted MR image reveals a focus of dark signal (*arrow*) at the gray-white junction of the right frontal lobe consistent with hemorrhagic shearing injury. (**b**) T2-weighted image shows abnormal bright signal within the splenium (*arrow*) of the corpus callosum. (**c**) Diffusion-weighted image and (**d**) corresponding ADC map show restricted diffusion in the same area (*circle*). (**e**) 3D color tractography demonstrates disruption of the commissural fibers at the posterior inferior margin of the splenium of the corpus callosum. (Reprinted with permission from Le TH, Mukherjee P, Henry RG, et al. Diffusion tensor imaging with three-dimensional fiber tractography of traumatic axonal shearing injury: an imaging correlate for the posterior callosal "disconnection" syndrome: case report. Neurosurgery. Jan 2005;56(1):189)

sparing of the underlying white matter. Regions of the brain that are in close contact with the rough inner surfaces of the skull are typically affected. Regions within the temporal lobes (above the petrous bone and posterior to the greater sphenoid wing) and the frontal lobes (above the cribriform plate, orbital roof, and lesser sphenoid wing) are the most commonly affected. Contusions are also common subjacent to depressed skull fractures. Contusions along the parasagittal convexity are less common. The cerebellum is infrequently involved (Gentry 1996).

On CT, hemorrhagic contusions appear as mottled areas of high density within the superficial gray matter (Fig. 2.19). They may be surrounded by larger areas of low density from associated vasogenic edema. As the contusion evolves, a "salt and pepper" pattern of mixed areas of hypodensity and hyperdensity is characteristic. Non-hemorrhagic contusions appear as

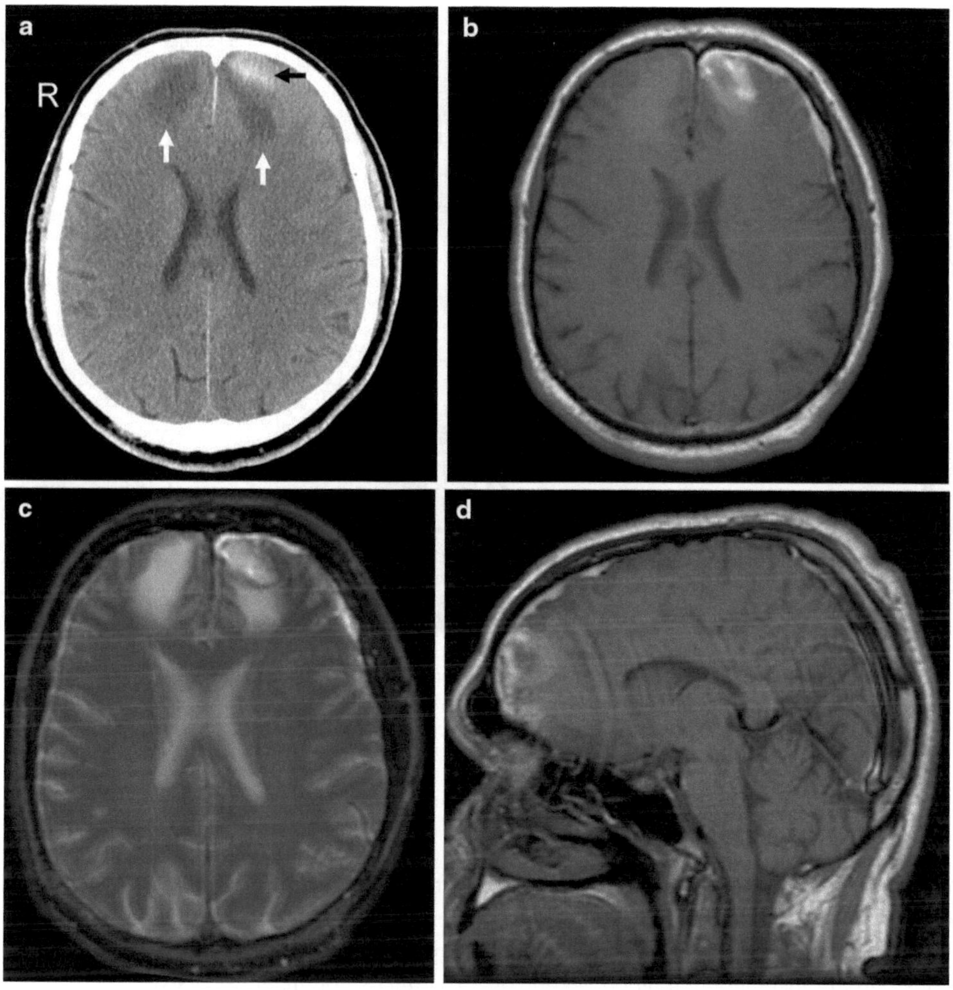

Fig. 2.19 Contusion on CT and MRI. (**a**) Axial CT shows an amorphous high-density area within the left orbitofrontal lobe consistent with an acute contusion (*horizontal arrow*). Bilateral frontal lobe low attenuation (*vertical arrow*) represents either vasogenic edema and/or non hemorrhagic contusion. (**b**) Follow-up axial T1-weighted MR image shows corresponding high signal due to the presence of methemoglobin. A thin left SDH is also noted. (**c**) Axial T2-weighted image shows the left hemorrhagic contusion of mixed high and dark signal, while the bilateral frontal non-hemorrhagic contusions versus vasogenic edema are more homogenous in appearance. (**d**) Sagittal T1-weighted MR image displays an area of left inferior frontal surface contusion, in addition to the more superior contusion and the left SDH seen in (**b**)

low density areas and can be difficult to detect initially until the development of sufficient edema. Due to its superficial location, the cortical contusion can be difficult to detect on CT, especially in the presence of beam hardening streak artifacts.

MRI can provide better delineation of contusions than CT since the skull does not distort the MR images. In addition, different MR techniques allow for emphasis on blood products at different ages (Hesselink et al. 1988). On MRI, contusions appear as ill-defined areas of variable signal intensity on both T1- and T2-weighted images, depending on the age of the lesions. Since contusions mainly involve the surface of the brain, they may have a "gyral" morphology. An old contusion commonly evolves into a wedge-shaped area of peripheral encephalomalacia with the broad base facing the skull. Therefore, it can mimic an old ischemic infarction.

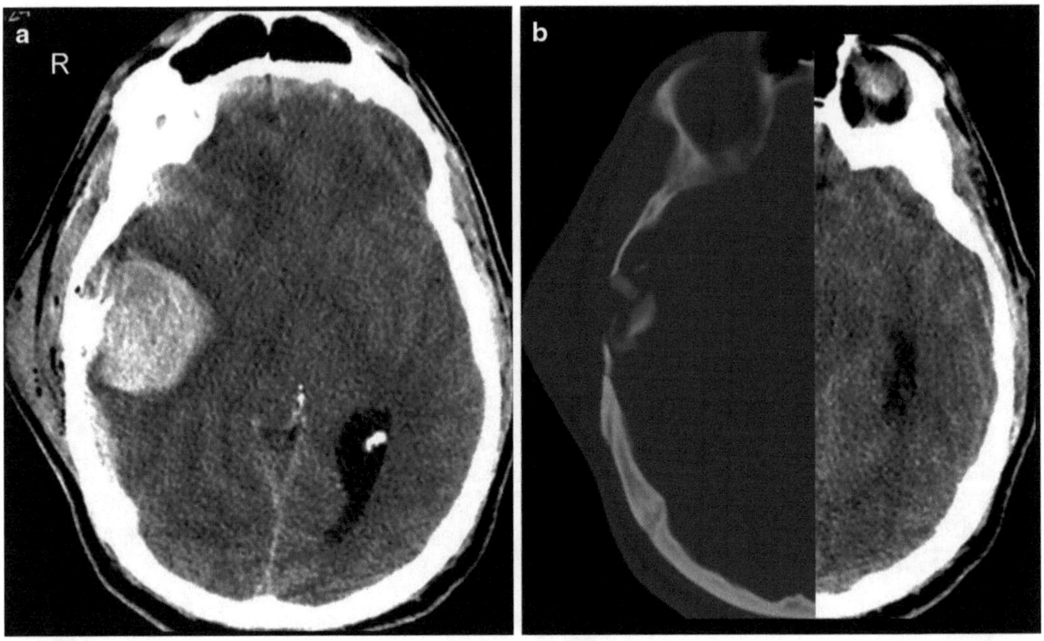

Fig. 2.20 ICH and skull fractures. (**a**) Non-contrast axial CT image, from a patient who sustained a snowboarding accident, shows a large round right posterior frontal intra-axial high attenuation mass due to an acute intracerebral hematoma. There is marked adjacent scalp soft-tissue swelling. (**b**) CT image, displayed in bone window, reveals a comminuted depressed skull fracture

Intracerebral Hematoma

The *intracerebral hematoma* (ICH) can develop from microcavitation or shear-induced hemorrhage of small intraparenchymal blood vessels or from expansion and coalescence of adjacent cortical contusions. In essence, the latter mechanism suggests that contusion and hematoma can be the same entity. Like contusions, ICHs frequently involve the frontotemporal white matter. Intracerebral hematomas are often associated with skull fractures and other primary intracranial injuries, including contusions and DAI, especially in patients who are unconscious at the time of injury. Several characteristic differences between the contusion and the hematoma should be noted. The ICH is usually more well defined and tends to have less surrounding edema than the cortical contusion. Intracerebral hematomas are often located deeper in the brain than cortical contusions. The intracerebral hematoma is the most common cause of clinical deterioration in patients who have experienced a lucid interval after the initial injury (Reilly et al. 1975). Delayed hemorrhage is a common cause of clinical deterioration during the first several days after head trauma (Soloniuk et al. 1986).

On CT, the acute intracerebral hematoma appears as a rounded hyperdense mass (Fig. 2.20). As the hematoma evolves, a low density rim, due to edema and pressure necrosis, can be observed. Contrast ring-enhancement can be seen within a subacute hematoma because of the proliferation of new capillaries lacking a complete blood–brain barrier. The enhancing subacute hematoma can be difficult, if not impossible, to differentiate from an abscess, infarct, or neoplasm without accurate clinical history or novel imaging methods such as MRS or DWI. The imaging findings of the chronic intracerebral hematoma are nonspecific, but involvement of the orbitofrontal and anteroinferior temporal lobes is typical.

On occasion, approximately 1–4 days following the onset of the initial trauma, delayed intracerebral hematomas can occur in areas that

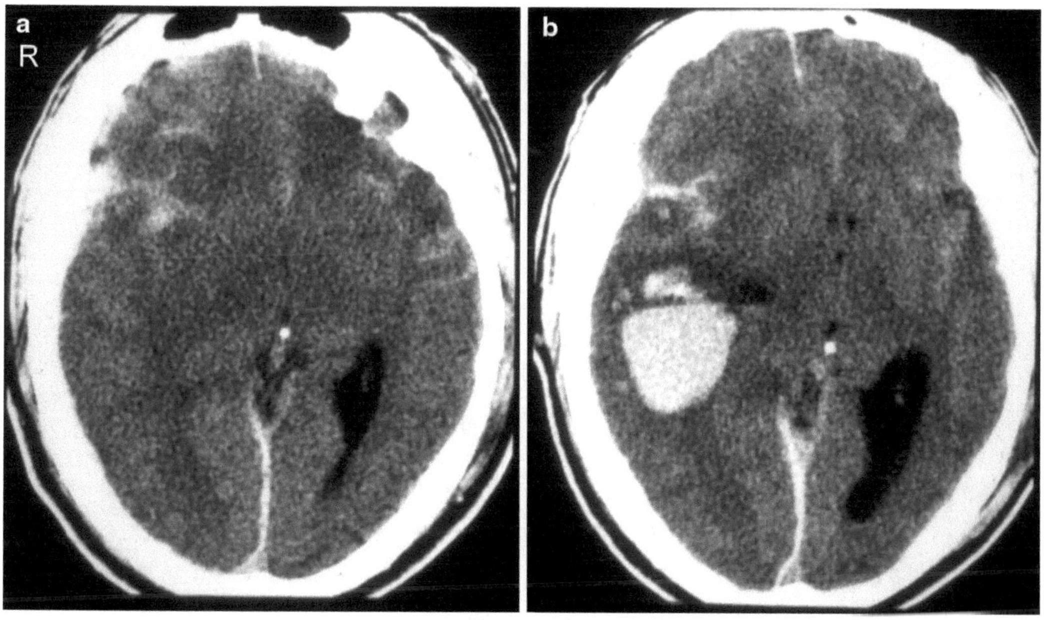

Fig. 2.21 "Delayed" intracerebral hematoma. (**a**) Noncontrast axial CT scan on admission demonstrates bilateral frontotemporal subarachnoid hemorrhages, right-to-left midline shift, and effacement of the right occipital horn, but without focal mass lesion. (**b**) The 4-h follow-up study reveals interval development of a large right temporal hematoma in the area of prior mass effect. (Reprinted with permission from Gean AD. Imaging of head trauma. Philadelphia, PA: Williams & Wilkins-Lippincott; 1994, p. 185)

previously demonstrated focal contusions on CT or MRI (Lipper et al. 1979; Nanassis et al. 1989). These delayed hematomas tend to occur in multiple lobar locations and are associated with a poor prognosis (Fig. 2.21). The proposed pathogenesis is due to reperfusion hemorrhage secondary to vasospasm with subsequent vasodilation or hypotension with subsequent hypertension, and may be further exacerbated by an underlying coagulopathy.

Encephalomalacia

Encephalomalacia is a nonspecific imaging finding but can develop in areas from either primary or secondary injury. It appears as a focal well-defined area of tissue loss with compensatory dilatation of the ipsilateral ventricle and sulci, and/or presence of old blood products. Macrocystic encephalomalacia follows CSF signal intensity on both CT and MR. Microcystic encephalomalacia appears as low signal intensity on T1-weighted MR images and high intensity on T2-weighted and FLAIR images.

Vascular Injury

Vascular injuries can lead to both intra- and extra-axial injuries, including hematomas and SAH. Traumatic vascular injuries can result from blunt or penetrating trauma and include arterial dissection, pseudoaneurysm, and arteriovenous fistula. Vascular injuries are often related to skull base fractures. The internal carotid artery is the most commonly affected vessel. The injury usually occurs at sites of relative fixation, where the internal carotid artery enters the carotid canal at the base of the petrous bone and at its exit from the cavernous sinus beneath the anterior clinoid process.

Arterial Dissection

A traumatic *arterial dissection* develops when there is incomplete disruption of the vessel wall with formation of a subintimal or intramural hematoma. The dissection is often best detected with T1-weighted MR images with fat suppression where the hematoma appears as a bright "crescent sign" (Fig. 2.22a). The affected vessel

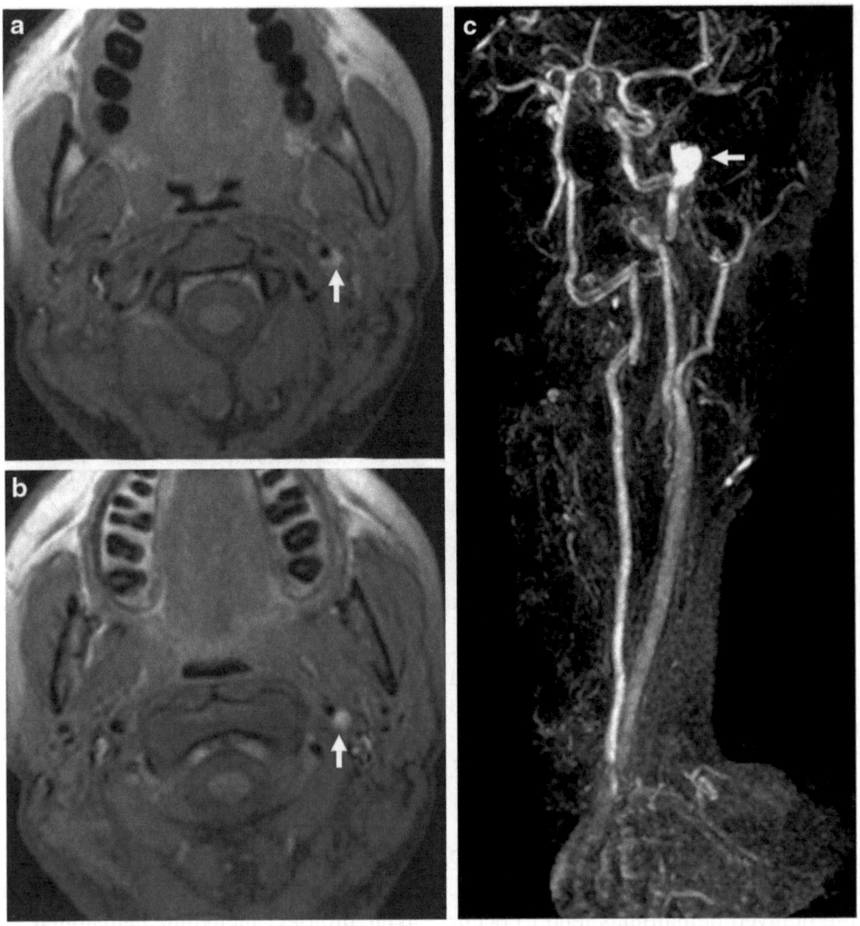

Fig. 2.22 Arterial dissection and pseudoaneurysm. (**a**) Axial T1-weighted with fat suppression image demonstrates a left common carotid artery high intensity rim due to an intramural hematoma from a focal dissection (*arrow*). (**b**) Image superior to the focal dissection shows a round extra-luminal high-density focus (*arrow*). (**c**) MRA of the neck shows a lobular "mass" protruding from the vessel, compatible with a pseudoaneurysm (*arrow*)

may appear irregular with relatively smaller caliber. Absence of the normal vascular flow void and abnormal flow-related enhancement secondary to slow flow, intraluminal thrombus, or vessel occlusion may be identified on MRI and MRA. A watershed and/or embolic parenchymal infarction (secondary injury) supplied by the injured vessel may occur.

Conventional catheter angiography has been traditionally considered to be the gold standard for confirmation and delineation of the vascular dissection, and it can also reveal associated vasospasm and pseudoaneurysm. However, MR angiography and CT angiography are increasing being used as noninvasive screening tools in patients with suspected vascular injury. In addition, because catheter angiography only demonstrates the caliber of the patent lumen, MR and CTA can identify a dissected vessel that may appear "normal" on catheter angiography. MR and CT are equally sensitive for the detection of intramural hematoma and subintimal flap, but CTA is more sensitive in depicting vertebral artery pseudoaneurysms (Vertinsky et al. 2008).

Pseudoaneurysm

Pseudoaneurysms are rare in adults but account for 11% of all pediatric aneurysms, although the overall incidence of aneurysms in pediatrics is relatively lower than in adults (Hardwood-Nash

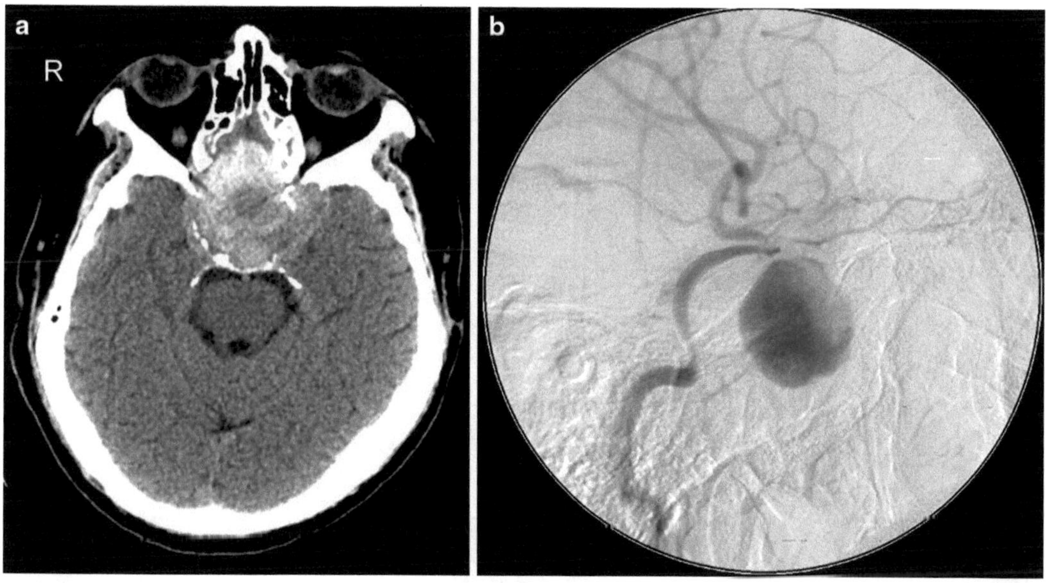

Fig. 2.23 Giant pseudoaneurysm. (**a**) Non-contrast axial CT image shows a large mixed low and high attenuation suprasellar mass. (**b**) Corresponding catheter cerebral angiogram from a selective left ICA injection shows a large mass partially filled with contrast arising from the left ICA, compatible with a partially thrombosed pseudoaneurysm

and Fritz 1976; Dubey et al. 2008). Typically, the wall of the pseudoaneurysm is actually an encapsulated hematoma in communication with the artery. On occasion, the adventitia may still be intact. Nevertheless, the wall of the pseudoaneurysm provides little support, and hence it has a propensity to hemorrhage. The pseudoaneurysm can also arises from a focal dissection ("*dissecting pseudoaneurysm*") (Fig. 2.22b, c). On imaging, the pseudoaneurysm frequently has an irregular contour and a wide neck. Thrombosis within the pseudoaneurysm manifests as a rounded mass with concentric laminated rings of heterogeneous signal intensity, consistent with thrombus in various stages of evolution (Fig. 2.23). The size of a partially thrombosed pseudoaneurysm is underestimated on conventional angiography because the angiogram only depicts the patent portion of the lesion. MRI and CT can better reveal the true extent of a partially thrombosed pseudoaneurysm than angiography. In the absence of thrombosis or turbulent flow, the pseudoaneurysm appears as a round area of signal void on both T1- and T2-weighted images. Pulsation within the pseudoaneurysm shows phase artifacts on MRI, a helpful imaging clue to the presence of a vascular lesion.

Arteriovenous Fistula

The traumatic *arteriovenous fistula* is a direct communication between an artery and a vein. The *carotid cavernous fistula* (CCF) is a direct communication between the cavernous portion of the internal carotid artery and the adjacent cavernous sinus venous plexus (Fig. 2.24). Traumatic CCF typically results from a full-thickness arterial injury, and can occur following either blunt or penetrating TBI. A CCF is also thought to be preceded by a traumatic pseudoaneurysm of the internal carotid artery. Classic imaging features of the CCF include engorgement of the cavernous and petrosal sinuses and a dilated tortuous ipsilateral superior ophthalmic vein. When the superior ophthalmic vein exceeds 4 mm in diameter, a CCF should be suspected. Other imaging findings include enlarged extraocular muscles, proptosis, retrobulbar fat stranding, pre-septal soft tissue swelling, and an ipsilateral convex cavernous sinus. These findings may even be bilateral and symmetric because venous channels

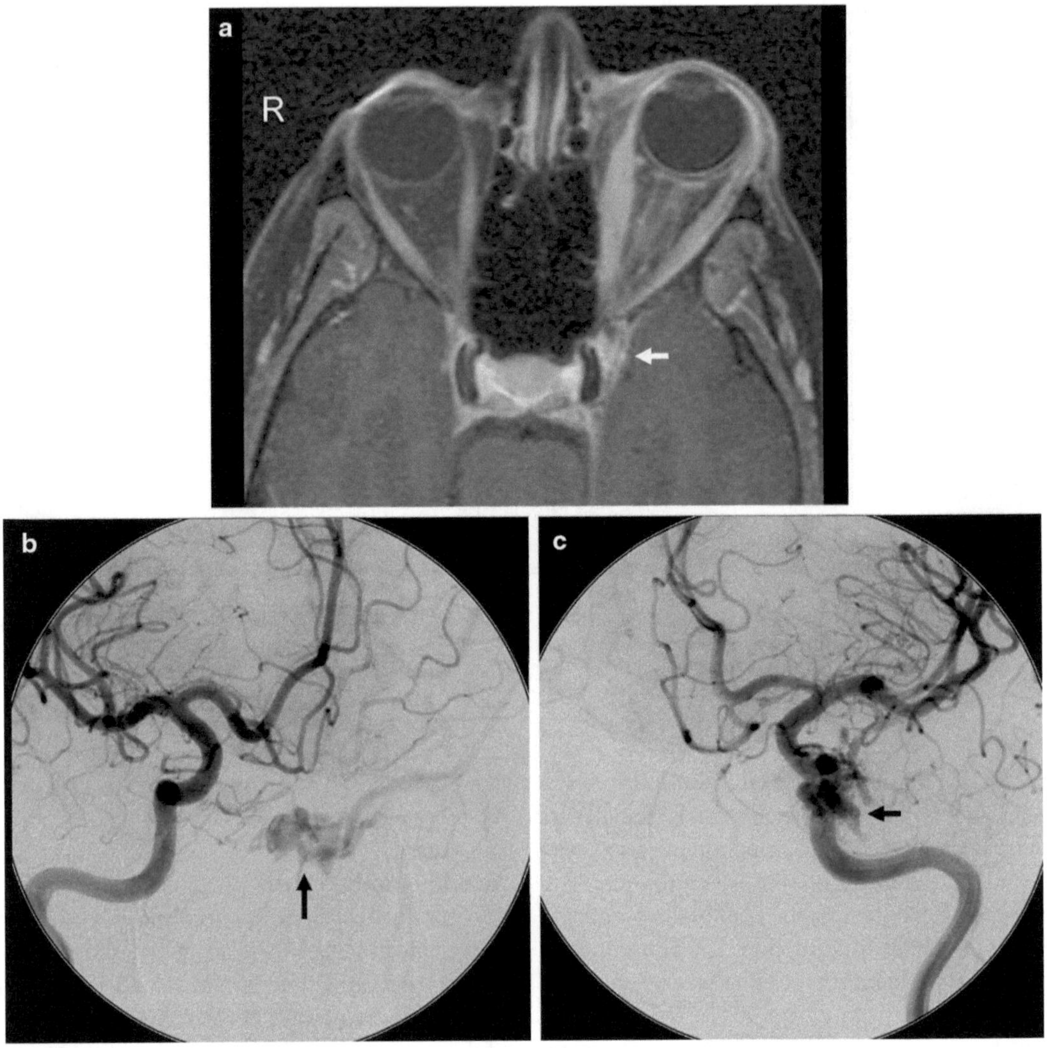

Fig. 2.24 Left CCF. (**a**) Axial T1-weighted post-contrast with fat suppression image demonstrates left proptosis, enlargement of the left extraocular muscles, and slight asymmetric fullness of the left cavernous sinus. (**b** and **c**) Catheter cerebral angiogram from selective right (**b**) and left (**c**) ICA injections show abnormal filling of the left cavernous sinus, confirming a left CCF (*arrow*)

connect the cavernous sinuses. In severe cases, intracranial venous hypertension can lead to brain edema and hemorrhagic venous infarction. Skull base fractures, especially those involving the sphenoid bone, should alert the clinicians to search for associated cavernous carotid injury. Patients can present weeks or even months after the initial trauma. Therefore, a CCF can be overlooked if a detailed clinical history and ophthalmic examination are not performed.

The *dural arteriovenous fistula* (DAVF) is most often caused by laceration of the middle meningeal artery with resultant meningeal artery to meningeal vein fistulous communication (Fig. 2.25). Because the fistula generally drains via the meningeal veins, the injured middle miningeal artery rarely leads to the formation of an EDH. Patients are often asymptomatic or present with nonspecific complaints such as tinnitus.

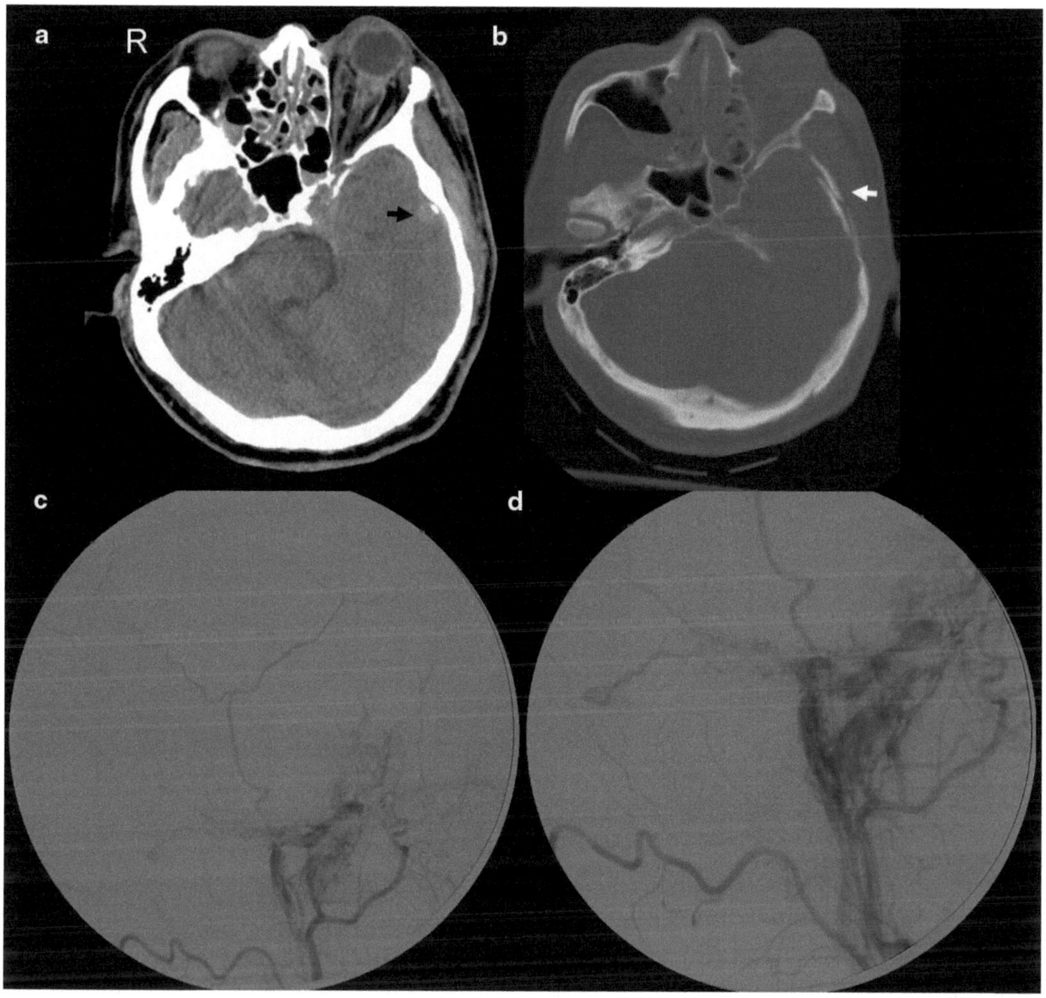

Fig. 2.25 Dural arteriovenous fistula (DAVF). (**a**) Axial CT image displayed in "soft tissue window" shows a small, round, dense, left temporal extra-axial focus (*arrow*). There is also left orbital proptosis and retrobulbar soft tissue stranding. (**b**) Corresponding "bone window" image shows a fracture of the squamosal portion of the left temporal bone (*arrow*). (**c** and **d**) Images from an external carotid artery catheter angiogram in the lateral projection show an abnormal blush of contrast due to a dural AVF with filling of the middle meningeal vein via the middle meningeal artery. (Reprinted with permission from Le TH and Gean AD. Neuroimaging of traumatic brain injury. Mt Sinai J Med. 2009;76:145–162)

Acute Secondary Injury

Cerebral Swelling

Cerebral swelling refers to an increase in cerebral volume which can develop from an increase in tissue blood volume (*hyperemia*) or an increase in tissue fluid (*cerebral edema*). Cerebral edema can be further divided into five major subtypes: vasogenic, cytotoxic, hydrostatic, hypo-osmotic, and interstitial. Among these subtypes, vasogenic edema is the most common in TBI. Hyperemia and vasogenic edema are thought to be the result of cerebral dysautoregulation. Cytotoxic edema is believed to occur secondary to tissue hypoxia. Hydrostatic edema occurs from a sudden increase in intravascular pressure, and can be seen with sudden decompression of a focal mass. Hypo-osmotic edema is caused by a decrease in serum osmolality, with subsequent efflux of fluid from the intravascular to the extravascular space. Interstitial edema occurs from movement of fluid into the periventricular space secondary to obstructive hydrocephalus.

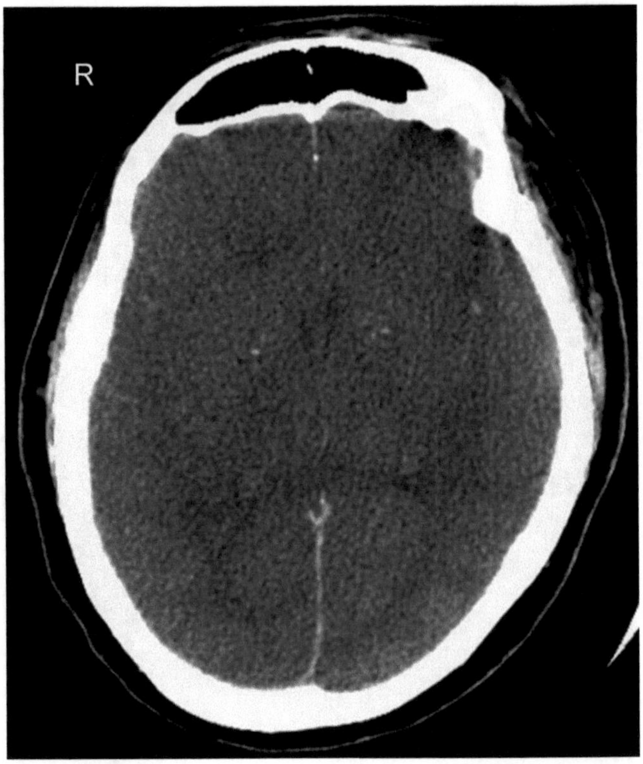

Fig. 2.26 Cerebral edema and DAI. Non-contrast axial CT image demonstrates diffuse effacement of the cerebral sulci and diffuse loss of gray-white matter differentiation due to diffuse cerebral edema. Multiple foci of shear hemorrhages within the left temporal lobe are also visible, indicating acute hemorrhagic DAI

Effacement of the cerebral sulci and cisterns, as well as compression of the ventricles, are typical imaging findings (Fig. 2.26). In cytotoxic edema, the gray-white differentiation is lost, which is in contrast to hyperemia and vasogenic edema where the gray-white differentiation is preserved. Even with cytotoxic edema, the cerebellum and brainstem are usually spared and may appear hyperintense relative to the affected cerebral hemispheres.

Brain Herniation

Traumatic *brain herniation* refers to displacement of brain tissue from one compartment to another secondary to mass effect produced either by primary or secondary injuries. The compartmentalization is based on the dural partitions and skull openings. In *subfalcine* herniation, the cingulate gyrus is displaced across the midline under the falx cerebri and above the corpus callosum (Figs. 2.8b and 2.10a). Compression of the ipsilateral ventricle due to mass effect and enlargement of the contralateral ventricle due to obstruction of the foramen of Monro can be seen on imaging. In *uncal* herniation, the medial temporal lobe is displaced over the free margin of the tentorium. Effacement of the lateral aspect of the suprasellar cisterns is an important early clue indicating the presence of uncal herniation. In *transtentorial* herniation, the brain herniates either upward or downward. Upward herniation occurs when portions of the cerebellum and vermis displace through the tentorial incisura. In posterior fossa downward herniation, the cerebellar tonsils displace through the foramen magnum. Downward herniation of the cerebrum manifests as effacement of the suprasellar and perimesencephalic cisterns. Inferior displacement of the calcified pineal gland is another clue for the presence of downward herniation. *External* herniation occurs when elevated ICP is combined with a skull defect (Figs. 2.8b and 2.28b). External herniation is observed more frequently due to an increased use of decompressive craniectomies. With all types of brain herniation, the underlying culprit must be corrected in a timely fashion to prevent further secondary injury.

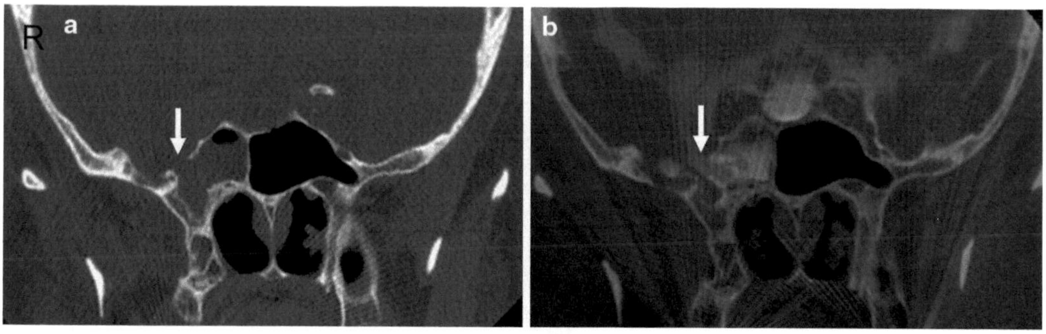

Fig. 2.27 CSF leak. (**a**) Coronal CT image shows a bony defect of the right sphenoid sinus (*arrow*). (**b**) Coronal CT image from a cisternogram shows leakage of contrast into the right sphenoid sinus through the bony defect. (Reprinted with permission from Le TH and Gean AD. Neuroimaging of traumatic brain injury. Mt Sinai J Med. 2009;76:145–162)

Ischemia and Infarction

Ischemia and infarction can result from vascular injury, diffuse increase in ICP, cytotoxic cerebral edema, or focal compressive mass effect on cerebral vasculature by herniation or hematoma. With subfalcine herniation, the anterior cerebral arteries (ACA) are displaced to the contralateral side, trapping the callosomarginal branches of the ACA, leading to ACA infarction. In severe uncal herniation, displacement of the brainstem can compress the contralateral cerebral peduncle and the posterior cerebral artery (PCA) against the tentorium ("*Kernohan's notch*"), leading to peduncular infarction and/or PCA infarction. Tonsillar herniation can cause ischemia in the territory of the posterior inferior cerebellar artery.

Chronic Secondary Injury

Hydrocephalus

Traumatic *hydrocephalus* develops due to impaired CSF reabsorption at the level of the arachnoid villi (*communicating hydrocephalus*) or due to intraventricular obstruction (*non-communicating hydrocephalus*), usually at the level of the cerebral aqueduct. Mass effect from brain herniation or a hematoma can also cause non-communicating hydrocephalus via compression of the aqueduct, foramen of Monro, or ventricular outflow foramina. Hydrocephalus commonly develops as a complication of prior SAH or IVH. On imaging, the ventricles are dilated, the sulci may be effaced, and periventricular transependymal interstitial edema may occur.

Cerebralspinal Fluid Leak

The *cerebrospinal fluid (CSF) leak* occurs from a dural tear and an associated skull base fracture. The dural tear results in communication between the intra- and extra-dural spaces. Communication between the subarachnoid space and middle ear, in association with a ruptured tympanic membrane, causes CSF otorrhea. Similarly, communication between the subarachnoid space and the paranasal sinuses causes CSF rhinorrhea. In patients with recurrent meningeal infections, a CSF leak should be suspected. CSF leaks are often difficult to localize. Radionuclide cisternography is highly sensitive for the detection of CSF leak (Curnes et al. 1985). However, CT scanning with intrathecal contrast is often required for detailed anatomic localization of the defect (Fig. 2.27) (La Fata et al. 2008).

Blast-Induced Injury

Blast induced TBI is brain injury generated by an explosion. Blast-induced TBI deserves special emphasis since it is considered the "*signature wound of the current war on terror*" (Neuroscience 2008) due to an increasing use of improvised explosive devices (IEDs) in terrorist and insurgent activities. Blast injuries can be classified as *primary, secondary, tertiary, or quaternary*. *Primary blast injuries* are due to an over-pressurization shock wave. The brain, surrounded by cerebral fluid, is especially susceptible to primary blast

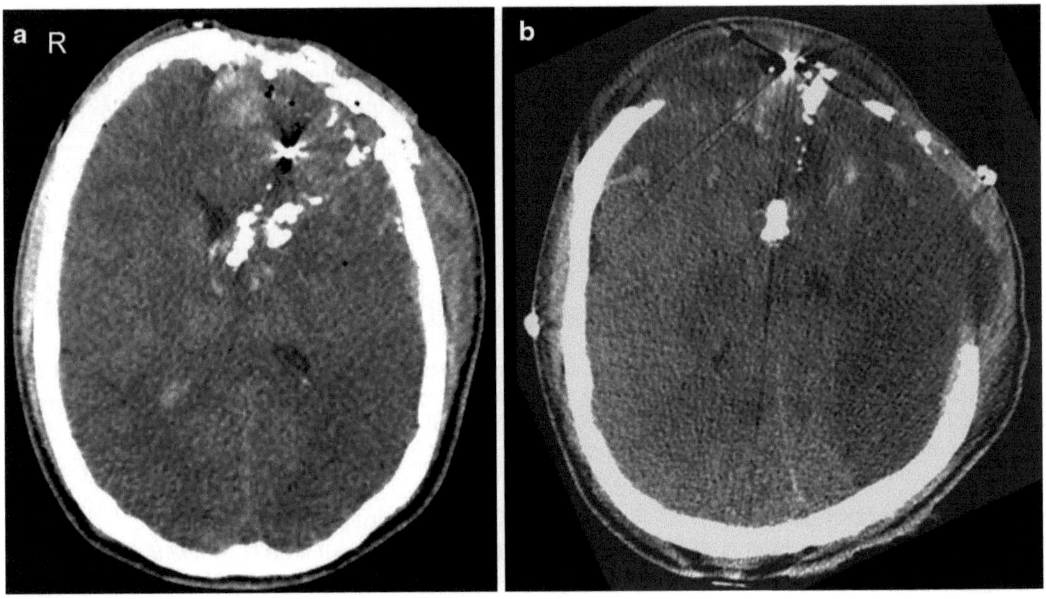

Fig. 2.28 Blast-induced TBI. (**a**) Non-contrast axial CT images show multiple metallic fragments, comminuted left frontal fractures, left frontal pneumocephalus, and left frontal scalp soft-tissue swelling. High-density collection within the occipital horn of the right lateral ventricle indicates acute IVH. (**b**) Follow-up CT, performed after decompressive craniectomy, reveals left frontal external herniation. There is diffuse decrease in attenuation of the left frontal lobe and loss of gray-white differentiation from secondary ischemic injury. There is also diffuse effacement of the cerebral sulci from cerebral edema. Bilateral anterior frontal low attenuation also indicates ischemic changes in these regions

injury (Elsayed 1997; Elsayed et al. 1997; Mayorga 1997). *Secondary blast injuries* are caused by bomb fragments and other objects propelled by the explosion, resulting in penetrating injuries. *Tertiary blast injuries* result when a person becomes a missile and is thrown against other objects. Therefore, tertiary blast injuries are similar to those that occur in blunt trauma. *Quaternary blast injuries* are all other injuries not included in the first three classes. The manifestation of blast injury on the brain is usually a combination of the different classes of blast injury (Fig. 2.28). Brain injuries acquired from the explosion often develop cerebral edema, subarachnoid hemorrhage, and vasospasm (Fig. 2.29).

Summary

Diagnosis and management of TBI requires a multi-disciplinary approach. The goals of imaging in TBI involve identifying treatable injuries, assisting in the prevention of secondary damage, and providing useful prognostic information. While progress in medical imaging technology has resulted in an increase in multiple imaging methods, leading to improvement in early detection of TBI and adding useful prognostic information, CT still remains the imaging modality of choice in the acute setting because it is fast, widely accessible, and has few contraindications. MRI is indicated in the acute setting if the neurologic findings are unexplained by the CT findings. MRI is preferred over CT for subacute and chronic TBI because of its superior sensitivity to older blood products and to both gray and white matter injury. Novel MRI methods, such as DWI, SWI, MRS, MTI and perfusion MRI, further improve the sensitivity of MRI in detecting TBI lesions, and can add valuable prognostic information. PET and MSI show promise in the evaluation of TBI, although their availability is limited due to cost. Continuing research and development in imaging will enhance our understanding of the pathophysiological manifestations of brain trauma and further improve clinical management of TBI.

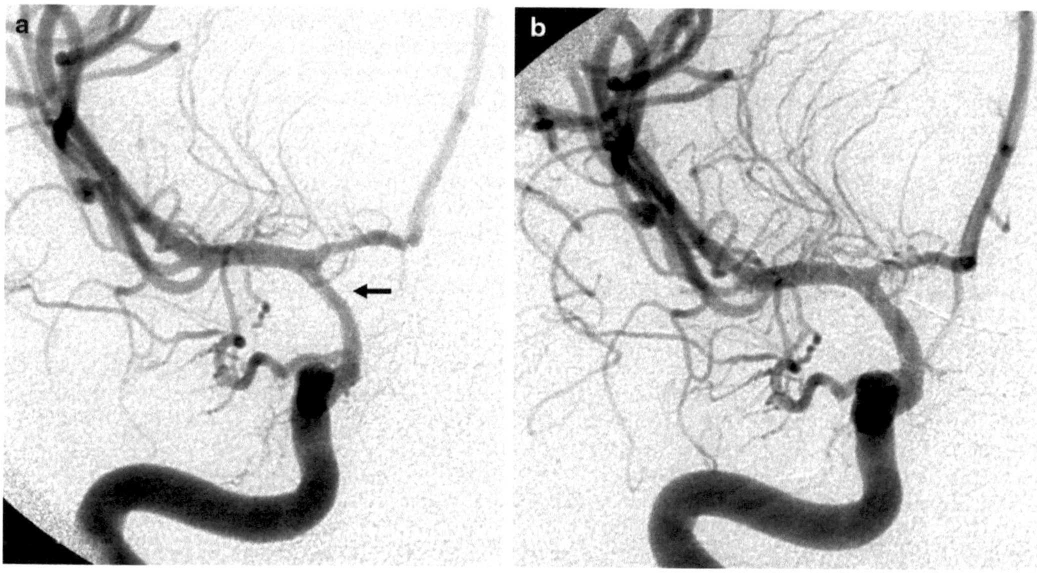

Fig. 2.29 Blast-induced vasopasm pre- and post-angioplasty. (**a**) Catheter cerebral angiogram from a selective left ICA injection, of the same patient in Fig. 2.28, shows mild narrowing and irregularity of the supraclinoid left ICA (*arrow*) due to vasospasm. (**b**) Follow-up angiogram post-angioplasty shows improvement in the irregularity and narrowing. (Courtesy of Rocco Armonda, M.D., Washington Hospital Center, Washington, DC)

Acknowledgments We thank the residents, fellows, and attendings from the Neuroradiology Section of the University of California, San Francisco for their continuing effort to submit interesting cases to the teaching file server (http://tfserver.ucsf.edu). Some of the cases presented in this article were the product of their contributions.

References

Adams J. Pathology of nonmissile head injury. Neuroimaging Clin N Am. 1991;1:397–410.

Adams JH, Graham DI, Gennarelli TA, Maxwell WL. Diffuse axonal injury in non-missile head injury. J Neurol Neurosurg Psychiatry. 1991;54(6):481 3.

Al-Nakshabandi NA. The swirl sign. Radiology. 2001; 218(2):433.

Arfanakis K, Haughton VM, Carew JD, Rogers BP, Dempsey RJ, Meyerand ME. Diffusion tensor MR imaging in diffuse axonal injury. AJNR Am J Neuroradiol. 2002;23(5):794–802.

Ashikaga R, Araki Y, Ishida O. MRI of head injury using FLAIR. Neuroradiology. 1997;39(4):239–42.

Awasthi D. Civilian gunshot wounds to the head. Proceedings of the American Association of Neurological Surgeons. San Francisco; 1992.

Babikian T, Freier MC, Tong KA, et al. Susceptibility weighted imaging: neuropsychologic outcome and pediatric head injury. Pediatr Neurol. 2005;33(3): 184–94.

Bell RS, Loop JW. The utility and futility of radiographic skull examination for trauma. N Engl J Med. 1971;284(5):236–9.

Bergsneider M, Hovda DA, McArthur DL, et al. Metabolic recovery following human traumatic brain injury based on FDG-PET: time course and relationship to neurological disability. J Head Trauma Rehabil. 2001;16(2):135–48.

Briggs M. Traumatic pneumocephalus. Br J Surg. 1974;61(4):307–12.

Coles JP, Fryer TD, Smielewski P, et al. Incidence and mechanisms of cerebral ischemia in early clinical head injury. J Cereb Blood Flow Metab. 2004a;24(2): 202–11.

Coles JP, Fryer TD, Smielewski P, et al. Defining ischemic burden after traumatic brain injury using 15O PET imaging of cerebral physiology. J Cereb Blood Flow Metab. 2004b;24(2):191–201.

Conturo TE, Lori NF, Cull TS, et al. Tracking neuronal fiber pathways in the living human brain. Proc Natl Acad Sci USA. 1999;96(18):10422–7.

Curnes JT, Vincent LM, Kowalsky RJ, McCartney WH, Staab EV. CSF rhinorrhea: detection and localization using overpressure cisternography with Tc-99m-DTPA. Radiology. 1985;154(3):795–9.

Dubey A, Sung WS, Chen YY, et al. Traumatic intracranial aneurysm: a brief review. J Clin Neurosci. 2008; 15(6):609–12.

Elsayed NM. Toxicology of blast overpressure. Toxicology. 1997;121(1):1–15.

Elsayed NM, Gorbunov NV, Kagan VE. A proposed biochemical mechanism involving hemoglobin for blast overpressure-induced injury. Toxicology. 1997;121(1): 81–90.

Enterline DS, Kapoor G. A practical approach to CT angiography of the neck and brain. Tech Vasc Interv Radiol. 2006;9(4):192–204.

Fobben ES, Grossman RI, Atlas SW, et al. MR characteristics of subdural hematomas and hygromas at 1.5T. AJR Am J Roentgenol. 1989;153(3):589–95.

Frigon C, Jardine DS, Weinberger E, Heckbert SR, Shaw DW. Fraction of inspired oxygen in relation to cerebrospinal fluid hyperintensity on FLAIR MR imaging of the brain in children and young adults undergoing anesthesia. AJR Am J Roentgenol. 2002;179(3): 791–6.

Garnett MR, Blamire AM, Corkill RG, Cadoux-Hudson TA, Rajagopalan B, Styles P. Early proton magnetic resonance spectroscopy in normal-appearing brain correlates with outcome in patients following traumatic brain injury. Brain. 2000a;123(Pt 10):2046–54.

Garnett MR, Blamire AM, Rajagopalan B, Styles P, Cadoux-Hudson TA. Evidence for cellular damage in normal-appearing white matter correlates with injury severity in patients following traumatic brain injury: a magnetic resonance spectroscopy study. Brain. 2000b;123(Pt 7):1403–9.

Gean AD, Kates RS, Lee S. Neuroimaging in head injury. New Horiz. 1995;3(3):549–61.

Gennarelli TA, Thibault LE, Adams JH, Graham DI, Thompson CJ, Marcincin RP. Diffuse axonal injury and traumatic coma in the primate. Ann Neurol. 1982;12(6):564–74.

Gentry LR. Head trauma. In: Atlas SW, editor. Magnetic resonance imaging of the brain and spine. 2nd ed. Philadelphia, PA: Lippincott-Raven; 1996. p. 611–47.

Gentry LR, Godersky JC, Thompson B, Dunn VD. Prospective comparative study of intermediate-field MR and CT in the evaluation of closed head trauma. AJR Am J Roentgenol. 1988;150(3):673–82.

Gomori JM, Grossman RI, Goldberg HI, Zimmerman RA, Bilaniuk LT. Intracranial hematomas: imaging by high-field MR. Radiology. 1985;157(1):87–93.

Greenberg J, Cohen WA, Cooper PR. The "hyperacute" extraaxial intracranial hematoma: computed tomographic findings and clinical significance. Neurosurgery. 1985;17(1):48–56.

Haacke EM, Xu Y, Cheng YC, Reichenbach JR. Susceptibility weighted imaging (SWI). Magn Reson Med. 2004;52(3):612–8.

Hackney DB. Skull radiography in the evaluation of acute head trauma: a survey of current practice. Radiology. 1991;181(3):711–4.

Hardwood-Nash DC, Fritz CR. Neuroradiology in infants and children. St. Louis, MO: CV Mosby; 1976.

Haydel MJ, Preston CA, Mills TJ, Luber S, Blaudeau E, DeBlieux PM. Indications for computed tomography in patients with minor head injury. N Engl J Med. 2000;343(2):100–5.

Hesselink JR, Dowd CF, Healy ME, Hajek P, Baker LL, Luerssen TG. MR imaging of brain contusions: a comparative study with CT. AJR Am J Roentgenol. 1988;150(5):1133–42.

Huisman TA, Sorensen AG, Hergan K, Gonzalez RG, Schaefer PW. Diffusion-weighted imaging for the evaluation of diffuse axonal injury in closed head injury. J Comput Assist Tomogr. 2003;27(1):5–11.

Inglese M, Makani S, Johnson G, et al. Diffuse axonal injury in mild traumatic brain injury: a diffusion tensor imaging study. J Neurosurg. 2005;103(2):298–303.

Jagoda AS, Cantrill SV, Wears RL, et al. Clinical policy: neuroimaging and decisionmaking in adult mild traumatic brain injury in the acute setting. Ann Emerg Med. 2002;40(2):231–49.

Jennett B, Adams JH, Murray LS, Graham DI. Neuropathology in vegetative and severely disabled patients after head injury. Neurology. 2001;56(4): 486–90.

Kato T, Nakayama N, Yasokawa Y, Okumura A, Shinoda J, Iwama T. Statistical image analysis of cerebral glucose metabolism in patients with cognitive impairment following diffuse traumatic brain injury. J Neurotrauma. 2007;24(6):919–26.

Kinuya K, Kakuda K, Nobata K, et al. Role of brain perfusion single-photon emission tomography in traumatic head injury. Nucl Med Commun. 2004;25(4): 333–7.

Kumbhani SR, Purcell DD, Gean AD. Contrast extravasation within a traumatic epidural hematoma: have we been missing something? Paper presented at: American Society of Neuroradiology 47th annual meeting & NER Foundation symposium 2009. Vancouver, Canada; 16–21 May, 2009.

La Fata V, McLean N, Wise SK, DelGaudio JM, Hudgins PA. CSF leaks: correlation of high-resolution CT and multiplanar reformations with intraoperative endoscopic findings. AJNR Am J Neuroradiol. 2008;29(3): 536–41.

Le TH, Gean AD. Neuroimaging of traumatic brain injury. Mt Sinai J Med. 2009;76(2):145–62.

Le TH, Mukherjee P, Henry RG, Berman JI, Ware M, Manley GT. Diffusion tensor imaging with three-dimensional fiber tractography of traumatic axonal shearing injury: an imaging correlate for the posterior callosal "disconnection" syndrome: case report. Neurosurgery. 2005;56(1):189.

Lee H, Wintermark M, Gean AD, Ghajar J, Manley GT, Mukherjee P. Focal lesions in acute mild traumatic brain injury and neurocognitive outcome: CT versus 3T MRI. J Neurotrauma. 2008;25(9):1049–56.

Lewine JD, Davis JT, Sloan JH, Kodituwakku PW, Orrison Jr WW. Neuromagnetic assessment of pathophysiologic brain activity induced by minor head trauma. AJNR Am J Neuroradiol. 1999;20(5): 857–66.

Lewine JD, Davis JT, Bigler ED, et al. Objective documentation of traumatic brain injury subsequent to mild head trauma: multimodal brain imaging with MEG, SPECT, and MRI. J Head Trauma Rehabil. 2007; 22(3):141–55.

Lindenberg R, Freytag E. The mechanism of cerebral contusions. A pathologic-anatomic study. Arch Pathol. 1960;69:440–69.

Lipper MH, Kishore PR, Girevendulis AK, Miller JD, Becker DP. Delayed intracranial hematoma in patients with severe head injury. Radiology. 1979;133(3 Pt 1): 645–9.

Liu AY, Maldjian JA, Bagley LJ, Sinson GP, Grossman RI. Traumatic brain injury: diffusion-weighted MR imaging findings. AJNR Am J Neuroradiol. 1999; 20(9):1636–41.

Masters SJ. Evaluation of head trauma: efficacy of skull films. AJR Am J Roentgenol. 1980;135(3):539–47.

Mayorga MA. The pathology of primary blast overpressure injury. Toxicology. 1997;121(1):17–28.

Menon DK. Brain ischaemia after traumatic brain injury: lessons from 15O2 positron emission tomography. Curr Opin Crit Care. 2006;12(2):85–9.

Messori A, Polonara G, Mabiglia C, Salvolini U. Is haemosiderin visible indefinitely on gradient-echo MRI following traumatic intracerebral haemorrhage? Neuroradiology. 2003;45(12):881–6.

Mittl RL, Grossman RI, Hiehle JF, et al. Prevalence of MR evidence of diffuse axonal injury in patients with mild head injury and normal head CT findings. AJNR Am J Neuroradiol. 1994;15(8):1583–9.

Mori S, van Zijl P. Fiber tracking: principles and strategies—a technical review. NMR Biomed. 2002;15: 468–80.

Munoz-Sanchez MA, Murillo-Cabezas F, Cayuela-Dominguez A, Rincon-Ferrari MD, Amaya-Villar R, Leon-Carrion J. Skull fracture, with or without clinical signs, in mTBI is an independent risk marker for neurosurgically relevant intracranial lesion: a cohort study. Brain Inj. 2009;23(1):39–44.

Nakashima T, Nakayama N, Miwa K, Okumura A, Soeda A, Iwama T. Focal brain glucose hypometabolism in patients with neuropsychologic deficits after diffuse axonal injury. AJNR Am J Neuroradiol. 2007;28(2):236–42.

Nanassis K, Frowein RA, Karimi A, Thun F. Delayed post-traumatic intracerebral bleeding. Delayed post-traumatic apoplexy: "Spatapoplexie". Neurosurg Rev. 1989;12 Suppl 1:243–51

Bhattacharjee Y. Neuroscience. Shell shock revisited: solving the puzzle of blast trauma. Science. 2008;319(5862):406–8.

Newton MR, Greenwood RJ, Britton KE, et al. A study comparing SPECT with CT and MRI after closed head injury. J Neurol Neurosurg Psychiatry. 1992;55(2): 92–4.

Niogi SN, Mukherjee P, Ghajar J, et al. Extent of microstructural white matter injury in postconcussive syndrome correlates with impaired cognitive reaction time: a 3T diffusion tensor imaging study of mild traumatic brain injury. AJNR Am J Neuroradiol. 2008;29(5):967–73.

Noguchi K, Ogawa T, Seto H, et al. Subacute and chronic subarachnoid hemorrhage: diagnosis with fluid-attenuated inversion-recovery MR imaging. Radiology. 1997;203(1): 257–62.

Orrison WW, Gentry LR, Stimac GK, Tarrel RM, Espinosa MC, Cobb LC. Blinded comparison of cranial CT and MR in closed head injury evaluation. AJNR Am J Neuroradiol. 1994;15(2):351–6.

Pruthi N, Balasubramaniam A, Chandramouli BA, et al. Mixed-density extradural hematomas on computed tomography-prognostic significance. Surg Neurol. 2009;71(2):202–6.

Purvis JT. Craniocerebral injuries due to missiles and fragments. Head injury conference proceedings. Philadelphia; 1966.

Reilly PL, Graham DI, Adams JH, Jennett B. Patients with head injury who talk and die. Lancet. 1975; 2(7931):375–7.

Siebert E, Bohner G, Dewey M, et al. 320-slice CT neuroimaging: initial clinical experience and image quality evaluation. Br J Radiol. 2009;82(979): 561–70.

Sinson G, Bagley LJ, Cecil KM, et al. Magnetization transfer imaging and proton MR spectroscopy in the evaluation of axonal injury: correlation with clinical outcome after traumatic brain injury. AJNR Am J Neuroradiol. 2001;22(1):143–51.

Soloniuk D, Pitts LH, Lovely M, Bartkowski H. Traumatic intracerebral hematomas: timing of appearance and indications for operative removal. J Trauma. 1986; 26(9):787–94.

Stiell IG, Lesiuk H, Wells GA, et al. Canadian CT head rule study for patients with minor head injury: methodology for phase II (validation and economic analysis). Ann Emerg Med. 2001a;38(3):317–22.

Stiell IG, Lesiuk H, Wells GA, et al. The Canadian CT Head Rule Study for patients with minor head injury: rationale, objectives, and methodology for phase I (derivation). Ann Emerg Med. 2001b;38(2):160–9.

Stiell IG, Wells GA, Vandemheen K, et al. The Canadian CT Head Rule for patients with minor head injury. Lancet. 2001c;357(9266):1391–6.

Teasdale G, Jennett B. Assessment of coma and impaired consciousness. A practical scale. Lancet. 1974;2(7872): 81–4.

Tong KA, Ashwal S, Holshouser BA, et al. Hemorrhagic shearing lesions in children and adolescents with posttraumatic diffuse axonal injury: improved detection and initial results. Radiology. 2003;227(2): 332–9.

Tong KA, Ashwal S, Holshouser BA, et al. Diffuse axonal injury in children: clinical correlation with hemorrhagic lesions. Ann Neurol. 2004;56(1):36–50.

Vertinsky AT, Schwartz NE, Fischbein NJ, Rosenberg J, Albers GW, Zaharchuk G. Comparison of multidetector CT angiography and MR imaging of cervical artery dissection. AJNR Am J Neuroradiol. 2008;29(9): 1753–60.

Wintermark M, van Melle G, Schnyder P, et al. Admission perfusion CT: prognostic value in patients with severe head trauma. Radiology. 2004;232(1):211–20.

Wintermark M, Sesay M, Barbier E, et al. Comparative overview of brain perfusion imaging techniques. Stroke. 2005;36(9):e83–99.

Woodcock Jr RJ, Short J, Do HM, Jensen ME, Kallmes DF. Imaging of acute subarachnoid hemorrhage with a fluid-attenuated inversion recovery sequence in an animal model: comparison with non-contrast-enhanced CT. AJNR Am J Neuroradiol. 2001;22(9): 1698–703.

Youn SW, Kim JH, Weon YC, Kim SH, Han MK, Bae HJ. Perfusion CT of the brain using 40-mm-wide detector and toggling table technique for initial imaging of acute stroke. AJR Am J Roentgenol. 2008;191(3): W120–6.

Zee CS, Go JL. CT of head trauma. Neuroimaging Clin N Am. 1998;8(3):525–39.

Zimmerman RA, Bilaniuk LT, Bruce D, Dolinskas C, Obrist W, Kuhl D. Computed tomography of pediatric head trauma: acute general cerebral swelling. Radiology. 1978;126(2):403–8.

Neurocognitive Assessment of mTBI

3

W. Huw Williams, Seb Potter, Helen J. Ryland, Philip Yates, James Tonks, and Adam Reuben

Abstract

The effects of Mild Traumatic Brain Injury (mTBI) typically resolve within days or weeks. However, a significant group of patients can report Persistent Concussional Symptoms (PCS). They may report a range of symptoms weeks, months and years post-injury. This review presents an overview of the pathogenesis, diagnosis and treatment options for mTBI and PCS, in adults and children. At early phases, post-injury, there are associations between neurological signs and symptoms, and neuropsychological functions and self-reported symptoms. However, over time, such associations become less coherent, and psychological issues become particularly relevant. Post-traumatic stress factors appear particularly important. We provide a biopsychosocial framework within which factors that predict such symptoms can be understood. An accurate diagnosis is critical for appropriate management of symptoms at various points post-injury.

Keywords

mTBI • Mild traumatic brain injury • PCS—post-concussional syndrome • PTSD—post-traumatic stress disorder • Biopsychosocial framework • Neuropsychology

W.H. Williams, Ph.D. (✉) • H.J. Ryland • J. Tonks, Ph.D., D.Clin.Psy.
School of Psychology, University of Exeter, Exeter, UK
e-mail: w.h.williams@ex.ac.uk

S. Potter, D.Clin.Psych.
Lishman Brain Injury Unit, South London & Maudsley NHS Foundation Trust, London, UK

P. Yates, D.Clin.Psy., C.Psychol.
School of Psychology, University of Exeter, Exeter, UK

Department of Psychological Medicine, Devon Partnership NHS Trust, Exeter, UK

A. Reuben, M.B.B.S.
Emergency Medicine, Royal Devon and Exeter Hospital, Exeter, UK

Introduction

Mild traumatic brain injury (mTBI) is a major public health issue globally. Around 80% of all TBIs are mild in nature and can be a major cause of disability leading to cognitive, mood and behavioural disorders (Fleminger and Ponsford 2005). For most people, injured symptoms usually resolve within days or weeks. Yet some argue that between 5 and 20% of those injured may be expected to have some ongoing problems—persistent Post-Concussional Syndrome (PCS)—weeks or months later (Kraus and Chu 2005;

J.W. Tsao (ed.), *Traumatic Brain Injury: A Clinician's Guide to Diagnosis, Management, and Rehabilitation*,
DOI 10.1007/978-0-387-87887-4_3, © Springer Science+Business Media, LLC 2012

Ruff and Weyer Jamora 2009). The provenance of such ongoing problems is controversial. Indeed, a formulation of a survivor's "current status" post-injury is a challenge as there is a lack of clarity as to whether certain signs, symptoms and cognitive functions are reliable post-concussion sequelae (see Williams et al. 2010). Neurological symptoms and signs and associated neurocognitive dysfunction are key indicators of injury severity and subsequent recovery trajectory. We provide an overview of assessment for neurocognitive functions in mTBI and later PCS, and consider the issues which may influence testing. We argue how the outcome post-mTBI must be seen as that determined by biopsychosocial factors, whereby there can be, at early phases, associations between neurological signs and symptoms, and neuropsychological functions and self-reports, but, over time, psychosocial issues become particularly relevant in explaining symptoms. An accurate diagnosis is crucial for appropriate management of symptoms at various points post-injury.

Definitions of mTBI and PCS

There are various terms used, often interchangeably, for the type of injury and subsequent forms of symptoms associated with mTBI and PCS. In this review, we use the term mTBI for the initial injury and PCS for persistent symptoms following such injury (over weeks, months and years). The immediate symptoms of mTBI/concussion include headache, dizziness and nausea as well as physical signs which may include unsteady gait, slurred speech, poor concentration and slowness when answering questions (McCrory et al. 2005). A loss of consciousness (LOC) (e.g. Glasgow Coma Scale (GCS) score of 13 or above) is considered a mild injury. However, amnesia, especially post-traumatic amnesia (PTA), has been proposed as either an additional or an alternative diagnostic criterion to LOC, in conjunction with confusion (Alexander 1995). Indeed, a recent study indicated that PTA was a more effective measure of severity of mTBI than GCS in the context of predicting behavioural outcomes at 6 months post-injury (Tellier et al. 2009). Even where there is an absence of PTA and/or LOC, neurocognitive abnormalities may be detected in the immediate aftermath of a suspected concussion (McCrea et al. 2002). The presence of such features and other concussion symptoms (e.g. diplopia) can be used to grade immediate "concussion" (see Cantu 1998; Colorado Medical Society 1991; American Academy of Neurology 1997).

For determining PCS, there are The International Classification of Diseases (ICD) section F07.2 (post-concussional syndrome) diagnostic criteria and The Diagnostic and Statistical Manual of the American Psychiatric Association (DSM-IV) research classification (e.g. Carroll et al. 2004a). There is significant agreement between the two sets of criteria for general symptoms (Boake et al. 2004). However, in DSM, objective cognitive impairment and disturbance in social or occupational functioning are required (McCauley et al. 2007). Furthermore, within the ICD-10 (WHO 1992) criteria, there is no point at which symptoms can be regarded as persistent while DSM-IV specifies 3 months.

Rates and Risks for Injury

The yearly incidence of TBI in western countries (e.g. the USA and the UK) is around 180–250 per 100,000 people (see Yates et al. 2006). As noted, the overwhelming majority of head injuries are mild with estimates ranging as high as 90% (McMillan 2001). Risk factors for injury are age (early childhood, males in adolescence and young adulthood and females in older age), urban dwelling and lower socio-economic level (see Yates et al. 2006). Major causes include road accidents, falls, sporting injury, assaults, etc., and the age-related aspects of these causes are well documented. In non-sporting injuries, alcohol and/or drug influence is a key factor (Kolakowsky-Hayner and Kreutzer 2001). In non-western areas, rates are likely to be very high (see Hyder et al. 2007). The global effect of TBIs as a disease—with various degrees of burden—is argued to be highly underestimated and to be likely to increase substantially in the future (Hyder et al. 2007).

Consequences of mTBI/PCS

mTBI is "classically defined as an essentially reversible syndrome without detectable pathology" (Ommaya and Gennarelli 1974, p. 633). It is often noted that recovery following mTBI is rapid—with most acute symptoms resolving within hours, and then, typically, a person being symptom free by around 10 days (McCrea et al. 2003).

However, as noted above, an mTBI and/or concussion can be graded for severity and more complicated cases may be associated with differential outcomes—as we shall see, in particular, delayed recovery.

Typically, the more severe injuries occur from greater rotational acceleration–deceleration forces involved in the impact (Guskiewicz et al. 2000). Following impact, a neurometabolic cascade ensues (Giza and Hovda 2001). The short-term effects can include a lack of electro-chemical activity, haemorrhaging and axonal shearing, especially in the frontal temporal lobe area, although in mTBI these early deficits may largely resolve themselves (Lezak 2004). mTBI, therefore, tends to be characterised by the dysfunction and not destruction of neurons (Iverson 2005). Caution is, though, still warranted regarding signs of greater impact.

An indication of mTBI having long-term biological consequences was suggested in a population-based study of all people born in Denmark. In this study, it was shown that there was a two-fold increased risk of epilepsy after a mild brain injury (Christensen et al. 2009). However, there is lack of clarity on how such biological indicators are associated with outcomes. For example, serum markers of brain injury such as S100B (a calcium-binding protein) are thought to be useful for predicting initial acute severity of TBI, but it is argued that there is only a weak association between marker levels and concussion symptoms (see Bazarian et al. 2006). Indeed, it has been noted that normal levels of S-100B marker are helpful but abnormal levels tend not to predict the outcome (Iverson et al. 2006).

As noted, is possible that around 15% of those with mTBI may have ongoing problems (Ruff et al. 1996). In one study in Glasgow, the UK, 47% of young people and adults with mild head injuries experienced moderate to severe disability at 1 year post-injury (Thornhill et al. 2000). A further study in Glasgow of children with mTBI also showed high levels of disability—with 43% of the sample having problems 1 year post-injury (Limond et al. 2009). However, these participants, although noted as having a "mild" injury, may have had more "complicated" injury as they were typically hospitalized for observation for over a day. Other studies have found that neuro-behavioural sequelae are significant at over 2 years post-injury for TBI of milder severity. Hawley et al. (2004a, b) found that children with mild TBI were significantly more anxious compared to controls, and that behavioural and school-related problems were reported by families of mildly injured children as well as moderate and severely injured children at just over 2 years post-injury. As we explore further, below, there is some evidence that younger age at injury may be a risk factor for worse outcomes. However, factors accounting for this are not well explicated.

There is much debate, therefore, over whether persistent symptoms are "driven" by neurological or psychological factors, and what role there is for pre-morbid issues (Alexander 1995; Lishman 1988; Carroll et al. 2004b). As we shall explore, outcomes are highly variable across population groups studied (such as general patient groups versus those being monitored within sports), and in terms of whether there are links between actual physical injury and various symptoms and problems experienced later on.

Considerations Regarding Neurocognitive Testing

Neurocognitive functions are those abilities that are supposed to be present in certain areas of the brain for performing mental operations important for daily life. That is—key thinking skills linked to certain brain area. If the brain is affected, then these systems could be compromised. The following are key functions relevant to mTBI: executive functions—a set of cognitive abilities that control and regulate volitional activities, such as planning, organising, self-awareness, impulse control and other self-regulatory functions; sustained attention—the ability to maintain consistent behavioural responses over time to specific stimuli during an ongoing repetitive task; divided attention—the ability to respond to two or more different tasks at the same time; and memory—the ability to encode, store and retrieve information within various time frames from the original encoding experience. There are two main reasons for neurocognitive assessment for concussion—to determine the presence of neurocognitive symptoms for early diagnosis of mTBI (in terms of severity and potential duration of injury) and to monitor recovery over days, weeks, months or even years later (Barth et al. 1989; Macciocchi et al. 1996; Davis et al. 2009). In the latter, there may be identification of lasting neurocognitive sequelae.

In the domain of testing for concussion symptoms, there are studies involving general patient group—typically those presenting to emergency departments (EDs)—and studies of particular risk groups—usually those involved in contact sports. There are also, increasingly, studies of military personnel—who are at particular risk of injury (e.g. from bomb blasts; see Hoge et al. 2008).

Over the past 20 years, the area of sports concussion management has provided much of the research base for informing clinical assessment practice in mTBI. Systems developed in this arena are being generalised to other groups (e.g. military; (and see Veterans and Dept. of Defense 2009)). The guiding principle of such testing is to ensure that those injured are taken out of the "game" until they are free of concussion symptoms and are therefore "fit" to resume play. The neurocognitive assessment forms part of a general review conducted to assess for concussion. Typically, athletes are tested out of season (baseline) and are then re-tested if they suffer a concussion/mTBI. They are, therefore, their own controls, and a significant deterioration from baseline suggests that the concussion has led to neurocognitive dysfunction which is not resolved. Where there are no baselines, performance would be compared to a representative control group. The neurocognitive element of the review may, therefore, provide a straightforward "cleared" (i.e. not showing neurocognitive symptoms) to resume, but may also indicate problems (if, on repeat testing, they do not achieve their baseline performance). In such circumstances, a review is needed of the person's fitness to return to the activity, and possible counselling regarding paced return to play (see McCrory et al. 2009). It is important to note, though, that a recent study indicated a high level of concussed athletes returned to play prematurely under AAN and Prague return-to-play guidelines (Yard and Comstock 2009).

Testing needs to be specific, sensitive, reliable and valid for identifying mTBI/PCS (Iverson et al. 2005). Validity is the accuracy of the measurement or the extent to which the test is measuring what it is purported to be measuring. Sensitivity and specificity refer to the likelihood of identifying either genuine positives or negatives, respectively. Sensitivity is the probability that someone in the category of interest (in this case, mTBI) is identified by the test. Conversely, if a test has a high level of specificity, it will reliably predict those who do have the condition versus those who do not have the condition. Reliability refers to the consistency of the measurement or the extent to which the test provides approximately the same result on each occasion it is used under the same set of conditions with the same participants. Test–retest reliability is especially important with regard to the use of baseline testing in sport when diagnosing concussion following head injury. This can be estimated by comparing the results of a test on the same population carried out at different times—e.g. using a correlation coefficient. However, such repeat testing can lead to practice effects, whereby the participant performs better in subsequent tests due to having "learned" from the previous experience (Collie et al. 2003).

Where it is known that a test is vulnerable to practice effect, then Reliable Change Indices (RCI) can be used to calculate what improvement would be expected from a person from baseline to post-concussional testing, and what adjustment is needed to take account of such supposed improvement (Hinton-Bayre and Geffen 2002). The RCI is calculated by use of a control group to establish the average change between tests and an additional correction is made for test variability and reliability using an error term which produces a standard score (*Z*). Furthermore, use of alternate versions of tasks can limit practice effects (Collie et al. 2001).

Neurocognitive Assessment: Development of Methodology

Recovery of neurocognitive functions following concussion has been extensively examined within the paradigm of "return-to-play" studies in sports (see Barth et al. 1989; Macciocchi et al. 1996; Echemendia et al. 2001). These studies allow for large-scale prospective, repeat, follow-up and retrospective analyses of athletes at risk of concussion. Typically, as we note above, there are baseline measures available for athletes which provide an individual benchmark for monitoring performance.

Initially, neuropsychological tests were "paper and pencil" tests that could take between 4 and 6 h to administer. This was because symptoms of concussion were considered highly variable and multiple tests were needed to identify possible cognitive deficits (Echemendia et al. 2001). As the focus of interest became refined, shorter versions of testing procedures were developed. These were found sensitive to the mild cognitive problems indicative of acute concussion—such as attention and complex memory (Barth et al. 1989; Macciocchi et al. 1996; Boll and Barth 1983; Hughes et al. 2004). Importantly, the tests were more effective than subjective reports in distinguishing between the injured and the non-injured at 48 h post-injury (e.g. Echemendia et al. 2001). The tasks frequently employed in "paper and pencil" testing include tests, such as Digit Span (Lezak 1995) which tests working memory with mental rotation, Speed of Comprehension and Language Processing (Lezak 1995) which tests general cognitive level and speed of processing, Trail-Making Tests A and B (Lezak 1995) which test sustained and divided attention, Stroop Color and Word (Lezak 1995) which tests executive skills (especially inhibition) and Symbol Digit Modalities Test (SDMT), a measure of visual-spatial and motor speed and accuracy (Smith 1982).

More recently, computerised tests have been developed which offer distinct advantages over conventional methods (e.g. Campbell et al. 1999). Computerised systems provide an accurate measurement of reaction times (RTs) for the high-level forms of cognitive functioning that tend to be compromised following a concussion (Pellman et al. 2004). Standardised presentation of stimuli or random presentations of a large number of alternate forms provide improved test–retest reliability (Schatz and Browndyke 2002). Various packages have been developed including Immediate Post-Concussion Assessment and Cognitive Testing (ImPACT) (Maroon et al. 2000), a computerised neuropsychological test battery designed to measure a range of cognitive functions including attention and processing speed. Other software packages designed to be used to diagnose post-concussional cognitive deficits in sports include HeadMinder™ (see Erlanger et al. 1999) and CogSport™ (Cogstate 1999). CogState Sport™ measures simple and complex attention, reaction times and accuracy, as well as memory and problem solving ability (Schatz and Zillmer 2003) to create a composite score. This score then determines pass or failure (caution versus good/all clear). The tasks involve single playing cards or playing cards presented in multiples.

Computerised testing is also less vulnerable to practice effects compared to traditional testing, although such effects have been shown for these types of systems if tests are serially repeated on the same day on a normal population (see Collie et al. 2003). However, the main effect for practice occurs within the first few repetitions of the tasks, and then performance tends to become more stable (i.e. reaches a plateau) thereafter (Falletti et al. 2006).

Two of the other key advantages of computerised testing are with regard to practical and logistical limitations. Administration of traditional neuropsychological tests requires one-to-one supervision as well as interpretation by a qualified person. In contrast, computerised testing can be carried out with less immediate supervision, remotely, and with individuals and groups simultaneously. We note, though, that testing processes may be undertaken by technicians but that this ideally should be under the supervision and/or guidance of an appropriately qualified psychologist—typically a clinical neuropsychologist. Indeed, interpretation of test results should preferably be carried out by a clinical neuropsychologist, although this may vary from country to country depending upon differing levels of training and availability (Echemendia et al. 2009). This is particularly important as such automated procedures may lead to the assumption that the computer can diagnose concussion and that those carrying out clinical evaluations may adopt a passive rather than an active role (Schatz and Putz 2006). It is important, in testing, to be aware of and take account of a range of factors that may influence testing (Schatz and Putz 2006) and that, as we have noted, test results are only part of the overall "data set" for formulating a clinical picture of an individual's functioning. Computerised tests may also lack some of the breadth and flexibility possible using traditional testing methods (Gualtieri and Johnson 2008). Consequently, while computerised testing may be increasingly used, traditional methods continue to have an important role to play, especially in a more individualised setting.

It is also worth noting that, while computerised testing is becoming available across a host of platforms for delivery, the use of technology may be lesser or greater among different groups within a society (Russell et al. 2003). Therefore, the attitude of the person being tested towards technology, especially if apprehensive, may lead to a poorer performance.

Iverson et al. (2005) examined the construct validity of ImPACT™ with the SDMT (Smith 1982). They found that the SDMT correlated most highly with the Processing Speed and Reaction Time composites from ImPACT™ suggesting that both tests are measuring a similar underlying construct. CogSport™ has been evaluated on 300 professional Australian football players as well as hundreds of healthy controls across a wide range of ages (Makdissi et al. 2001).

The Use of "Self-Rating" Scales in Assessment

Important information for assessment of mTBI/PCS would be gained from subjective accounts of patients/participants. We shall discuss later particular issues to be aware of that may influence reporting of symptoms. One of the main methods of gaining information, relevant to testing, is that of the use of standardised scales.

There is a range of scales available for assessment of mTBI/PCS (see Alla et al. 2009 for a review of those used in acute assessment sports). Some are "embedded" within neurocognitive testing systems (e.g. within ImPACT™, there is a 22-item scale), and there are "stand-alone" scales, such as the Rivermead PCS Questionnaire (see King et al. 1995). These scales typically contain items that address somatic, affective and cognitive symptoms. The structure of symptoms in mTBI/PCS in cognitive, emotional and physical domains is relatively consistent across a variety of studies using different questionnaires and in different populations, whereby symptoms are separate but are also associated (Potter et al. 2006). That is, there can be a "single-factor solution" (i.e. one consistent overall score) but analysis can also be undertaken of sub-groups of symptoms (Lannsjö et al. 2009). However, there is considerable consistency in symptom reporting across a range of PCS checklists and questionnaires—that is—they seem to be measuring the same underlying phenomena (Alla et al. 2009).

Although PCS has typically been associated with mTBI, individuals with moderate and severe TBIs can experience similar difficulties (e.g. Oddy et al. 1985). Also an analogous constellation of symptoms have been shown in non-brain-injured trauma controls (e.g. Meares et al. 2008; McLean et al. 2009): for example, in one prospective study, while 58% of people with mTBI met the criteria for PCS at 1 month post-injury, so did 34% of orthopaedic controls (Bazarian et al. 1999). Overlap of symptoms with other clinical populations is also considerable, including individuals with depression (e.g. Iverson and Lange 2003), chronic pain (Smith-Seemiller et al. 2003) and chronic whiplash symptoms (Haldorsen et al. 2003). And subjective cognitive difficulties within those with mTBI/PCS may—in turn—be associated with comorbid anxiety, depression and fatigue (Stulemeijer et al. 2008).

It is important to note, though, that group differences may emerge with mTBI/PCS individuals compared to others. It has been found that mTBI individuals, for example, report higher levels of subjective cognitive difficulties compared to individuals with chronic pain (Smith-Seemiller et al. 2003) or orthopaedic controls (Gerber and Schraa 1995). The presence and severity of symptoms on such measures are not trivial due to their association with quality of life (e.g. Stålnacke 2007) and return to work (e.g. Nolin and Heroux 2006). Therefore, assessment of the severity and impact of symptoms (rather than their presence or absence) using scales such as the Rivermead PCS is indicated.

Neuropsychological Functions Post-mTBI

Sports Studies

There are many sports "return-to-play" studies that show that a single concussive episode may have little lasting neurocognitive consequence (Wall et al. 2006; and see Williams et al. in press). A meta analytic review of neuropsychological testing of concussion in sports by Belanger and Vanderploeg (2005) identified 21 of 69 studies between 1970 and 2004 (key inclusion criteria including a control or baseline comparison). They reported mild-to-moderate effect of concussion in the first 24 h on global measures and larger deficits on memory (acquisition and delayed). However, there was, typically, full resolution by 7–10 days post-injury. They did note, however, that practice effects—particularly in the context of "comparison to baseline" studies—may be linked to an underestimate of concussion effects. Also studies in which prior head injury cases were excluded had smaller effect sizes than those that had not excluded such athletes. These findings suggest that prior "head injury" may be associated with greater cognitive sequelae. McCrea et al. (2003) followed up a concussed group ($n=94$) and an uninjured control group ($n=56$) of American college football players selected from a cohort of 1,631. They were tested at pre-season, then immediately after injury, at 3 h post-injury, and then again at 1, 2, 3, 5, 7, and 90 days post-injury. By 7 days, basic assessment on the SAC showed no significant group effect between a non-concussed and concussed group. Mild impairments in cognitive processing speed and verbal memory were noted for the concussed athletes at 2 and 7 days post-injury, and verbal fluency was still affected in the concussed group at 7 and 90 days post-injury. There was no evidence of other "lingering symptoms" at 90 days. Also, importantly, they noted that 10% of players needed more than a week for symptoms to resolve.

Studies using computerised systems have shown similar significant recovery trajectory, but also variation in outcome. Iverson et al. (2006) followed up concussed athletes ($n=30$) from baseline at 1–2 days, 3–7 days and 1–3 weeks post-injury using the ImPACT™. The athletes' scores on a range of measures (memory, speed, reaction time) were significantly reduced at day 1. Significant improvements had occurred by 5 days post-injury, although at 10 days post-injury, 37% of athletes had two or more composite scores that were lower than those of pre-season. Pre-existing head injury or presence of headaches (possibly indicating more complicated initial injury) was suggested as associated with compromised recovery. Collins et al. (1999) also found, in a sample of 393 American Football players, that a history of multiple concussions was associated with lowered neurocognitive performance in divided attention and visuo-motor speed.

Traditional neuropsychological testing has provided further support for the cumulative effects of concussion. Wall et al. (2006) showed that jockeys with repeated "historical" (more than 3 months since) concussions were less efficient on tasks of executive functions and attention compared to those with a single concussion. Younger age accounted for much of the variance in decrement in attention, suggesting that younger age of injury, or repeat injury within a shorter time span, may be an important consideration. Other studies have not shown that repeat injury leads to cumulative effects on neurocognitive performance (Collie et al. 2006). A recent meta-analysis—which identified 10 relevant studies from 123 between 1970 and 2009—by Belanger et al. (2010) indicated that two or more mTBIs had "little overall association with cognitive performance several months later, although there is a small association with poorer performance on delayed memory and executive measures" (p. 5). They note, though, that the clinical significance of these effects was unclear.

The effects of repeat concussion, therefore, remain unclear (see Williams et al. 2010). Recent guidance on management of sports concussion notes "modifiers" that may be associated with worse outcomes (or delayed recovery), such as prior concussion, especially where the injuries have occurred within a short timescale, greater-than-1 min LOC, longer duration and severity of initial symptoms, as well as the greater amount of symptoms, concussive convulsions, younger age, presence of other conditions such as depression, a high level of risk associated with the sport as well as risky behaviour within the sport and finally use of medications such as psychoactive drugs or anticoagulants (McCrory et al. 2009).

Comparisons Between Sports and Patient Groups

There are key differences between sports populations and general patient groups. There may not, therefore, be direct comparators to patient populations. Sports people may "downplay" symptoms and have a strong motivation to return to play (Ruff and Weyer Jamora 2009). Also, athletes who are at risk may well be assessed as being concussed for relatively minor disturbances in consciousness within protocols in place for safety in sports. In patient groups, there is much greater heterogeneity of issues to consider: range of pre-morbid factors (educational, socio-economic, etc.), injury variables (mechanisms, forces, etc.) and degree of support available. A major difference between sports and general populations is that, in the latter, there are typically no baseline measures available. Therefore, the interpretation of test scores is based on the normative data provided by publishers—which inherently lowers sensitivity and specificity of injury detection.

Patient Studies

One early, well-controlled patient study—comparing 22 participants with mTBI versus 19 uninjured matched controls—revealed that single minor head injury was associated with mild but "probably clinically non-significant difficulties at 1 month after injury" (Dikmen et al. 1986). This applies especially to those without any compromising pre-existing conditions. Neurocognitive problems included problems with concentration and new learning, but these were not present at 1 year post-injury.

A meta-analytic review of neurocognitive studies (from 1970 to 2004) of patients with mTBI by Belanger and Vanderploeg (2005) identified 39 of 133 studies that met the key criteria (participants sought medical attention and there was grading of severity of injury). Of eight cognitive domains assessed in "selected" samples, problems were mostly confined to verbal fluency (executive skills) and delayed memory. In those who were "unselected", there was no difference to controls at 90 days post-injury, although litigation appeared to be a moderating factor. Another meta-analysis by Schretlen and Shapiro (2003) indicated that cognitive performance of mTBI patients could not be distinguished from matched controls at 1 month post-injury. Such trends lend support to the notion that recovery tends to be "complete" by 3 months (see Binder 1997; also see Frencham et al. 2005). Pertab et al. (2009) noted caution though, as it may be that lasting neurocognitive deficits can be found within sub-sets of neuropsychological measures—suggesting that some participants may have ongoing neurocognitive sequelae.

How early "complicating" factors relate to neuropsychological functions has been recently explored. Shreedy et al. (2006) investigated prediction of post-concussion symptoms using an ED assessment that examined neuropsychological and balance deficits and pain severity of 29 concussed individuals. Thirty participants with minor orthopaedic injuries and 30 ED visitors were recruited as control subjects. Concussed and orthopaedically injured participants were followed up by telephone at 1 month to assess symptom severity. In the ED, concussed subjects performed worse on some neuropsychological tests and had impaired balance compared to controls. They also reported significantly more post-concussive symptoms at follow-up. Neurocognitive impairment, pain and balance deficits were all significantly correlated with severity of post-concussion symptoms. The findings suggest that a combination of variables assessable in the ED may be useful in predicting which individuals will suffer persistent post-concussion problems. Brief short-form traditional assessments have continued to be studied in the literature. Shores et al. (2008) examined whether administering the Revised Westmead Post-traumatic Amnesia (PTA) Scale (R-WPTAS) in addition to the GCS would increase diagnostic accuracy in the early identification of cognitive impairment in patients with mTBI. Data were collected from 82 consecutive participants with mTBI who presented to the ED of a level-one trauma centre in Australia. A matched sample of 88 control participants who attended the ED for reasons other than head trauma was also assessed. All patients were assessed using the GCS, R-WPTAS and a battery of neuropsychological tests. Patients with mTBI scored poorly compared with control patients on all measures. The R-WPTAS showed greater concurrent validity with the neuropsychological measures than the GCS and significantly increased prediction of patients with mTBI who had cognitive impairment. The R-WPTAS also significantly improved diagnostic accuracy in identifying patients with mTBI who may have PTA. Administration took less than 1 min, and since early identification of a patient's cognitive status facilitates management decisions, it was recommended for routine use whenever the GCS is used.

The emerging literature on recovery in childhood will be discussed in greater detail below. However, for now, we wish to note that for children recovery is complex and tends not to be characterised by problems with neurocognitive functioning per se but rather with neuro-behavioural difficulties. Indeed, Hawley et al. (2004a, b) showed that for those injured between 5 and 15 years, with a mean of 2.2 years post-injury, there was no evidence to suggest a threshold of injury below which the risk of late sequelae could be safely discounted, although the risks increase with severity.

Relationships Between Neurological and Neurocognitive Functions

Whether mTBI leads to reliable changes in cognitive status associated with particular forms of injury (severity, location, etc.) is addressed in studies, where neuroradiological and neurocognitive data can be linked. There is emerging evidence linking neurocognitive dysfunction to neuro-imaging findings post-mTBI. We shall now review the strength of such relationships. A study of a group of patients with "day-of-injury" CT scans showing "abnormalities" (hence "complicated"), compared to uncomplicated, showed that complicated mTBI was associated with worse performance for executive and attention functions. A further study of 20 complicated mTBI (based on GCS falling between 13 and 15 and/or CT scan results) and "uncomplicated" matched patients revealed that the complicated mTBI patients performed worse on memory tasks (visual reproduction and verbal learning) (Lange et al. 2009). MRI scanning provides for more "fine-grained" imagery of brain systems. An MRI study of neuropsychological functions in 30 mTBI patients compared to matched controls indicated that patients with traumatic lesions performed more poorly on neurocognitive tasks within 4 days of injury compared to those with non-specific lesions or no lesions (Kurca et al. 2006).

Performance was worse for concentration and attention.

It appears that neurocognitive recovery follows a variable time course. A study by Hughes et al. (2004) revealed that patients identified as complicated by MRI were also found to have neuropsychological dysfunction, with memory, attention and executive functions being impaired. Interestingly, however, there was no difference in terms of whether those with normal or abnormal scans returned to work or not. A recent study by Kwok et al. (2008) of "complicated" patients (abnormal CT scan within 24 h of injury) at 1 and 3 months post-injury compared to non-patient controls indicated that the complicated group were poor on speed, attention (both sustained and divided) and executive functions at the time of 1 month, but, by 3 months, speed and divided attention were much improved. Sustained attention and executive functions were not fully resolved, however. In a similar study by Hofman et al. (2001), further evidence of coherence between neurological functions and neurocognition over time has been found. In their MRI with single-photon emission CT (SPECT) study, it was found that 57 and 61% of their 21 and 18 patients (GCS on average 14.48) had abnormalities on MRI and SPECT imaging, respectively, within 5 days after injury. Moreover, there was associated brain atrophy at 6 months[63]. Those with complicated mTBI were slower on reaction time tasks.

Functional imaging studies have provided further evidence of systems implicated in mTBI. In an fMRI study of 18 mTBI patients up to 1 month post-injury, there were significant changes in activation patterns (McAllister et al. 2001). The patient group, compared to controls, had differential activation patterns—in bilateral frontal and parietal areas—on working memory tasks under moderate load. An fMRI study of working memory task with concussed athletes (15 "symptomatic" participants who had sustained their last injury from 1 to 14 months previously) revealed differential activity patterns compared to a control group (Chen et al. 2004). They had weaker activity in areas related to self-monitoring—such as prefrontal cortex. Chen and colleagues conducted fMRI imaging for working memory task on athletes 1 month post-injury who had self-rated for severity of symptoms—(a "low" ($n=9$) symptoms group and a "moderate" ($n=9$) symptoms group, and a control group). The moderate group showed less activation in the ROI identified in controls for the tasks—the dorsolateral prefrontal cortex. Both concussed groups had increased activation in the left temporal area (Chen et al. 2007). These findings suggest that it may be possible to detect physiological changes in neurological systems linked to changes in cognitive functions.

Associations between neurological activation and cognition have recently been investigated with transcranial magnetic stimulation (TMS) and electroencephalogram (EEG) over a 30-year period. In this study, 19 former athletes who had sustained concussions 30 years prior to testing were compared to 21 healthy, uninjured athletes. The concussed group performed poorer on tasks of memory and response inhibition (that is, stopping oneself from doing something). Also, athletes with a history of concussion showed significant P3a latency delays and amplitude reductions compared to controls. The duration of the Cortical Silent Period (CSP) on TMS was also reported to be significantly longer in the concussed group—which may indicate change in motor cortical excitability (De Beaumont et al. 2009).

Such studies, therefore, indicate that "complicated" mTBI may be predicted on the basis of neurologic evidence and tracked by neurocognitive testing. However, there are important limitations that relate to a number of these studies. First, across most studies, there is insufficient information as to whether those who display any abnormality or differential activation pattern may have had pre-morbid factors relevant to such functions. It is known, for example, that ADHD may be a risk factor for early head injury (Keenan et al. 2008). Second, particularly at long term post-injury, there is a possibility that participants were inaccurate in their reports on the severity and number of mTBIs. Third, numbers of participants tend to be low, and retention rates low, which leads to concerns over the representativeness of the groups studied.

There are also contrasting findings. A 1-year prospective study in Norway of 115 patients with Mild, Moderate and Severe TBI found that the Mild group reported greater PCS symptoms at 3 months but not at 1 year post-injury (Sigurdardottir et al. 2009). Also, at 3 months—there was no difference in the Mild group between those meeting the PCS criteria on the basis of any inter-cranial pathology—detected by MRI.

Psychological Processes Mediating Outcomes

Persistence of symptoms may, then, be due to residual neurological injury. However, given the lack of consistent association among neurological status, neurocognitive function and self-reports, there is a clear role for consideration of a wider array of issues—particularly psychosocial—in the maintenance, and, indeed possibly, genesis, of problems in the longer term. In this context, it is worth noting that, while factors such as female gender and previous psychiatric history (see Carroll et al. 2004a) have been linked to poorer outcome, much of the literature has been critiqued both conceptually and methodologically (see Carroll et al. 2004b), with failures to replicate significant findings being noted: limitations can include issues around consistency of mTBI definitions, unclear or heterogeneous populations, use of cross-sectional rather than longitudinal study designs and questions around potential recall and recruitment biases.

To provide a more comprehensive understanding of the roles of various biological, psychological and social factors in accounting for outcomes, diathesis-stressor models have been proposed. These combine both "organic" and "psychogenic" factors to account for PCS post-mTBI (Kay 1993; Alexander 1995; Jacobson 1995: King 2003; Wood 2004). Lishman (1988) provided an early version of this model by noting how early biological mechanisms may be responsible for initial PCS symptoms, but "vicious cycles" of psychological factors may be responsible for their persistence. King (2003) provided a model positing a number of potential "windows of vulnerability", such as early worries about symptom longevity and various coping styles which may influence symptoms. There have been recent advances in explicating psychological reactions to trauma that may have a significant role in PCS symptomology. Also, there has been evidence to show that patients may misattribute subjective phenomena as due to mTBI. For example, as we shall discuss below, mood symptoms associated with Post-traumatic Stress Disorder (PTSD) could be mistaken for PCS (Hoge et al. 2008).

Psychological Reaction

There are elevated rates of psychiatric co-morbidity in PCS groups (Ruff and Jurica 1999). This may be a response to persisting effects of brain injury on cognition and associated limitations in functioning but could be a psychological reaction to the trauma event. PTSD has recently been shown to develop post-TBI (e.g. King 1997; Bryant and Harvey 1999). It had been thought that a loss of memory for the event would be a protective factor for PTSD post-TBI. However, a number of studies have shown that PTSD does occur after mild, and even moderate to severe, TBI (see Williams et al. 2003). Potential mechanisms for such post-traumatic stress (PTS) have been identified—such as islands of memory, external causal attributions, etc. (see McMillan et al. 2003 for a review). Rates of PTSD after TBI vary hugely—from 0% prevalence through to 48% in one review (Harvey et al. 2003). Moreover, there has been ambiguous evidence as to whether amnesia may be a protective factor (Gil et al. 2005; Caspi et al. 2005; Bryant et al. 2009) or not (e.g. Greenspan et al. 2006). Very recently, a large-scale study of 920 trauma patients in Australia by Bryant and colleagues showed that mTBI patients were more likely to develop PTSD compared to non-TBI controls, but that longer PTA was a protective factor (Bryant et al. 2009).

In a recent retrospective review of the US soldiers returning from Iraq, post-concussional symptoms were elevated in individuals exposed to mTBI compared with other injuries, but PTSD (along with depression) emerged as a major factor mediating the relationship between the two (Hoge et al. 2008). Belanger et al. (2010) also recently identified a role for PTSD in symptomology post-mTBI. In their study of mTBI and moderate to severe TBI patient groups ($n = 225$: 97% were active duty or veteran military personnel), those with mTBI endorsed more symptoms than the moderate to severe groups. However, when controlling for variance due to the effect of PTSD, the mTBI group was no longer different from the other groups (across all three domains of affective, somatic and cognitive domains). It is important to note, though, in this context, that the relationship between PTSD and PCS is complicated by overlapping domains and other methodological issues (Chalton and McMillan 2009). For example, it is questioned whether PTSD measures can be sensitive to the effects of non-traumatic stressors, and whether responses may reflect personality traits such as negative affectivity (Shapinsky et al. 2005). Questions, therefore, persist around PTSD and other psychiatric disorders, such as depression in relation to mTBI, their relationship with pre-injury psychiatric status and the extent to which they moderate or mediate the interaction between an injury and PCS. However, evolving stress (e.g. reactions to changed life situations and circumstances) and distress (including depression, as well as a potential range of anxiety disorders rather than PTSD exclusively) in the days, weeks and months after mTBI seem likely to be important factors in the formation and maintenance of PCS.

Attributions and Expectations

There are various ways in which subjective biases can influence reporting of symptoms, and even moderate test performance. Individuals with persistent PCS may under-report normal "post-concussional" symptoms they experienced prior to their head injury—the "Good Old Days" phenomena (Iverson et al. 2010). Even the act of reading vignettes related to head injury has been shown to lead to uninjured controls expecting post-concussional symptoms (Mittenberg et al. 1992). Suhr and Gunstad (2005) demonstrated the phenomena of how expectation can influence test performance. They administered neurocognitive measures (memory, attention and executive functioning) to two groups of undergraduates who had reported a history of mTBI. One group were made aware of their "head injury" and what kinds of cognitive effects occurred post-head injury prior to testing ("diagnosis threat" group). This group showed significantly worse performance on a number of neurocognitive measures. Whittaker and colleagues and others (e.g. Fenton et al. 1993; King et al. 1999; Meares et al. 2006) suggested that psychological mechanisms may play a role in influencing later symptoms early on after injury. They examined the extent to which perceptions of symptoms on the Revised Illness Perception Questionnaire (Moss-Morris et al. 2002) within the first 3 weeks after mTBI predicted the presence of persistent symptoms at 3 months after injury. They found that individuals who initially viewed their injury as having serious and persisting negative consequences had greater symptomology at 3 months.

Involvement in medico-legal or compensation claims may lead to expectations to be moderated (Binder and Rohling 1996; Carroll et al. 2004a) with the possibility of symptoms being maintained. Individuals being involved in tort as compared to no-fault insurance claims following motor vehicle incidents have been shown to be subject to slower recovery (Cassidy et al. 2004). Also, there is evidence that at least a proportion of individuals with persisting difficulties after mTBI can show evidence of at least suboptimal effort on formal neurocognitive assessment (Larrabee 2003; Mooney et al. 2005). However, it is also important to consider how involvement in a medico-legal action—with repeated rehearsal of symptoms and an emphasis on blame and culpability (see Lishman 1988; Jacobson 1995)—may play a role. And it is important to consider the roles that comorbid issues, such as anxiety and pain, have on cognitive performance (e.g. Radanov et al. 1999; Nicholson et al. 2001), for example by distracting attention form the "task in hand".

Children and Adolescents

With regard to children, the literature is relatively underdeveloped compared to that for adults with mTBI. As we have noted above, there is some evidence of problems in children post-mTBI. However, the evidence base is not strong, and there are methodological problems with a range of studies (see Carroll et al. 2004a, b), particularly with regard to lack of control groups and consideration of pre-morbid and non-injury factors. In general, as Carroll et al. (2004a, b) noted: "Where post-concussion symptoms are present, they are usually transient in nature". In their review of a wide range of studies, they note that there are often pre-morbid issues and poverty factors that are linked to worse outcomes (Carroll et al. 2004a, b). However, as also noted above, there have been some recent studies suggesting a higher level of disability than expected (Limond et al. 2009).

A study by Wrightson et al. (1995) provides interesting insights into how such problems may occur. They followed up pre-school children who had mTBI soon after injury and then at 6 months and a year. There was an orthopaedic control group. They found no differences after injury on a range of cognitive tasks. But, at 6 months and then at 1 year, the children with scored less well on tasks measuring visual problem solving. There was also an association with further injury. A prospective, longitudinal follow-up at 23 years post-injury study by Hessen and colleagues (Hessen et al. 2007) identified PTA as a particularly important factor in mTBI in childhood injuries. They tested 45 and 74 adults who had injuries 23 years previously as children or adults, respectively. Those who had injuries in childhood, and had a PTA of half an hour or more, were found to have vulnerability to chronic, mild, neuropsychological dysfunction. They note that here was no control group, but they had taken account of pre-injury factors in analysis. Cognitive outcomes, and the effect of advice giving, were investigated by Ponsford et al. (1999). They found that initial symptoms had resolved by 3 months, but children with previous "head injury" or learning difficulty had ongoing problems. On a related theme, cognitive reserve—a resilience issue—was examined in a study by Fay et al. (2009). They found that children with lower cognitive ability with complicated mTBI (determined by MRI) were especially prone to cognitive symptoms. The needs of children and families were addressed by Hawley (2003) who found that across severity of TBI there were significant problems associated with anxiety over time with no significant resolution of problems when comparing mTBI and moderate to severe TBI groups. Recent work by Anderson et al. (2009) provides an important heuristic for understanding these differential effects of childhood injuries (Anderson et al. 2005). They have referred to the need to consider the early vulnerability model of recovery from brain injury in childhood and suggest that age of injury and age at testing are important factors in the context of neuro-plasticity and crowding effects (see Anderson et al. 2009). Family functioning variables are also strong mediators of outcome both pre- and post-injury (Yeates and Taylor 2005) and these have to be considered as part of a wider biopsychosocial assessment protocol.

Tonks et al. (2011) have studied a range of mediating variables of recovery from various forms of Acquired Brain Injury in childhood—including age of injury, underlying cognitive factors and socio-emotional functioning. This work suggests that there are associations between hyperactive behaviour and speed of processing deficits in children between the ages of 8–10 years, and there are significant links between hyperactivity and difficulties in establishing peer relationships for children aged 10–15 years. In the samples used in these studies, some children had milder traumatic brain injuries, although we note that they may well not be fully representative of the majority of children mTBI due to selection biases. In general, this work points to the need to incorporate not only self-report and cognitive testing measures into assessment schedules but also to widen the pool of enquiry to psychosocial domains and consider additional more subtle executive assessment measures of social and emotional processing and inference (e.g. of another's "Theory of Mind"

(TOM) shown by expressions of emotion). In the child literature, assessments such as the Strengths and Difficulties Questionnaire (Goodman 1996) provide well-standardised reliable data on the child in both family and school settings with child, teacher and parent reporting options. It provides measurement for emotional symptoms, conduct problems, inattention, peer relationships and pro-social behaviour. Child versions of the measures such as The Awareness of Social Inference Test (TASIT) (McDonald et al. 2006) are not forthcoming at present, although Baron-Cohen et al. (1997) has routinely used similar measures with children with Autism Spectrum Disorder (ASD) to determine abilities such as Theory of Mind and empathy. The development and refinement of measures that are sensitive to mTBI groups would be important for children, who appear to develop subtle executive and higher level cognitive and socio-behavioural difficulties.

Summary and Conclusions

mTBI may be best seen as a spectrum disorder, with the "dosage" of injury setting a context for recovery and/or resolution of symptoms. Neurocognitive functions appear to recover rapidly early on. Studies linking radiographic neuroanatomic data and neurocognitive functions suggest functional changes in brain activation which may resolve readily but that there may be structural changes—particularly evident in "complicated" cases. In such cases, delayed recovery (at 3 months to a year) may be anticipated. There appears to be concordance between neurological findings and neurocognitive functions early after injury, but, with time, such associations dissipate. Subjective complaints also appear to become less "tied" to neurocognitive functions over time. The role of psychosocial factors in symptomology is coming under increased scrutiny, with such issues as PTSD and expectations being identified as influential in predicting outcomes. Compared to adults, assessment of children and adolescents is complicated by the dynamics of neurocognitive development and significant contextual factors. It is crucial, therefore, that assessments are undertaken not only to identify neurocognitive processing, but also such issues, with careful monitoring over return to activities. With a better understanding of the multiple causal variables that interplay in mTBI and PCS, patients and relatives may be given better advice to ensure that recovery is maximised.

References

Alexander MP. Mild traumatic brain injury: pathophysiology, natural history and clinical management. Neurology. 1995;45:1253–60.

Alla S, Sullivan SJ, Hale L, McCrory P. Self-report scales/checklists for the measurement of concussion symptoms: a systematic review. Br J Sports Med. 2009;43:i3–12.

American Academy of Neurology. Practice parameter: the management of concussion in sports (summary statement). Neurology. 1997;48:581–5.

American Psychiatric Association. Diagnostic and statistical manual of mental disorders: DSM-IV. 4th ed. Washington, DC: American Psychiatric Association; 1994.

Anderson V, Catroppa C, Morse S, Haritou F, Rosenfeld J. Outcome fomr mild head injury in young children: a prospective study. J Clin Exp Neuropsychol. 2001;23:705–17.

Anderson V, Spencer Smith M, Leveneter R, Coleman L, Anderson P, Williams J, Greenham M, Jacobs R. Childhood brain insult: can age at insult help us predict outcome? Brain. 2009;132:45–56.

Anderson V, Catroppa C, Morse S, Haritou F, Rosenfeld J. Functional plasticity or vulnerability after early brain injury? Pediatrics. 2005;116:1374–82.

Baron-Cohen S, Jolliffe T, Mortimore C, Robertson M. Another advanced test of theory of mind: evidence from very high functioning adults with autism or Asperger Syndrome. J Child Psychol Psychiatry. 1997;38:813–22.

Barth JT, Alves WM, Ryan TV, Macciocchi SN, Rimel RW, Jane JA, Nelson WE. Mild head injury in sports: neuropsychological sequelae and recovery of function. In: Levin HL, Eisenberg HM, Benton AL, editors. Mild head injury. New York, NY: Oxford University Press; 1989.

Bazarian JJ, Blyth B, Cimpello L. Bench to bedside: evidence for brain injury after concussion—looking beyond the computed tomography scan. Acad Emerg Med. 2006;13:199–214.

Bazarian JJ, Wong T, Harris M, Leahey N, Mookerjee S, Dombovy M. Epidemiology and predictors of post-concussive syndrome after minor head injury in an emergency population. Brain Inj. 1999;13:173–89.

Belanger H, Kretzmer T, Vanderploeg RD, et al. Symptom complaints following combat-related traumatic brain injury: relationship to traumatic brain injury severity and posttraumatic stress disorder. J Int Neuropsychol Soc. 2010;16(1):194–9.

Belanger HG, Vanderploeg RD. The neuropsychological impact of sports-related concussion: a meta-analysis. J Int Neuropsychol Soc. 2005;11:34–57.

Binder LM. A review of mild head trauma. Part II: clinical implications. J Clin Exp Neuropsychol. 1997;18: 432–57.

Binder LM, Rohling ML. Money matters: a meta-analytic review of the effects of financial incentives on recovery after closed-head injury. Am J Psychiatry. 1996;153:7–10.

Boake C, McCauley SR, Levin HW, Contant CF, Song JX, Brown SA, Goodman HS, Brundage SI, Diaz-Marchan PJ, Merritt SG. Limited agreement between criteria-based diagnoses of postconcussional syndrome. J Neuropsychiatry Clin Neurosci. 2004;16:493–9.

Boll TJ, Barth JT. Mild head injury. Psychiatr Dev. 1983;3:263–75.

Bryant RA, Creamer M, O'Donnell M, Sillove D, Clark CR, McFarlane AC. Post-traumatic amnesia and the nature of post-traumatic stress disorder after mild traumatic brain injury. J Int Neuropsychol Soc. 2009;15(6):862–7. doi:10.1017/S1355617709990671.

Bryant RA, Harvey AG. Postconcussive symptoms and posttraumatic stress disorder after mild traumatic brain injury. J Nerv Ment Dis. 1999;187:302–5.

Campbell KA, Rohlman DS, Storzbach D, Binder LM, Anger WK, Kovera CA, Davis KL, Grossman SJ. Test–retest reliability of psychological and neurobehavioural tests self-administered by computer. Assessment. 1999;6:21–32.

Cantu RC. Return to play guidelines after a head injury. Clin Sports Med. 1998;17:45–60.

Carroll LJ, Cassidy JD, Peloso PM, Borg J, von Holst H, Holm L, Paniak C, Pépin M. Prognosis for mild traumatic brain injury: results of The WHO Collaborating Centre Task Force on mild traumatic brain injury. J Rehabil Med. 2004a;36:84–105.

Carroll LJ, Cassidy JD, Holm L, Kraus J, Coronado VG. Methodological issues and research recommendations for mild traumatic brain injury: the WHO Collaborating Centre Task Force on mild traumatic brain injury. J Rehabil Med. 2004b;S43:113–25.

Caspi Y, Gil S, Ben-Ari IZ, Koren D, Aaron-Peretz J, Klein E. Memory of the traumatic event is associated with increased risk for post traumatic stress disorder: a retrospective study of patients with traumatic brain injury. J Loss Trauma: Int Perspect Stress Coping. 2005;1532-5032:319–35.

Cassidy JD, Carroll LJ, Cote P, Holm L, Nygren A. Mild traumatic brain injury after traffic collisions: a population based cohort study. J Rehabil Med. 2004;43:15–21.

Chalton LD, McMillan TM. Can 'partial' PTSD explain differences in diagnosis of PTSD by questionnaire self-report and interview after head injury? Brain Inj. 2009;23:77–82.

Chen J-K, Johnston KM, Frey S, et al. Functional abnormalities in symptomatic concussed athletes: an fMRI study. Neuroimage. 2004;22:68–82.

Chen JK, Johnston KM, Collie A, McCrory P, Ptito A. A validation of the post-concussion symptom scale in the assessment of complex concussion using cognitive testing and functional MRI. J Neurol Neuropsychol Psychiatry. 2007;78:1231–8.

Christensen JC, Pedersen MG, Pedersen CB, Sidenius P, Olsen J, Vestergaard M. Long term risk of epilepsy after traumatic brain injury in children and young adults: a population based cohort study. Lancet. 2009. doi:10.1016/S-1470-6736(09) 60214-2. Published on-line.

Cogstate. Cogsport (Computer Software). Parkville: Cogstate Ltd.; 1999.

Collie A, Darby DG, Maruff P. Computerised cognitive assessment of athletes with sports related head injury. Br J Sports Med. 2001;35:297–302.

Collie A, Makdissi M, Maruff P, et al. Cognition in the days following concussion: comparison of symptomatic athelets. J Neurol Neurosurg Psychiatr 2006;77:241–5.

Collie A, Maruff P, McStephen M, Darby DG. Psychometric issues associated with computerised neuropsychological assessment of concussed athletes. Br J Sports Med. 2003;37:556–9.

Collins MW, Grindel SH, Lovell MR, Dede DE, Moser DJ, Phalin BR, Nogle S, Wasik M, Cordry D, Klotz Daugherty M, Sears SF, Nicolette G, Indelicato P, McKeag DB. Relationship between concussion and neuropsychological performance in college football players. J Am Med Assoc. 1999;282:964–70.

Colorado Medical Society. Report of the sports medicine committee: guidelines for the management of concussion in sports. Denver, CO: Medical Society; 1991.

Davis GA, Iverson GL, Guskiewicz KM, Ptito A, Johnston KM. Contributions of neuroimaging, balance testing, electrophysiology and blood markers to the assessment of sport-related concussion. Br J Sports Med. 2009;43:i36–45.

De Beaumont L, Théoret H, Mongeon D, Messier J, Leclerc S, Tremblay S, Ellemberg D, Lassonde M. Brain function decline in healthy retired athletes who sustained their last sports concussion in early adulthood. Brain. 2009;132:695–708.

Defense and Veterans Brain Injury Center Consensus Conference (2008). The acute management of concussion/mild traumatic brain injury (mTBI) in the deployed setting. 31 July and 1 August 2008, Washington, DC.

Dikmen S, McLean A, Temkin N. Neuropsychological and psychosocial consequences of minor head injury. J Neurol Neurosurg Psychiatry. 1986;49:1227–32.

Echemendia RJ, Herring S, Bailes J. Who should conduct and interpret the neuropsychological assessment in sports-related concussion? Br J Sports Med. 2009;43: i32–5.

Echemendia RJ, Putakian M, Mackin SR, Julian L, Shoss N. Neuropsychological test performance prior to and following sports-related mild traumatic brain injury. Clin J Sport Med. 2001;11:23–31.

Erlanger D, Feldmand D, Kutner K. Concussion resolution index. New York, NY: Headminder Inc.; 1999.

Falletti MG, Maruff P, Collie A, Darby DG. Practice effects associated with the repeated assessment of cognitive function using the CogSport battery at 10-minute, one week and one month test-re-test intervals. J Clin Exp Neuropsychol. 2006;28:1095–112.

Fay, Yeates, Taylor et al. (2009).

Fenton G, McClelland R, Montgomery A, MacFlynn G, Rutherford W. The postconcussional syndrome: social antecedents and psychological sequelae. Br J Psychiatry. 1993;162:493–7.

Fleminger S, Ponsford J. Long term outcome after traumatic brain injury. Br Med J. 2005;331:1419–20.

Frencham KA, Fox AM, Maybery MT. Neuropsychological studies of mild traumatic brain injury: a meta-analytic review of research since 1995. J Clin Exp Neuropsychol. 2005;27:334–51.

Gerber DJ, Schraa JC. Mild traumatic brain injury: searching for a syndrome. J Head Trauma Rehabil. 1995;10:28–40.

Gil S, Caspi Y, Ben-Ari IZ, Koren D, Klein E. Does memory of a traumatic event increase the risk for post traumatic stress disorder in patients with traumatic brain injury? A prospective study. Am J Psychiatry. 2005; 162:963–9.

Giza CC, Hovda DA. The neurometabolic cascade of concussion. J Athl Train. 2001;36:228–35.

Gualtieri CT, Johnson LG. A computerized test battery sensitive to mild and severe brain injury. Medscape J Med. 2008;15:90.

Goodman R. The strengths and difficulties questionnaire: a research note. J Child Psychol Psychiatry. 1996;38: 581–6.

Greenspan AL, Stringer AY, Phillips VL, Hammond FM, Goldstein FC. Symptoms of post-traumatic stress: intrusion and avoidance 6 and 12 months after traumatic brain injury. Brain Inj. 2006;20(7):733–42. 1362-301x.

Guskiewicz KM, Weaver NL, Padua DA, Garrett WE. Epidemiology of concussion in collegiate and high school football players. Am J Sports Med. 2000;28:643–50.

Haldorsen T, Waterloo K, Dahl A, Mellgren SI, Davidsen PE, Molin PK. Symptoms and cognitive dysfunction in patients with the late whiplash syndrome. Appl Neuropsychol. 2003;10:170–5.

Harvey AG, Bryant RA, Tarrier N. Cognitive behaviour therapy for post traumatic stress disorder. Clin Psychol Rev. 2003;23(3):501–22.

Hawley CA, Ward AB, Long J, Owen DW, Magnay AR. Prevalence of traumatic brain injury amongst children admitted to hospital in one health district: a population-based study. Injury. 2004a;34:256–60.

Hawley CA, Ward AB, Magnay AR, Long J. Outcomes following childhood head injury: a population. J Neurol Neurosurg Psychiatry. 2004b;75:737–42.

Hessen E, Nestvold K, Anderson V. Neuropsychological function 23 years after Mild traumatic brain injury: a comparison of outcome after paediatric and adult head injuries. Brain Inj. 2007;21:963–79.

Hinton-Bayre AD, Geffen G. Severity of sports-related concussion and neuropsychological test performance. Neurology. 2002;59:1068–70.

Hofman PA, Stapert SZ, van Kroonenburgh MJ, Jolles J, de Kruihk J, Wilmink JT. MR imaging, single-photon emission CT, and neurocognitive performance after mild traumatic brain injury. Am J Neuroradiol. 2001;22:441–9.

Hoge CW, McGurk D, Thomas JL, Cox AL, Engel CC, Castro CA. Mild traumatic brain injury in US soldiers returning from Iraq. N Engl J Med. 2008;358: 453–63.

Hughes DG, Jackson AL, Mason DL, Berry E, Hollis S, Yates DW. Abnormalities on magnetic resonance imaging seen acutely following mild traumatic brain injury: correlation with neuropsychological tests and delayed recovery. Neuroradiology. 2004;46:550–8.

Hyder AA, Wunderlich CA, Puvanachandra P, Gururaj G, Kobusingye OC. The impact of traumatic brain injuries: a global perspective. NeuroRehabilitation. 2007; 22:341–53.

Iverson GL, Lange RT, Brooks BL, et al. "Good Old Days" bias following mild traumatic brain injury. Clin Neuropsychol. 2010;24(1):17–37.

Iverson GL, Lange RT, Gaetz M, Zasler ND. Mild TBI. In: Zasler ND, Katz DI, Zafonte RD, editors. Brain injury medicine: principles and practice. New York, NY: Demos Medical Publishing; 2006.

Iverson GL, Lovell MR, Collins MW. Validity of ImPACT for measuring attention and processing speed following sports-related concussion. J Clin Exp Neuropsychol. 2005;27:683–9.

Iverson GL, Lange RT. Examination of "post-concussion-like" symptoms in a healthy sample. Appl Neuropsychol. 2003;10(3):137–44.

Iverson GL. Outcome from mild traumatic brain injury. Curr Opin Psychiatry. 2005;18:301–17.

Jacobson RR. The post-concussional syndrome: physiogenesis psychogenesis and malingering, an integrative model. J Psychosom Res. 1995;39:675–93.

Kashluba S, Casey JE, Paniak C. Evaluating the utility of ICD-10 diagnostic criteria for postconcussion syndrome following mild traumatic brain injury. J Int Neuropsychol Soc. 2006;12:111–8.

Kay T. Neuropsychological treatment of mild traumatic brain injury. J Head Trauma Rehabil. 1993;8:74–85.

Keenan HT, Hall GC, Marshall SW. Early head injury and attention deficit hyperactivity disorder: retrospective cohort study. BMJ. 2008;337:a1984.

King NS. Post-concussion syndrome: clarity amid the controversy? Br J Psychiatry. 2003;183:276–8.

King NS. Post-traumatic stress disorder and head injury as a dual diagnosis: "islands" of memory as a mechanism. J Neurol Neurosurg Psychiatry. 1997;62:82–4.

King NS, Crawford S, Wenden FJ, Caldwell FE, Wade DT. Early prediction of persisting post-concussion symptoms following mild and moderate head injuries. Br J Clin Psychol. 1999;38:15–25.

King NS, Crawford S, Wenden RJ, Moss NEG, Wade DT. The Rivermead Post Concussion Symptoms Questionnaire: a measure of symptoms commonly experienced after head injury and its reliability. J Neurol. 1995;9:1432–59.

Kolakowsky-Hayner SA, Kreutzer JS. Pre-injury crime, substance abuse, and neurobehavioural functioning after traumatic brain injury. Brain Inj. 2001;15:53–63.

Kurca E, Sivak S, Kucera P. Impaired cognitive functions in mild traumatic brain injury patients with normal and pathologic magnetic resonance imaging. Neuroradiology. 2006;48:661–9.

Kraus JF, Chu LD. Epidemiology. In: Silver JM, McAllister TW, Yudofsky SC, editors. Textbook of traumatic brain injury. Washington, DC: American Psychiatric Publishing; 2005.

Kwok FY, Lee TMC, Leung CHS, Poon WS. Changes of cognitive functioning following mild traumatic brain injury over a 3-month period. Brain Inj. 2008; 22(10):740–51.

Lange R, Iverson GL, Franzen M. Neuropsychological functioning following complicated vs. uncomplicated mild traumatic brain injury. Brain Inj. 2009;23(2):83–91.

Lannsjö M, af Geijerstam JL, Johansson U, Bring J, Borg J. Prevalence and structure of symptoms at 3 months after mild traumatic brain injury in a national cohort. Brain Inj. 2009;23:213–9.

Larrabee GJ. Detection of malingering using atypical performance patterns on standard neuropsychological tests. Clin Neuropsychol. 2003;7:410–25.

Lezak M. Neuropsychological Assessment. Oxford University Press; 1995.

Lezak MD. Neuropsychological assessment. 4th ed. Oxford: Oxford University Press; 2004.

Limond J, Dorris L, McMillan TM. Quality of life in children with acquired brain injury: parent perspectives 1–5 years after injury. Brain Inj. 2009;23:617–22.

Lishman WA. Physiogenesis and psychogenesis in the 'post-concussional syndrome'. Br J Psychiatry. 1988;153:460–9.

McAllister TW, Sparling MB, Flashman LA, Guerin SJ, Mamourian AC, Saykin AJ. Differential working memory load effects after mild traumatic brain injury. Neuroimage. 2001,14:1004–12.

Macciocchi SN, Barth JT, Alves W, Rimel RW, Jane JA. Neuropsychological functioning and recovery after mild head injury in collegiate athletes. Neurosurgery 1996;39:510–4.

Makdissi M, Collie A, Maruff P, Darby DG, Bush A, McCrory P, Bennell K. Computerised cognitive assessment of concussed Australian Rules footballers. Br J Sports Med. 2001;35:354–60.

Maroon JC, Lovell MR, Norwig J, Podell K, Powell JW, Hartl R. Cerebral concussion in athletes: evaluation and neuropsychological testing. Neurosurgery. 2000;47:659–72.

McCauley SR, Boake C, Pedroza C, Brown SA, Levin HS, Goodman HS, Merritt SG. Correlates of persistent postconcussional disorder: DSM-IV criteria versus ICD-10. J Clin Exp Neuropsychol. 2007;30:360–79.

McCrea M, Guskiewicz KM, Marshall SW, Barr W, Randolph C, Cantu RC, Onate JA, Yang J, Kelly JP. Acute effects and recovery time following concussion in collegiate football players. J Am Med Assoc. 2003;290:2556–63.

McCrea M, Kelly JP, Randolph C, Cisler R, Berger L. Immediate neurocognitive effects of concussion. Neurosurgery. 2002;50:1032–42.

McCrory P, Meeuwisse W, Johnston K, Dvorak J, Aubry M, Molloy M, Cantu R. Consensus statement on concussion in sport: the 3rd international conference on concussion in sport held in Zurich, November 2008. Clin J Sports Med. 2009;19:185–200.

McCrory P, Johnston K, Meeuwisse W, Aubry M, Cantu R, Dvorak J, Graf-Baumann T, Kelly J, Lovell M, Schamasch P. Summary and agreement statement of the 2nd international conference on concussion in sport, Prague 2004. Br J Sports Med. 2005;39: 196–204.

McDonald S, Bornhofen C, Shum D, Long E, Saunders C, Neulinger K. Reliability and validity of the awareness of social inference test (TASIT): a clinical test of social perception. Disabil Rehabil. 2006;28:1529–42.

McLean SA, Kirsch NL, Tan-Schriner CU, Sen A, Frederiksen S, Harris RE, Maixner W, Maio RF. Health status, not head injury, predicts concussion symptoms after minor head injury. Am J Emerg Med. 2009;27:182–90.

McMillan TM, Williams WH, Bryant R. Post-traumatic stress disorder and traumatic brain injury: a review of causal mechanisms, assessment, and treatment. Neuropsychol Rehabil. 2003;13(1 & 2):149–64.

McMillan TM, Errors in diagnosing post-traumatic stress disorder after traumatic brain injury. Brain Inj. 2001;15:39–46.

Meares S, Shores EA, Taylor AJ, Batchelor J, Bryant RA, Bagueley IJ, Chapman J, Gurka J, Dawson K, Capon L, Marosszeky JE. Mild traumatic brain injury does not predict acute postconcussion syndrome. J Neurol Neurosurg Psychiatry. 2008;79:300–6.

Meares S, Shores EA, Batchelor J, Bryant RA, Bagueley IJ, Chapman J, Gurka J, Marosszeky JE. The relationship of psychological and cognitive factors and opioids in the development of the postconcussion syndrome in general trauma patients with mild traumatic brain injury. J Int Neuropsychol Soc. 2006;12:792–801.

Mittenberg W, DiGuilio DV, Perrin S, Bass AE. Symptoms following mild head injury: expectation as aetiology. J Neurol Neurosurg Psychiatry. 1992;55:200–4.

Mooney G, Speed J, Sheppard S. Factors related to recovery after mild traumatic brain injury. Brain Inj. 2005;19:975–87.

Moss-Morris R, Weinman J, Petrie K, Horne R, Cameron L, Buick D. Revised illness perception questionnaire. Psychol Health. 2002;17:1–16.

Nicholson K, Martelli MF, Zasler N. Does pain confound interpretation of neuropsychological test results? NeuroRehabilitation. 2001;16:225–30.

Nolin P, Heroux L. Relations among sociodemographic, neurologic, clinical and neuropsychologic variables, and vocational status following mild traumatic brain injury: a follow-up study. J Head Trauma Rehabil. 2006;21(6):514–26.

Oddy M, Coughlan T, Tyerman A, Jenkins D. Social adjustment after closed head injury: a further follow-up seven years after injury. J Neurol Neurosurg Psychiatry. 1985;48:564–8.

Ommaya AK, Gennarelli TA. Cerebral concussion and traumatic unconsciousness: correlation of experimental and clinical observations on blunt head injuries. Brain. 1974;97:633–54.

Pellman EJ, Lovell MR, Viano DC, Casson IR, Tucker A. Concussion in professional football: neuropsychological testing—part 6. Neurosurgery. 2004;57:1290–3.

Pertab JL, James KM, Bigler ED. Limitations of mild traumatic brain injury meta-analyses. Brain Inj. 2009;23(6):498–508.

Ponsford J, Willmott C, Rothwell A, Cameron P, Ayton G, Nelms R, Curran C, Ng KT. Cognitive and behavioral outcome following mild traumatic head injury in children. J Head Trauma Rehabil. 1999;14:360–72.

Potter S, Leigh E, Wade D, Fleminger S. The Rivermead post concussion symptoms questionnaire. J Neurol. 2006;253:1603–14.

Radanov BP, Bicik I, Dvorak J, Antinnes J, von Schulthess GK, Buck A. Relation between neuropsychological and neuroimaging findings in patients with late whiplash syndrome. J Neurol Neurosurg Psychiatry. 1999;66:485–9.

Ruff RM, Weyer Jamora C. Myths and mild traumatic brain injury. Psychol Inj Law. 2009;2:34–42.

Ruff RM, Jurica P. In search of a unified definition for mild traumatic brain injury. Brain Inj. 1999;13(12):943–52.

Ruff RM, Camenzuli L, Mueller J. Miserable minority: emotional risk factors that influence the outcome of a mild traumatic brain injury. Brain Inj. 1996;10:551–66.

Russell M, Goldberg A, O'Connor K. Computer-based testing and validity: a look back into the future. Assess Educ. 2003;10:279–93.

Schatz P, Zillmer EA. Computer-Based assessment of sports-related concussion. Appl Neuropsychol. 2003;10:42–7.

Schatz P, Putz BO. Cross-validation of measures used for computer-based assessment of concussion. Appl Neuropsychol. 2006;13:151–9.

Schatz P, Browndyke J. Applications of computer-based neuropsychological assessment. J Head Trauma Rehabil. 2002;17:395–410.

Schretlen DJ, Shapiro AM. A quantitative review of the effect of traumatic brain injury on cognitive functioning. Int Rev Psychiatry. 2003;15:341–9.

Shapinsky AC, Rapport LJ, Henderson MJ, Axelrod BN. Civilian PTSD scales: relationships with trait characteristics and everyday distress. Assessment. 2005;12(2):220–30.

Shores EA, Lammél A, Hullick C, Sheedy J, Flynn M, Levick W, Batchelor J. The diagnostic accuracy of the Revised Westmead PTA Scale as an adjunct to the Glasgow Coma Scale in the early identification of cognitive impairment in patients with mild traumatic brain injury. J Neurol Neurosurg Psychiatry. 2008;79:1100–6.

Shreedy J, Geffen G, Donnelly J, Faux S. Emergency department assessment of mild traumatic brain injury and prediction of post-concussion symptoms at one month post injury. J Clin Exp Psychol. 2006;28:755–72.

Sigurdardottir S, Andelic N, Roe C, Jerstad T, Schanke A-K. Post-concussion symptoms after traumatic brain injury at 3 and 12 months post-injury: a prospective study. Brain Inj. 2009;23(6):489–97.

Smith A. Symbol digit modalities test manual. Los Angeles, CA: Western Psychological Services; 1982.

Smith-Seemiller L, Fow NR, Kant R, Franzen MD. Presence of post-concussion syndrome symptoms in patients with chronic pain vs. mild traumatic brain injury. Brain Inj. 2003;17:199–206.

Stulemeijer M, van der Werf SP, Borm GF, Vos PE. Early prediction of favorable recovery six-months after mild traumatic brain injury. J Neurol Neurosurg Psychiatry. 2008;79:936–42.

Stålnacke B-M. Community integration, social support and life satisfaction in relation to symptoms 3 years after mild traumatic brain injury. Brain Inj. 2007;21(9):933–42.

Suhr JA, Gunstad J. Further exploration of the effect of "diagnosis threat" on cognitive performance in individuals with mild head injury. J Int Neuropsychol Soc. 2005;11(1):23–9.

Tellier A, Marshall SC, Wilson KG, Smith A, Perugini M, Gilmour Stiell I. The heterogeneity of mild traumatic brain injury: where do we stand? Brain Inj. 2009;23:879–87.

Thornhill S, Teasdale GM, Murray GD, McEwen J, Roy CW, Penny KI. Disability in young people and adults one year after head injury: prospective cohort study. Br Med J. 2000;320:1631–5.

Tonks J, Yates PJ, Williams WH, Slater AM, Frampton IJ. Cognitive correlates of psychosocial outcome following traumatic brain injury in early childhood; comparisons between groups of children aged under and over 10 years of age. Clin Child Psychol Psychiatry. 2011;16(2):185–94.

Veterans Affairs and Dept. of Defense (2009) Clinical practice guideline for management of concussion/mild traumatic brain injury, The Management of Concussion/mTBI working Group, Office of Quality & Performance & Quality Management, VA, Washington, DC v. 1.0.

Wall SE, Williams WH, Cartwright-Hatton S, Kelly TP, Murray J, Murray M, Owen A, Turner M. Neuropsychological dysfunction following repeat concussion in jockeys. J Neurol Neuropsychiatry Psychiatry. 2006;77:518–20.

Williams WH, Potter S, Ryland H. Mild traumatic brain injury and post concussion symptoms: a neuropsychological perspective. J Neurol Neurosurg Psychiatry. 2010;81:1116–22.

Wood RLl. Understanding the 'miserable minority': a diathesis-stress paradigm for post-concussional syndrome. Brain Inj. 2004;18:1135–53.

World Health Organisation. The ICD-10 classification of mental and behavioural disorders: clinical descriptions and diagnostic guidelines. 10th ed. Geneva: World Health Organisation; 1992.

Wrightson P, McGinn V, Gronwall D. Mild head injury in preschool children: evidence that it can be associated with a persisting cognitive defect. J Neurol Neurosurg Psychitary. 1995;59:375–80.

Yard EE, Comstock RD. Compliance with return to play guidelines following concussion in US high school athletes, 2005–2008. Brain Inj. 2009;23: 888–98.

Yates PJ, Williams WH, Harris A, Round A, Jenkins R. An epidemiological study of head injuries in a UK population attending an emergency department. J Neurol Neurosurg Psychiatry. 2006;77:699–701.

Yeates KO, Taylor HG. Neurobehavioural outcomes of mild head injury in children and adolescents. Pediatr Rehabil. 2005;8:5–16.

Management of Moderate and Severe TBI

4

Scott A. Marshall, Randy Bell, Rocco A. Armonda, and Geoffrey S.F. Ling

Abstract

The management of moderate and severe traumatic brain injury (TBI) is a complex and developing practice in the acute neurosciences. The management of such, from the field phase of illness to the tertiary definitive medical and surgical management of TBI, is discussed. Clinical syndromes and radiographic examples of brain injury are presented, along with a current review of the literature in the early critical care phase of moderate and severe brain injury management. We discuss an algorithm for managing the challenging patient, and discuss areas of needed future research.

Keywords

Traumatic brain injury • Osmotic therapy • Intracerebral hypertension • Decompressive craniectomy • Brain code • Herniation syndromes • Therapeutic hypothermia • Pharmacologic coma

S.A. Marshall, M.D. (✉)
Neurology and Critical Care, San Antonio Military Medical Center, Brooke Army Medical Center, Fort Sam Houston, TX 78234, USA

Department of Neurology, Uniformed Services University of the Health Sciences, Bethesda, MD 20814, USA
e-mail: scott.a.marshall1@us.army.mil

R. Bell, M.D. • R.A. Armonda, M.D.
Department of Surgery (Neurosurgery), Uniformed Services University of the Health Sciences, Bethesda, MD 20814, USA

G.S.F. Ling, M.D., Ph.D., F.A.A.N.
Neurology and Critical Care, San Antonio Military Medical Center, Brooke Army Medical Center, Fort Sam Houston, TX 78234, USA

Department of Neurology, Uniformed Services University of the Health Sciences, Bethesda, MD 20814, USA

Department of Surgery (Neurosurgery), Uniformed Services University of the Health Sciences, Bethesda, MD 20814, USA

Critical Care Medicine for Neurology, Anesthesiology, and Surgery, Uniformed Services University of the Health Sciences, Bethesda, MD 20814, USA

J.W. Tsao (ed.), *Traumatic Brain Injury: A Clinician's Guide to Diagnosis, Management, and Rehabilitation*, DOI 10.1007/978-0-387-87887-4_4, © Springer Science+Business Media, LLC 2012

Introduction

The spectrum of traumatic brain injury (TBI) is mild, moderate, or severe. Severity is based largely on the presenting Glasgow Coma Scale Score (GCS) (Table 4.1). Patients with *mild* TBI have an admission GCS of ≥13. This is often referred to as concussion. These patients may have experienced a brief (<30 min) loss of consciousness, and presenting complaints include headache, confusion, and amnesia (The Management of Concussion in Sports (Summary Statement) 1997). Guidelines suggest appropriate Neurological evaluation with concomitant neuroimaging with CT or MR after any concussion with loss of consciousness (The Management of Concussion in Sports (Summary Statement) 1997). The spectrum of presentation of mild TBI is broad and its long-term sequelae is referred to as post-concussion syndrome, the discussion of which is beyond the scope of this chapter. *Moderate* TBI is defined as an admission GCS of 9–12, and is usually associated with prolonged loss of consciousness, abnormal neuroimaging, and neurological deficit (Geocadin et al. 2004). Patients with moderate TBI will require hospitalization and may need neurosurgical evaluation or intervention. Patients with GCS scores of 8 or less have significant neurological injury and are classified as having *severe* TBI. Typically, These patients have abnormal neuroimaging such as a CT scan with skull fracture or intracranial hemorrhage (ICH) (Stiver et al. 2009). Such patients require rapid evacuation to the trauma center and admission to the intensive care unit (ICU) for immediate airway control, mechanical ventilation, neurosurgical evaluation, and intracranial pressure monitoring. These classifications have prognostic, monitoring, and treatment implications (Contant et al. 2001). The initial goals in the management of a patient who sustains a moderate or severe TBI are to provide clinical stability, arrest any element of ongoing injury, preserve neurological function, and prevent medical complications secondary to severe trauma. The presence of a brain injury must be suspected in any case of severe trauma and followed closely using appropriate out-of-hospital treatment algorithms. Next, TBI patients should be triaged and evacuated to a trauma center or appropriate hospital environment with available specialized neurological care, such as neurosurgery and neurointensivist care. After that, once clinically stable, TBI patients move into a posture of early rehabilitation, initially in the acute care setting, and eventually to a brain injury rehabilitation center.

Table 4.1 Glasgow Coma Scale (Blumenfeld & Manley 2002)

Best motor response (M)	
Follows commands	6
Localizes to pain	5
Withdrawal to pain	4
Flexor posturing	3
Extensor posturing	2
No response	1
Best verbal response (V)	
Oriented, alert	5
Confused, appropriate	4
Disoriented, inappropriate	3
Incomprehensible speech	2
No response	1
Best eye opening (E)	
Opens eyes spontaneously	4
Opens eyes to voice	3
Opens eyes to pain	2
No response	1

Clinical Evaluation

The clinical examination of a patient with a suspected TBI has both prognostic and management implications, especially in the early treatment of TBI. An organized team approach is essential to appropriate management. This begins in the out-of-hospital or field setting with the first responder and continues to the trauma center or tertiary hospital, where good clinical decisions made in the acute period are essential for optimal outcome. The Guidelines for Field Management of Combat-Related Head Trauma and Advanced Trauma Life Support (ATLS) are both primary resources for military and civilian providers who treat TBI. The Brain Trauma Foundation publishes other guidelines related to head injury which are also helpful, including guidelines for the surgical management of TBI and pre-hospital management of TBI (available at http://braintrauma.org). After ensuring that the ABCs (airway, breathing, and circulation) are cared for, the provider should make a rapid initial neurological evaluation, especially determining the patient's GCS score (Table 4.1) (Teasdale and Jennett 1974; American College of Surgeons 2004). The GCS score is important for triage and is a quantifiable measure of impairment which can help decide early management sequences. This initial exam also helps prognosticate the outcome of moderate and severe TBI and penetrating TBI (pTBI) (Surgical Management of Penetrating, Brain injury 2001; Perel et al. 2008).

Initial Emergency Department and Field Management

It is crucial that emergency management personnel evaluate and address the ABCs to optimize cerebral oxygenation and perfusion. The brain can tolerate severe hypoxia for a very limited period, and it is well established that the duration and severity of hypoxia and hypotension in this critical early period have dramatic consequences on the ultimate clinical outcome (Povlishock et al. 2007; Marion et al. 1997). Thus, the goals of early resuscitation are to ensure adequate oxygen saturation (>90%) and avoid hypotension (SBP <90 mmHg). Airway protection is needed in most moderate to severe TBI patients, and in many of these, ventilation support may also be required. Although many studies have failed to show a mortality benefit from early intubation, attention should be paid to maintaining normoxemia to mild hyperoxemia as recent work has shown extreme hyperoxemia to be associated with an increased risk of mortality in severe TBI (David et al. 2009). Attention to circulation starts with hemorrhage control followed by fluid resuscitation with isotonic crystalloid solution or blood products, depending upon the clinical setting.

The head should be kept in midline position, the head of bed elevated to 30°, and the cervical spine should be immobilized with a rigid neck collar. This will protect the cervical spine until cleared, and allow for optimal venous drainage in order not to aggravate any developing intracranial hypertension. An occult cervical spine injury is assumed in all TBI patients with altered mental status or blunt injury above the clavicle until ruled out by radiographic imaging (American College of Surgeons 2004). Spinal injuries concomitant with TBI are not uncommon, as a recent retrospective review of head injury casualties from the wars in Iraq and Afghanistan included a 16% incidence of spinal column trauma of various types (Bell et al. 2009).

Examination and Secondary Survey

The ATLS secondary survey examination includes a more detailed but rapid neurologic evaluation (Table 4.2). Examining the patient and detailing the extent of impairment are essential. Ideally, this can be accomplished in the emergency department in advance of sedation and/or paralysis for endotracheal intubation and other procedures. The diagnosis of TBI is made on history and physical examination with subsequent neuroimaging providing helpful supportive information of hypothesis testing and guiding further medical and surgical management. In evaluating a trauma patient, it is also important to remember that altered mental status or obtundation due to other causes, including impaired ventilation, oxygenation, hypoperfusion, glycemic derangement, or toxin exposure, may be complicating the examination in addition to occult or obvious head injury. These conditions must be considered during the initial evaluation (American College of Surgeons 2004).

Table 4.2 Focused Neurologic Exam in TBI

Specific tests	Examination pearls
Mental Status Evaluation testing Orientation, language evaluation, and overall level of consciousness	May be accessed quickly or indirectly while attending to other injuries
Cranial Nerves (CNs) CN I: Olfaction CN II: Vision CN III, IV, VI: Vertical and horizontal eye movements and identification of specific CN impairment, if any CN V, VII: Corneal reflex and facial symmetry to painful stimuli (grimace) CN VIII: Evaluation of hearing loss and rapid assessment of integrity of tympanic membrane (TM) CN IX, X: Gag or cough (if intubated) response CN XI: Sternocleidomastoid (SCM) or trapezius movement CN XII: Tongue protrusion	CNs should be documented in every TBI patient CN I: Not usually assessed unless mild TBI CN II: Pupil reactivity and presence of blink to threat (BTT) or field cut on confrontational testing CN III, IV, VI: CN III and VI deficits often associated with increased ICP or transtentorial herniation events; may test with oculocephalics *only if c-spine is cleared* CN V, VII: Corneal reflex testing more sensitive for subtle reactivity with cotton wisp than with saline drops CN VIII: Gross testing and inspection indicated; always inspect TM prior to external canal irrigation with cold water for caloric testing CN IX, X: Commonly tested with in-line suction via the endotracheal tube CN XI: Ensure that C-spine is cleared prior to SCM testing CN XII: Important midline command which, along with forced eye closure, may be the only command followed during emergence from coma
Motor evaluation of spontaneous movements, movements to pain, or strength on commanded movements in a cooperative patient	When administering pain for a motor response, give a stimulus in an area where a withdrawal, localization, or flexion response will be distinct movements from each other (i.e., the axilla or the inner thigh)
Sensory testing with pain sensation and temperature, vibration and position sense in cooperative patients	Pinprick sensation in the neck, arms, trunk, and legs with evaluation of perception of via grimace or localization in the stuporous patient
Deep tendon reflexes (DTRs) in the arms, legs, and Babinski (extensor plantar) responses	DTRs provide an objective exam finding which can help confirm the presence of a lateralizing exam in an uncooperative patient
The cerebellar exam in the cooperative patient is done by evaluation of simple dysmetria of the arms and legs with finger-nose-finger and heel-shin testing	Difficult to accurately assess in the comatose, moribund, or uncooperative patient

Neuroimaging and Vasospasm

Advanced neuroimaging is needed for the complete evaluation of moderate and severe TBI patients. Acutely, CT imaging of the brain will generally provide sufficient information for the initial clinical management, with MRI offering finer delineation of traumatized neuroanatomy. Brain MRI can be quite helpful during the evaluation of TBI, but should not be used in the imaging of acute pTBI from metallic projectiles due to the risk of heat and movement of retained foreign bodies by the MRI's high magnetic field (Surgical Management of Penetrating 2001). MRI should also not be used outside of the setting of overall clinical hemodynamic and airway stability. If a vascular injury is suspected, then catheter cerebral angiography is recommended. The incidence of vasospasm in the setting of blast-related pTBI is high, approaching 50% (Armonda et al. 2006). Thus, it is recommended that patients with acute pTBI from explosives undergo regular noninvasive vascular assessment via transcranial Doppler, or invasive angiography for definitive diagnosis and potentially for interventional revascularization procedures (Armonda et al. 2006).

Herniation Syndromes

Patients with severe TBI who develop intracranial hypertension may progress to a cerebral herniation event. Awareness of the clinical manifestations of increased intracranial pressure is paramount to managing the patient with TBI. The skull is a fixed and rigid container almost completely filled with blood, brain, and cerebrospinal fluid (CSF). Any increase in volume from hemorrhage or edema is initially compensated by displacement of blood or CSF. Herniation occurs when these compensatory mechanisms are exceeded, which manifests clinically in a variety of neurologic syndromes.

Subfalcine Herniation

Subfalcine herniation is lateral shift of one frontal lobe into the contralateral side. It can occur with any degree of midline shift (MLS). The most common clinical manifestations are increasing lethargy and, occasionally, neurological deficits related to compromised flow to one or both anterior cerebral arteries (ACAs). Unilateral ACA compromise classically causes weakness of the contralateral lower extremity, although involvement of the proximal arm and shoulder has been reported (Brazis et al. 2007).

Uncal Herniation

Uncal, or lateral transtentorial, herniation occurs when a supratentorial mass pushes the mesial temporal lobe and uncus anteriorly and downward through the tentorial opening between the ipsilateral aspect of the midbrain and the tentorium. The Kernohan's notch phenomenon, with hemiparesis ipsilateral to the side of the supratentorial lesion, is a potentially false localizing sign which may present after uncal herniation (Brazis et al. 2007). Classically, a unilaterally large pupil and subsequent third nerve palsy may signal this phenomenon. Radiographic findings of uncal herniation may be seen (Fig. 4.1a) with resulting midbrain Duret hemorrhages (Fig. 4.1b, c) and midbrain ischemia (Fig. 4.1d) secondary to compromised blood flow to paramedian midbrain perforator vessels (Brazis et al. 2007). Although significant, the presence of Duret hemorrhages and a good neurologic outcome are not mutually exclusive (Stiver et al. 2009).

Central Herniation

Central herniation is downward movement of the brainstem by pressure from the supratentorial brain components. Early findings with central herniation include cranial nerve (CN) VI palsy manifesting as lateral gaze deficits, which can be unilateral or bilateral. Like uncal herniation, if this progresses, the clinical trial of a CN III palsy (including an ipsilateral nonreactive dilated pupil), coma, and posturing can occur. Posterior cerebral artery (PCA) infarctions can occur with ongoing central or uncal herniation due to compression of the PCA as it passes upwards over the tentorial notch (Blumenfeld and Manley 2002). These can be unilateral or bilateral.

Extracranial Herniation

Extracranial herniation occurs when brain tissue breeches through a skull defect. Most commonly, this occurs after craniectomy as the brain can shift through the surgical site (see Fig. 4.2), or can result from severe trauma. Extracranial herniation can occur in over 20% of postsurgical TBI patients, and essentially represents therapeutic decompression of intracranial hypertension. Unfortunately, complications of extracranial herniation can manifest to include venous infarctions and cerebral cortex lacerations. Some have reported that large, rather than small, craniectomies may help to minimize complications from extracranial herniation (Yang et al. 2008).

Paradoxical Herniation

A less reported type of herniation phenomenon is paradoxical herniation, which has occurred during lumbar cistern drainage in the setting of a craniectomy. Counterintuitively, paradoxical herniation manifests by downward movement of brain in the setting of an overall *lowered* intracerebral pressure (ICP) (Vilela 2008). Only a handful of cases are reported, although this can likely occur in the setting of sodium dysregulation and hypernatremia. Remote cerebellar hemorrhages may be seen with paradoxical herniation. If the herniation event was precipitated by lumbar puncture, some have reported that an emergent blood patch provided reversal of the herniation syndrome (Muehlschlegel et al. 2009).

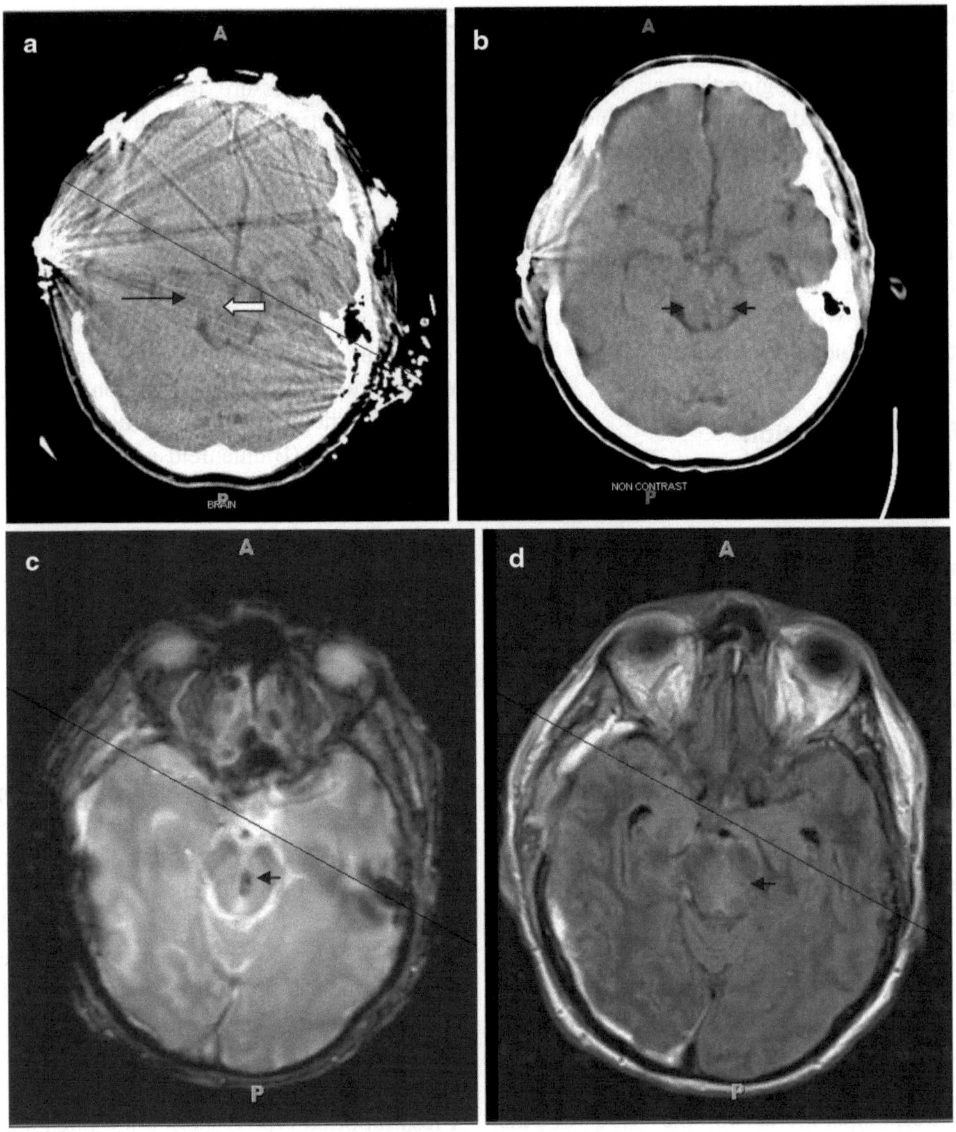

Fig. 4.1 (**a**) Uncal herniation: Note the lateral displacement of the uncus (*black arrow*) and compression of midbrain structures (*white arrow*). (**b**) Duret hemorrhages of the midbrain tegmentum (*arrows*) on HCT of the same patient days later. (**c**) Duret hemorrhages (*arrow*) in same location seen on GRE sequence MRI. (**d**) Duret hemorrhages and ischemic change on FLAIR MRI of the central midbrain (*arrow*)

Tonsillar Herniation

Tonsillar herniation occurs from displacement downward of the cerebellar tonsils into the foramen magnum and compression of the medulla. This can manifest as sudden death from apnea or hemodynamic changes due to compression of medullary respiratory and homeostatic centers. Posterior fossa hematomas with CSF outflow obstruction from the fourth ventricle may result in an acute hydrocephalus (Blumenfeld and Manley 2002). A posterior fossa hematoma or fourth ventricular dilation, distortion, or obliteration requires urgent neurosurgical evaluation for possible intervention to include suboccipital craniectomy (Bullock et al. 2006).

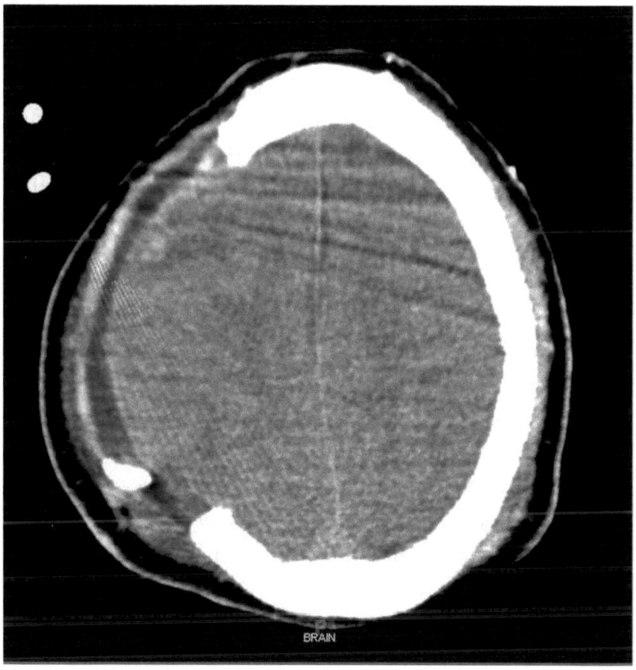

Fig. 4.2 Extracranial herniation through craniectomy defect

Upward Herniation

Upward herniation is movement of brain cephalad through the tentorium into the cranium resulting in brainstem compression. Typically, this occurs with excessive or overzealous therapeutic CSF drainage from an extraventricular drain. The clinical presentation of upward herniation is not well described, although a decrease in a patient's level of consciousness progressing to an obtunded, apneic patient can be expected.

Definitive Management of TBI

Criteria for Intensive Care Unit Admission

After initial emergency care, patients with moderate and severe TBI require close neurological and physiological monitoring. This is best done in the ICU, where monitors and advanced clinical practice nurses are present. Improved outcomes are demonstrated when specialized neurological intensive care teams guide management by employing evidence-based care (Patel et al. 2002). If present, other traumatic injuries may require management from colleagues in trauma surgery, and orthopedic, craniofacial, and other specialists, and this can be facilitated by a team approach in the neurologic ICU.

In this critical injury period, the best measure of efficacy of treatment or worsening of condition is the neurologic examination. Thus, regular clinical neurological examination by skilled practitioners comfortable with neurologic exam skills is needed. In the acute period, it may be as often as every hour and then less frequently if the patient remains stable. ICP and cerebral perfusion pressure (CPP) measurements should be made continuously if an ICP monitor is indicated. However, even in the presence of ICP monitoring, the importance of the clinical examination and neurological assessment cannot be overstated. The period with the highest risk for deterioration is in the first few days after TBI, which can be due to a number of factors, including concomitant critical illness. A common cause is the conversion to traumatic intracerebral hemorrhage (tICH) from a non-hemorrhagic contusional injury. This is reported to occur within the first 9 h after injury, with the peak period of cerebral edema occurring from 48 to 96 h after TBI

(Narayan et al. 2008). Thereafter, it wanes and there is clinical improvement with better ICP control (Ling and Marshall 2008). A more liberal examination paradigm by critical care staff may be reasonable to adopt after this period.

Use of Published Clinical Guidelines

As stated above, the overriding concept of management of the moderate and severe TBI patient is the prevention of secondary injury. In the initial hours after the inciting trauma, this involves mitigating elevations in ICP, tICH, cerebral edema, and hypoxia or other metabolic derangements. Treatment guidelines for the management of severe TBI published by the Brain Trauma Foundation have been instrumental in improving care through guiding therapy with evidence-based recommendations (Povlishock et al. 2007). Guidelines are also available for the pre-hospital management of severe TBI, field management of combat-related head trauma, and surgical management of traumatic brain injury, and all four sets of guidelines can be obtained online from the Brain Trauma Foundation (2011) (http://braintrauma.org).

Ventilation and Airway Management

Ensuring adequate oxygenation and appropriate ventilation of the head-injured patient is vital. Oxygenation and ventilation goals should be to maintain adequate oxygenation with the partial pressure of oxygen in arterial blood (PaO_2) remaining above 60 mmHg, and avoidance of either hypocarbia or hypercarbia by maintaining a partial pressure of carbon dioxide in the blood (PCO_2) in the 30–39 mmHg range (Povlishock et al. 2007; Warner et al. 2008). Avoidance of hypoxemia or extreme hyperoxemia (PaO_2>487 mmHg) is crucial (David et al. 2009). In the field, oxygen saturation should be ≥90%. Hypoxic episodes with saturations lower than this are associated with worse outcome (McHugh et al. 2007). Absolute indication for inserting an artificial airway is a GCS score of 8 or less or suspicion that the patient's ability to ventilate or protect his or her airway is compromised. Oral endotracheal intubation is preferred. Nasotracheal intubation is not advocated in the setting of any significant head trauma as there is significant potential for increasing ICP due to nares' stimulation as well as occult skull fracture which may be worsened by nasopharyngeal manipulation (Stiver and Manley 2008). A clinician may control PCO_2 in intubated patient. As increased ICP is correlated with hypercapnea, likewise clinicians should be aware that overaggressive hyperventilation should be avoided due to the potential for decreased cerebral perfusion and even ischemia at $PCO_2 \leq 25$ mmHg (Povlishock et al. 2007). It may represent a better goal to avoid even approaching this level of PCO_2 for more than a very short period of time. Newer ventilator management strategies, such as Airway Pressure Release Ventilation (APRV), aimed at improving oxygenation at the expense of ventilation, require further study for use in the setting of head injury, and must be used with caution due to the possibility of hypercapnea. It is suggested to monitor capnography in patients ventilated on rescue modes of ventilation with known head injury.

Hemodynamic Management

The objective of hemodynamic therapy in TBI is to ensure adequate brain perfusion. The specific treatment goals are systolic blood pressure (SBP) ≥90 mmHg, CPP≥60 mmHg, and euvolemia (Povlishock et al. 2007). CPP represents the mean arterial pressure (MAP) minus ICP. Although CPP is neither a direct measure of cerebral blood flow nor of regional cerebral flow, it is indicative of the overall adequacy of global brain perfusion, especially in the context of high ICP.

Blood pressure management may be challenging in head-injured patients. Often, the patient is in hemorrhagic shock due to polytrauma injuries which accompany the head injury. Hypotension is common and is independently associated with poor outcome and mortality from TBI (Chesnut et al. 1993; Schreiber et al. 2002; Chesnut and

Marshall 1993). An SBP<90 mmHg has an especially deleterious effect. When compared to hypoxia, low SBP is associated relatively with an even worse outcome (Barton et al. 2005). With head injury, the ability of the neurovasculature to autoregulate is impaired, and thus regional cerebral blood flow becomes directly dependent on systemic blood pressure (Stiver and Manley 2008). Experimental models show that the injured brain is highly susceptible to even subtle ischemic states (Jenkins et al. 1989). It is, therefore, imperative to avoid even short episodes of hypotension after TBI.

Hemostasis of the obvious soft tissue head wound can be obtained with out-of-hospital dressings such as Hemacon® or Quik Clot®, which have been used extensively in the military trauma setting. Crystalloid fluids are used for fluid resuscitation in the field phase of TBI and polytrauma treatment. Later, blood products may be transfused as needed. From the wars in Afghanistan and Iraq, it has been reported that hemorrhagic shock is best treated with red blood cells and plasma using a 1:1 ratio based on volume (Holcomb et al. 2007; Gonzalez et al. 2007). Colloid and hypotonic fluids are relatively contraindicated in TBI due to the fact that colloid fluids containing albumin have been shown to increase the risk of mortality when given in the setting of brain trauma (Myburgh et al. 2007). Hypotonic fluids, such as 1/2 Normal Saline (NS) and Lactated Ringer's, have the potential of exacerbating cerebral edema and should be avoided (Stiver and Manley 2008). Overall fluid balance of head-injured patients is also important. TBI patients who were fluid balance negative by approximately 600 cm^3 had worse proximal outcomes in a recent study (Clifton et al. 2002).

CPP goals are initially met with intravenous fluids, but if adequate MAPs cannot be maintained with intravenous fluids alone, vasoactive pharmacologic agents may be considered. Norepinephrine and phenylephrine are preferred as they have the least effect on cerebral vasomotor tone. If vasopressors are being used, then continuous hemodynamic monitoring is needed with both a central venous pressure catheter and a peripheral arterial pressure catheter (Ling and Marshall 2008). Aggressive use of vasopressor agents has been associated with increased incidence of acute respiratory distress syndrome (ARDS); however, this complication potentially could have been the result of exceeding CPP levels of 70 mmHg (Contant et al. 2001).

Intracerebral Pressure Management

The management of ICP is paramount in neurocritical and neurosurgical care. If ICP progresses unchecked, it will culminate in cerebral herniation, discussed earlier in this chapter. Conservative measures should be instituted in every moderate to severe TBI patient so as to minimize increasing ICP. Such simple interventions include raising the head of the bed to 30°, keeping the head midline, avoiding any circumferential neck dressings for wound hemostasis or securing the endotracheal tube, and avoiding placement of internal jugular (IJ) central venous lines into the dominant IJ. All of these will optimize venous outflow from the head. The Trendelenburg position should not be used for central access and line insertion for treatment of an acute exacerbation of increased ICP as placing the patient into this position may serve to increase ICP further (Raslan and Bhardwaj 2007). In this setting, emergency line placement should not include central lines that require Trendelenburg positioning.

Goals for ICP Treatment

The goal of ICP for the brain-injured patient is to maintain normal intracranial pressure. This is generally less than 20 cmH_2O or 15 mmHg. However, there is data to suggest that elevations over 25 mmHg are associated with poor outcome, and thus interventions should be aimed at reducing ICP to less than this amount. Current guidelines recommend instituting measures to control ICP when pressures of 20 mmHg are reached, and aggressive means employed to prevent ICP elevations over 25 mmHg (Povlishock et al. 2007). One must keep in mind the achievable CPP based on MAP and ICP during therapy, as many interventions to decrease ICP may also have systemic effects on peripheral hemodynamics. The maintenance of a CPP of at least 60 mmHg is strongly recommended (Povlishock et al. 2007). This is often accomplished with the use of vasopressor agents, although complications including higher incidence of ARDS may result from overshooting the goal CPP to greater than 70 mmHg with vasopressors and intravenous fluids, as discussed earlier in this chapter (Contant et al. 2001).

Indications for ICP Monitoring

All severe TBI patients with a strong suspicion of increased ICP should have an ICP monitor placed. There are a number of options that include intraventricular catheter (IVC), also known as an extraventricular drain (EVD), intraparenchymal fiber-optic monitor, subdural bolt, and epidural fiber-optic catheters. The most invasive is the EVD. It provides the most accurate measurement of ICP as it is placed into the third ventricle which is almost at the center of the cranial vault. It is also the most consistently reliable and it can be zeroed after insertion. The other methods are less invasive as they either require only minimal or no penetration of brain parenchyma. As closed systems, they have a lower incidence of infection but, unfortunately, also are subject to measurement drift as they cannot be zeroed externally once placed. Another benefit of the EVD is that it provides a treatment option for ICP management. Thus, the IVC is best referred to as an EVD, as it can be used for CSF removal and this avoids confusion with nomenclature (Povlishock et al. 2007). If hydrocephalus is seen on CT, an EVD is the best option.

Clear indications exist for placing an ICP monitor. If the patient has a GCS $\leq$ 8 (after resuscitation) and an acute abnormality on CT such as tICH, compression of the basal cisterns, and evidence of contusion or herniation, then an ICP monitor should be placed (Povlishock et al. 2007). If a patient has two of the following—SBP $\leq$ 90 mmHg, motor posturing on exam, and/or age $\geq$40 years—then an ICP monitor should likewise be placed or strongly considered (Povlishock et al. 2007). Typically, a neurosurgeon places these devices. However, there is evidence that with proper training, placement of an EVD or other ICP monitors can be done safely by neurointensivists (Ehtisham et al. 2009; Harris et al. 2002). It should be stated that this is not yet a mainstream practice, and that access to the cranial vault should be obtained only with close neurosurgical oversight and advanced training in these procedures. Other monitoring devices, such as brain tissue oxygenation monitors, microdialysis catheters, and jugular venous saturation monitors, can be used to tailor therapy, but widespread or routine application of these devices is not recommended at this time pending further study of variables which may be manipulated and subsequent outcome with the help of the information these monitors provide (Povlishock et al. 2007).

Medical Treatment Options for ICP Management

Initial medical intervention for elevated ICP usually includes avoidance of exacerbating factors, such as fever, seizures, hyperglycemia, or hypercarbia. The next line of therapy involves pharmacologic creation of an osmotic gradient causing movement of water from intracellular and extracellular compartments of the brain into the vasculature, where it reduces the volume of the overall cranial compartment (Raslan and Bhardwaj 2007). Several agents have been used for this purpose in the past, but currently mannitol and hypertonic saline (HTS) are the mainstays of hyperosmolar therapy.

Mannitol

Mannitol should be given intravenously via a peripheral or central intravenous line at a dose of 0.25–1.0 g/kg. Small doses of mannitol (0.25 g/kg) have been shown to effectively reduce ICP in patients with TBI (Marshall et al. 1978). Earlier data shows that mannitol use in TBI correlates with decreased ICP and improvements in cerebral blood flow and CPP (Stein et al. 2008). Past recommendations for mannitol to be given as bolus infusions rather than continuous are no longer supported. Still, in common clinical practice, a single bolus dose is most widely used (Povlishock et al. 2007). So long as serum osmolality is followed closely, additional doses of mannitol can be given. A serum osmolality of 320 mOsm/L is generally accepted as treatment end point, although some investigators advocate that slightly higher levels can be obtained with caution (Diringer and Zazulia 2004).

Hypertonic Saline

Another option for hyperosmolar therapy is HTS. Studies using 7.5 and 23.4% HTS provide evidence of efficacy. Recent evidence supports the use of bolus doses of 30–60 ml of 23.4% HTS to emergently reverse a herniation event (Koenig et al. 2008). An additional benefit of using 23.4% HTS is that its ameliorative effect on ICP lasts longer than that of mannitol (Ware et al. 2005). When used, 23.4% HTS must be administered via a central venous line over 10–15 min to prevent phlebitis and hypotension, respectively. A commonly used initial treatment goal is to achieve serum sodium levels 145–155 mEq/L, which is equivalent to a serum osmolality of 300–320 mOsm/L in most patients (Raslan and Bhardwaj 2007). Recent evidence shows 23.4% HTS to be effective in reducing ICP by a mean value of 8.3 mmHg when given for ICP >20 mmHg and can increase CPP values by 6 mmHg when pre-treatment values are <70 mmHg (Rockswold et al. 2009). A continuous intravenous infusion of 2 or 3% HTS can be used to maintain high serum osmolality and does not have the issues of causing systemic hypotension as does higher concentrations of saline. When using 2 or 3% saline, it is suggested that the fluid be made as a 50:50 mix of sodium chloride and sodium acetate so as to prevent hyperchloremic metabolic acidosis. At a 2% concentration, HTS can be given through a peripheral intravenous catheter, but at 3% or higher, it should be given via a central line due to its potential to cause phlebitis. Other published recommendations have suggested that 3% saline can be safely administered peripherally or via intraosseous access (US Army Institute of Surgical Research 2011). Infusion rate is set based on the particular patient's intravascular needs. Typically, a maintenance rate of 75 cc/h is used. However, these solutions can be administered in 250-cc boluses to treat episodes of intracranial hypertension or as a volume expander to treat systemic hypotension.

If continuous infusions of hypertonic saline are used, serum sodium should be monitored every 6 h or more frequently. Rapid drops in serum sodium are to be avoided so as not to precipitate cerebral edema (Szaflarski et al. 2010). Care must be taken when increasing serum sodium levels from hyponatremic states to avoid central pontine myelinolysis (CPM). Dehydration must likewise be avoided (Clifton et al. 2002). Generally, HTS therapy is maintained for the first 4–7 days after injury, and after the peak edema period elapses, HTS infusions can be switched to normal saline or terminated while observing the serum sodium level for the slow return to normonatremia.

Other Pharmacologic Agents to Reduce ICP

If ICP remains poorly controlled after the efforts described above, then induced pharmacologic coma can be considered. The postulated effect of pharmacologic coma on ICP is through reduction of cerebral metabolism, measured by the cerebral metabolic rate of oxygen ($CMRO_2$) with concomitant reductions in cerebral blood flow and reduced tissue oxygen demand. The most commonly used agent for pharmacological coma is pentobarbital. This drug can be administered intravenously at a loading dose of 5 mg/kg, followed by an infusion of 1–3 mg/kg/h. There is a higher dose regimen that begins with an intravenous loading dose of 10 mg/kg over 30 min followed by 5 mg/kg/h infusion for 3 h, followed by 1 mg/kg/h titrated to therapeutic goals, which are either burst suppression on continuous electroencephalography (EEG) monitoring or a reduction in ICP (Ling and Marshall 2008). If burst suppression is not obtained with this dose, then a smaller loading dose and increased rate can be given until a satisfactory EEG tracing is seen or ICP is controlled. Recall that additional loading doses must be part of any increase in barbiturate therapy, as only increasing the continuous infusion rate will not affect ICP, EEG, or serum levels for some time. Other barbiturates may be used including the much shorter acting thiopental, whose half-life of 5 h is suited for short-term therapy of elevations in ICP (Raslan and Bhardwaj 2007). Thiopental doses of 200–500 mg can be given via bolus intravenous push while monitoring for hypotension. Use of this medication is reserved for patients with a definitive airway. In the USA, the supply of thiopental is currently problematic and this medication is not currently widely available (Medscape News Today 2011).

Another option for pharmacological coma is propofol, which is given at an intravenous loading dose of 2 mg/kg, followed by a titrated infusion of up to 100 mcg/kg/min. The use of propofol for this clinical indication is controversial. In terms of efficacy, a study using propofol for ICP reduction showed a failure of an improvement in 6-month outcome benefit (Kelly et al. 1999). Long-term and high-dose propofol infusions have been associated with the development of propofol infusion syndrome, which consists of renal failure, rhabdomyolysis, hyperkalemia, myocardial failure, metabolic acidosis, lipemia, hepatomegaly, and death. The mechanism for this is not fully understood, but significant caution must be used in any infusion over 5 mg/kg/h or treatment lasting longer than 48 h (Povlishock et al. 2007). If propofol is to be used, then similarly to pentobarbital therapy, continuous EEG monitoring is helpful as the therapeutic goal will be burst suppression and/or ICP control.

Hyperventilation and Induced Hypothermia

Hyperventilation for ICP reduction may also be considered, but only as an emergent, temporary intervention. Prolonged hyperventilation has been clearly associated with exacerbation of cerebral ischemia (Marion et al. 1995). Short durations of hyperventilation are acceptable as a temporizing measure until other (surgical, hyperosmolar, metabolic) means of managing increased ICP are available. If hyperventilation is continued for longer than 12 h, metabolic compensation negates the ameliorative effects of respiratory alkalosis caused by a hypocapnic state and continued hyperventilation may be harmful. The recommended goal for a chronic PCO_2 is 35–40 mmHg, but during an impending herniation event, hyperventilation will acutely lower PCO_2, as well as ICP, within seconds. The current recommended PCO_2 is to strictly avoid levels below 25 mmHg (Povlishock et al. 2007; Stiver and Manley 2008).

Induced hypothermia for TBI remains controversial but promising. Recent animal data shows promise for induced hypothermia with improved neurophysiologic metrics in an asphyxial brain injury model (Jia 2008). There is also data in brain trauma that induced mild hypothermia (33–35°) may improve outcomes as far out as 2 years post-head injury (Qiu et al. 2005). Current use of prophylactic hypothermia for treatment of ICP in severe TBI is a second-tier therapy but may be helpful in refractory intracranial hypertension. If utilized, modalities of induction of hypothermia include skin-applied gel cooling systems and intravenous methods, as well as traditional air-circulating cooling blankets, iced gastric lavage, and surface ice packing (Raslan and Bhardwaj 2007). Unlike induced hypothermia, the goal of maintaining normothermia and avoiding hyperthermia in TBI patients, however, remains strongly recommended (Maas et al. 2008). The potential coagulopathic and antiplatelet effects of hypothermia should be considered, especially in the setting of hemorrhagic TBI (Mossad et al. 2007; Valeri et al. 1987; Michelson et al. 1994; Watts et al. 1998; Polderman 2004).

The Brain Code

When ICP elevation becomes an emergency or is persistently outside of established goals, an important change in the neurological exam is manifest, or a herniation event occurs, a brain code should be performed. This term has gained popularity and many feel that a codified approach to a herniation event or other acute elevation in ICP is best managed via a treatment algorithm, similar to an ACLS protocol. This may encourage non-neurologist or non-neurosurgeon ICU practitioners to develop a standardized approach to such emergencies (Qureshi 2008). An example of one such algorithmic approach to the management of elevated ICP is presented in Fig. 4.3.

Clinical Approach for Treating Elevated ICP

An approach that may be followed involves initial treatment of elevations in ICP with confirmation that the waveform and ICP reading is accurate. Seizure activity must be ruled out if suspected. Brain CT imaging should be considered in any new manifestation of increased ICP without explanation. Maneuvers, such as repositioning the head to midline using the head of Bed to 30 degrees, establishing normothermia, and cessation of suctioning or other noxious stimuli, may help lower temporary spikes in ICP. If this is unsuccessful and the ICP is felt to be accurate, a brief period of hyperventilation of intubated patients may be performed. If central access exists, then 30 cm^3 of 23.4% HTS may be given via a central line over 10–15 min. Alternatively, mannitol may be given via a peripheral line. The dose of mannitol chosen depends on the clinical situation. If a herniation event has manifested, then 1 g/kg is given. If a less severe clinical situation exists, then lower doses such as 0.25–0.5 g/kg may be used. In a herniation event, central access should be readied, likely with the placement of a femoral central venous catheter to avoid the placement of the patient in Trendelenburg position to gain jugular vein access, which may elevate ICP (Raslan and Bhardwaj 2007). It is reasonable in any patient with moderate or severe TBI and concerns for elevated ICP to have central venous access placed early, either in the subclavian or femoral veins.

If ICP continues to be elevated after these maneuvers, then additional HTS can be given as well as further boluses of mannitol, treating up to a serum osmolality of approximately 320 mOsm/L. Standing infusions of HTS such as 3% can be started or increased, with goal sodium values that may exceed 160 mEq/L. Further medical management includes use of bolus doses of propofol and thiopental and consideration given to pharmacologic coma, induced hypothermia, or surgical intervention as discussed in the next section.

Surgical Treatment Options

Extraventicular Drains

As discussed above, if acute hydrocephalus, with or without obstructive hydrocephalus, is complicating the clinical picture, then the placement of an EVD may be indicated. Guideline-based recommendations detailed earlier in this chapter give indications for ICP monitoring, and also the choice of the monitor is influenced by the need for therapeutic intervention with direct CSF drainage (Povlishock et al. 2007). If there is any concern for increasing or clinically relevant hydrocephalus on imaging, an EVD should be considered as the initial surgical option for treating increased ICP.

Decompressive Craniectomy

Decompressive craniectomy (DC) is an emerging clinical approach to the early intervention and management of TBI. The reported experience to date is conflicting. In a study of 57 young patients with severe TBI (age <50), early decompressive craniectomy was associated with a good outcome, defined as social rehabilitation, in 58%. The authors reported a relatively low mortality of less than 20% (Guerra et al. 1999). A retrospective French study was able to show a similar outcome in only 25% of severe TBI patients (Albanese et al. 2003). Older data from the Trauma Coma Data Bank has suggested that even though radiographic improvement occurred, there is no significant improvement on patient outcome after craniectomy (Munch et al. 2000). One of the difficulties in interpreting the available data is the lack of agreement as to how the procedure is to be performed, e.g., release the dura

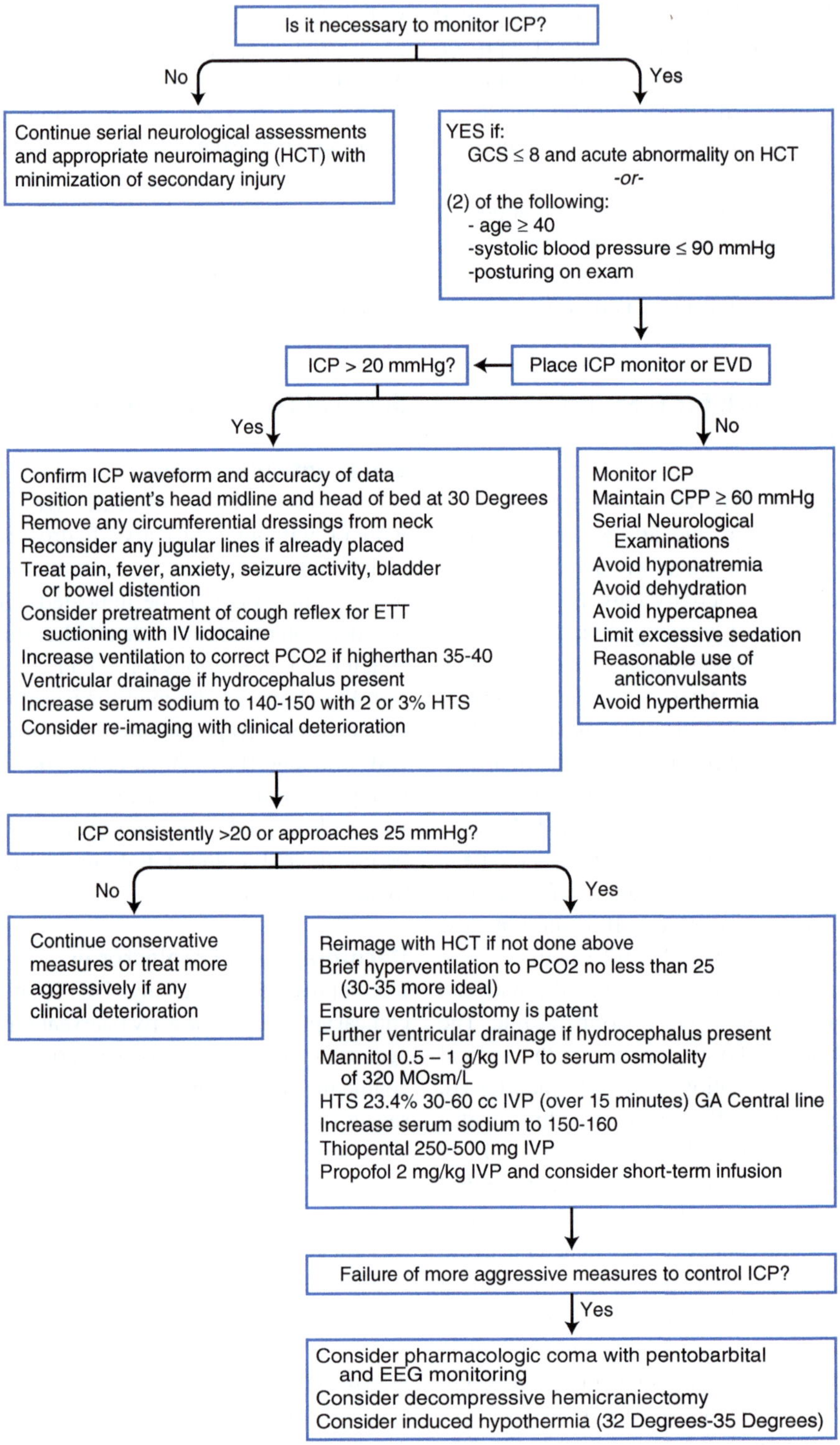

Fig. 4.3 An Example of a Brain code Algorithm

or not, timing of surgery, cutoff age, and TBI severity on presentation (Pompucci et al. 2007).

Currently, two trials enrolling an estimated combined number of 600 patients are completed (Current Controlled Trials 2011). The Randomized Evaluation of Surgery with Craniectomy for Uncontrollable Elevation of Intra-Cranial Pressure (RESCUEicp) and the decompressive craniectomy (DECRA) trials together may better elucidate the role of DC in severe TBI. RESCUEicp is the larger of the two, and is a multicenter trial in Europe comparing decompressive craniectomy to medical management in TBI. The recently reported DECRA trial completed a smaller enrollment over 8 years and was conducted in Australia, New Zealand, and Saudi Arabia (Cooper et al. 2011). Although several methodological confounders exist with DECRA, the study outcome of Extended Glasgow Outcomes Score (GOSE) was not supportive of bilateral DC in the setting of diffuse TBI. The DECRA protocol included patients aged 15–59, with majority of male patients and an average age of 24. A major concern with DECRA is the baseline characteristics of the two intervention groups, with a significant difference in the number of patients with bilateral nonreactive pupils given bilateral DC compared with the medically managed patients. The subsequent potential for the surgical arm to have worse proximal outcome from this selection bias is clear. When this difference in the two groups was controlled for, the statistical significance in the outcome of the study is lost. Certainly, this study offers insight on the continuing debate over the role of DC in TBI, and may predict outcome after bilateral DC in a finite subset of patients given an uncommon operation (Chi 2011). RESCUEicp is completed and results are expected to be published soon (Current Controlled Trials 2011).

The US Military Neurosurgical experience in Operation Enduring Freedom and Operation Iraqi Freedom supports early hemicraniectomy for treating some cases of severe TBI with concerns for imminent elevations in ICP, whether from penetrating, blunt injury, or blast induced (Schlifka 2010). In a recent paper comparing GCS of patients at the time of head trauma and at discharge, TBI patients who underwent a craniectomy had a lower initial GCS than those who underwent craniotomy, but at discharge their GCS was not significantly different. This implies that although these patients were worse initially, they improved after DC to the point where they appeared indistinguishable from those who initially presented with a better neurologic exam (Armonda et al. 2006). A more recent study has shown similar findings, with mean follow-up outcome of 11 months ascertained by use of the GOSE (Howard et al. 2008). In this retrospective review, 12 of the 18 survivors of severe TBI treated with decompressive craniectomy had a favorable outcome. DC may be a practical, though aggressive, approach to ICP management. Future studies on larger cohorts of patients and with more rigorous study design may either support or refute this practice.

Other Considerations

Anticonvulsants

TBI patients are at risk for both early (less than 7 days) and late (more than 7 days) post-traumatic seizures. This risk is worsened by tICH. A seizure in the acute phase can exacerbate the injury. Phenytoin, a well-established antiepileptic drug (AED), has been shown to be beneficial in reducing the risk of seizures during the first week after TBI (Temkin et al. 1995; Temkin 2001). Carbamazepine, phenobarbital, and valproate are also effective AEDs (Temkin 2001). Unfortunately, no AED has been shown to prevent the development of late post-traumatic seizures. Studies have shown that when followed for 15 years after TBI, approximately 50% of patients will develop late seizures. As 50% will not, the recommended approach is to stop AED therapy after the first 7 days and only reinstitute treatment should late seizures manifest (Povlishock et al. 2007). Additionally, the potential for cognitive and other side effects of phenytoin in other types of vascular neuropathology makes prolonged prophylactic use of this medication less attractive (Naidech et al. 2005). If a patient requires intravenous medications, alternatives to phenytoin and fosphenytoin are valproate and levetiracetam. Intravenous lacosamide is now available, but to date reports have not been published for its use in the setting of TBI (Clinical Trials 2011). Levetiracetam has not undergone a rigorous human clinical TBI trial but has been shown to be highly effective in preclinical TBI models and limited human study (Wang et al. 2006; Szaflarski et al. 2010).

There is little evidence to support or refute the use of AEDs for prevention of post-pTBI seizures. The risk of seizure following pTBI is much higher than nonpenetrating TBI, and thus AEDs are prescribed by most providers. The guideline recommendation is to use AEDs during the first 7 days after pTBI and then discontinue. Should the patient suffer a late seizure, the AED therapy can restarted. Therapeutic options are phenytoin, fosphenytoin, carbamazepine, valproate, or phenobarbital (Surgical Management of Penetrating 2001). Currently in clinical practice, levetiracetam is commonly used in this setting.

Venous Thromboembolism Prophylaxis

Other important considerations include prevention of secondary complications of critical illness, including venous thromboembolism (VTE), gastric stress ulcers, and decubitus ulcers. Immobilized patients are at high risk for developing deep venous thrombosis (DVT) with subsequent VTE. The optimal approach for VTE/DVT prophylaxis in severe TBI complicated by ICH is uncertain. Sequential compression devices (SCDs) on the lower extremities are minimally invasive and are not associated with worsening intracranial hemorrhage. Thus, they should be placed as soon as possible if no contraindications exist, such as known DVT or loss of skin integrity from burns or trauma. The optimal timing of introduction of unfractionated or low-molecular-weight heparin for VTE prophylaxis in head trauma is less clear. However, if there are no contraindications to heparin use, then treatment should be started as soon as possible, ideally within the first 36 h after injury (Rogers et al. 2002). The routine placement of inferior vena cava (IVC) filters is controversial, and placement is currently supported only by a low-level recommendation in patients with a GCS < 8 and contraindications to anticoagulation (Rogers et al. 2002; Marion 1998).

Gastric Ulcer Prophylaxis and Skin Breakdown

Gastric stress ulcers may be prevented using either H2 antagonists or proton pump inhibitors (PPIs). Recall that the literature is currently illuminating concerns with the indiscriminate use of PPIs and the possibilities of drug–drug interactions; thus, consideration of alternative means of gastric ulcer prophylaxis should be made in the uncommon event that a patient with TBI must be maintained on an antiplatelet regimen (Juhasz et al. 2009). Either one of these medications should be used for gastric stress ulceration prophylaxis in severe TBI patients, although the tendency for H2 blockers to cause thrombocytopenia may limit their usefulness (Ropper et al. 2004). Prevention of skin breakdown is a concern in all severely injured trauma patients, and care must be taken to reduce the likelihood of decubitus ulcers through frequent repositioning, vigilant nursing care, and good skin hygiene practices.

Future Directions

The potential benefit of induced hypothermia in TBI has been discussed above, and this remains an area of great interest. In addition, preclinical data from the 1980s suggested an improved outcome in female rats given progesterone following experimental models of brain injury (Attella et al. 1987). Elevated levels of progesterone have been proposed to offer neuroprotective properties from the development of cerebral edema. As further data began to accumulate, interest in the potential therapeutic benefit of progesterone therapy in TBI has grown (Roof et al. 1993; Stein et al. 2008). There are two ongoing clinical trials studying the potential outcome benefit of progesterone therapy in TBI. ProTECT III (Progesterone for Traumatic Brain Injury, Experimental Clinical Trial III) and SyNAPSE (Study of the Neuroprotective Activity of Progesterone in Severe Traumatic Brain Injury) have a planned enrollment of over 1,100 patients each and may delineate the role of this potential therapy in TBI (Clinical Trials 2011). Other ongoing work in moderate and severe TBI includes hyperbaric oxygen therapy, tranexamic acid

Ketamine for invisdel ICP, recombinant human erythropoietin, and enhanced oxygen-carrying molecules such as Oxycyte perflurocarbon as neuroprotective agents or therapeutic adjuncts in the medical management of TBI (Herzig et al. 2009; Maas et al. 2010).

Summary

Medical and surgical management of the moderate and severe TBI patient is challenging. The field and hospital care of TBI are largely confined to supportive efforts to minimize secondary injury for optimal neurologic recovery. This is accomplished through maintaining brain perfusion, controlling ICP, and preventing morbidity associated with critical illness. As new pharmacologic and medical approaches are introduced, there will be increasing opportunity to better manage these patients and enhance their long-term neurologic outcomes.

References

Albanese J, Leone M, Alliez JR, et al. Decompressive craniectomy for severe traumatic brain injury: evaluation of the effects at one year. Crit Care Med. 2003;31:2535–8.

American College of Surgeons. Advanced trauma life support, program for doctors. 11 ed. Chicago; 2004.

Anesthesiologists ask FDA to okay importation of sodium thiopental. Medscape News Today. http://www.medscape.com/viewarticle/737303. Accessed 19 June 2011.

Armonda RA, Bell RS, Vo AH, et al. Wartime traumatic cerebral vasospasm: recent review of combat casualties. Neurosurgery. 2006;59:1215–25.

Attella MJ, Nattinville A, Stein DG. Hormonal state affects recovery from frontal cortex lesions in adult female rats. Behav Neural Biol. 1987;48:352–67.

Barton CW, Hemphill JC, Morabito D, et al. A novel method of evaluating the impact of secondary brain insults on functional outcomes in traumatic brain-injured patients. Acad Emerg Med. 2005;12:1–6.

Bell RS, Vo AH, Neal CJ, et al. Military traumatic brain and spinal column injury: a 5 year study of the impact blast and other military grade weaponry on the central nervous system. J Trauma. 2009;66(4 suppl): S104–11.

Blumenfeld H, Manley GT. Neuroanatomy through clinical cases. Sunderland, MA: Sinauer Associates; 2002.

Brazis PW, Masdeu JC, Biller J. Localization in clinical neurology. Baltimore, MD: Lippincott Williams & Wilkings; 2007.

Bullock MR, Chesnut R, Ghajar J, et al. Surgical management of traumatic parenchymal lesions. Neurosurgery. 2006;58(3 suppl):S25–46.

Chesnut RM, Marshall LF. Management of severe head injury. 3rd ed. New York, NY: Raven Press; 1993.

Chesnut RM, Marshall LF, Klaubeer MR, et al. The role of secondary brain injury in determining outcome from severe head injury. J Trauma. 1993;24:216–22.

Chi J. Craniectomy for traumatic brain injury: results from the DECRA trial. Neurosurgery. 2011;68:n19–20.

Clifton GL, Miller ER, Choi SC, et al. Fluid thresholds and outcome from severe brain injury. Crit Care Med. 2002;30:739–45.

Clinical Trials. http://clinicaltrials.gov. Accessed 19 Dec 2011.

Clinical Trials. http://www.clinicaltrials.gov. Accessed 19 June 2001.

Contant CF, Valadka AB, Gopinath SP, et al. Adult respiratory distress syndrome: a complication of induced hypertension after severe head injury. J Neurosurg. 2001;95:560–8.

Cooper DJ, Rosenfeld JV, Murray L, et al. Decompressive craniectomy in diffuse traumatic brain injury. N Engl J Med. 2011;364:1493–502.

Current Controlled Trials. http://controlled-trials.com/. Accessed 28 Nov 2011.

David DP, Meade W, Sise MJ, et al. Both hypoxemia and extreme hyperoxemia may be detrimental in patients with severe traumatic brain injury. J Neurotrauma. 2009;26:2217–23.

Diringer MN, Zazulia AR. Osmotic therapy: fact and fiction. Neurocrit Care. 2004;1:219–33.

Ehtisham A, Taylor S, Bayless L, et al. Placement of external ventricular drains and intracranial pressure monitors by neurointensivists. Neurocrit Care. 2009; 10:241–7.

Geocadin R, Bhardwaj A, Mirski M, et al. Traumatic brain injury. Totowa, NJ: Humana Press; 2004.

Gonzalez EA, Moore FA, Holcomb JB, et al. Fresh frozen plasma should be given earlier to patients requiring massive trasfusion. J Trauma. 2007;62:112–9.

Guerra WK, Gaab MR, Dietz H, et al. Surgical decompression for traumatic brain swelling: indications and results. J Neurosurg. 1999;90:187–96.

Harris CH, Smith RS, Helmer SD. Placement of intracranial pressure monitors by non-neurosurgeons. Am Surg. 2002;68:787–90.

Herzig SJ, Howell MD, Ngo LH, et al. Acid-suppressive medication use and the risk of hospital-acquired pneumonia. JAMA. 2009;307:2120–8.

Holcomb JB, McMullin NR, Pearse L, et al. Causes of death in U.S. special operations forces in the global war on terrorism. Ann Surg. 2007;245:986–91.

Howard JL, Cipolle MD, Anderson M, et al. Outcome after decompressive craniectomy for the treatment of severe traumatic brain injury. J Trauma. 2008;65(2): 380–5.

Jenkins LW, Moszynshi K, Lyeth BG, et al. Increased vulnerability of the mildly traumatized rat brain to cerebral ischemia: the use of controlled secondary ischemia as a research tool to identify common or different mechanisms contributing to mechanical and ischemic brain injury. Brain Res. 1989;477:211–24.

Jia X. Improving neurological outcomes post-cardiac arrest in a rat model: immediate hypothermia and quantitative EEG monitoring. Resuscitation. 2008;90:1042–52.

Juhasz M, Herszenyi L, Tulassay Z. Current Standings of the proton pump inhibitor and Clopidogrel Co-therapy: review on evolving field with the eyes of the gastroenterologist. Digestion. 2009;81(1):10–5.

Kelly DF, Goodale DB, Williams J, et al. Propofol in the treatment of moderate and severe head injury: a randomized, prospective double-blinded pilot trial. J Neurosurg. 1999;90:1042–52.

Koenig MA, Bryan M, Lewin III JL, et al. Reversal of transtentorial herniation with hypertonic saline. Neurology. 2008;70:1023–9.

Ling GS, Marshall SA. Management of traumatic brain injury in the intensive care unit. Neurol Clin. 2008; 26:409–26.

Maas AI, Stocchetti N, Bullock R. Moderate and severe traumatic brain injury in adults. Lancet Neurol. 2008;7:728–41.

Maas AIR, Roozenbeek B, Manley GT. Clinical trials in traumatic brain injury: past experience and current developments. Neurotherapeutics. 2010;7:115–26.

Marion DW. Head and spinal cord injury. Neurol Clin. 1998;16:485–502.

Marion DW, Firlik A, McLaughlin MR. Hyperventilation therapy for severe traumatic brain injury. New Horiz. 1995;3:439–47.

Marion DW, Penrod LE, Kelsey SF, et al. Treatment of traumatic brain injury with moderate hypothermia. N Engl J Med. 1997;336:540–6.

Marshall LF, Smith RW, Rauscher LA, Shapiro HM. Mannitol dose requirements in brain-injured patients. J Neurosurg. 1978;48:169–72.

McHugh GS, Engel DC, Butcher I, et al. Prognostic value of secondary insults in traumatic brain injury: results from the IMPACT study. J Neurotrauma. 2007; 24:287–93.

Michelson AD, MacGregor H, Barnard MR, et al. Hypothermia-induced reversible platelet dysfunction. Thromb Haemost. 1994;71:633–40.

Mossad EB, Machado S, Apostolakis J. Bleeding following deep hypothermia and circulatory arrest in children. Semin Cardiothorac Vasc Anesth. 2007; 11:34–46.

Muehlschlegel S, Voetsch B, Sorond FA. Emergent epidural blood patch: lifesaviing treatment of paradoxical herniation. Arch Neurol. 2009;66:670–1.

Munch E, Horn P, Schurer L, et al. Management of severe traumatic brain injury by decompressive craniectomy. Neurosurgery. 2000;47:315–22.

Myburgh J, Cooper DJ, Finfer S, et al. Saline or albumin for fluid resuscitation in patients with traumatic brain injury. NEJM. 2007;357:874–84.

Naidech AM, Kreiter KT, Janjua N, et al. Phenytoin exposure is associated with functional and cognitive disability after subarachnoid hemorrhage. Stroke. 2005;36:583–7.

Narayan RK, Maas AI, Marshall LT, et al. Traumatic ICH Study Group. Recombinant factor VIIA in traumatic intracerebral hemorrhage: results of a dose-escalation clinical trial. Neurosurgery. 2008;62:776–86.

Patel HC, Menon DK, Tebbs S, et al. Specialist neurocritical care and outcome from head injury. Intensive Care Med. 2002;28:547–53.

Perel P, Arango M, Clayton T, et al. Predicting outcome after traumatic brain injury: practical prognostic models based on large cohort of international patients. BMJ. 2008;336:425–9.

Polderman KH. Application of therapeutic hypothermia in the intensive care unit. Opportunities and pitfalls of a promising treatment modality-part 2: practical aspects and side effects. Intensive Care Med. 2004;30(5):757–69.

Pompucci A, Bonis PD, Pettorini B. Decompressive craniectomy for traumatic brain injury: patient age and outcome. J Neurotrauma. 2007;24:1182.

Povlishock JT, Bratton SL, Randall M, et al. Guidelines for the management of severe traumatic brain injury. J Neurotrauma. 2007;24 suppl 1:S21–5.

Qiu WS, Liu WG, Shen H, et al. Therapeutic effect of mild hypothermia on severe traumatic head injury. Chin J Traumatol. 2005;8:27–32.

Qureshi AI. SJI. More evidence supporting a brain code protocol for reversal of transtentorial herniation. Neurology. 2008;70:990–1.

Raslan A, Bhardwaj A. Medical management of cerebral edema. Neurosurg Focus. 2007;22:E12.

Rockswold GL, Solid CA, Paredes-Andrade E, et al. Hypertonic saline and its effect on intracranial pressure, cerebral perfusion pressure, and brain tissue oxygen. Neurosurgery. 2009;65:1035–41.

Rogers FB, Cipolle MD, Velmahos G, et al. Practice management guidelines for the prevention of venous thromboembolism in trauma patients: the EAST practice management guidelines work group. J Trauma. 2002;53:142–64.

Roof RL, Duvdevani R, Stein DG. Gender influences outcome of brain injury: projesterone plays a protective role. Brain Res. 1993;607:333–6.

Ropper AH, Gress DR, Diringer MN, et al. Neurological and neurosurgical intensive care. 4th ed. Philadelphia, PA: Lippincott Williams & Wilkins; 2004.

Schlifka B. A neurosurgical perspective. J Trauma. 2010;62:S103–4.

Schreiber MA, Aoki N, Scott BG, et al. Determinants of mortality in patients with severe blunt head injury. Arch Surg. 2002;137:285–90.

Stein DG, Wright DW, Kellermann AL. Does progesterone have neuroprotective properties? Ann Emerg Med. 2008;51:164–72.

Stiver SI, Manley GT. Prehospital management of traumatic brain injury. Neurosurg Focus. 2008;33(3 suppl):S228–40.

Stiver SI, Gean AD, Manley GT. Survival with good outcome after cerebral herniation and Duret hemorrhage caused by traumatic brain injury. J Neurosurg. 2009; 110:1242–6.

Surgical management of penetrating Brain injury. J Trauma 2001:S16–25.

Szaflarski JP, Sangha KS, Shutter LA. Prospective, randomized, single-blinded comparative trial of intravenous levetiracetam versus phenytoin for seizure prophylaxis. Neurocrit Care. 2010;12(2):165–72.

Teasdale G, Jennett B. Assessment of coma and impaired consciousness: a practical scale. Lancet. 1974;2:81–4.

Temkin NR. Antiepileptogenesis and seizure prevention trials with antiepileptic drugs: meta-analysis of controlled trials. Epilepsi. 2001;42:515–24.

Temkin NR, Haglund MM, Winn HR. Causes, prevention, and treatment of post-traumatic epilepsy. New Horiz. 1995;3:518–22.

The Brain Trauma Foundation. http://braintrauma.org. Accessed 22 Nov 2011.

The management of concussion in sports (summary statement). Report of the quality standards subcommittee. Neurology 1997;48:581–5.

US Army Institute of Surgical Research. Joint Trauma System: clinical practice guidelines. www.usaisr.amedd.army.mil/cpgs.html (2011). Accessed 22 Nov 2011.

Valeri CR, Feingold H, Cassidy G, et al. Hypothermia-induced reversible platelet dysfunction. Ann Surg. 1987;205:175–81.

Vilela MD. Delayed paradoxical herniation after a decompressive craniectomy: case report. Surg Neurol. 2008;69:293–6.

Wang H, Gao J, Lassiter TF, et al. Levetiracetam is neuroprotective in murine models of closed head injury and subarachnoid hemorrhage. Neurocrit Care. 2006;5:71–8.

Ware ML, Nemani VM, Meeker M, et al. Effects of 23.4% sodium chloride solution in reducing intracranial pressure in patients with traumatic brain injury: a preliminary study. Neurosurgery. 2005; 57:727–36.

Warner KJ, Cuschieri J, Compass MK, et al. Emergency department ventilation effects outcome in severe traumatic brain injury. J Trauma. 2008;64:341–7.

Watts DD, Trask A, Soeken K, et al. Hypothermic coagulopathy in trauma: effect of varying levels of hypothermia on enzyme speed, pletelet function and fibrinolytic activity. J Trauma. 1998;44:846–54.

Yang XF, Wen L, Shen F, et al. Surgical complications secondary to decompressive craniectomy in patients with a head injury: a series of 108 consecutive cases. Acta Neurochir (Wien). 2008;150:1241–7.

Sports Concussion

5

Sharon R. Weeks and Jack W. Tsao

Abstract

An estimated 300,000 sports concussions are suffered in the USA every year, frequently as the result of full contact sports such a football and boxing. As these concussions can have serious and long-term consequences, a complete understanding of their causes and effects is critical for both clinical care as well as public health awareness and prevention. In this chapter, we discuss the etiology and sequelae of sports concussions, offer a summary of the guidelines on triage and treatment of these injuries, and survey the existing literature for areas of future research.

Keywords

Sports concussions • Treatment guidelines • Head injury • Neurological injury • Cognition

Introduction

Concussions, or mild traumatic brain injuries, are a persistent problem in athletic competition. Full contact sports, such as football and boxing, report the highest incidence of sports concussions, but the injuries are also frequently reported in other sports, including soccer, hockey, lacrosse, and basketball. With an estimated 300,000 sports-related concussions occurring in the USA every year (Sosin et al. 1996), defining, assessing, and treating these injuries have become critical questions for physicians, coaches, and players alike. Recent evidence that repeated concussions can have long-term or even fatal effects has raised policy questions for diagnosis and return-to-play guidelines. Increased participation in athletics at both the high school and collegiate levels has resulted in more and more youths being exposed to concussion risks (National Federation of State High School Associations 2006). The increase in participation and competition also means that elite athletes are sometimes subject to the effects of multiple concussions over many years of

S.R. Weeks, B.A.
Department of Orthopedics & Rehabilitation,
Walter Reed Army Medical Center, Washington, DC, USA

J.W. Tsao, M.D., D.Phil., F.A.A.N. (✉)
Traumatic Brain Injury Programs (M96), Wounded, Ill, & Injured Directorate, US Navy Bureau of Medicine and Surgery, Washington, DC, USA

Department of Neurology, Uniformed Services University of the Health Sciences, Bethesda, MD, USA
e-mail: Jack.tsao@med.navy.mil

J.W. Tsao (ed.), *Traumatic Brain Injury: A Clinician's Guide to Diagnosis, Management, and Rehabilitation*,
DOI 10.1007/978-0-387-87887-4_5,

athletic competition prior to their professional or even college careers. Some neurocognitive testing has been developed to attempt to assess the damage caused by these injuries and to categorize injury severity and necessary treatment. However, recent discoveries in some deceased National Football League (NFL) players of chronic traumatic encephalopathy (CTE, tau protein deposition in brain tissue) highlight that there is much to learn. In this chapter, we review the literature of sports concussions etiology and sequelae, highlight the areas of interest for future research, and present a culmination of the literature's guidelines on triage and treatment for both youths and adults.

Etiology and Symptoms of Sports Concussions

The etiology of sports concussions varies from sport to sport, but common mechanisms of injury include rotational acceleration (shearing), linear acceleration (compressive and tensile stresses on axons), carotid artery injuries, and deceleration on impact (Cantu 1996; Lampert and Hardman 1984). Sports with the greatest chance of causing catastrophic head injury are football, gymnastics, ice hockey, and wrestling (Cantu and Mueller 1990).

Boxing carries especially high risks of concussions since injury is a goal of the sport; in contrast to football, concussion is an objective of boxing rather than a competitive risk (Ryan 1987). Additionally, as boxers are subject to numerous (and sometimes rapidly consecutive) blows to the head, whether concussive or sub-concussive, these athletes often demonstrate a range of neurological defects (Corsellis 1973). A longitudinal study of 484 amateur boxers revealed statistically significant correlations between the number of bouts completed before the baseline examination and changes in memory, visual-spatial ability, and perceptual/motor ability 2 years later (Stewart et al. 1994). Another study of 41 boxers and 27 control subjects revealed that boxers performed worse on psychometric tests than controls; furthermore, boxers with more bouts performed worse than less experienced boxers (Kemp et al. 1995). Additionally, controls had fewer aberrations in cerebral perfusion than boxers, as detected by PET scanning. Finally, an estimated 9–25% of boxers develop "punch drunk syndrome," or CTE, discussed later in this chapter (Ryan 1987).

Another sport of particular interest is football, in which the nature of the sport and the frequency of impact with other players are of considerable concern. The popularity of the sport across ages and regions of the country also contributes to the public health concern; one insurance company reported that rates of injury in organized high school football were double those of the general population (DeLee and Farney 1992). It has been estimated that as many as 1.5 million young men participate in American football at the high school and collegiate levels alone. An estimated 1.2 million football-related injuries are sustained annually; concussions account for as many as 5% of all these injuries (Saal 1991; Zemper 1989; Canale et al. 1981; DeLee and Farney 1992). These injuries were largely the result of direct competition; a 2-year study of over 6,000 football players found that the rate of injury was 8.6 times higher in games than in practice, consistent with previous reports in other sports (Zemper 1989).

Recognition of head injury is obvious when there is a loss of consciousness. However, over 90% of head injuries in sports fall into the category of mild concussions, those in which there is no loss of consciousness (LOC) (Cantu 1986, 1991). The resulting difficulty in sideline diagnoses, in addition to internal and external pressures on a player to return to play, has been a difficult challenge for the medical community. In addition to LOC (which may or may not occur with a mild concussion), immediate effects of concussions include vacant stare, delayed verbal and motor responses, confusion and inability to focus attention, disorientation, slurred or incoherent speech, gross observable incoordination, disproportionate emotions, and memory deficits (Kelly and Rosenberg 1998).

As the brain is possibly the most variable of human organs in its response to external stimuli or insult (McKeag 2003), it should come as no surprise that the presentation of concussed athletes varies significantly from individual to individual.

Table 5.1 Risk factors for concussive injury

High risk	Medium risk	Low risk
Focal neurologic findings	Initial GCS score of 15	Currently asymptomatic
Asymmetric pupils	Brief LOC	No other injuries
Skull fracture on clinical examination	Post-traumatic amnesia	No focal deficits on examination
Multiple trauma	Vomiting	Normal pupils
Serious, painful, distracting injuries	Headache	No change in consciousness
External signs of trauma above the clavicles	Intoxication	Intact orientation/memory
Initial GCS score of 14 or 15		Initial GCS score of 15
Loss of consciousness		Accurate history
Post-traumatic confusion/anemia		Trivial mechanism
Progressively worsening headache		Injury more than 24 h ago
Vomiting		No or mild headache
Post-traumatic seizure		No vomiting
History of bleeding disorder/anticoagulation		No preexisting high-risk factors
Recent ingestion of intoxicants		
Unreliable/unknown history of injury		
Previous neurologic diagnosis		
Previous epilepsy		
Suspected child abuse		
Age older than 60 years or younger than 2 years		

This table adapted with permission from Marx J, Hockberger R, Walls R, et al., editors. Rosen's emergency medicine: concepts and clinical practice. 6th ed. Mosby; 2006, p. 349–82; Copyright Elsevier (2006)

In addition to individual differences, contributing factors to varying presentations include biomechanical forces involved and the athlete's prior history of injury, among others (Lovell 2009). Concussed individuals commonly describe headaches, disorientation, confusion, or amnesia. Nausea and emesis are also common (Heegaard 2007). In children, symptoms typically include restlessness, lethargy, confusion, or irritability. The adult symptoms are classically thought to suggest intracranial lesions. However, the data supporting this conclusion are sparse; the need for additional diagnostic tests after a thorough neurological examination, including detailed mental status examination, depends upon the individual's risk factors (Table 5.1) (Heegaard 2007). In fact, it has been reported that less than 1% of patients with minor head trauma have surgically significant lesions (Narayan 1994). The consequences of a concussive event can last for several days. McCrea et al. (2003) found that concussed football players continue to show acute symptoms for at least 5 days, cognitive impairments for up to 7 days, and balance effects for up to 5 days after injury.

Lasting Effects of Sports Concussion

The lasting effects of sports concussions were first highlighted in the public eye in the early 1990s when NFL players Al Toon and Merrill Hoge retired from the league because of prolonged post-concussion syndrome. Some reviews report an incidence of post-concussive syndrome of approximately 10–20% of concussed athletes (Lovell 2009). Symptoms of the syndrome include headache, dizziness, anxiety, and impaired cognition and memory (Rutland-Brown et al. 2006). These symptoms affect more than 58% of patients 1 month following their injury (Bazarian and Atabaki 2001) and 15% of patients 1 year following injury (Rutherford et al. 1979). The presence of headache, nausea, and dizziness during the acute head injury assessment can be predictive of post-concussive syndrome as the presence of all three is associated with a 50% likelihood of PCS at 6 months post-injury; an absence of all three symptoms is associated with only a 28% likelihood.

Additionally, research has long suggested that the effects of sports concussions can extend far out from the time of injury. Gronwall and Wrightson (1975) originally reported over 30 years ago that the rate at which young adults processed information was reduced more in those subjects who had suffered two concussions compared to those who had been concussed only once. It has also been long suspected that sustaining one concussion increases the risk of additional concussions (Salcido and Costich 1992; Annegers et al. 1980). One study of over 15,304 player-seasons examined high school and collegiate football players prospectively over a 2-year period and reported that the relative risk for repeat concussions in individuals with a history of concussion is 5.8 times greater than for individuals with no history (Zemper 2003). Recent studies in high school and collegiate athletes have also shown that cumulative effects may result from three or more concussive episodes. Collins et al. (2002) found that athletes with three or more concussions were more likely to experience on-field LOC (6.7 times more likely), anterograde amnesia (3.8 times), and confusion (4.1 times) after a subsequent concussion. Guskiewicz et al. (2003) found an association between the reported number of previous concussions and the likelihood of incident concussion during follow-up of 4,251 player-seasons. The study additionally found that players who reported a history of three or more previous concussions were three times more likely to have an incident concussion than players with no concussive history. Similarly, players with two previous concussions were 2.8 times more likely to have an incident concussion, and those with one previous concussion, 1.5 times more likely. These findings are supported by animal studies that show a neurochemical and metabolic cascade that detrimentally affects cognitive functions for up to 2 weeks after a concussive injury (Hovda et al. 1995, Giza and Hovda 2001). Studies of high school and collegiate athletes showed with ImPACT testing (an automated neurocognitive test battery) that there were no detectable cumulative effects of only one or two previous concussions (Iverson et al. 2006), but marked effects in athletes with three or more concussions (Iverson et al. 2004). These discoveries highlight the need for adequate treatment and prevention strategies in the sports world.

A discovery of considerable concern to athletes at all levels has been the reports of "second impact syndrome." Initially reported in 1984 (Saunders and Harbaugh 1984), there have since been several other reports of this syndrome in the literature (Kelly et al. 1991; Cantu and Voy 1995). In these cases, athletes suffer a concussion, usually mild, and sometimes, but not always, with LOC. After returning to play within a few days, they experience a second head injury, which may be very minor, that results in subsequent collapse, a semicomatose state, and respiratory failure. The malignant brain swelling that causes these symptoms is often fatal and has only been reported in teenage athletes. The confinement of this syndrome to such a youthful population may indicate an increased risk for SIS in the developing brain. Alternatively, another hypothesis is if the syndrome is due to a genetic mutation with low prevalence, the reporting of SIS exclusively in teenagers may be due to a combination of this low prevalence and the age structure of populations in contact sports. These cases show that repeated mild brain injuries occurring within a short period of time can be catastrophic or fatal, and highlight a need for proper initial diagnosis, increased education, and vigilance surrounding athletes with head injuries.

One of the more severe consequences of the multiple concussions that can be suffered by an athlete over the course of a career is CTE. This condition, first described by Harrison Martland (1928) as dementia pugilistica, is characterized by early symptoms of slight mental confusion, a slowing of muscular movements, hesitancy in speech, and hand tremors. In time, these symptoms become more severe and progressive; they include speech and gait disturbance, pyramidal tract dysfunction, memory impairment, extrapyramidal features, behavior or personality changes, and psychiatric disease (Jordan 1993, 1998; Jordan et al. 1997; Unterharnscheidt 1970). Corsellis first identified the neuropathology of this syndrome in the brains of 15 deceased boxers, 8 of whom were world or national champions (Corsellis 1973). Through autopsy, he found that the neuropathology of CTE was characterized by septum pellucidum, degeneration of substantia nigra, septal fenestration, cerebellar scarring, diffuse neuronal loss, and prominent neurofibrillary tangles, now known to be composed of tau protein. The syndrome has recently become an issue of increased public interest when the first documented case of long-term neurodegenerative changes in a retired professional NFL player consistent with CTE was published (Omalu et al. 2005). Since that study, the group has reported neuropathological changes associated with CTE in six former professional football players. As this issue gains more attention, an ongoing prospective research study, the C.O.N.T.A.C.T. research program (Consent to Offer Neural Tissue of Athletes with Concussive Trauma) has been developed. This study involves more than 150 former athletes, including 40 retired NFL players and 3 active NFL players. All participant athletes have agreed to be interviewed annually by phone throughout their lives and, upon their death, will donate their brains to be examined by the Center for the Study of Traumatic Encephalopathy (CSTE), an independent academic research center located at the Boston University School of Medicine (BU CSTE 2010).

Differences Due to Age and Developmental Level

Age differences in concussion diagnosis and management were not often considered until recent studies appeared to reveal marked differences in the way youths and adults respond to and recover from concussions. Multiple studies have now shown that high school athletes require more time to recover cognitive performance than college athletes (Sim et al. 2008; Pellman et al. 2006), in spite of the fact that college athletes had a greater prior incidence of concussion which typically slows recovery (Field et al. 2003). Lovell and colleagues (2003, 2004) also revealed a heightened vulnerability to concussion in younger athletes (ages 13–17), proposing that the currently accepted return-to-play guidelines for adults may be too liberal for adolescents. It has been proposed that the immature brain's sensitivity to glutamate (Pickles 1950), a neurotransmitter involved in the metabolic cascade following concussion, may partly explain these differences in recovery time (Lovell 2009). It is also possible that youths may undergo more prolonged and diffuse cerebral swelling after traumatic injury, so are thus more at risk for secondary injury, partly explaining why SIS has only been reported in youths (McCrory et al. 2005). Whatever the reason, these new findings suggest that clinicians exercise caution in returning young athletes to play following a concussion or concussive symptoms.

Triage and Treatment

It should be noted that most people recover successfully from a concussion with no noticeable long-term effects. McCrea et al. (2003) found that 91% of concussed football players had returned to their pre-injury baselines within a week following injury. The severe conditions that can result from sports head injuries in a small but noteworthy number of cases, however, highlight the necessity of taking concussions seriously and being conservative in return-to-play guidelines.

Concussive sports injuries have encouraged the development of easy-to-administer neurocognitive tests that can be given on the sidelines of a playing field immediately after a suspected concussion to guide return-to-play decisions. Of those reported in the literature, the SAC, the Standardized Assessment of Concussion, is possibly the most popular and well studied. This assessment takes approximately 5 min to administer (and requires no prior experience in neuropsychological testing) and consists of four components: orientation, immediate memory, concentration, and delayed recall (McCrea et al. 1997). An assessment of strength, sensation, and coordination is included as is the documentation of LOC, retrograde amnesia, and post-traumatic amnesia. The total composite score on the exam was sufficient to differentiate between non-concussed controls and those players who had suffered even mild concussions. A study of this test

Table 5.2 Immediate assessments for concussion

Assessment	SAC	MACE	Maddocks questions
Orientation	Month, date, day of the week, year, time	Month, date, day of the week, year, time	Which field are we at? Which team are we playing?
Immediate memory	Recall a list of five words immediately, three trials	Recall a list of five words immediately, three trials	
Concentration	Reverse strings of digits (3–6 digits in length)	Reverse strings of digits (3–6 digits in length)	Who is your opponent at present?
	Reverse the months of the year	Reverse the months of the year	Which half/period is it? How far into the half is it?
Delayed recall	Recall a list of five words 5 min later	Recall a list of five words 5 min later	Which side scored the last touchdown/goal/point?
Neurologic screening	Recollection of injury, strength, sensation, coordination	Pupil size and reactivity, speech fluency and word finding, pronator drift, gait and coordination	Which team did we play last week?
Exertional Measures	40-yard sprint, 5 sit-ups, 5 push-ups, 5 knee bends	None	Did we win last week?

The SAC and Maddocks questions are typically used for sideline assessments for sports injuries; the MACE was developed for battlefield screening for military personnel suspected of concussion. Adapted from McCrory et al. 2009; Coldren et al. 2010; Maddocks et al. 1995

in 141 high school football players demonstrated that more demanding cognitive measures utilized could be sensitive enough for the detection of mild concussions to determine benching and return-to-play decisions (McCrea et al. 1997). These findings were later supported by a larger study of 568 high school and college football players (McCrea et al. 1998). Normative data from more than 2,500 male and female junior high, high school, college, and professional athletes has shown that the SAC is reliable over repeated administrations and is free of significant gender effects. It is also acceptable for use at all competitive and educational levels (McCrea et al. 2000). In addition to the SAC, the Second International Symposium on Concussion Prague 2004 developed another sideline assessment, the Sport Concussion Assessment Tool (SCAT) (McCrory et al. 2005). This tool was created by combining several common tools into one standardized test; it includes a neurologic screening, cognitive and memory assessments, and queries symptoms, LOC, convulsive activity, and balance problems. However, this tool has not been tested for reliability and validity. This tool was recently updated to include the calculation of the SAC score as well as the Maddocks questions for sideline concussion assessment (McCrory et al. 2009; Maddocks et al. 1995). These tools have been used by the military to develop the Military Acute Concussion Evaluation (MACE) which is used by combat medics on the battlefield to evaluate service members in whom a concussion is suspected (Coldren et al. 2010). The MACE uses many of the same examination tasks as the SAC and also includes collection of demographic and injury incident details. The SAC, MACE, and Maddocks questions are summarized in Table 5.2.

Neuropsychological testing is also becoming common among sports health professionals. The wide range of tests available show sensitivity to concussion impairments and include both paper and pencil tests as well as computerized assessments. Conventional tests include the Trail Making Tests A and B (Reitan and Wolfson 1985), Digit Symbol Substitution Test (Weschler 1944), Controlled Oral Word Association (COWA) test (Benton and Hamsher 1976), Hopkins Verbal Learning Test (Shapiro et al. 1999), and the Stroop Word Color Test (Golden and Freshwater 2002). Computerized tests developed

Table 5.3 Conventional tests for assessment of mild head injury

Assessment	Description
Trail Making Tests A and B	Part A involves drawing lines between 25 numbered circles, in sequential order, which are randomly arranged. Part B requires subjects to connect circles containing the letters A through L and numbered 1 through 13 by drawing lines alternating between numbers and letters in sequential order. Subjects are instructed immediately on their mistakes and continue from the last correct circle. The test takes approximately 5–10 min to complete. The test evaluates information processing speed, visual scanning ability, integration of visual and motor functions, letter and number recognition and sequencing, and the ability to maintain two different trains of thought
Digit symbol substitution test	Paper–pen test consisting of digit-symbol pairs followed by a list of digits. The subject writes as many of the corresponding symbols on the list of digits as possible within the allowed time. Is sensitive to brain damage
Hopkins Verbal Learning Test—Revised	Verbal learning and memory test requiring the use of both working and episodic memory. Subjects are asked to recall a repeated list of words several times. The words fall into discrete categories. Learning ability and total immediate recall and delayed recall are recorded
Controlled Oral Word Association (COWA)	Spoken word test. The examinee has 1 min to name as many words as possible that begin with particular letters. Examinee is then given 1 min to name as many animals as possible. This test is a measure of verbal fluency, specifically for letters, requiring initiation and maintenance, both considered to be aspects of frontal lobe function
Stroop Word Color Test	Provides diagnosis of brain dysfunction, and the evaluation of stress, personality cognition, and psychopathology. Assesses cognitive flexibility, resistance to interference from outside stimuli, creativity, and psychopathology by requiring subject to read through words, name ink colors of symbols, and name ink colors of color words that do not match. Five minutes to administer
Automated Neuropsychological Assessment Metrics (ANAM)	Computer-administered neuropsychological battery. Specifically designed for military use. Consists of nine subtests and a questionnaire of symptoms. Assesses energy-fatigue level, predominant mood state, visuo-motor response timing, visual search, sustained attention, working memory, processing efficiency, computational skills, spatial processing, and visuo-spatial working memory
Braincheckers	Computer-administered neuropsychological battery. Consists of six subtests and a questionnaire of symptoms. Assesses energy-fatigue level, predominant mood state, visuo-motor response timing, visual search, sustained attention, working memory, processing efficiency, computational skills, spatial processing, fronto-executive functioning, and visuo-spatial working memory
CogState Sport	Battery of four card-based games. Assesses psychomotor function, processing speed, visual attention/vigilance, visual learning, and memory
Headminder Cognitive Stability Index (CSI)	Web-based neurocognitive test protocol. Subtests relevant to general cognitive screening techniques. Adaptable for repeatable, longitudinal assessments. Ten subtests; 30 min in length
CNS Vital Signs	Computerized neurocognitive test battery. Comprised seven tests: verbal and visual memory, finger tapping, symbol digit coding, the Stroop Test, a test of shifting attention, and the continuous performance test. Sensitive to malingerers and patients with conversion disorder. Suitable as a screening instrument
Immediate Post-Assessment of Concussion Test (ImPACT)	Computerized neuropsychological test battery. Six individual cognitive test modules assess cognitive functioning, including attention, memory, reaction time, and processing speed. Modules include word memory, design memory, X's and O's, symbol match, color match, and three letters. Composite scores are derived in the areas of memory, reaction time, and processing speed

included the Automated Neuropyschological Assessment Metrics (ANAM) (Jones et al. 2008), CogState Sport (2008), Headminder Cognitive Stability Index (CSI) (Erlanger et al. 2002), Braincheckers (Elsmore et al. 2007), CNS Vital Signs (Gualtieri and Johnson 2006), and Immediate Post-Assessment of Concussion Test (ImPACT) (Iverson et al. 2003) (Table 5.3).

The popularity of these tests has increased in light of research that shows a need to test higher cognitive functioning, rather than relying on reports of LOC and amnesia. One study reported that the presence of amnesia, not brief LOC, was most predictive of post-injury difficulties measured at 3 days after injury (Collins et al. 2003). Another study similarly found that impairment of

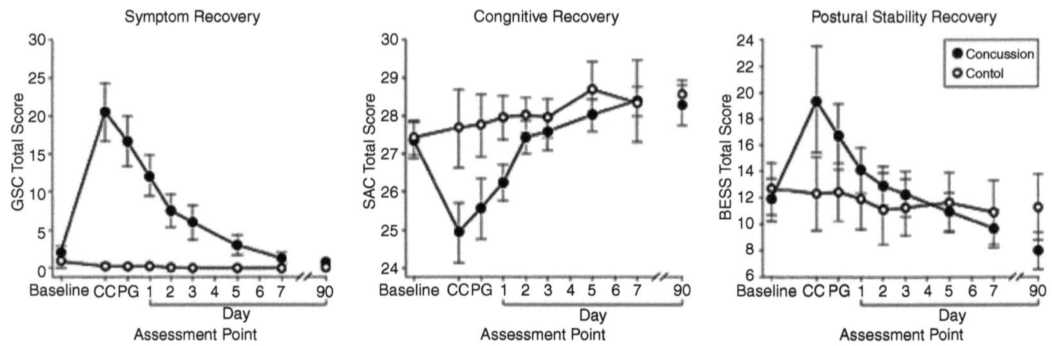

Fig. 5.1 Symptom, cognitive, and postural stability recovery in concussion and control participants. Higher scores on the Graded Symptom Checklist (GSC) indicate more severe symptoms; lower scores on the Standardized Assessment of Concussion (SAC) indicate poorer cognitive performance; and higher scores on the Balance Error Scoring System (BESS) indicate poorer postural stability. Error bars indicate 95% confidence intervals. CC indicates time of concussion; *PG* postgame/postpractice. On the BESS, multiple imputation was used to estimate means and 95% confidence intervals for control participants for the CC and PG assessments

immediate recall was much more frequent than disorientation and suggested that evaluating cognitive function and disability by asking the concussed athlete to state the day, time, month, and year may not be the most clinically useful evaluation task (Pellman et al. 2004—part III). A third study again found that athletes reporting memory problems following injury had significantly more symptoms, longer duration of symptoms, and significantly decreased performance on neurocognitive testing (Erlanger 2003). These results indicate that the conventional focus on LOC and disorientation as predictors for severity of a concussion may be misplaced. This type of evaluation of memory and immediate recall is of critical importance in sports concussions, where prolonged LOC is even less frequent than in other concussive events (where it is rare to begin with and occurs in less than 10% of concussive injuries) (Collins et al. 2003).

McCrea and colleagues (2003) published an important report on their NCAA concussion study which prospectively examined 1,631 football players from 15 US colleges. Their findings showed that injured athletes experienced the most severe symptoms immediately after a concussion, followed by a curve of recovery over 5–7 days, often needing full 7 days to return to baseline and control levels for clinical symptoms, longer than the 5 days needed to return to normal cognitive functioning (Fig. 5.1). This large cohort study supported the clinical experience of many professionals and contributed scientific evidence to return to play guidelines that suggest a gradual reintroduction to sport over the course of several days to weeks, depending on the severity of injury.

In spite of growing research and interest in addressing sports concussions, there is little consensus in the field on when and how to return athletes with head injuries to play. Hunt and Asplund (2010) suggest that whatever assessment tools are used, they include a cognitive assessment, some measure of balance testing, and a self-reported symptom assessment. Many guidelines promote allowing athletes to recover from all symptoms before testing so as to prevent learning effects. In the US military, exercise to a target heart rate is recommended prior to repeat neurocognitive testing to assess whether clinical symptoms, such as headache, have fully resolved (DVBIC 2007). Many institutions have started mandating baseline neurocognitive testing for athletes at risk for head injury so as to obtain an individualized standard in the event of a concussion. These pre-season baselines,

Table 5.4 Zurich guidelines, graduated return-to-play protocol

Rehabilitation stage	Functional exercise at each stage of rehabilitation	Objective of each stage
No activity	Complete physical and cognitive rest	Recovery
Light aerobic exercise	Walking, swimming, or stationary cycling, keeping intensity to 70% of maximum predicted heart rate; no resistance training	Increase heart rate
Sport-specific exercise	Skating drills in hockey, running drills in soccer, no head impact activities	Add movement
Noncontact training drills	Progression to more complex training drills, e.g., passing drills in football and ice hockey; may start progressive resistance training	Exercise, coordination, and cognitive load
Full-contact practice	Following medical clearance, participate in normal training activities	Restore athlete's confidence and functional skills
Return to play	Normal game play	

Athlete should continue to the next level if asymptomatic at the current level. Generally, each step should take 24 h so that an athlete would take approximately 1 week to proceed through the full rehabilitation protocol once asymptomatic at rest and with provocative exercise. If any post-concussion symptoms occur while in the stepwise program, then the patient should drop back to the previous asymptomatic level and try to progress again after a further 24-h period of rest has passed. Adapted with permission from McCrory et al. Consensus statement on concussion in sport. J Athletic Training 2009;44(4):434–48

therefore, account for any co-morbidities that may affect testing, such as learning disabilities, previous concussion history, medication usage, and mental conditions.

The decision about when to return an athlete to play without limitations is an issue of considerable importance in the sports medicine field, given the potential for external or internal pressures on an athlete to return prematurely. There are many published guidelines in the literature, which are based largely on clinical experience and expertise in the field rather than on rigorous studies. Most guidelines currently recommend a gradual, stepwise return to full activity once the athlete has become asymptomatic. Injured athletes are returned to rest or must return to a previous step if they exhibit any symptoms with increased activity. The guidelines proposed by the Third International Conference on Concussion in Sport, in Zurich, Switzerland, in November 2008 (McCrory et al. 2009) improved upon the guidelines previously presented by the same conference in Vienna (Aubry et al. 2002) and Prague (McCrory et al. 2005). The recommendations of the Zurich conference are presented in Table 5.4.

Additionally, the research on the effect of multiple concussions has prompted clinicians to differentiate return-to-play guidelines based on the severity of the concussion and the athlete's concussion history. Guidelines by Cantu are presented in Table 5.5 (2001). The concussion grades referenced in these guidelines include Grade 1, no loss of consciousness and post-traumatic amnesia (PTA) or post-concussive symptoms lasting less than 30 min; Grade 2, LOC less than 1 min and PTA or post-concussive symptoms 30 min to 24 h in duration; and Grade 3, LOC lasting more than 1 min or PTA lasting longer than 24 h with post concussion signs or symptoms lasting longer than 7 days (Cantu 2001). This system is revised from his previous grading system (Cantu 1986) based on the evidence from prospective studies on PTA and persistence of post-concussive symptoms. Several other grading systems for concussion also exist in the literature. Commonly cited are the Colorado Medical Society (Report of the Sports Medicine Committee 1990), the American Academy of Neurology (Kelly and Rosenberg 1997; Jordan et al. 1989; Ommaya 1985; Nelson and Jane 1984; Roberts 1992), and Torg Grading Systems for Concussion (1991).

Table 5.5 Cantu guidelines for return to play after concussion

	First concussion	Second concussion	Third concussion
Grade 1 (mild)	May return to play if asymptomatic for 1 week	Return to play in 2 weeks if asymptomatic at that time for 1 week	Terminate season; may return to play next season if asymptomatic
Grade 2 (moderate)	Return to play after asymptomatic for 1 week	Minimum of 1 month; may return to play then if asymptomatic for 1 week; consider terminating the season	Terminate season; may return to play next season if asymptomatic
Grade 3 (severe)	Minimum of 1 month; may return to play if asymptomatic for 1 week	Terminate season; may return to play next season if asymptomatic	

Note: Asymptomatic means no headache, dizziness, or impaired orientation, concentration, or memory during rest or exertion. Reprinted from Clin Sports Med 1998;17:56. Cantu RC. Return-to-play guidelines after a head injury, with permission from Elsevier

Neuroimaging and Concussions

CT and MRI remain the imaging technique of choice for initial assessment of acute head injury for skull fractures and intracranial hemorrhage while MRI is standard of care for evaluation of subacute or chronic traumatic brain injury (Tuong and Gean 2009). However, the study of the neuroimaging of concussions has not been thoroughly explored as most mTBIs that result in concussion do not result in abnormalities that can be detected by computed tomography (CT) and standard MRI imaging studies (DiFiori and Giza 2010). Research has suggested that less than 10% of patients with minor head injuries have positive CT findings and less than 1% require neurosurgical intervention (Jeret et al. 1993).

The reliance on neurocognitive testing and symptom checklists for concussion diagnosis has motivated clinicians and researchers in the field to use advanced imaging techniques to better quantify and define structural injuries in the brain following concussion. Possible techniques with increased sensitivity over traditional neuroimaging studies include diffusion tensor MRI (DTI), functional MRI (fMRI), magnetic resonance spectroscopy (MRS), and positron emission tomography (PET). DTI provides a measurement modality for white matter integrity and connectivity. Functional MRI offers the opportunity to receive real-time feedback on cerebral metabolism and brain activation patterns during specific cognitive or motor tasks. MRS and PET alike provide images that indicate functional cerebral metabolism. All of these modalities, however, require relatively long collection times and, with the exception of PET, require post-imaging data processing. These technologies are not currently used in clinical assessments of sports concussion, but following investigation of their sensitivity and specificity, may soon serve to estimate injury severity.

Prevention

Prevention of sports-related concussion can be encouraged through further education of players, coaches, and referees as well use of research-based guidelines by sports health professionals. To take the sport of football as an example, Mueller and Schindler (1989) noted that coaches and referees must do a better job of emphasizing and enforcing the rules against using the head as an initial contact point. This rule protects the impacted player by decreasing the contributing torso mass of the tackling player, resulting in lower effective mass and lower force on the impacted player and thus lowering the risk of concussion (Viano and Pellman 2005). This is particularly important as a study of NFL players found no concussions in striking players, only impacted players, making it particularly important to decrease the force on the impacted player

(Pellman et al. 2003). The difference in force translates directly to a difference in peak head acceleration, which was found to have a statistical correlation to whether a collision resulted in a concussed or an uninjured player (Pellman et al. 2003).

Areas for Future Research

Public interest in sports concussions has increased research in the area, but many details about the mechanisms, etiologies, and best treatments remain topics of current research. Both large-scale studies and anecdotal evidence from practitioners indicate that the great variability in the human brain between individuals significantly contributes to concussion incidence and resolution. As a result, further research will explore the effects of co-morbidities and predisposing factors, both hereditary and environmental. Additionally, while neuropsychological tests have improved to provide better recommendations to practitioners on return to play and the need for further assessment, these tests must continue to be validated in different populations and potentially incorporate new technologies to facilitate ease of administration and evaluation.

Conclusion

The complex and wide-ranging presentations of concussions make the careful study and care of concussed athletes an important issue for the medical community. With recent studies showing the potential long-term effects and increased future risk for concussed athletes, it is our hope that the increase in awareness among the public and medical professionals will lead to evidence-based practices in diagnosing and treating concussed athletes. Since concussion is perhaps the single most common form of brain injury, it is imperative that both health providers and sports professionals receive education and develop an understanding of the risks, prevention, diagnosis, and treatment of sports concussions.

References

1981–82–2004–05 NCAA sports sponsorship and participation rates report. National Collegiate Athletic Association. http://www.ncaa.org/library/research/participation_rates/1982-2005/1982_2005_participation_rates.pdf. Accessed 27 March 2007.

Annegers JF, Grabow JD, Kurland LT, Laws Jr ER. The incidence, causes, and secular trends of head trauma in Olmsted County, Minnesota, 1935–1974. Neurology. 1980;30:912–9.

Aubry M, Cantu R, Dvorak J, et al. Summary and agreement statement of the First International Conference on Concussion in Sport. Vienna 2001. Recommendations for the improvement of safety and health of athletes who may suffer concussive injuries. Br J Sports Med. 2002;36:6–10.

Bazarian JJ, Atabaki S. Predicting postconcussion syndrome after minor traumatic brain injury. Acad Emerg Med. 2001;8:788–95.

Benton AL, Hamsher KD. Multilingual aphasia examination. Iowa City: University of Iowa Press; 1976.

Boston University Center for the Study of Traumatic Encephalopathy. "Brain Donation Registry." http://www.bu.edu/cste/our-research/brain-donation-registry/. Accessed 22 Mar 2010.

Canale ST, Cantler ED, Sisk TD, Freeman BL, 3rd. A chronicle of injuries of an American intercollegiate football team. Am J Sports Med. 1981;9:384–9.

Cantu RC. Guidelines for return to contact sports after a cerebral concussion. Physician and Sportsmed. 1986;14:10.

Cantu RC. Minor head injuries in sports. In: Dyment PG, editor. Adolescent medicine: state of the art reviews. Philadelphia, PA: Hanley & Belfus; 1991.

Cantu RC, Voy R. Second impact syndrome: a risk in any contact sport. Physician Med. 1995;23:27–34.

Cantu RC. Head injuries in sport. Br J Sports Med. 1996; 30:289–96.

Cantu RC, Mueller F. Catastrohpic spine injury in football 1977–1989. J Spinal Disord. 1990;3:227–31.

Cantu RC. Posttraumatic retrograde and anterograde amnesia: pathophysiology and implications in grading and safe return to play. J Athletic Training. 2001;36: 244–8.

CogState Sport. (2008). Our Tests. http://www.cogstate.com/go/sport/. Accessed 25 March 2010.

Coldren RL, Kelly MP, Parrish RV, Dretsch M, Russell ML. Evaluation of the military acute concussion evaluation for use in combat operations more than 12 hours after injury. Mil Med. 2010;175:477–81.

Collins MW, Lovell MR, Iverson GL, Cantu RC, Maroon JC, Field M. Cumulative effects of concussion in high school athletes. Neurosurgery. 2002;51:1175–81.

Collins MW, Iverson GL, Lovell MR, et al. On-field predictors of neuropsychological and symptom deficit following sports-related concussion. Clin J Sport Med. 2003;13:222–9.

Corsellis JAN, Bruton CJ, Freeman-Browne D. The aftermath of boxing. Psychological Medicine. 1973;3: 270–303.

Defense and Veterans Brain Injury Center (DVBIC). Consensus Conference on the Acute Management of Concussion/Mild Traumatic Brain Injury (mTBI) in the Deployed Setting. 31 July and 1 August 2008, Washington, DC. http://www.dvbic.org/Providers/TBI-Clinical-Tools-%281%29.aspx. Accessed 19 Mar 2010.

DeLee JC, Farney WC. Incidence of injury in Texas high school football. Am J Sports Med. 1992;20:575–80.

DiFiori J, Giza C. New techniques in concussion imaging. Curr Sports Med Rep. 2010;9;35–9.

Elsmore TF, Reeves DL, Reeves AN. The ARES test system for palm OS handheld computers. Arch Clin Neuopsychol. 2007;22 Suppl 1:S135–44.

Erlanger DM, Kaushik T, Broshek D, Freeman J, Feldman D, Festa J. Development and validation of a web-based screening tool for monitoring cognitive status. J Head Trauma Rehabil. 2002;17:458–76.

Erlanger D, Kausik T, Kantu R, Barth JT, et al. Symptom-based assessment of the severity of concussion. J Neurosurg. 2003;98:34–9.

Field M, Collins MW, Lovell MR, et al. Does age play a role in recovery from sports-related concussion? A comparison of high school and collegiate athletes. J Pediatr. 2003;142:546–53.

Giza CC, Hovda DA. The neurometabolic cascade of concussion. J Athl Train. 2001;36:228–35.

Golden C, Freshwater SM. Stroop color and word test. Wood Dale, IL: Stoelting Co; 2002.

Gronwall D, Wrightson P. Cumulative effect of concussion. Lancet. 1975;2:995–7.

Gualtieri CT, Johnson LG. Reliability and validity of a computerized neurocognitive test battery, CNS Vital Signs. Arch Clin Neuropsychol. 2006;21:623–43.

Guskiewicz KM, McCrea M, Marshall SW, et al. Cumulative effects associated with recurrent concussion in collegiate football players: the NCAA Concussion Study. JAMA. 2003;290:2549–55.

Heegaard W, Biros M. Traumatic brain injury". Emerg Med Clin North Am. 2007;25:655–78, viii.

Hovda DA, Lee SM, Smith ML, et al. The neurochemical and metabolic cascade following brain injury: moving from animal models to man. J Neurotrauma. 1995;12: 903–6.

Hunt T, Asplund C. Concussion assessment and management. Clin Sports Med. 2010;29:5–17.

Iverson GL, Lovell MR, Collins MW. Interpreting change on ImPACT following sport concussion. Clin Neuropsychol. 2003;17:460–7.

Iverson G, Gaetz M, Lovell M. Cumulative effects of concussion in amateur athletes. Brain Inj. 2004;18: 433–43.

Iverson GL, Brooks BL, Lovell MR, Collins MW. No cumulative effects for one or two previous concussions. Br J Sports Med. 2006;40:72–5.

Jeret JS, Mandell M, Anziska B, Lipitz M, Vilceus AP, Ware JA, et al. Clinical predictors of abnormality disclosed by computed tomography after mild head trauma. Neurosurgery. 1993;32:9–15.

Jones WP, Loe SA, Krach SK, Rager RY. Automated neuropsychological assessment metrics (ANAM) and Wookcock-Johnson III tests of cognitive ability: a concurrent validity study. Clin Neuropsychol. 2008;22: 305–20.

Jordan B, Relkin N, Ravdin L. Apolipoprotein E epsilon 4 associated with chronic traumatic brain injury in boxing. JAMA. 1997;278:136–40.

Jordan B. Genetic susceptibility to brain injury in sports: a role for genetic testing in athletes? Phys Sportsmed. 1998;26:25–6.

Jordan B, editor. Medical aspects of boxing. Boca Raton, FL: CRC Press; 1993.

Jordan B, Tsairis PT, Warren RF, editors. Sports neurology. Gaithersburg, MD: Aspen Publishers; 989. p. 227.

Kelly JP, Nichols JS, Filley CM, Lillehei KO, Rubinstein D, Kleinschmidt-DeMasters BK. Concussion in sports: guidelines for the prevention of catastrophic outcome. JAMA. 1991;266:2867–9.

Kelly JP, Rosenberg JH. The diagnosis and management of concussion in sports. Neurology. 1997;48:575–80.

Kelly JP, Rosenberg JH. The development of guidelines for the management of concussion in sports. J Head Trauma Rehabil. 1998;13:53–65.

Kemp PM, Houston AS, Macleod MA, Pethybridge RJ. Cerebral perfusion and psychometric testing in military amateur boxers and controls. J Neurol Neurosurg Psychiatry. 1995;59:368–74.

Lampert PW & Hardman JM. Morphological changes in brains of boxers. *JAMA*. 1984;251:2676–9.

Lovell M. The management of sports-related concussion: current status and future trends. Clin Sports Med. 2009;28:95–111. http://medicine.tums.ac.ir/fa/Users/farzin_halabchi/Journal%20Club/18.8.88/Review%20Article%20Dr.%20Vakili%2018.8.

Lovell MR, Collins MW, Iverson GL, et al. Recovery from mild concussion in high school athletes. J Neurosurg. 2003;98:296–301.

Lovell MR, Collins MW, Iverson GL, et al. Grade 1 or "ding" concussions in high school athletes. Am J Sports Med. 2004;32:460–7.

Maddocks DL, Dicker GD, Saling MM. The assessment of orientation following concussion in athletes. Clin J Sport Med. 1995;5:32–3.

Martland H. Punch Drunk. JAMA. 1928; 91:1103–7.

McCrea M, Kelly JP, Randolph C, Kluge J, Bartolic E, Finn G, Baxter B. Standardized assessment of concussion (SAC): on-site mental status evaluation of the athlete. J Head Trauma Rehabil. 1998;13:27–35.

McCrea M, Kelly JP, Kluge J, Ackley B, Randolph C. Standardized assessment of concussion in football player. Neurology. 1997;48:586–8.

McCrea M, Kelly JP, Randolph C. Standardized assessment of concussion (SAC): manual for administration, scoring and interpretation. 2nd ed. Waukesha, WI: CNS Inc.; 2000.

McCrory P, Johnston K, Meeuwisse W, Aubry M, Cantu R, Dvorak J, Graf-Baumann T, Kelly J, Lovell M, Schamasch P. Summary and agreement statement of the 2nd International Conference on Concussion in Sport, Prague 2004. Br J Sports Med. 2005;39:196–204.

McCrory P, Meeuwisse W, Johnston K, Dvorak J, Aubry M, Molloy M, Cantu R. 3rd International Conference on Concussion in Sport Held in Zurich, November 2008. Clin J Sport Med. 2009;19:185–200.

McCrea M, Guskiewicz KM, Marshall SW, Barr W, Randolph C, Cantu RC, Onate JA, Yang J, Kelly JP. Acute effects and recovery time following concussion in collegiate football players: the NCAA concussion study. JAMA. 2003;290:2556–63.

McKeag D. Understanding sports-related concussion: coming into focus but still fuzzy. JAMA. 2003;290: 2604–5.

Mueller FO, Schindler RD. Annual Survey of Football Injury Research 1931–1988. Prepared for American Football Coaches Association, National Collegiate Athletic Association, National Federation of State High School Associations, American Football Coaches Association: Orlando, FL; February 1989.

Narayan R. Closed head injury. In: Rengachary SS, Ellenbogen RG, editors. Principles of neurosurgery. London: Wolfe; 1994. p. 235–92.

National Federation of State High School Associations. Participation in high school sports increases again; confirms NFHS commitment to stronger leadership. http://www.nfhs.org/web/2006/09/participation_in_high_school_sports_increases_again_confirms_nf.aspx. Accessed 23 March 2007.

Nelson WE, Jane JA, Gieck JH. Minor head injury in sports: a new system of classification and management. Physician Sportsmed. 1984;12:103–7.

Omalu BI, DeKosky ST, Minster RL, et al. Chronic traumatic encephalopathy in a National Football League player. Neurosurgery 2005; 57(1):128–34.

Ommaya AK. Biomechanics of head injury: experimental aspects. In: Nahum AM, Melvin J, editors. Biomechanics of trauma. Norwalk, CT: Appleton & Lange; 1985. p. 245–69.

Pellman EJ, Viano DC, Tucker AM, Casson IR, Waeckerle JF. Concussion in professional football: reconstruction of game impacts and injuries. Neurosurgery. 2003;53: 799–814.

Pellman EJ, Powell JW, Viano DC, et al. Concussion in professional football: epidemiological features of game injuries and review of the literature – part 3. Neurosurgery. 2004;54:81–97.

Pellman E, Lovell MR, Viano DC, et al. Concussion in professional football: recovery of NFL and high school athletes assessed by computerized testing-Part 12. Neurosurgery. 2006;58:263–4.

Pickles W. Acute general edema of the brain in children with head injuries. N Engl J Med. 1950;242:607–11.

Reitan RM, Wolfson D. The Halstead–Reitan Neuropsycholgical Test Battery: Therapy and clinical interpretation. Tucson, AZ: Neuropsychological Press; 1985.

Report of the Sports Medicine Committee. Guidelines for the Management of Concussion in Sports. Denver, CO: Colorado Medical Society; 1990 (revised May 1991).

Roberts WO. Who plays? Who sits? Managements concussions on the sidelines. Physician Sportsmed. 1992;20:66–76.

Rutherford WH, Merrett JD, McDonald JR. Symptoms at one year following concussion from minor head injuries. Injury. 1979;10:225–30.

Rutland-Brown W, Langlois J, Thomas K, Lily Y. Incidence of traumatic brain injury in the United States. J Head Trauma Rehabil. 2006;21:544–8.

Ryan AJ. Intracranial injuries resulting from boxing: a review (1918–1985). Clin Sports Med. 1987;6:31–40.

Saal JA. Common American football injuries. Sports Med. 1991;12:132–147.

Salcido R, Costich JF. Recurrent traumatic brain injury. Brain Inj. 1992;6:293–8.

Saunders RL, Harbaugh RE. The second impact in catastrophic contact-sports head trauma. JAMA. 1984;252:538–9.

Shapiro AM, Benedict RH, Schretlen D, Brandt J. Construct and concurrent validity of the Hopkins Verbal Learning Test-Revised. Clin Neuropsychol. 1999;13:348–58.

Sim A, Terryberry-Spohr L, Wilson KR. Prolonged recovery of memory functioning after mild traumatic brain injury in adolescent athletes. J Neurosurg. 2008;108: 511–6.

Sosin DM, Sniezek JE, Thurman DJ. Incidence of mild and moderate brain injury in the United States, 1991. Brain Inj. 1996;10:47–54.

Stewart WF, Gordon B, Selnes O, Bandeen-Roche K, Zeger S, Tusa RJ, et al. Prospective study of central nervous system function in amateur boxers in the United States. Am J Epidemiol. 1994;139:573–88

Torg JS. Athletic Injuries to the head, neck and face. St Louis, MO: Mosby-Year Book; 1991. p. 226.

Tuong HL, Gean AD. Neuroimaging of traumatic brain injury. Mt Sinai J Med. 2009,76:145–62.

Unterharnscheidt FJ. About boxing: review of historical and medical aspects. Tex Rep Biol Med. 1970;28:421–95.

Viano DC, Pellman EJ. Concussion in professional football: biomechanics of the striking player – part 8. Neurosurgery. 2005;56:266–80.

Weschler D. The measurement of adult intelligence. Baltimore, MD: William & Wilkins Co; 1944.

Zemper ED. Injury Rates in a National Sample of College Football Teams: A Two-Year Prospective Study. Physician Sports Med. 1989; 17:100–13.

Zemper ED. Two-year prospective study of relative risk of a second cerebral concussion. Am J Phys Med Rehabil. 2003;82:653–9.

Blast-Related Concussion

6

Carson Lawall

Abstract

Blast-related concussion is a serious problem faced by providers in both the military and civilian setting. Blast may cause injury to the central nervous system by several mechanisms including the primary blast wave, secondary penetrating or blunt trauma, tertiary effects of being projected by the blast and blunt or crushing trauma, quaternary effects from exposures due to the explosion, and the experience of the traumatic event may have psychological sequelae that can result in prolonged symptoms. While the mechanism is significantly different, the outcomes and treatment of blast-related concussion are similar to that of other mechanisms.

Keywords

Blast • Concussion • Blast-related concussion • Post-traumatic stress disorder • PTSD • Primary blast injury • Explosive injury • Post-concussive symptoms • Post-concussive syndrome • PCS

Introduction

Neurological sequelae of blast-related injury have been described in medical literature as early as World War I (WWI) (Hertz 1915), as at the time exposure to blast injuries was prevalent and on a scale not before seen. Soldiers engaged in trench warfare were subjected to frequent artillery and mortar attacks, and an estimated 60% of the deaths in that war were due to shrapnel. In this setting, several soldiers would describe events consistent with a concussion (Jones et al. 2007). The diagnosis of "shell shock" was an attempt to describe cases where the patients had neurological symptoms in the context of a blast exposure, but could not be linked to an organic lesion. Shell shock was originally thought to be a neurological lesion directly caused by compressive forces from the blast wave, but as time progressed there grew concern that the symptoms may have been more psychological rather than organic in nature (Jones et al. 2007). It has been historically recognized that both physical and psychological factors may play a role in symptomatology following concussion (Cramer et al. 1948). This observation continues to this day and

C. Lawall, M.D. (✉)
Naval Medical Center San Diego,
San Diego, CA, USA
e-mail: Carsonlawall@gmail.com

J.W. Tsao (ed.), *Traumatic Brain Injury: A Clinician's Guide to Diagnosis, Management, and Rehabilitation*, DOI 10.1007/978-0-387-87887-4_6, © Springer Science+Business Media, LLC 2012

continues to engender debate. In clinical practice both in the theater of war and in following patients who have returned from the battlefield, it does appear that both physical and psychological factors are important in the symptoms seen after a blast-related concussion. The diagnostic difficulties in regard to concussion and the overlap of psychological symptoms have also been described in the past, as well as concerns about the sensitivity and specificity of the available diagnostic tests (Cramer et al. 1948). This also continues today despite the array of medical technology at our disposal.

Given changes to the tactics on the modern battlefield and improvements in personal protective equipment, body armor, and vehicles protecting against injuries that would have previously been fatal (Nyein et al. 2010; Wilk et al. 2010), concussion due to blast injury has become a major concern for those caring for patients both in the combat environment and after soldiers return home. While determining the number of concussions that occur in a theater of war does have some methodological issues, the number of patients who have suffered a concussion while deployed in Operation Enduring Freedom/ Operation Iraqi Freedom is estimated to be between 225 and 370,000 (Hoge et al. 2008; Hoge et al. 2009; Luethcke et al. 2011; Elder and Cristian 2009; Rosenfeld and Ford 2010). Of those injured, many are due to blast exposure which may account for up to 78% of injuries to service members in Iraq and Afghanistan (Belanger et al. 2009, 2011). Given the large numbers of patients involved, this represents a significant long-term health concern (Ling and Ecklund 2011).

Historical Perspective

Injury due to blast exposure is by no means a problem specific to modern warfare. In many ways, there are parallel experiences seen with the conflicts in Iraq and Afghanistan in comparison to the trench warfare seen in WWI. In all three conflicts, blast exposure is the primary means of injury to soldiers, albeit in WWI, the explosives were generally delivered by artillery and mortars (Jones et al. 2007), and in current conflicts explosive injury is most often delivered by the improvised explosive device (IED) (Ling and Ecklund 2011).

An estimated 60% of deaths in WWI were due to shrapnel wounds (Jones et al. 2007), which suggests that explosive exposures accounted for a large proportion of the injuries sustained by soldiers, similar to the wars in Iraq and Afghanistan. In WWI patients exposed to shelling and blasts reported symptoms of headaches, amnesia, difficulty concentrating, dizziness, tinnitus, and sensitivity to noise. Many of these patients by today's definition would meet clinical criteria for concussion (Jones et al. 2007; Defense and Veterans Brain Injury Center 2011). This constellation of symptoms, combined with blast exposure, was termed "shell shock." Originally the symptoms were thought to be due to a structural lesion caused by the compressive forces of the blast wave (Jones et al. 2007; Elsayed 1997), and based on descriptions of cases, some exposures did appear to cause structural damage leading to neurological deficits (Hertz 1915). However, as understanding evolved, it became clear that some patients who did not have concussions, had minor injuries, or were not involved in blasts had similar symptoms and in most cases symptoms could not be linked to an organic lesion. As the symptoms are common to multiple disorders, various explanations for their occurrence appeared. Research into the stresses of trench warfare yielded more information and contributed to further observations that many patients with shell shock did not actually have significant exposures to blasts (Jones et al. 2007). Despite research, resources, and attempts at treatment in forward areas, shell shock remained a common phenomenon. It has been estimated that 10% of battle casualties were categorized as shell shock or neurasthenia in WWI. One seventh of all discharges from the British army were due to shell shock, and 32,000 war pensions were awarded for shell shock, which increased with time as it became popularized in the public. Involvement of the lay media in support of individual veterans distorted policy and research by an emotional public (Jones et al. 2007).

In WWII, to avoid the epidemic of shell shock, the term was actually banned, but the common symptoms experienced by soldiers continued. In 1939 the term post-concussional syndrome was introduced to describe the symptom complex. In WWII, it was also recognized that distinguishing symptoms caused from blast-concussion versus another etiology was difficult both clinically and with the available diagnostic testing. At the time, diagnostic testing was largely in the form of X-rays, pneumoencephalogram, and electroencephalogram, which were neither sensitive nor specific for the diagnosis of disorders related to concussion (Hoge et al. 2008; Jones et al. 2007).

Soldiers also were much more likely to attribute symptoms to shell shock as there was no stigma attached to the diagnosis. Patients and the public could identify with the condition, which was considered to be a neurological diagnosis, and not feel that a negative label was implied by the description. This may have benefitted patients by encouraging them to seek help; however, it may also have led to mistreatment if symptoms were attributed to concussion or shell shock, when other causes of such symptoms could be treated more appropriately (Jones et al. 2007).

Understanding some of the history of blast-related injury may be helpful in interpreting some of the issues today. Interestingly, there appear to be several parallels. There is still stigma associated with psychological conditions, and in the military, where admitting anxiety or fears may be viewed as weakness, attributing symptoms to mild traumatic brain injury (TBI) is a much less stigmatizing option (Jones et al. 2007; Elder and Cristian 2009). Unfortunately, while it may be less stigmatizing, it is clear that beliefs about concussion and brain injury may actually affect recovery. Strongly held beliefs about brain injury or brain damage may play a role in maintenance of symptoms (Jones et al. 2007; Hoge et al. 2009; Ropper and Gorson 2007). Today there is also a great deal of media coverage and clearly an emotional component in the debate about the consequences of concussion and blast-related concussion which may cloud the issue, and at times can create difficulties in discussing symptoms and prognosis with patients as the information available in the lay media, as well as commonly held opinions, are not necessarily consistent with what has been demonstrated in the medical literature (Hoge et al. 2009). There is also an increased focus in the military on forward treatments of concussion in the form of diagnostic imaging available in the theater of war, increased number of specialists in neurology, and specialized concussion recovery centers. Just as it has in the past, diagnosis of concussion and post-concussive symptoms continues to be complicated by reliance on clinical symptoms, which have overlap with several other disorders including post-traumatic stress disorder (PTSD), depression, and migraine (Jones et al. 2007; Hoge et al. 2008; Hoge et al. 2009; Luethcke et al. 2011; Belanger et al. 2009; Howe 2009; Elder and Cristian 2009; Rosenfeld and Ford 2010; Belanger et al. 2011; Tsao 2010). Diagnostic tests, such as physical examination and computed tomography (CT) scanning, are not sensitive in making the diagnosis of concussion (and by definition must be normal in the setting of concussion), and newer modalities such as magnetic resonance imaging (MRI) have limited clinical use at this time due to issues with specificity and sensitivity, even in moderate and severe TBI (Skandsen et al. 2011; Weiss et al. 2007; MacDonald et al. 2011; McCrory et al. 2009). Finally, many of the problems and frustrations that complicate treatment of concussion and blast-related concussion today have also created difficulty in the past (Jones et al. 2007; Elder and Cristian 2009).

Pathophysiology

Explosive blast may cause injury to the body via several different mechanisms (Table 6.1) (Ling and Ecklund 2011). The mechanisms leading to injury are divided into primary effects from the blast wave, secondary effects caused by projectiles/flying debris from the blast causing blunt or penetrating injuries to the body, tertiary effects from the body being thrown from the blast, and quaternary effects such as burns, asphyxia, and/or toxic exposures from the blast as well as exacerbation of previous illnesses

Table 6.1 Immediate effects of blasts and explosions

Primary—Direct effects (e.g., overpressurization and underpressurization), rupture of tympanic membranes, pulmonary damage, rupture of hollow viscera
Secondary—Penetrating trauma, fragmentation Injuries
Tertiary—Effects of structural collapse and persons being thrown by the blast wind, crush injuries and blunt trauma, penetrating or blunt trauma, fractures and traumatic amputations, open or closed brain injuries
Quaternary—Burns, asphyxia, and exposure to toxic inhalants

Adapted from DePalma et al. NEJM 2005

(Howe 2009; Elder and Cristian 2009; DePalma et al. 2005; Belanger et al. 2011).

The primary mechanism is due to the blast wave and overpressurization (Belanger et al. 2009; Howe 2009; Elder and Cristian 2009; DePalma et al. 2005; Belanger et al. 2011). The blast wave propagates from the point of detonation and dissipates with distance from the source. The blast wave is followed by a blast wind behind the initial shock wave, and is initially directed away from the blast, then as the energy dissipates, reverses back to the point of detonation and causes underpressure. Injury results from barotruama, which is a difference between pressure, either overpressurization or underpressurization, of the outer surfaces of the body and the internal organs (Howe 2009; Elder and Cristian 2009). As the blast wave strikes an object, part of the blast wave is reflected back to the source and part of the blast wave is deflected away, but the majority of the energy is absorbed and propagated through the body. The energy propagates through the body as a high frequency stress wave and a low frequency shear wave. The high frequency stress wave may cause damage to tissue by implosion, spalling (cavitation caused by reflection of the blast wave at the interface of materials with different density/acoustic impedance), or by pressure differentials. The low frequency shear wave results from compression of the body wall and structures underneath. The blast wave itself may cause damage to internal structures and the brain parenchyma without external injury (Kocsis and Tessler 2009). Distance from the point of detonation is also an important factor as blast waves in an outdoor setting dissipate by the cubed root of the distance from the source. Those closest to the source will have significantly more overpressure effects than those at a distance (Howe 2009), and those in enclosed structures may have more injuries as a result of barotraumas than those in open spaces due to reflection of the wave off structures and multiple wave effects (DePalma et al. 2005; Ling and Ecklund 2011; Elsayed 1997).

Air-filled organs and air–fluid interfaces are the most susceptible areas to blast wave damage (Howe 2009; Elder and Cristian 2009; Kocsis and Tessler 2009; Elsayed 1997). The tympanic membrane, lungs, and GI tract are especially susceptible, with the tympanic membrane being the most easily injured with even minor increases in pressure (Howe 2009; Elsayed 1997). Physical pathological changes to the brain seen in TBI are frequently associated with pathological changes in other organs (Kocsis and Tessler 2009). While the tympanic membrane is cited as the most frequently injured structure in a blast wave injury, rupture of the tympanic membrane is only partially helpful in determining the potential for injury to the brain or other organs (Harrison et al. 2009; Xydakis et al. 2007). There are some conflicting data as to the association of tympanic membrane rupture with blast-related concussion. Tympanic membrane rupture is associated with loss of consciousness in blast exposure (Howe 2009; Xydakis et al. 2007), but is not sensitive as a marker for primary blast injury to the body. In a study of 167 patients exposed to blasts in Iraq, tympanic membrane rupture had only a 50% sensitivity as a biomarker for other primary blast injury, although it was fairly specific with an 87% specificity in determining if there was sufficient force from the blast to cause injury to other organs (Harrison et al. 2009). By inference, the brain, which does not have air–fluid interfaces, may be more resistant to blast wave phenomena affecting the tympanic membrane (Howe 2009; Kocsis and Tessler 2009), but in clinical experience the majority of patients with concussion (most often grade I or II concussion by American Academy of Neurology criteria) due to blast do not have damage to the tympanic membrane, which demonstrates the limits of its clinical utility as a biomarker for central nervous system (CNS) injury. This is also complicated by the fact that simple ear protection may prevent injury to the tympanic membrane in blasts that otherwise would have enough energy to have caused more severe injuries (Howe 2009).

Secondary and tertiary injuries are most likely similar to injuries sustained by other mechanisms of head trauma leading to concussion. Secondary injuries from objects projected from the blast may cause penetrating or blunt trauma (Belanger et al. 2009; Howe 2009; DePalma et al. 2005), and one would expect a similar pattern of injury to the CNS. Tertiary injuries result from being thrown by the blast into other objects and, again, one would expect an injury pattern similar to that seen in other mechanisms (Howe 2009).

Quaternary injuries are due to exposure to burns, chemicals, and additional variables which may occur in the setting of blast exposure (Howe 2009; DePalma et al. 2005). Conventional military ordinance releases light/electromagnetic, acoustic, and thermal energy as well as toxic fumes. The effect of these variables on the brain may be difficult to predict and may be different in each exposure, and the magnitude of effect is difficult to determine in the setting of other injuries. (Ling and Ecklund 2011). Patients may have a contribution from one or all four injury subtypes, each of which may contribute to the overall pattern of injury (Elder and Cristian 2009), and further complicate distinction from blast-related injury primarily from the blast wave itself, and nonblast injuries.

One additional consideration is the environment in which the injury occurred. Blast injury in the combat setting is unlikely to occur in isolation. Frequently, service members are exposed to a blast when under extreme stress. While an IED blast may occur in isolation, it is not uncommon that the blast occurs when under direct or indirect enemy fire, or an IED is a prelude to a more coordinated attack. Those involved are often in life-threatening situations and are not only exposed to potentially deadly fire from enemy combatants, but also may have suffered other wounds, be involved in vehicle accidents or fires, have to care for the wounds of their comrades, may see disturbing wounds suffered by comrades or the enemy, may have friends die in the attack, and may be forced to return fire and kill enemies. Each of these factors may have additional psychological consequences and likely contribute to symptoms seen after concussion.

Pathology

The pathology of blast-related concussion is largely described in animal models as concussion/mild TBI, in humans not a fatal injury. There are some limitations in interpretation of these findings as there are significant structural differences in mouse, rat, rabbit, or pig models that may lead to differences in how blast waves affect or propagate through the brain. Also, many models use high blast pressures on anesthetized animals which may be less consistent with mild injury, although there is evidence that even modest blast pressures may cause effects in the CNS (Elder and Cristian 2009). One must be careful in interpreting data as in animals a more severe (moderate or severe TBI) may have resulted from the exposure, which would be more difficult to distinguish clinically in an animal model. Mild blast injury in one study was considered to be an exposure to a shockwave that caused 5% mortality in animals in a supine position and no lethality in the prone position although many of the injuries sustained were to the lung and liver (Koliatsos et al. 2011). While this is considered mild, it may represent a significant injury.

Animal studies suggest that blast waves may have structural effects on the brain and have demonstrated alterations in physiology as well as microscopic structure following blasts (Elder and Cristian 2009; Koliatsos et al. 2011; Rosenfeld and Ford 2010). In a porcine model, following a blast there is transient flattening of the EEG and brief apnea suggestive of effects on the brainstem. In a mouse model, the most common structures injured as seen in pathological evaluations were the cerebellar white matter, the internal capsule, the cerebral peduncles, and pyramidal fibers in the pons and medulla, but again, based on the protocol the severity of injury was likely greater than that seen in mild TBI. Microscopically, one may see expanded perineuronal spaces, cytoplasmic vacuoles, myelin deformation, and axonoplasmic shrinkage (Elder and Cristian 2009). The findings in these models is felt to be most closely related to diffuse axonal injury (Elder and Cristian 2009; Kocsis and Tessler 2009; Koliatsos et al. 2011). There may also be temporary evidence of abnormal axonal transport after blast exposure in rats, which may contribute to the physical findings seen in these animals (Elder and Cristian 2009). In mouse models, after a blast exposure there is evidence of abnormal social interaction with other mice and behavioral changes; however, these often improve with time, and in one study, 2 weeks after the exposure the mice showed the same interactions as mice exposed to a sham blast experience (Koliatsos et al. 2011). There may also be some evidence that pathological changes may not be permanent and improve in time, which may parallel clinical improvement in time in animal models (Rosenfeld and Ford 2010; Kaur et al. 1995).

Unfortunately, there is very little data in regard to pathological consequences of concussion/mild TBI due to blast in humans (Elder and Cristian 2009). Mild TBI is not a fatal condition and there is little data to describe pathological chances seen in humans acutely after a blast.

Much data in regard to the immediate pathological consequences in humans is from moderate or severe TBI (Elder and Cristian 2009). In patients who have died as a result of blast injury, microscopic parenchymal or leptomeningial hemorrhages are the most commonly described finding. This can be seen throughout the cerebral white matter, in the corpus callosum, and in the basal ganglia. In a description of nine soldiers who died as a result of an atmospheric blast, with no evidence of external trauma, there was evidence of hyperemia in the brain and leptomeninges, and both microscopic hemorrhages, as well as in some cases larger hemorrhages, contusions, and in one case a laceration of the cerebellum with extensive hemorrhage (Kocsis and Tessler 2009). Unfortunately, much of the data in regard to these pathological findings is based on rather old case series and did not describe findings consistent with diffuse axonal injury, although since microhemorrhages are seen in diffuse axonal injury, one may postulate that diffuse axonal injury may have been present in these cases as well (Kocsis and Tessler 2009). Given limited data in the setting of mild TBI, one could expect similar pathologic findings in humans and animal models, and likely similar changes in time, but making definitive conclusions at this time is not possible.

Symptoms

Patients with blast-related concussion experience many of the same symptoms experienced by those who have suffered a concussion by other means. Symptoms such as headache, dizziness, vertigo, imbalance, difficulty concentrating, alteration in consciousness, confusion, seeing "stars," feeling "dazed," brief post-traumatic amnesia, loss of consciousness, blurry vision or transient double vision, nausea, vomiting, and/or insomnia are common to both blast- and nonblast-related concussion (Elder and Cristian 2009; Belanger et al. 2011; Ropper and Gorson 2007).

In blast-related concussion patients commonly also complain of ear pain, hearing loss, and tinnitus.

Acutely, there may also be some psychological symptoms that also may present as many patients report a sensation of time slowing down, a near out-of-body experience, tunnel vision, diminished hearing, difficulty understanding, and confusion which may be related more to the experience than due to physical trauma (Hoge et al. 2009), which further complicates diagnosis and treatment. Confusion in the setting of extreme stress, combat, injuries, threat of physical injury, sleep deprivation, and rapid change in sensory environment (from calm, quiet, to loud, smoke-filled, and chaotic) may be mistaken for symptoms caused by head trauma (Hoge et al. 2009). Blast-related concussion may have more psychological sequelae and may have a stronger association with PTSD (Rosenfeld and Ford 2010), but this also may occur in nonblast-related concussion.

It is also important to be vigilant for other injuries in the setting of blast exposure. As discussed before, it is possible to have injuries without evidence of external trauma (Kocsis and Tessler 2009), and rupture of the tympanic membrane is not sensitive as a biomarker for additional injuries due to blast wave trauma (Xydakis et al. 2007; Harrison et al. 2009; DePalma et al. 2005). A good clinical exam is often sufficient in evaluating for other areas of trauma, but laboratory evaluation and imaging (often in the form of CT) are helpful, especially if there are unexplained symptoms or findings on exam suggestive of other injuries.

Of note, in the literature there is discussion of concern about soldiers ignoring symptoms in order to return to the fight. Often these statements are found in the introduction of the papers discussing concussion/mild TBI (Marion et al. 2010). To the author's knowledge there is no study that examines the incidence of over- or under-reporting of post-concussive symptoms in the deployed setting. While this does occur, clinical experience in Kandahar Afghanistan from December 2010 to May 2011 is that under-reporting symptoms is actually quite infrequent, and the opposite appears to be more common. This may be an artifact of observations at the NATO Role III hospital in Kandahar (a referral center for more complex cases), but in this setting it is a small minority of patients that minimize somatic symptoms in order to return to combat. Most patients accurately report their symptoms and express concern that their experience is properly documented. A significant proportion over represent symptoms or have nonphysiologic findings such as past pointing or gait disturbance or a decline in the MACE (Military Acute Concussion Evaluation, a battlefield concussion assessment tool modeled after the Standard Assessment of Concussion used on sports sidelines) score despite improvement in overall level of consciousness. Frequently, over representation of symptoms is transient in the first few days after an injury and resolves spontaneously. This is simply an observation, but one could theorize that this may be a result of changing perceptions of symptoms, feelings of reassurance as they recover, or a result of validation once a patient has been heard and their injury is recognized. A second minority (albeit a minority that can take a disproportionate amount of time and attention) actively continue to over-represent symptoms for secondary gain.

An interesting finding has also been described in relation to cognitive complaints after concussion in patients in the Veteran's Affairs medical system after returning from deployment. Cognitive complaints are out of proportion to the findings on objective cognitive measures (Spencer et al. 2010). Perception of symptoms may be affected by recall bias, increased sensitivity to symptoms, misattribution of symptoms, or emotional factors that may lead to perception of cognitive dysfunction despite normal objective measures (Hoge et al. 2009; Howe 2009; McCrea et al. 2009). Minimization of symptoms absolutely occurs, but it is the least common of these presentations despite popular discussion to the contrary (Marion et al. 2010).

Diagnosis

Diagnosis is based on clinical history and physical exam. Currently, there are no accepted radiologic or laboratory tests to diagnose concussion (Hoge et al. 2009; Elder and Cristian 2009). Imaging acutely with CT is helpful in evaluating for more severe injuries or immediately life-threatening problems associated with blast injury, but is not sensitive for the diagnosis of concussion. By some criteria, if there is a lesion seen on neuroimaging the event is no longer considered a concussion/mild TBI, but instead is graded as a moderate or severe brain injury (McCrea et al. 2009). MRI is a promising method of diagnosis and is more sensitive than CT in detecting parenchymal damage to the brain in TBI (Weiss et al. 2007), but more research is needed in determining its utility for TBI. Standard MRI modalities may not be sensitive enough to detect injury sustained in a concussion/mild TBI, and while newer modalities such as functional MRI and diffusion tensor imaging (DTI) appear to be more sensitive (Jantzen 2010; Niogi and Mukherjee 2010), there are still questions about the clinical interpretation of these findings (Jantzen 2010). In a recent study of US service members who sustained a blast-related concussion in Iraq or Afghanistan, DTI was able to detect abnormalities in 18 of 63 patients with normal CT scans, however, while this is more sensitive, it still only detected abnormalities in 29% of patients with clinically determined concussion (MacDonald et al. 2011). The authors concluded that while this may demonstrate some evidence of axonal injury in patients with blast-related concussion, the diagnosis of concussion remains clinical as the majority of the patients with concussion did not have a definite abnormality on DTI (MacDonald et al. 2011). While there are some imaging findings suggestive of poor outcomes in severe TBI (such as bilateral brainstem lesions or posterior brainstem lesions), MRI is not predictive of outcome in moderate TBI, and may not be predictive in all cases of severe TBI (Skandsen et al. 2011; Weiss et al. 2007). As the imaging findings are far less conspicuous, if present at all, in concussion/mild TBI, one would expect that interpretation of findings in mild TBI would be more difficult and less predictive of outcome.

Documenting the details about the event is helpful in determining the level of injury, the severity (mild, moderate, or severe TBI), and may be helpful in the future to determine changes in treatment as more is discovered about concussion. It is also helpful in communicating the extent of the injury to other providers (Elder and Cristian 2009). In the military setting, a commonly used test is the MACE. The MACE is based on the Standardized Assessment of Concussion (SAC) often used in sports (Coldren et al. 2010), and consists of three parts—history and symptom evaluation, cognitive score, and a brief neurological examination. The MACE is helpful in that it creates a consistent framework for the evaluation of a patient suspected to have sustained a recent concussion and is fairly simple; however, it has not been clinically validated (Defense and Veterans Brain Injury Center 2011). In theater, much of the focus has been on the cognitive score, but it is the clinical history that is more important in making the diagnosis of concussion. Patients with an alteration of consciousness after a head injury should have at least one positive answer on the MACE clinical history portion. The cognitive score may serve as a measure of severity; however, in practice it appears to be less helpful. A MACE cognitive score of less than 25 out of a possible 30 is considered abnormal and consistent with an injury. However, clinical experience in theater has shown that patients with a concussion by clinical criteria and post-concussive symptoms frequently score better than 25/30, and conversely some patients without a concussion score less than 25/30. A study using the MACE for soldiers in Iraq found that the MACE exam if administered more than 12 h from the injury was neither sensitive nor specific and was not clinically useful (Niogi and Mukherjee 2010). The MACE exam is helpful in providing consistency in evaluation, and the history portion should catch patients that meet clinical criteria for concussion (clinical history remains the standard for the diagnosis of concussion), but the conclusions one can make from the cognitive score are very limited.

Clinical criteria for concussion are inclusive and vary based on the source (Niogi and Mukherjee 2010). The US Department of Defense uses the definition of concussion proposed by the Mild Traumatic Brain Injury Section of the American Congress of Rehabilitation Medicine (Ling and Ecklund 2011; Coldren et al. 2010) with the addition a fifth criterion of the finding of the absence of an intracranial lesion on imaging (Table 6.2). Concussion is defined as a traumatically induced structural injury and/or physiological disruption of brain function as a result of an external force that is indicated by new onset or worsening of at least one of the following clinical signs immediately following the event:

1. Any period of loss or decreased level of consciousness
2. Any loss of memory for events immediately before or after the injury
3. Any alteration of mental state at the time of the injury
4. Neurological deficits that may or may not be transient
5. Absence of intracranial lesion (Defense and Veterans Brain Injury Center 2011; Ling and Ecklund 2011; Coldren et al. 2010)

Table 6.2 The Department of Defense and Department of Veteran Affairs Traumatic Brain Injury Task Force Criteria for mild TBI/concussion

A traumatically induced structural injury and/or physiological disruption of brain function as a result of an external force that is indicated by new onset or worsening of at least one of the following clinical signs immediately following the event: 1. Any period of loss or decreased level of consciousness 2. Any loss of memory for events immediately before or after the injury 3. Any alteration of mental state at the time of the injury 4. Neurological deficits that may or may not be transient 5. Absence of intracranial lesion

Table 6.3 The AAN concussion grading criteria

(No concussion/mTBI)—No alteration in consciousness
Concussion, Grade I—No loss of consciousness, alteration of consciousness <15 min
Concussion, Grade II—No loss of consciousness, alteration of consciousness >15 min
Concussion, Grade III—Any loss of consciousness (this is sometimes divided into brief or prolonged)
Brief concussion, Grade III—Loss of consciousness lasting seconds
Prolonged concussion, Grade III—Loss of consciousness lasting minutes or more

Concussion is graded in severity as well (Table 6.3). Grade I concussion is an alteration in consciousness after the event lasting for less than 15 min. Grade II concussion is an alteration in consciousness after the event lasting more than 15 min. Grade III concussion is divided into Brief Concussion, Grade II with a loss of consciousness lasting seconds, and Prolonged Concussion, Grade III with a loss of consciousness lasting minutes or more (Ropper and Gorson 2007; Ling and Ecklund 2011). In the setting of the theater of combat and blast-related concussion, grading of the concussion unfortunately is not very helpful in directing treatment, as generally patients are not returned to duty until they are symptom free, regardless of the concussion grade. Grading may have some utility as a descriptor of the event, creating a contextual framework when approaching the patient and managing expectations, and is sometimes used administratively in the military, but in clinical care the grade of concussion does not change management as patients are treated supportively until symptom resolution. While the mechanism is different, and patients are returned to full duty as opposed to returned to play in competitive sport, this is consistent with the Zurich Consensus Statement on Concussion in Sport, and the AAN position statement on sports concussion in October 2010, which recommends that athletes do not return to play until symptom free and are evaluated by a neurologist or provider experienced in the treatment of concussion (American Academy of Neurology Website 2011; McCrory et al. 2009).

Diagnosis of concussion/mild TBI based on clinical criteria is complicated because symptoms reported may be biased, forgotten, misattributed to concussion but caused by other factors, or confused with psychological symptoms that may not represent physical injury to the brain (Jones et al. 2007; Hoge et al. 2008; Hoge et al. 2009; Luethcke et al. 2011; Belanger et al. 2009; Howe 2009; Elder and Cristian 2009; Rosenfeld and Ford 2010; Belanger et al. 2011; Tsao 2010). While there are difficulties in making a diagnosis based on clinical history, as an observation by this author in treating patients in both the deployed setting and after patients have returned from deployment, it appears that patients in most cases are able to provide a detailed history of the event, despite concerns about memory issues in close relation to the event (Hoge et al. 2008; Hoge et al. 2009). It is best to obtain history as soon as possible, but in comparing experience with service members in Afghanistan and interviews with service members once they have returned to their home base, most are able to provide a reliable history. Issues such as brief loss of consciousness versus post-traumatic amnesia with no loss of consciousness are difficult to determine in both settings, as is determining the duration of post-traumatic amnesia, but in most cases patients are able to provide a fairly reliable estimate that is generally consistent with the observations of their medics and medical providers as they are transported from point of injury to higher levels of care. This observation has been consistent for neurologists both at NATO Role III

Multi-National Medical Unit in Kandahar, Afghanistan and the Craig Joint Theater Role III Hospital in Bagram, Afghanistan.

Treatment

The treatment of blast-related concussion is similar to that of concussion due to other mechanisms. The mainstay of treatment is rest and targeted treatment of clinical symptoms. Patients frequently report worsening of symptoms with exertion and appear to improve faster when allowed (or ordered) to rest, but supporting data overall is quite limited at this time. Gradual return to activity is encouraged (McCrea et al. 2009). Similar to findings in collegiate athletes after concussion, the period of recovery is variable for patients (McCrea et al. 2003), even those exposed to the same explosive blast, so in general patients are followed until their symptoms remit or improve, then are returned to light activity before returned to full activity. Frequently provocative testing is performed before return to full activity to ensure there is not a relapse of symptoms with vigorous activity. Avoidance of re-injury while the patient is symptomatic and likely recovering from the injury, is also important (Ling and Ecklund 2011) and while second impact syndrome is controversial, and generally seen in the pediatric population, it is conceivable a second concussion during a vulnerable period after a previous injury could have more concerning consequences (McCrea et al. 2009; Ling and Ecklund 2011).

Education is also very important in the treatment of blast-related concussion. As concussion is very common, especially in young service members, who very frequently were (or are still) active in sports. It helps to explain that the concussion suffered as a result of a blast has a similar recovery pattern to any other concussion they or a friend may have had from a sports injury, and that one would not expect long-term, persistent symptoms. There does not appear to be a significant difference in outcome between concussion cause by blast exposure and that caused by other mechanisms (Luethcke et al. 2011; Belanger et al. 2009; Howe 2009; McCrea et al. 2009; Belanger et al. 2011; Wilk et al. 2010). It helps to create an expectation for full recovery (Hoge et al. 2009; Ropper and Gorson 2007). Discussion of the common symptoms may normalize the experience and reassure the patient. It may also be helpful to address the likelihood of other stressors contributing to symptoms, as in most cases the blast was both a physically and psychologically traumatic experience. Education may decrease the incidence of post-concussive symptoms at 6 months (Ropper and Gorson 2007; Mittenberg et al. 2001). In a review of several studies conducted in Finland, the Netherlands, Great Britain, New Zealand, the USA and Canada which examined early interventions after concussion, it was consistently found that education about symptoms of post concussive syndrome, reassurance, and reattribution of the symptoms to a benign cause (concussion) were effective in preventing long-term symptoms (Mittenberg et al. 2001). The terms "concussion," "mild traumatic brain injury," and "mTBI" used interchangeably (Hoge et al. 2008, 2009; Ling and Ecklund 2011), but the diagnostic label and management of expectations are important (Hoge et al. 2009; Howe 2009; McCrea et al. 2009; Lippa et al. 2010). "Concussion" suggests an event that has occurred in the past, and a clinical state, whereas "mild traumatic brain injury" implies a pathological state (Hoge et al. 2009; Ling and Ecklund 2011) that may be ongoing, or permanent "brain damage." Many patients can identify with having a concussion and have a positive perception of their likely recovery. Fewer patients can identify with having a brain injury of any type, and generally do not have positive expectations for recovery.

By observation, addressing somatic symptoms does appear to improve recovery. Treatment of symptoms in relation to blast-related concussion is no different than treatment of these symptoms from nonblast concussion, or these symptoms in isolation. Headaches are quite common after a blast exposure and are frequently the factor that limits return to activity. It is ideal to take a detailed history of headache to determine if it is similar to a primary headache syndrome such as tension or migraine. Treatment of post-traumatic headache is no different than treating a primary headache syndrome. Most post-traumatic headaches have several features in common with migraine and tend to respond to migraine medications, including prophylactic medications such as tricyclic antidepressants and abortive medications such as nonsteroidal anti-inflammatory medications and triptans (Tsao 2010), although if there are features suggestive of a different headache syndrome, it may be helpful to change the treatment strategy accordingly. It is recommended that narcotics are avoided for treatment of post-concussive headaches (Ropper and Gorson 2007; Tsao 2010).

Sleep disturbances are very common after blast-related head injury, likely due to a combination of factors including environment, acute stress, and the injury itself. Frequently if the sleep disturbance is addressed, headaches and cognitive symptoms also improve. Sleep hygiene is the most important factor, and unfortunately is one of the most difficult to address in the setting of ongoing combat operations. Rest in a quiet environment is key, along with avoidance of video games and energy drinks very commonly used by service members. Amitriptyline appears to be especially helpful in treating headache and sleep disorders after a blast-related concussion if pharmacological treatment is required, but other agents such as Benadryl, Mirtazapine, Melatonin, Zolpidem, and Temazaepam have also been helpful for short-term treatment.

Tinnitus, hearing loss, and tympanic membrane rupture are very common after blast-related concussion. Tympanic membrane rupture generally will heal on its own. If there are concerns for infection, one can start a 7-day course of ciprofloxacin otic drops, but in most cases antibiotics are not needed. Patients should avoid getting water or foreign objects in the ear. If the tympanic membrane does not heal in 60–90 days, consider referral to an otolaryngologist for further evaluation. Hearing is also frequently impaired. Treatment is supportive, and in most cases hearing improves. If not improved in 60–90 days consider audiology evaluation. Unfortunately, there is no accepted treatment for tinnitus. Treatment of tinnitus is supportive.

Balance dysfunction frequently occurs in the acute setting after the blast. Immediately after the blast, patients frequently have difficulty maintaining their balance with running or walking, but often recover even with just brief rest. Recovery of vestibular function is generally very rapid, so it is uncommon for it to persist until neurological evaluation in theater. With subjective complaints of dizziness, it is also very uncommon to find any deficits on a general neurological exam. Most patients appear to improve in 3–7 days, which is consistent with data from sports literature (McCrea et al. 2003; Guskiewicz 2011).

Cognitive complaints generally improve with time. Treatment is supportive as there is limited data for pharmacological treatments after concussion. Most patients report resolution of cognitive symptoms within 1–2 weeks from the injury which appears consistent with data from sports literature (McCrea et al. 2009; McCrea et al. 2003). There also appears to be some subjective component to cognitive dysfunction that may be due to event recall bias, mood disorders, stress, or anxiety (Iverson and Lange 2003). Subjective complaints of cognitive dysfunction also appear to be more prominent than those measured on formal neuropsychological testing available in theater, which is also consistent with the findings of subjective cognitive dysfunction in patients who have returned from deployment evaluated in the Veteran's Affairs system (Spencer et al. 2010).

Acute stress and mood disorders are very important contributors to continued symptoms after concussion (Hoge et al. 2008; Hoge et al. 2009; Howe 2009; McCrea et al. 2009; Rosenfeld and Ford 2010; Iverson and Lange 2003; Lippa et al. 2010). Treatment of acute stress symptoms, PTSD, and mood disorders is no different in a patient with a history of concussion than one without a prior history. Referral to a combat stress provider, psychologist, or psychiatrist may be helpful if symptoms are not well managed in the primary care setting. Early intervention to treat acute stress symptoms is recommended (Rosenfeld and Ford 2010; Belanger et al. 2011).

Prevention of blast injury with personal protective equipment may also be helpful in the future. Interestingly, shielding, at least in rodent models and in computer models, may provide some protection in blast exposure (Nyein et al. 2010; Koliatsos et al. 2011), but the practical application at this time is not yet clear.

Return to Duty

After a blast-related concussion in combat, it is important to determine when a patient is safe to return to duty. Similar to literature in sport-related concussion, service members exposed to blast or other mechanism of injury are generally not returned to duty unless symptom free (American Academy of Neurology Website 2011; McCrory et al. 2009). There may be situations where the patient must return to duty due to a combat situation, prior to resolution of symptoms but this is very strongly avoided, and uncommon. Service members are encouraged to rest by medics, corpsman, and/or primary care providers trained in the treatment of concussion, adhering to clinical practice guidelines for the treatment of concussion, (Defense and Veterans Brain Injury Center 2011) and if symptoms persist or a patient has concerning findings, they are referred to specialty concussion center and/or a neurologist in the theater of operation for further evaluation or imaging. Patients are evaluated by the specialty provider as needed, and referred for additional testing as indicated by clinical history or findings on exam. As determined by the theater neurologist or specialty provider, if indicated, patients may be additionally evaluated by a physical therapist for musculoskeletal complaints or balance issues in relation to the event, an occupational therapist to ensure the patient will be able to perform once returned to duty and tolerate the physical stresses associated with their duty, and a neuropsychologist or psychologist trained in cognitive testing if there are cognitive issues after the injury. Psychiatry, psychology, and Combat stress providers may also be utilized in the treatment of patients with concussion when there is a significant component of acute stress reaction (ASR) or PTSD. Prior to return to duty patients are tested with provocative testing to determine if symptoms return with exertion. Patients with persistent symptoms are instructed to rest, then gradually return to activity before provocative testing and return to duty, and are not returned to full duty until they do well on provocative testing and are symptom free at baseline, or have returned to their premorbid baseline (as in the case of patients with preexisting migraine or other symptoms that may appear similar to post-concussive symptoms) (Defense and Veterans Brain Injury Center 2011).

Outcomes

While the mechanism of injury in blast-related concussion is significantly different than non-blast-related concussion, outcomes after the injury, regardless of mechanism, appear to be similar (Luethcke et al. 2011; Belanger et al. 2009; Belanger et al. 2011; Wilk et al. 2010). Patients with blast-related and nonblast-related concussion had similar cognitive outcomes and symptomatic outcomes regardless of mechanism (Luethcke et al. 2011; Belanger et al. 2009; Belanger et al. 2011; Wilk et al. 2010). There has not been a significant association between blast mechanism and post-concussive symptoms (Belanger et al. 2011; Wilk et al. 2010; Fear et al. 2009).

Post-concussive symptoms are more common in patients who are preoccupied with brain damage or have worsening of symptoms with exertion (Ropper and Gorson 2007) reinforcing the role of education in the treatment of concussion. Post-concussion symptoms may also be more common in women than in men, which has been seen in both in the civilian (Bazarian et al. 2010) and the military population (Fear et al. 2009). While there are some theories as to why this observation occurs, the reasons for this are unclear, and are especially difficult to understand given female subjects in animal models of concussion appear to fare better than their male counterparts (Bazarian et al. 2010). Compensation and litigation are frequently cited as risk factors for continued post-concussion symptoms or post-concussion syndrome (PCS) (Hoge et al. 2009; Howe 2009; McCrea et al. 2009; Holm et al. 2005), which does present a difficult problem in the military population as compensation, even if not consciously, is an issue as patients with concussion are allowed to rest, leave the combat area, are sometimes awarded medals for the injury, and may be eligible for monetary compensation for the injury when they leave the military. All of these factors are potentially producing incentive for the continued reporting of symptoms. Post-concussive symptoms are also not well associated with head injury or concussion, and can occur in patients who have not had head injuries (Howe 2009; Belanger et al. 2011; Wilk et al. 2010; Fear et al. 2009; Boake et al. 2005; Iverson and Lange 2003). Several investigations have found that post-concussive symptoms are much more closely associated with PTSD than with a history of concussion (Hoge et al. 2008; Hoge et al. 2009; Howe 2009; Rosenfeld and Ford 2010; Belanger et al. 2011; Lippa et al. 2010).

Despite the poor association between concussion and post-concussive symptoms, and stronger association between post-concussive symptoms and psychiatric comorbidity, there are some symptoms that may be more strongly related to concussion. Hoge et al., in a 2008 study of US soldiers returning from Iraq, did find that concussion with loss of consciousness was associated with a higher risk of headache (Hoge et al. 2008). Blast-related concussion may have some additional associated symptoms as well. Wilk et al. (2010) found that blast-induced concussion with loss of consciousness (but not without loss of consciousness) was more likely to be associated with tinnitus and headache at 3 and 6 months after deployment, and Belanger et al. (2011) found hearing loss was associated with blast injury, but was otherwise not related to increased risk of physical post-concussion complaints. In fact there was a significant inverse relationship between blast mechanism and cognitive complaints in the study (Wilk et al. 2010). This has not been entirely consistent between studies, but many studies show that blast exposure may have a higher associated risk of PTSD (Luethcke et al. 2011; Belanger et al. 2009; Rosenfeld and Ford 2010; Belanger et al. 2011). PTSD was very prevalent at a rate of approximately 40% in the population of US soldiers returning from Iraq, evaluated in the Hoge study in 2008 (Hoge et al. 2008).

This is also noted observationally in the deployed setting. The experience in Kandahar, Afghanistan at the Role III Multinational Medical Unit, Neurology Clinic, consists of over 200 consecutive patients with concussion/mTBI evaluated from December 2010 to June 2011. The data have not been fully evaluated at the time of publication, but the majority of patients evaluated were exposed to primary blast without brain injury from other mechanisms, a second group of patients suffered from primary and tertiary blast injuries which may have contributed to the injury. A smaller number of patients suffered from concussion due to other mechanisms. Unfortunately, determining the contribution of quaternary blast injury does not appear to be possible at this time as there are no doubt exposures with each blast, but the exposure varies considerably. Clinical observations in Afghanistan have been largely consistent with the current body of literature. There does not appear to be a good dose–response relationship between blast exposure and persistent symptoms. It is not an infrequent occurrence that 2–6 service members will require treatment after a single blast. Service members involved in the same blast may report very different symptoms or duration of symptoms. Also, it is not uncommon that soldiers closer to the blast, some close enough to suffer fragmentation injuries, have less symptoms than those further from the blast, and sometimes fewer post-concussive symptoms than patients who did not meet clinical criteria for concussion in the same blast. Currently, in between the two neurology providers in Kandahar Air field, the return to duty rate has been between 93 and 97% which also appears to be consistent with the sports literature in resolution of post-concussive symptoms (McCrea et al. 2009; McCrea et al. 2003).

Overall, the different mechanism of injury and potentially different patterns of injury in the brain, do not result in significantly different functional outcomes, and similar to other mechanisms of injury, most patients return to baseline within a month of the concussion (Belanger et al. 2011).

Conclusion

Concussion due to blast wave exposure has been recognized as a source of potential injury to soldiers, and also has been recognized as a significant problem since the First World War. Military physicians historically faced many of the issues that we also face today. Patients exposed to an explosive blast may have injury to the brain through several mechanisms including the primary blast wave, secondary effects from projectiles causing blunt or penetrating trauma, tertiary effects from projection of the body from the blast, and quaternary effects due to other factors in the blast exposure. Limited conclusions can be made based largely on animal data and data from more severe brain injury, but there are likely microscopic changes that do occur in the brain parenchyma as a result of blast injury. These changes appear to improve with time, as do the clinical findings associated with blast-related concussion. The events and experience surrounding the blast exposure may also be important in pathology of concussion as large studies have shown that PTSD and depression are important contributors to long-term symptoms. Several factors may contribute to symptoms after blast-related concussion, and it is likely that both physical and psychological components contribute to the overall clinical picture. Perceptions of disability and expectations for recovery are important factors in recovery. While the mechanism of injury is different than concussion suffered in sports and other blunt trauma, clinical outcome is more closely associated with the severity of the injury rather than the mechanism of injury. Persistent symptoms are most likely associated with comorbid conditions or associated factors (Howe 2009; McCrea et al. 2009), and the overall prognosis, with return to normal baseline function after concussion, is quite good. As with other mechanisms of concussion, treatment remains is based on clinical diagnosis of an injury, rest, education, and symptomatic therapy for somatic symptoms such as headache, dizziness, and sleep disorders.

References

American Academy of Neurology Website. http://www.aan.com/globals/axon/assets/7913.pdf. Accessed 8 Jul 2011.

Bazarian JJ, Blyth B, Mookerjee S, Hua H, McDermott MP. Sex difference in outcome after mild traumatic brain injury. J Neurotrauma. 2010;27:527–39.

Belanger HG, Kretzmer T, Yoash-Gantz R, Picket T, Tupler LA. Cognitive sequelae of blast-related versus other mechanisms of brain trauma. J Int Neuropsychol Soc. 2009;15:1–8.

Belanger HG, Proctor-Weber Z, Kretzmer T, Kim M, French LM, Vanderploeg RD. Symptom complaints following reports of blast versus non-blast mild tbi: does mechanism of injury matter? Clin Neuropsychol. 2011;1:iFirst–14.

Boake C, McCauley SR, Levin HS, Pedroza C, Contant CF, Song JX, Brown SA, Goodman H, Brundage SI, Diaz-Marchan PJ. Diagnostic criteria for postconcussional syndrome after mild to moderate traumatic brain injury. J Neuropsychiary Clin Neurosci. 2005;173(3):350–6.

Coldren RL, Kelly MP, Parish R, Dretsch M, Russell ML. Evaluation of the Military Acute Concussion Evaluation for use in combat operations more than 12 hours after injury. Mil Med. 2010;175(7):477–81.

Cramer F, Paster S, Stephernson C. Cerebral injuries due to explosion waves; blast concussion. Arch Neurol Psychiatry. 1948;60(1):101–3.

Defense and Veterans Brain Injury Center. http://www.dvbic.org. Accessed 1 Feb 2011.

DePalma RG, Burris DG, Champion HR, Hodgson MJ. Blast injuries. N Engl J Med. 2005;352:1335–42.

Elder GA, Cristian A. Blast-related mild traumatic brain injury: mechanisms of injury and impact on clinical care. Mt Sinai J Med. 2009;76:111–8.

Elsayed NM. Toxicology of blast overpressure. Toxicology. 1997;121:1–15.

Fear NT, Jones E, Groom M, Greenberg N, Hull L, Hodgetts TJ, Wessely S. Symptoms of post concessional syndrome are non-specifically related to mild traumatic brain injury in UK Armed Forces personnel on return from deployment in Iraq: an analysis of self-reported data. Psychol Med. 2009;39:1379–87.

Guskiewicz KM. Balance assessment in the management of sport-related concussion. Clin Sports Med. 2011;30:89–102.

Harrison CD, Bebarta VS, Grant GA. Tympanic membrane perforation after combat blast exposure in Iraq: a poor biomarker for primary blast injury. J Trauma. 2009;67(1):210–1.

Hertz A. Paresis and involuntary movements following concussion caused by a high explosive shell. Proc R Soc Med. 1915;8 (Neurol Sect):83–4.

Hoge CW, McGurk D, Thomas JL, Cox AL, Engel CC, Castro CA. Mild traumatic brain injury in U.S. Soldiers returning from Iraq. N Engl J Med. 2008;358(5):453–63.

Hoge CW, Goldberg HM, Castro CA. Care of war veterans with mild traumatic brain injury—flawed perspectives. N Engl J Med. 2009;360(16):1588–91.

Holm L, Cassidy DJ, Carroll LJ, Borg J. Summary of the WHO Collaborative Centre for Neurotrauma Task Force on mild traumatic brain injury. J Rehabil Med. 2005;37:137–41.

Howe LLS. Giving context to post-deployment post-concussive-like symptoms: blast-related potential mild traumatic brain injury and comorbidities. Clin Neuropsychol. 2009;23:1315–37.

Iverson GL, Lange RT. Examination of "Postconcussion-Like" symptoms in a healthy sample. Appl Neuropsychol. 2003;10(3):137–44.

Jantzen KJ. Functional magnetic resonance imaging of mild traumatic brain injury. J Head Trauma Rehabil. 2010;25(4):256–66.

Jones E, Fear NT, Wessely S. Shell shock and mild traumatic brain injury: a historical review. Am J Psychiatry. 2007;164:1641–5.

Kaur C, Singh J, Lim KM, et al. The response of neurons and microglia to blast injury in the rat brain. Neuropathol Appl Neurobiol. 1995;21:369–77.

Kocsis JD, Tessler A. Pathology of blast-related brain injury. J Rehabil Res Dev. 2009;46(6):667–42.

Koliatsos VE, Cernak I, Xu L, Song Y, Savonenko A, Crain BJ, Eberhart CG, Frangakis CE, Melnikova T, Kim H, Lee D. Mouse model of blast injury to the brain: initial pathological neuropathological, and behavioral characterization. J Neuropathol Exp Neurol. 2011;70(5):399–416.

Ling GSF, Ecklund JM. Traumatic brain injury in modern war. Curr Opin Anesthesiol. 2011;24:124–30.

Lippa SM, Pastorek NJ, Benge JF, Thornton GM. Postconcussive symptoms after blast and nonblast-related mild traumatic brin injuries in Afghanistan and Iraq War Veterans. J Int Neuropsychol Soc. 2010;16:856–66.

Luethcke CA, Bryan CJ, Morrow CE, Isler WC. Comparison of concussive symptoms, cognitive performance, and psychological symptoms between acute blast-versus nonblast-induced mild traumatic brain injury. JINS. 2011;17:36–45.

MacDonald CL, Johnson AM, Cooper D, Nelson EC, Werner NJ, Shimony JS, Snyder AX, Raichle MF, Witherow JR, Fang R, Flaherty SF, Brody DL. Detection of blast-related traumatic brain injury in U.S. military personnel. N Engl J Med. 2011;362(22):2091–100.

Marion DW, Curley KC, Schwab K, Hicks RR, the mTBI Diagnostics Workgroup. Proceedings of the Military mTBI Diagnostics Workshop, St. Pete Beach, August 2010. J Neurotrauma 2011;28:517–26.

McCrea M, Guskiewicz KM, Marshall SW, Barr W, Randlolph C, Cantu RC, Onate JA, Yang J, Kelly JP. Acute effects and recovery time following concussion in collegiate football players: the NCAA concussion study. JAMA. 2003;290:2556–63.

McCrea M, Iverson GL, McAllister TW, et al. An integrated review of recovery after mild traumatic brain injury (MTBI): implications for clinical management. Clin Neuropsychol. 2009;23:1368–90.

McCrory P, Meeuwisse W, Johnston K, Dvorak J, Aubry M, Molloy M, Cantu R. Consensus statement on concussion in sport—The 3rd International Conference on concussion in sport, held in Zurich, November 2008. J Clin Neurosci. 2009;16:755–63.

Mittenberg W, Canyock EM, Condit D, Patton C. Treatment of post-concussion syndrome following mild head injury. J Clin Exp Neuropsychol. 2001;23:829–36.

Niogi S, Mukherjee P. Diffusion tensor imaging of mild traumatic brain injury. J Head Trauma Rehabil. 2010;25(4):241–55.

Nyein MK, Jason AM, Yu L, Pita CM, Joannopoulos JD, Moore DF, Radovitzky RA. In silico investigation of intracerebral blast mitigation with relevance to military traumatic brain injury. PNAS. 2010;107(48):20703–8.

Ropper AH, Gorson KC. Concussion. N Engl J Med. 2007;356:166–72.

Rosenfeld JV, Ford NL. Bomb blast, mild traumatic brain injury and psychiatric mobidity: a review. Injury. 2010;41:437–43.

Skandsen T, Kvistad KA, Solheim O, Lydersen S, Strand IH, Vik A. Prognostic value of magnetic resonance imaging in moderate and severe head injury: a prospective study of early MRI findings and one-year outcome. J Neurotrauma. 2011;28:691–9.

Spencer RJ, Drag LL, Walker SJ, Bieliauskas LA. Self-reported cognitive symptoms following mild traumatic brain injury are poorly associated with neuropsychological performance in OIE/OEF veterans. JRRD. 2010;47(6):521–30.

Tsao JW, editor. Traumatic brain injury. Continuum: Lifelong Learning Neurol 2010;16(6). Copyright © 2010 American Academy of Neurology.

Weiss N, Galanaud D, Carpentier A, Naccache L, Puybasset L. Clinical review: prognostic value of magnetic resonance imaging in acute brain injury and coma. Crit Care. 2007;11:230.

Wilk JE, Thomas JL, McGurk DM, Riviere LA, Castro CA, Hoge CW. Mild traumatic brain injury (concussion) during combat: lack of association of blast mechanism with persistent postconcussive symptoms. J Head Trauma Rehabil. 2010;25(1):9–14.

Xydakis MS, Bebarta VS, Harrison CD, Conner JC, Grant GA, Robbins AS. Tympanic-membrane perforation as a marker of concussion. N Engl J Med. 2007;357(8):830–1.

7

Sleep/Wake Disturbances in Mild Traumatic Brain Injury Patients

Michael Russo, Aimee L. Alphonso, and Ian C. Murphy

Abstract

The continued research and practice of sleep medicine has provided insights into brain physiology, novel diagnostic tools, and innovative treatment options for poorly understood diseases. Sleep is broken down into a circadian rhythm pattern characterized by the three stages: maintenance mechanisms of the NREM cycle and the oscillation of phasic and tonic movements in the REM cycle. Recently, traumatic brain injury has been shown to negatively impact these normal sleep/wake cycles and to increase significantly the risk of comorbid disease. The link between TBI and sleep disorders has been established through the use of subjective measures of sleep disturbance such as the Pittsburgh Sleep Quality Index and through objective analysis like polysomnography. Case studies demonstrate that clinicians' use of these types of assessments creates a more complete medical picture and treatment plan for TBI patients.

Keywords

Mild traumatic brain injury • Sleep disturbances • Excessive daytime sleepiness • Insomnia • Sleep disorders (care and treatment)

Introduction

Mild traumatic brain injury (mTBI) may disrupt both neuronal synaptic circuitry and glial myelin maintenance throughout the brain and brainstem. Because mechanisms for initiating and maintaining sleep as well as wake are distributed throughout the brain and brainstem, damage to either region is likely to impair some aspects of the sleep/wake system. TBI-related sleep/wake disorders may impair either or both nighttime sleep and daytime function. Insomnia, an inability to initiate and/or

M. Russo, M.D.
Department of Neurology,
Uniformed Services University of the Health Sciences,
Bethesda, MD, USA

A.L. Alphonso, B.S. (✉) • I.C. Murphy, B.A.
Department of Orthopedics & Rehabilitation,
Walter Reed National Military Medical Center,
Bethesda, MD, USA
e-mail: Aimee.alphonso@med.navy.mil

J.W. Tsao (ed.), *Traumatic Brain Injury: A Clinician's Guide to Diagnosis, Management, and Rehabilitation*,
DOI 10.1007/978-0-387-87887-4_7,

maintain sleep, is reported in up to 24% of the general population (Ohayon 2002) and in up to 84% of mTBI patients (Zeitzer et al. 2009). Excessive daytime sleepiness (EDS), a severe impairment of daytime alertness, is reported in up to 20% of the general population (Pagel 2009). In the mTBI population, EDS has been identified in up to 55% of patients (Orff et al. 2009). Prior to the onset or recognition of insomnia or EDS, subtle symptoms of sleep/wake disturbance may occur, including mild cognitive impairment, headaches and fatigue, appetite change, anhedonia, and mood instability. These commonly seen mTBI symptoms may be harbingers of incipient sleep/wake disturbances, and/or represent comorbid illnesses.

This chapter (1) discusses the anatomy and physiology of the sleep/wake initiation and maintenance systems; (2) suggests mechanisms whereby mTBI may precipitate specific sleep disorders; (3) presents illustrative case histories, and (4) discusses specific nonpharmacologic, pharmacologic, and experimental therapies.

Section 1: The Physiology of Sleep/Wake Systems

The relationships among sleep, wake, and traumatic brain injury (TBI) may best be understood by thinking of sleep/wake centers and their projections as a distributed network within the brain and brainstem. Normal sleep is divided into non-rapid eye movement (NREM) and rapid eye movement (REM) sleep. The stages are wake (W), Drowsy, N1 (NREM sleep stage 1—equivalent to light sleep), N2 (NREM sleep stage 2—equivalent to early slow-wave sleep), N3 (NREM stages 3 and 4—equivalent to deep sleep), and REM sleep; sleep is an active process that cycles at an ultradian* rhythm (a biological cycle occurring within a 24-h period) of about 90 min. Stage N1 is considered a transition between wake and sleep. It occurs upon falling asleep and during brief arousal periods, and usually accounts for 5–10% of total sleep time. Stage N2 occurs throughout the sleep period and represents 40–50% of total sleep time. Stage N3 is classically referred to as "delta wave sleep" and occurs mostly in the first third of the night.

Upon falling asleep, waking usually transitions into NREM sleep stage N1 quickly followed by N2. REM follows NREM sleep by about 90 min and occurs 4–5 times during a normal 8- to 9-h sleep period. The first REM period of the night may be less than 10 min in duration, while the last may exceed 60 min. In most healthy young adults, 8–8.4 h of sleep is considered fully restorative. In some cultures, total sleep often is divided into an overnight sleep period of 6–7 h and a mid-afternoon nap of 1–2 h.

Sleep is a state of unconsciousness in which the brain is relatively more responsive to internal than to external stimuli. During the transition from wake to sleep, the brain gradually becomes less responsive to visual, auditory, and other environmental stimuli. This reversal of relative external unresponsiveness as well as the predictable cycling of sleep assists in distinguishing sleep from other states of unconsciousness.

Historically, sleep was thought to be a passive state initiated through withdrawal of sensory input. Currently, withdrawal of sensory awareness is believed to be a factor in sleep in addition to an active initiation mechanism that facilitates brain withdrawal.

NREM Sleep

NREM sleep is controlled by complex initiation and maintenance mechanisms, the extent of which is not fully understood. Researchers speculate that the mechanism is governed by sleep-generating circuits with inputs from brainstem and hypothalamic neuronal groups. Within these circuits, sleep initiation may begin with the emergence of inhibitory signals from the anterior hypothalamic pre-optic nucleus directed caudally toward the brainstem reticular core and posterior hypothalamus. The pre-optic nucleus inhibits the histaminergic posterior hypothalamic tuberoinfundibular region through gamma aminobutyric acid (GABA) and probably acetylcholine (Eriksson et al. 2010).

The tuberoinfundibular region projects rostrally to the intralaminar nuclei of the thalamus and to the cerebral cortex. Inhibition of the tuberoinfundibular region is a critical step toward falling asleep because it results in functional disconnection between the brainstem and the more rostral thalamus and cortex. A decrease in ascending thalamic cholinergic transmissions occurs in association with decreasing cortical responsiveness. In addition to inhibiting higher cortical consciousness, the tuberoinfundibular tract projects caudally into the pontine reticular system and inhibits afferent transmissions from ascending cholinergic tracts.

NREM is an active state that is maintained partly through oscillations between the thalamus and the cortex. The three major oscillation systems are sleep spindles, delta oscillations, and slow cortical oscillations. Sleep spindles, a hallmark of stage N2 sleep, are generated by bursts of hyperpolarizing GABAnergic thalamic reticular neurons that inhibit thalamocortical projection neurons. As deafferentation spreads, corticothalamic projections back to the thalamus synchronize. As hyperpolarization of the thalamic reticular neurons progresses, delta waves are produced by interactions from both thalamic reticular and cortical pyramidal sources. Slow cortical oscillations are produced in neocortical networks by cyclic hyperpolarizations and depolarizations.

REM Sleep

REM sleep is characterized by muscle atonia, cortical activation, low-voltage synchronization of the EEG, and REMs. The sleep state is generated by mesencephalic and pontine cholinergic neurons; referred to as REM-on neurons. As REM sleep initiates, monoadrenergic locus ceruleus and serotonergic raphe neurons become inactive and are thereby referred to as REM-off neurons. REM is separated into both tonic and phasic characteristics.

Tonic Movements

Tonic muscle atonia is present throughout REM sleep and results from inhibition of alpha motor neurons by clusters of peri–locus ceruleus neurons, collectively referred to as the dorsolateral small cell reticular group. Projection of the presumed cholinergic dorsolateral small cell reticular group is through the medullary reticular formation, which projects through the ventrolateral reticulospinal tract to inhibitory spinal and bulbar interneurons. Glycinergic interneurons produce postsynaptic inhibition and hyperpolarization of the spinal alpha motor neurons. Tonic cortical activation with EEG desynchronization is promoted by projections from cholinergic lateral dorsal tegmental and pedunculopontine tegmental neurons to the thalamic nuclei. Other projections through brainstem reticular formation neurons are likely to be involved as well.

Phasic Movements

Phasic features of REM sleep include periodic skeletal muscle twitches, increased heart rate variability, pupil dilation, increased respiratory rate, phasic spikes, and REM. Phasic rapid eye movements are composed of lateral saccades generated in the paramedian pontine reticular formation and vertical saccades thought to be generated in the mesencephalic reticular formation.

Phasic pontine–geniculate–occipital (PGO) spikes are another neurophysiological feature of REM sleep. These spikes appear to be generated by lateral dorsal tegmental and pedunculopontine tegmental neuronal bursts. They are projected to the lateral geniculate and other thalamic nuclei, and then to the occipital cortex. PGO bursts precede REMs by several seconds, and increases in PGO bursts are seen after REM sleep deprivation.

Circadian Rhythms

Circadian sleep rhythm is one of the several intrinsic body rhythms modulated by the hypothalamus. Light is called a "zeitgeber," a German word meaning "time-giver," because it sets the suprachiasmatic clock. The suprachiasmatic nucleus sets the body clock to approximately 25 h, with both light exposure and schedule clues entraining to the 24-h cycle. The retinohypothalamic tract allows light cues to directly influence the suprachiasmatic nucleus. The nadir of the circadian sleep rhythm is in the early morning. The downswing in circadian rhythm prior to the nadir is thought to assist the brain in remaining asleep overnight for full restoration by preventing premature awakening. The morning upswing then facilitates awakening and through the day acts as a counterbalance to the progressive discharge of awake neuronal activity. After the circadian apex in the early evening, the downswing aids sleep initiation. This model explains the relatively steady cognitive function throughout wakefulness.

Body temperature cycles are ultradian rhythms also under hypothalamic control. Body temperature increases during the course of the day and decreases during the night. The temperature peaks and troughs are thought to mirror the sleep rhythm. People who are alert late in the evening (i.e., evening types) have body temperature peaks late in the evening, while those who find themselves most alert early in the morning (i.e., morning types) have body temperature peaks early in the morning.

Section 2: Sleep and Traumatic Brain Injury

In an early study of the relationships between sleep and TBI, Cohen et al. (1992) found that of motor vehicle accident patients in Tel Aviv, Israel:

- 73% of patients hospitalized with TBI complained of sleep problems
- 82% of the sleep problems were insomnia (difficulty initiating and/or maintaining sleep)
- 73% complained of excessive daytime somnolence

Cohen et al. (1992) was the first to recommend that *early evaluation and treatment of sleep disturbances (in TBI patients) must be considered an integral part of the rehabilitation process.* Although his recommendations were not widely appreciated at the time, his continued research has made them more widely accepted.

Current research has further supported this link between sleep disturbances and TBI using a military population. A retrospective review of 41 mTBI and 44 control patients revealed significant differences between the sleeping habits of the two groups. Ninety-eight percent of all mTBI patients reported at least one sleep-related complaint compared to 77% of all control patients (Cuff et al. 2009). Sleep complaints ranged from EDS to insomnia and nightmares. While this study represents a relatively small sample size, it demonstrates consistency with previous research, further emphasizing the relationship between TBI and disturbances to the normal sleep/wake cycle.

Selected Research on Sleep and TBI

TBI may impair judgment, concentration, working memory, and other prefrontal-mediated tasks through direct damage to the prefrontal regions and/or through sleep deprivation-related comorbid impairment. In a review of the sleep changes following acute brain injury (less than 2 weeks), George et al. (1981) and Ron et al. (1980) showed an increase in sleep onset latency, in light sleep, and in wakenings after sleep onset (WASO). These increases in sleep fragmentation were counterbalanced by decreases in REM sleep and decreases in slow wave sleep. After 2 weeks, in the subacute stage, the investigators noted a reversal of the earlier described architectural pathologies and noted improvement towards normal sleep architecture. Their findings led them to hypothesize that tracking sleep architecture could provide a prognostic tool.

The Effect of Sleep Deficits on Cognitive Function

In tasks requiring judgment, the chance of risky behaviors increases with increasing sleep deprivation (Brown et al. 1970). A potential explanation for this behavior in sleep-deprived mTBI patients is the occurrence of microsleep. Microsleep is defined as brief (several seconds) runs of theta or delta activities that break through the otherwise normal beta or alpha EEG of waking. Studies which use polysomnography to monitor sleep patterns demonstrate that microsleep impairs continuity of cognitive function prior to performance failure (Thomas et al. 1998; Welsh et al. 1998; Balkin et al. 2004). Thus, sleep intrusions are an important consideration for TBI patients who present with new onset blackout episodes that are not associated with convulsive movements. These patients may not recognize

STANFORD SLEEPINESS SCALE
An Introspective Measure of Sleepiness

Please select the statement that reflects how alert you feel at the moment

Degree of Sleepiness	Scale Rating
Feeling active, vital, alert, or wide awake	1
Functioning at high levels, but not at peak; able to concentrate	2
Awake, but relaxed; responsive but not fully alert	3
Somewhat foggy, let down	4
Foggy; losing interest in remaining awake; slowed down	5
Sleepy, woozy, fighting sleep; prefer to lie down	6
No longer fighting sleep, sleep onset soon; having dream-like thoughts	7

Fig. 7.1 The Stanford Sleepiness Scale (SSS). The SSS scale rating subjectively assesses how sleepy an individual is at the time of the assessment by asking the stage of alertness with which they would characterize his or her mood. A scale rating below 3 (3–7) indicates a significant sleep debt (Hoddes et al. 1973)

how sleepy they are and may fall asleep driving or during other equally dangerous situations. These patients will always complain of severe sleepiness when questioned.

To be sure, sleep deprivation is a relative concept. Small amounts of sleep loss (e.g., 1 h per night over many nights) have subtle cognitive costs, which appear to go unrecognized by the individual experiencing the sleep loss. More severe restriction of sleep for a week leads to profound cognitive deficits, which are similar to those seen in some stroke patients and which also appear to go unrecognized by the individual.

Tools for Analysis of Sleep Patterns

Subjective Measures of Sleepiness

Stanford Sleepiness Scale (Hoddes et al. 1973)

The Stanford Sleepiness Scale (SSS) is a subjective scale to assess the degree of sleepiness at the moment of testing and may be used to compare sleepiness from visit to visit. The patient is presented with seven statements and selects the one that best represents his/her current feelings (Fig. 7.1).

Epworth Sleepiness Scale (Johns 1991)

The Epworth Sleepiness Scale (ESS) subjectively measures sleepiness by asking how likely the individual is to fall asleep in specific, well-known situations. The Epworth Scale reflects the patient's self-assessment of sleepiness over the prior several days, weeks, or months (Fig. 7.2).

The Pittsburgh Sleep Quality Index (Buysse et al. 1989)

The Pittsburgh Sleep Quality Index (PSQI) (Fig. 7.3) assesses a larger range of sleep/wake symptoms and provides a more structured and detailed history of the wake/sleep problems than the ESS. The results enable the clinician to better focus a differential diagnosis. The PSQI asks for input by the bed partner or roommate, and, therefore, is of decreased value in individuals who sleep alone.

Objective Measures of Sleepiness/Wakefulness

Multiple Sleep Latency Test (Carskadon et al. 1986; Thorpy et al. 1992)

The Multiple Sleep Latency Test (MSLT) is an objective measure of sleepiness, performed the day following an adequate all night polysomnogram. At each of five, 20-min nap opportunities in a darkened room, the patient is instructed to let sleep occur. Sleep latency is the length in minutes from lights-off to any stage of sleep, measured by standard polysomnographic methods. Mild sleepiness is scored as a sleep latency of between 10 and 15 min, moderate sleepiness between 5 and 10 min, and severe sleepiness as less than 5 min.

THE EPWORTH SLEEPINESS SCALE

How likely are you to doze off or fall asleep in the following situations, in contrast to feeling just tired? This refers to your usual way of life *in the recent past.* Even if you have not done some of these things recently try to work out how they woul dhave affected you. Use the following scale to choose *the most appropriate number* for each situation:

0 = no chance of dozing
1= slight chance of dozing
2 = moderate chance of dozing
3 = high chance of dozing

Situation	**Chance of Dozing**
Sitting and reading	___________
Watching TV	___________
Sitting inactive in a public place (e.g. a theater or a meeting)	___________
As a passenger in a car for an hour without a break	___________
Lying down to rest in the afternoon when circumstances permit	___________
Sitting and talking to someone	___________
Sitting quietly after a lunch without alcohol	___________
In a car, while stopped for a few minutes in traffic	___________
Total Score	___________

Fig. 7.2 The Epworth Sleepiness Scale (ESS). The ESS subjectively assesses how sleepy an individual has been over the past month by asking how likely he or she is to fall asleep in eight common situations. The scores across the eight situations are summed to obtain the ESS score, with 0 being the lowest score and 24 the highest. Healthy, well-rested adults have Epworth scores in the 2–10 range. Idiopathic hypersomnia, narcolepsy, and obstructive sleep apnea patients have scores up to 23 and 24. The ESS score distinguishes individual and diagnostic groups over a wide range of daytime sleepiness (Johns 1991)

Maintenance of Wakefulness Test (Mitler et al. 1982)

The Maintenance of Wakefulness Test (MWT) is an objective measure of wakefulness performed the day following an adequate all-night polysomnogram. In a darkened room while in a semireclining position, the patient is instructed to attempt to remain awake during five, 40-min sessions. Mild sleepiness is scored as a sleep latency between 10 and 15 min, moderate sleepiness between 5 and 10 min, and severe sleepiness as less than 5 min.

Classification of Sleep Disorders

Long Sleeper

Long sleepers are defined as those requiring 9.5 h of sleep or more per night for well-rested daily function. If those individuals are restricted to less than optimum sleep time by lifestyle constraints such as school, work, or family, they will manifest with EDS and other associated symptoms of sleep deprivation. Behaviorally induced insufficient sleep syndrome (BISS) may be difficult to diagnose in these individuals as they may present with a history of apparently normal sleep quantity.

Environmental Sleep Disorder

The essential feature of the environmental sleep disorder is an adverse sleep environment, which may be overly warm, cold, cramped, loud, motion-filled, etc. The level of the noxious environmental stimulus is less important than its effect on the patient—that is, the same stimulus may disrupt one individual's sleep while barely impacting another individual's sleep. The clinical feature is a complaint of insomnia. The insomnia may not be recognized by the patient as being caused by a noxious environmental stimulus, and the EDS may occur in the presence of an apparently normal amount of time in bed. Identification and exorcism of the noxious environmental feature is both diagnostic and therapeutic.

THE PITTSBURGH SLEEP QUALITY INDEX (PSQI)

The following questions relate to your usual sleep habits during *the past month only*. Your answers should indicate the most accurate reply for the *majority* of days and nights in the past month.

1. What time do you usually go to bed? ________
2. How long (in minutes) does it take you to fall asleep? ________
3. What time do you usually get up in the morning? ________
4. How many hours do you usually sleep per night? ________
5. How often had you had trouble sleeping because (check the best response):

	Not during the past month	Less than once a week	Once or twice a week	Three or more times a week
Cannot go to sleep within 30 minutes	____	____	____	____
Wake up in the middle of the night or early morning	____	____	____	____
Have to get up to use the bathroom	____	____	____	____
Cannot breathe comfortably	____	____	____	____
Cough or snore loudly	____	____	____	____
Feel too cold	____	____	____	____
Feel too hot	____	____	____	____
Had bad dreams	____	____	____	____
Have pain	____	____	____	____

6. How would you rate your sleep quality overall?
   - Very good ________
   - Fairly good ________
   - Fairly bad ________
   - Very bad ________

7. How often have you taken medicine [prescribed or "over the counter"] to help you sleep?
   Not during the past month ______ Less than once a week______ Once or twice a week______ Three or more times a week ______

8. How often have you had trouble staying awake while driving, eating meals, or engaging in social activity?
   Not during the past month ______ Less than once a week______ Once or twice a week______ Three or more times a week ______

9. How much of a problem has it been for you to keep up enough enthusiasm to get things done?
   - No problem at all ________
   - Only a very slight problem ________
   - Somewhat of a problem ________
   - A very big problem ________

10. Do you have a bed partner or roommate?
    - No bed partner or roommate ________
    - Partner/roommate in other room ________
    - Partner in same room, but not same bed ________
    - Partner in same bed ________

If you have a roommate or bed partner, ask him/her how often in the past month you have had...

	Not during the past month	Less than once a week	Once or twice a week	Three or more times a week
Loud snoring	____	____	____	____
Long pauses between breaths while asleep	____	____	____	____
Legs twitching or jerking while asleep	____	____	____	____
Episodes of disorientation or confusion while asleep	____	____	____	____

Fig. 7.3 The Pittsburgh Sleep Quality Index (PSQI). The PSQI measures sleep quality over the previous month and discriminate between "good" and "poor" sleepers. The evaluation consists of 19 self-rated questions and 5 questions rated by the bed partner or roommate. The 19 self-rated items are scored on a range of 0–3 points, with 0 indicating "no difficulty" and 3 indicating "severe difficulty," and then combined to form seven "component scores." The seven components measure: (1) subjective sleep quality, (2) sleep onset latency, (3) sleep duration, (4) habitual sleep efficiency, (5) sleep disturbances, (6) sleeping medication use, and (7) daytime dysfunction. The seven component scores are added to yield one "global" score, with a range of 0–21 points. A global score greater than 5 indicates significant sleep disturbance (Buysse et al. 1989)

Inadequate Sleep Hygiene Disorder

Insomnia associated with poor sleep habits in the absence of other extrinsic or intrinsic causes of insomnia and excessive sleepiness leads one to consider Inadequate Sleep Hygiene Disorder. Because there are so many reasons for poor sleep habits, ruling out other more readily quantifiable causes of insomnia and EDS is essential. Similar to BISS, the habits composing the poor sleep hygiene may be voluntary, albeit unintended. However, unlike BISS, the time allotted to sleep may be completely sufficient. When both poor sleep habits and regularly decreased time in bed occur simultaneously, Inadequate Sleep Hygiene Disorder may be diagnosed as a secondary disorder.

Insomnia Due to a Drug or Substance

The essential feature of this disorder is an insomnia that can be related to a drug, substance, or drug withdrawal. Medications and withdrawal cause restlessness, insomnia and tiredness. An incomplete list of medications that may contribute to this disorder includes hypnotics, antihistamines, major tranquilizers, beta-blockers, over-the-counter medications containing alcohol, and medication withdrawal such as caffeine withdrawal. This syndrome occurs episodically when sleep is sufficiently disrupted or reduced and may be associated with the daytime use of a stimulant drug such as caffeine. For example, if a patient excessively drinks coffee all week and then stops or reduces intake on the weekend, sleepiness may manifest on weekends, even if the patient has increased the amount of weekend time in bed. Insomnia Due to a Drug or Substance may be diagnosed as a contributing diagnosis in Inadequate Sleep Hygiene Disorder.

Circadian Rhythm Sleep Disorders

Excessive sleepiness, insomnia, and functional impairment are essential components of circadian rhythm sleep disorders. Two of the circadian rhythm sleep disorders—Jet-lag type and shift-work type—are directly caused by exogenous factors. Jet-lag type is self-limiting and resolves with adjustment to the new time zone. Shift-work disorder, caused by inadequate recovery time between shifts at work, is not necessarily self-limiting and is often the cause of chronic sleep deprivation. Patients may experience pressure to remain awake during their scheduled sleep periods while performing work shifts desynchronized from the majority of their family and friends.

Insomnia Due to a Medical Condition

The essential feature of this disorder is insomnia clearly linked to an identifiable medical condition. Indolent health problems cause sleepiness by interfering with both quality and quantity of sleep. Pain, such as may be caused by headache syndromes, neuropathies, musculoskeletal disorders, trauma, or surgical interventions, can cause insomnia and result in sleep deprivation. Physical health problems such as asthma and mental health problems, including depression and post-traumatic stress disorder, can also lead to insomnia. Excessive sleepiness varies according to both the degree of sleep deprivation and the functional level of the medically impaired patient. Treatment of the medical condition and resolution of the insomnia should resolve the EDS.

Circadian Rhythm Disorder Due to a Medical Condition

Excessive sleepiness results from sleep deprivation associated with the impaired circadian rhythm-induced insomnia. Excessive sleepiness, insomnia, and functional impairment are essential components of all circadian rhythm sleep disorders, whether endogenous or exogenous.

Circadian Rhythm Disorder, Delayed Sleep Phase Type

Individuals with early rising times due to school, work, or other regular obligations and with delayed sleep phase circadian rhythm disorder complain of excessive sleepiness and insomnia. Unable to sleep at the time their families retire, and unable to fall asleep early enough to obtain enough restorative sleep, these patients function below optimal efficiency. Delayed sleep phase patients may respond initially to hypnotics but will most likely return to their late sleep times upon drug discontinuation or tolerance.

Sleep Disordered Breathing Disorders

Excessive sleepiness is a major presenting complaint in the sleep disordered breathing disorders and may be caused by the decreased quality and quantity of the fragmented sleep. Treatment of the underlying breathing disorder reduces the fragmented sleep and results in improved daytime alertness.

Sleep-Related Movement Disorders

Sleep-related movement disorders that significantly impair restorative sleep may result in EDS. Periodic limb movements of sleep often interrupts restorative sleep to the degree that complaints of daytime inattentiveness, easy fatigability, and excessive sleepiness interfere with daily functions. Dopamine agonists are often helpful in the treatment of the movement disorder. With improvement of the overnight sleep quality, the sleep deprivation symptoms resolve.

Chronic Traumatic Encephalopathy-Related Sleep Disorders

Chronic traumatic encephalopathy (CTE), also known as Dementia pugilistica, is characterized by motor, behavioral, and cognitive symptoms. Tremor, incoordination, Parkinsonian features usually appear early in the course of disease development. Behavioral changes include sleep disruption, most frequently insomnia. Volatility, agitation, and depression may develop. Usually progressive, the pathology develops from an accumulation of multiple head injuries, with many, if not most, being subclinical. The neuropathology demonstrates tau protein accumulations.

Case Studies

The growth in sleep medicine over the past few decades has offered new tools for physicians to assess disease. A patient's sleeping patterns can offer significant insight into ongoing disorders and improve prognostication of final outcomes. In order to create a complete clinical picture, physicians should take time to include nocturnal habits when recording patient history. The following studies represent instances where complaints of sleep disorders were indicative of serious neurological disease. Each case is presented with the patient's relevant medical history and an imaging study performed after sleep difficulties were identified. A summary of take home points concludes each of the three cases.

Case 1 The Auto Accident

Patient History

- Forty-nine-year-old man complains of weight loss and slowly evolving weakness for 10–15 years.
- Motor Vehicle Accident in 1985—went head first through windshield. Had brief loss of consciousness (LOC) with rapid return to fully alert and oriented. GCS 15. CT head normal.

Review of Symptoms

- *When asked*, reported sleep onset insomnia with daytime irritability but without EDS.
- After multiple negative workups, patient referred to neurology for head CT and neurologic workup.

Exam

- Emaciated. Hyperreflexia. Muscles atrophied; without fasciculations.

Imaging Studies

See Fig. 7.4.

Take-Home Points

Glasgow Coma Scale (GCS) score at the time of injury may not reflect degree of injury. Early neuroimaging may not show lesions. Sleep problems may not be spontaneously mentioned, and the provider must ask in order to fully assess a patient's medical condition.

Case 2 The Football Player

Patient History

- Thirty-nine-year-old active duty soldier referred for intractable headaches.

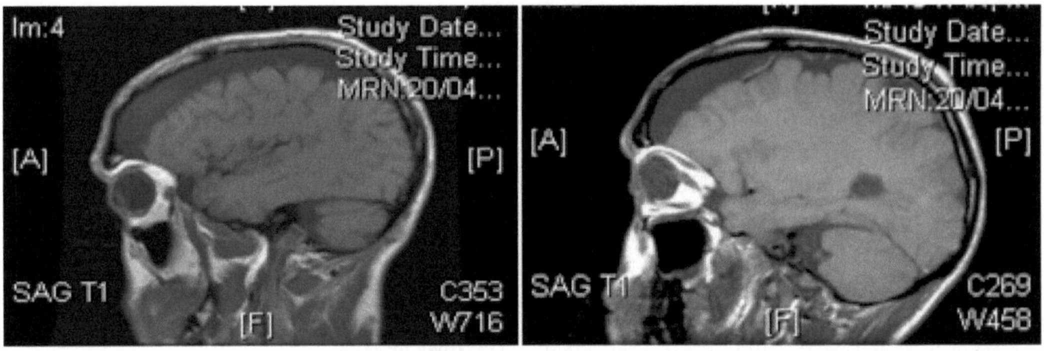

Fig. 7.4 Sagittal MRI shows large subdural hygromas bilaterally. Hypothesized etiology is that slowly evolving subdural hematomas formed following the 1985 injury. These subdural hematomas depressed motor regions causing sclerosis bilaterally of the primary motor regions. The hematomas eventually progressed to hygromas

- Constant headache after most recent injury (Nov 2008) when he used head as a battering ram during football game. Brief LOC, not hospitalized.
- Six concussions over 10 years, three without LOC, three with brief LOC. No nausea, vomiting, or seizures.
- Headaches:
  - Five year history of migraines.
  - After most recent injury—right-sided hemicranial stabbing pain, radiating into posterior neck; moderate to severe intensity all day, every day.
  - Denies: nausea, vomiting, photo/phonophobia, exercise intolerance.
- Denies: improvement with Imitrex or Excedrin.

Review of Symptoms

- *When asked,* complained of difficulty sleeping for 1 year.
- Snores loudly and awakens himself. Thrashes and jumps and moves during sleep. Feels sleepy and fatigued upon awakening and during days. Naps once or twice per day.
- Denies memory/concentration impairments.
- Admits to neck pain and occasional tingling sensation in hands.

Neurological Exam

Nonfocal.

Imaging

Normal head CT.

Differential Diagnosis

- *Headaches*—could be a primary or secondary symptom. Patient presents with an atypical migraine which could be the result of neuralgia, musculoskeletal pain, or cervical spine origin.
- *Insomnia*—Sleep onset insomnia, possibly psychophysiological (resulting from excessive and chronic worry prior to sleep).
- *Obstructive sleep apnea*—based on patient's report of loudly awakening himself.
- *REM sleep behavioral disorder*—could be the result of periodic limb movements, restless legs syndrome, or minor seizures.
- *Daytime sleepiness*—characterized as secondary hypersomnia resulting from any of the following: sleep deprivation, post-traumatic narcolepsy, post-traumatic encephalopathy, or early Dementia pugilistica.
- *TBI*—defined as "mild" because of brief LOC, normal neurological exam, normal CT, and no hospitalization.

Overnight Polysomnography Analysis

- Apnea Hypopnea Index (AHI)—34 (indicative of severe apnea), with desaturation episodes to 88% (abnormal).
- MSLT shows sleep onset latency of 6 min. No sleep onset REMs.
- MRI brain: white matter lesions in paramedian pons and right frontal regions (Fig. 7.5).

Diagnoses

1. Moderate TBI visualized on the MRI findings.

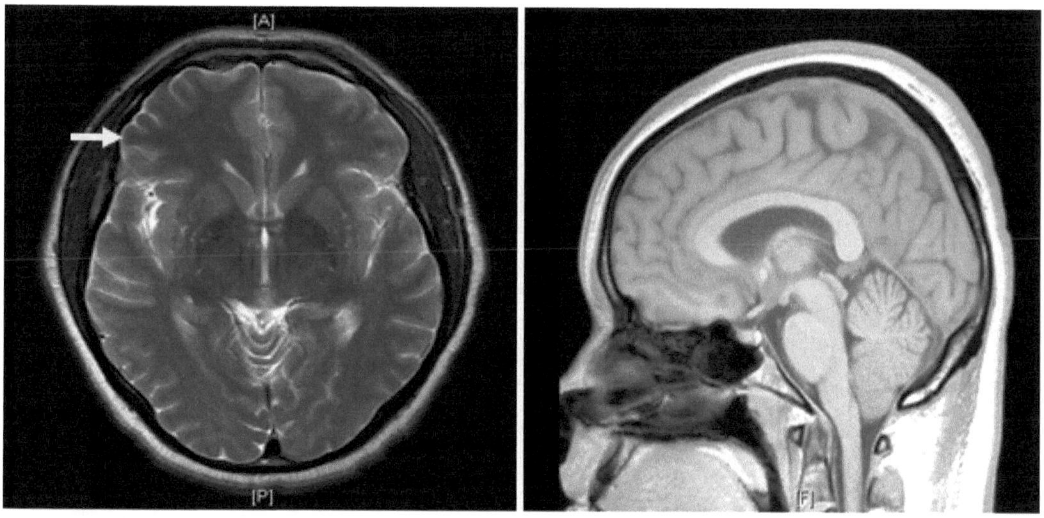

Fig. 7.5 On MRI, small white matter lesions are found in the right frontal area (*left*) and in the paramedian pons (*right*). These subtle macroscopic lesions most likely are the "tip of the iceburg" with significant microscopic damage disrupting the sleep/wake network

2. Post-traumatic obstructive sleep apnea due to the AHI of 34.
3. Sleep deprivation-related daytime sleepiness due to the poor sleep at night.
4. Insomnia: TBI-related psychophysiologic-type at sleep onset.

Take-Home Points

More than one type of sleep disorder may be diagnosed in an individual. Lesions may be found on MRI that are not found on CT. Because sleep problems may not be spontaneously mentioned, the provider must use directed questions in order to receive a complete patient history.

Case 3 The Boxer

Patient History

- Nineteen-year-old military boxer complaining of inability to sleep at night.
- Five concussions, several with LOC. Other less severe head injuries.

Review of Symptoms

- Has irresistible urge to sleep during days, and naps at work and before dinner.
- Has frequent nighttime awakenings for no particular reason.
- Vivid dreams, sometimes during daytime naps.

Neuro Exam

Positive—Nystagmus; Hyperreflexic Hoffman's; Clonus; Tremor.

CT Scan

Normal.

MRI

Multiple lesions throughout brain and brain stem (Fig. 7.6).

Differential Diagnosis

- *TBI*—defined as "moderate" because of MRI findings and history of LOC across several concussive episodes.
- *Motor systems damage*—presenting symptoms of hyperreflexia and tremor, which could be related to disease in the corticospinal tracts or basal ganglia.
- *Wake/sleep systems damage*
  - Sleepiness could be attributed to damage in the hypothalamus and basal forebrain.
  - Nystagmus may be the result of brainstem, midbrain, and pontine damage resulting in

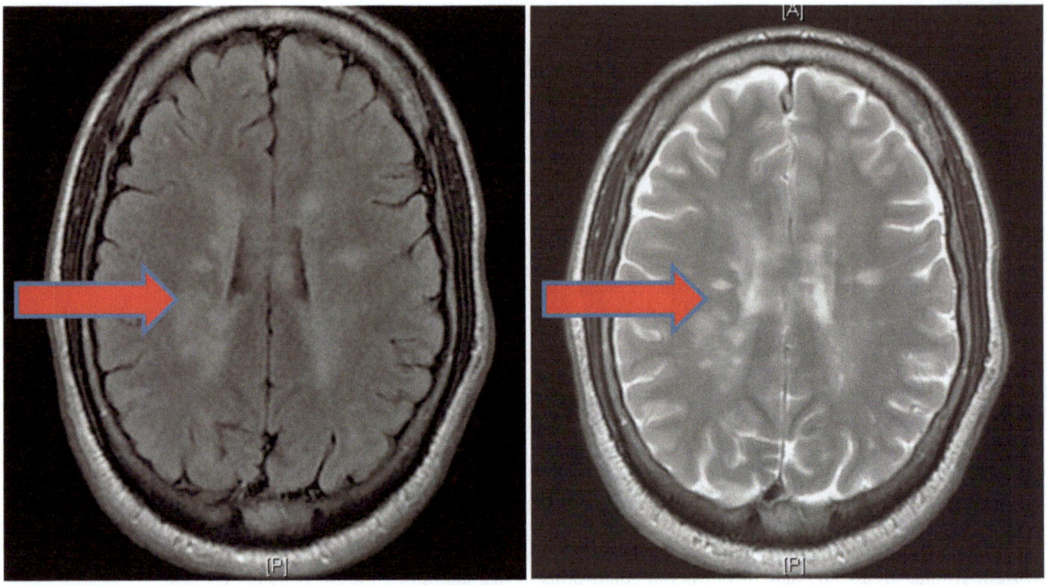

Fig. 7.6 On MRI (T1 and T2 images), white matter lesions are found throughout the left and right hemispheres and throughout the brainstem. These lesions resemble those seen in multiple sclerosis (MS). The lab evaluation for MS did not show oligoclonal bands. If deterioration continues, and the clinical definition of lesions in time and space are met, then the patient would also be given a diagnosis of multiple sclerosis

disruption of the medial longitudinal fasciculus and ascending reticular activating systems.

Overnight Polysomnography

- No apnea/hypopnea.
- Frequent arousals.

Multiple Sleep Latency Test

- Sleep onset latency 5 min.
- Three sleep onset REMs.

Diagnosis

- Post-traumatic narcolepsy.
- Clinical findings of sleep intrusions during day, hypnagogic (upon falling asleep) and hypnopompic (upon awakening) hallucinations, confirmed by MSLT.
- Suspected multiple sclerosis (MS), possibly post-traumatic in origin.

Take Home Points and Analysis

This patient developed post-traumatic narcolepsy, hypothetically through the inadequate production of the hypocretin/orexin neuropeptide and subsequent destabilization of the wake and sleep states. The patient with narcolepsy presents with sudden and inappropriate sleep onsets. The sleep is restorative, and upon awakening the patient feels refreshed. During the night, the patient cannot sustain the sleep state and awakens frequently. Other manifestations are the occurrence of early onset REM periods, often within 30 min of sleep onset. These early REM periods may also occur when the patient is falling asleep and appear to the patient as vivid hypnagogic hallucinations. When cataplexy is present, the normal atonia seen in REM sleep is disrupted and occurs inappropriately during the waking state. In response to sudden and strong emotion, most often spontaneous laughter, the patient with cataplexy may lose muscle tone. The loss may be mild, with jaw and abdomen muscles relaxing, or may be more severe, with hip and lower limb muscles relaxing. When the lower limbs are severely affected, the patient may fall to the ground, remaining conscious and alert. Cataplexy may develop if the atonia control network in the brainstem is disrupted.

Classification and Treatment of Sleep Disorders in TBI Patients

Excessive Daytime Sleepiness

EDS is one of the primary complaints reported by mTBI patients (Russo et al. 2009). EDS may be defined as sleepiness or unintentional sleep episodes occurring at undesirable or inappropriate times and locations. EDS may be associated with severe and moderate sleep deprivation. With sleep deprivation-associated sleepiness, sleep refreshes and adequate sleep satiates. Excessive sleepiness may also occur with apparently ample sleep, such as in the idiopathic and recurrent hypersomnias or in long sleepers deprived of adequate sleep time. In the hypersomnias, sleep is not refreshing and no amount of sleep satiates. TBI may cause hypersomnia in isolation or as part of a CTE syndrome.

Mild chronic sleep deprivation may also have effects apart from excessive sleepiness. Some patients report attention difficulties, loss of short-term memory or working memory problems, language difficulties, poor judgment and "unprofessionalism," irritability, moodiness, and confusion. Some of this may be described as feelings of lack of inhibition. Patients express that they feel tired and perform poorly, but they often deny feeling that they are about to fall asleep. Note that most patients seen for sleep deprivation-related complaints in clinical settings will manifest the effects of *chronic partial* sleep deprivation. Many of the symptoms of sleep deprivation overlap the symptoms of TBI. Treating the sleep deprivation will help resolve those symptoms due to poor sleep and distinguish those symptoms due to TBI.

Presenting Symptoms of TBI Patients

TBI patients report degrees of exhaustion, fatigue, and lack of physical energy. These common symptoms may be due to depression, anxiety, as well as chronic headaches. As sleep disorders occur frequently in TBI patients, these symptoms must also be appreciated as potentially due to sleep deprivation-related EDS. Exhaustion and fatigue affect emotional moods and may cause pessimism, sadness, stress, and anger. In some depressed patients, sleep deprivation can improve their mood and affect. Complaints of poor sleep and daytime drowsiness predominate. Some patients complain of clumsiness, lack of coordination, and weakness, while others complain of loss of energy, apathy, and feeling cold. Aldrich (1999) listed the following signs of drowsiness: eye rubbing, decreased blinking rate, glazed and unfocused eyes, slow eye movements, heavy eyelids with drooping, closed eyes, fidgeting, yawning, slumped posture, reduced activity, slack faces, head-nodding, and sleep-seeking behavior. With mild and moderate chronic sleep deprivation of between 4 and 6 h sleep per night, patients may report easy distractibility, tangentialism, short-term or working memory problems, word-finding difficulties, diminished judgment, increased risk-taking behaviors, increased irritability, increased moodiness, and indecisiveness.

Treatment Options for Sleep Disorders

Sleep Hygiene

The first step towards improving sleep should always be a review of sleep hygiene behaviors, followed by cognitive behavioral therapy. Behavioral modification should include the following standard recommendations, summarized in Fig. 7.7.

Pharmacological Treatment Options

Hypnotics

Medications are effective in the short-term treatment of insomnia, in nonpathologic sleeplessness, and in conditions where the environmental conditions are not conducive to desired sleep. For volitional sleep deprivation, drug therapy should not be a replacement for behavioral modification. In some situations to aid in altering behavior, short-term use of medication is an appropriate consideration. Table 7.1, modified from Mendelson (2005), discusses specific hypnotic medications.

(a) Physical Activity

- Associate the bed with sleep. Avoid watching TV, eating, and evoking perturbing emotions in bed. Associating the bed with activities other than sleep can prolong sleep latency.
- Take a short nap. A nap during the post-prandial, mid-afternoon circadian trough may not interfere with nighttime sleep and may improve alertness and performance. Short naps should be brief enough to avoid entering slow-wave sleep. Awakening from slow wave sleep is more difficult and sleep inertia effects may impair immediate post-awakening performance. If a longer nap is desired, awakening may be timed to occur from REM.
- Avoid vigorous exercise within two or three hours of bedtime, which may interfere with sleep induction. Exercise is best scheduled in the morning or afternoon.
- Establish a regular exercise routine. Healthy individuals who run or walk 40 minutes, three days a week, experience longer periods of deep sleep than less active individuals (Vitiello et al. 1994, 1996).
- Maintain the same bedtimeevery night and wake up at the same time every morning.
- Engage in a relaxing evening ritual to reduce stress. Rituals may include taking a hot bath or shower, performing stretches or meditation, or listening to quiet relaxing music. Repeat the stress reduction technique each evening in preparation for sleep induction.
- Record adjustments to bedtime and wake up time in a sleep diary.

(b) Oral Intake

- Avoid:
  - Fluids after 8 p.m. to reduce awakenings due to the urge to urinate
  - Nicotine, especially near bedtime and upon night awakenings
  - Caffeine intake 4-6 hours before bedtime.
  - Alcohol as a sleeping aid. Although alcohol is a depressant and may help to induce sleep, the subsequent metabolism causes a sleep-fragmenting withdrawal syndrome.
- Eat a light snack priorto sleep to prevent hunger from disturbing sleep.

(c) Sleep Environment

- Minimize noise, light, and temperature extremes during sleep by using ear plugs, window blinds, warm blankets, or air conditioning. White noise, natural sounds such as a gurgling brook, or non-vocal music may be helpful.
- Avoid sleeping with pets. Canine and feline wake/sleep hours differ from those of humans, and animal movements can awaken light sleepers.

Fig. 7.7 Nonpharmacological sleep hygiene interventions for sleep disorders. Recommendations include changes to (**a**) physical activity, (**b**) oral intake, and (**c**) sleep environment that may optimize the likelihood of sleep induction and duration

Special Use Sleep-Inducing Agents

Sodium oxybate (*Xyrem*). Significantly shortens the latency to sleep onset and rapidly induces deep sleep and decreases the occurrence of cataplexy in narcolepsy. The drug is started at 4.5 g divided into two doses: one at bedtime, one 4 h later and titrated to effect or 6–9 g per night. Sodium oxybate is a schedule III drug with moderate abuse potential. The company directly dispenses the medication to the patient after the patient and physician have been taught proper techniques for utilization. Common side effects may include depression and problems with bladder control.

Doxepine (*Sinequan, Silenor*). Low dose doxepin (3–6 mg) is approved by the FDA for the treatment of insomnia under the brand name Silenor. Doxepin inhibits the reuptake of serotonin and norepinephrine and is primarily used as an antidepressant. Dexepine is thought to exert its sedation effects through strong antagonism of H_1, H_2 receptors. Side effects associated with Silenor are rare, but the most common one is nausea.

Trazodone hydrochloride (*Desyrel*). Trazodone hydrochloride is a triazolopyridine derivative antidepressant unrelated to tricyclic, tetracyclic, or other known antidepressant agents. It is not FDA approved for the treatment of insomnia but is widely used off-label. Trazodone may be given at a starting dose of 50 mg nightly and raised to 100 mg nightly if necessary. In depression, it is used at much higher doses of up to 400 mg/day divided into three doses. Male patients should be warned about the possibility of priapism, and female patients should be warned that trazodone is not recommended for use during pregnancy.

Quetiapine (*Seroquel*). Quetiapine is not recommended for use in insomnia. Quetiapine is an antipsychotic agent with antagonism of dopamine, serotonin, and histamine receptors, and somnolence is reported in up to 50% of patients. If the patient has insomnia associated with schizophrenia, bipolar disorder, or psychotic depression, then Quetiapine may be considered for the primary FDA approved indication.

Combination Therapy

TBI-associated insomnia may be refractory to traditional cognitive behavioral therapies and to standard

Table 7.1 Pharmacokinetic properties and dosages of some hypnotic drugs used in the treatment of insomnia (modified from Table 36.1. Kryger, Roth, Dement. Principles and practice of sleep medicine, 4th ed., on-line; reproduced with permission from Elsevier)

Hypnotic drugs[a]	Half-life (h)	Onset of action (min)[b]	Pharmacologically active metabolites	Dose (mg)
Benzodiazepine hypnotics				
Quazepam (Doral)	48–120	30	*N*-Desalkyl (flurazepam)	7.5–15
Flurazepam (Dalmane)	48–120	15–45	*N*-Desalkyl (flurazepam)	15–30
Triazolam (Halcion)	2–6	2–30	None	0.125–0.25
Estazolam (ProSom)	8–24	Intermediate	None	1–2
Temazepam[c] (Restoril)	8–20	45–50	None	15–30
Loprazolam[d] (Dormonoct)	4.6–11.4	–	None	1–2
Flunitrazepam[d] (Rohypnol)	10.7–20.3	Short	*N*-Desmethyl (flunitrazepam)	0.5–1
Lormetazepam[d] (Loramet)	7.9–11.4	–	None	1–2
Nitrazepam[d] (Alodorm)	25 35	Intermediate	None	5–10
Nonbenzodiazepine hypnotics				
Eszopliclone (Lunesta)	6–9	Rapid	*N*-Desmethyl zopiclone	2–3 adult[e], 1–2 elderly
Eszopiclone (Estorra)[f]	5–7	Intermediate	None	2–3 adult, 1 elderly
Zolpidem (Ambien)	1.5–2.4	Rapid	None	5–10 (age >65 year)
Zopiclone[d] (Imovane)	5–6	Intermediate	None	3.75 (age >65 year)
Zaleplon (Sonata)	1	Rapid	None	5–10

[a]Citations for kinetic information are found in Maczaj M. Pharmacological treatment of insomnia. Drugs. 1993
[b]Derived from Smith CM, Reynard AM. Essentials of Pharmacology. Philadelphia, PA: WB Saunders; 1995. p. 228, and other sources
[c]Originally formulated as a hard capsule in the USA, concerns with kinetics and efficacy led to reformulation of the preparation to a soft gelatin capsule with characteristics comparable with those of other marketed benzodiazepines of its class
[d]Not available in the USA
[e]There is no FDA-recommended dose for this purpose. Doses are approximations of those often used in clinical practice
[f]Not yet on the market in the USA at the time of writing, the manufacturer has recently received an "approvable" letter from the FDA for 2 and 3 mg in adults and 1 mg in the elderly

insomnia monotherapy. If this is the case, then combination therapy may be considered. One recipe is to begin with trazodone 50 mg at dinner to induce sleepiness, then adding a hypnotic at bedtime to induce sleep. If sleep onset insomnia is the major form of insomnia to be treated, then most of the hypnotics may be considered. If both sleep onset and sleep maintenance insomnia are to be treated, then utilization at bedtime of a long acting hypnotic such as extended release zolpidem (Ambien CR) 12.5 mg or temezepam (Restoril) 30 mg may be considered.

Treatments for Alertness

Caffeine—(*"Stay Alert," "Jolt"*)—100 or 200 mg upon awakening and as needed. Effective about 3–4 h. Physiological manifestations, tolerance, withdrawal. Easy to obtain, large therapeutic window, essentially safe.

Modafinil (*Provigil*)—100 or 200 mg upon awakening. Novel drug with minimal physiological side effects. Effective about 4–6 h. (Schedule IV—low abuse potential.)

Armodafinil (*Nuvigil*)—150 or 250 mg upon awakening. *R*-enantiomer of modafinil. Effective 8–10 h. (Schedule IV—low abuse potential.)

Dextroamphetamine (Dexadrine)—10 or 20 mg upon awakening, physiological manifestations, effective 8–10 h or longer. (Schedule II—high abuse potential.) Tolerance, withdrawal.

Methylphenidate (*Ritalin, Ritalin SR*)—Methylphenidate may be started at 5 mg twice daily, upon awakening and at noon to increase attention and focus. Increases may be made in 5 mg/day increments, until effective, side effects outweigh benefits, or until a dose of 20 mg twice daily has been achieved.

Specific Diagnostic Categories

In TBI patients, excessive sleepiness may be caused by exogenous and/or endogenous factors and may be a symptom of sleep disorders, behavioral disorders, or physical disorders. *Exogenous factors* are those that arise from outside the body, including volitional, yet unintended, reductions in sleep time. Exogenous factors may lead to sleep deprivation-related sleep disorders, such as the extrinsic insomnias (e.g., inadequate sleep hygiene, behavioral, drug-induced), extrinsic circadian rhythm disorders (e.g., jet-lag, shift-work), and environmental sleep disorder.

Endogenous factors arise from within the body, such as those associated with medical disorders and pain syndromes. Endogenous sleep disorders that lead to EDS and sleep deprivation include the intrinsic insomnias, sleep-related breathing disorders, and intrinsic circadian rhythm disorders.

Disorders Associated with Exogenous Factors

Behaviorally induced insufficient sleep syndrome: In the 1990 and 1997 editions of the International Classification of Sleep Disorders (ICSD) Diagnostic and Coding manual, insufficient sleep syndrome were defined as the voluntary, albeit unintentional, curtailment of sleep to levels below those required to support normally alert wakefulness. In the ICSD 2005 edition, the name was revised to BISS. The primary complaint is excessive sleepiness, and the primary historical feature is shorter than required habitual sleep time. The patients usually attempt to make up sleep when possible, such as on weekends. If polysomnography or MSLT are performed, the results show at least moderate sleepiness (latency of <8–10 min) and highly efficient sleep (>90%). Ruling out other causes of sleepiness is essential. Increases in sleep time are both diagnostic and therapeutic. Lifestyle choices are often the direct cause of fatigue and sleeplessness, although with many lifestyle choices sleep deprivation is an acknowledged and inevitable component. For example, having a family is a lifestyle choice—with co-sleeping, nursing, and the immediate postpartum period all resulting in sleep deprivation. To be sure, the above description is an example of the classic volitional sleep deprivation syndrome, many more nuanced forms exist.

Physiological Consequences of TBI, EDS, and Sleep Deprivation

Sleep deprivation results in a broad spectrum of physiologic changes, including decreases in brain glucose metabolism (Thomas et al. 2000, 2003), decreases in core body temperature (Minors et al. 1999), alterations in immune system function (Moldofsky 1995; Balachandran et al. 2002; Spiegel et al. 2002), fluctuations in hormone levels (Spiegel et al. 2000; Orthmann et al. 2001; Spiegel et al. 2004; Taheri et al. 2004; Gangwisch et al. 2005), and increased heart rate variability (Montano et al. 2005).

As the function of sleep has not been fully determined, the absolute number of hours necessary to fulfill its function remains unknown. Short sleepers report full effectiveness with only 3–5 h of sleep per night, while long sleepers admit needing more than 8 h to perform effectively.

Cognitive performance—Among the most serious consequences of TBI-related sleep deprivation are insidious decrements in cognitive functions, both simple and complex such as situational awareness, judgment, and decision-making. These performance deficits result from selectively decreased metabolism in the prefrontal, parietal associational, and thalamic areas of the brain. Hypometabolism often persists in these areas and in some cases can become more pronounced across 48 and 72 h of sustained wakefulness (Thomas et al. 2003).

Speed before accuracy—With decreased sleep, higher-order cognitive tasks are affected early and disproportionately. Tests requiring both speed and accuracy demonstrate considerably slower speed before accuracy begins to fail (Horne and Pettitt 1985; Thorne et al. 1997, 1998; Belenky et al. 2003; Balkin et al. 2004). In chronic partial sleep deprivation studies, total sleep duration of 7 h per night over 1 week resulted in decreased speed in tasks of both simple reaction time and in more demanding computer-generated mathematical problem solving. Total sleep duration of 5 h per night over 1 week shows both decrease in speed and the beginning of accuracy failure (Balkin 2000).

Driving performance—The National Transportation Safety Board (NTSB) reports driver fatigue as a contributing cause of multiple automobile and truck accidents (SB03-15, SB04,-10, SB05-13). When total sleep time is reduced to 5 h per night over 1 week, increased lane deviations and increased speed variability are seen, while when total sleep time is reduced to 3 h per night, significantly increased accident rates occurred in driving simulator experiments (Balkin 2000; Belenky et al. 2003).

Visual performance—Acute sleep loss beginning at 19 h awake was associated with decreased ability to simultaneously appreciate peripheral and central visual stimuli, suggesting a transient sleep deprivation-induced visual simultanagnosia and peripheral neglect (Russo et al. 2004, 2005). During multiple consecutive days of partial sleep deprivation, group mean saccadic velocity showed consistent daily decreases Fig. 7.8 ordered according to the number of hours of sleep restriction (Russo et al. 2003). Groups that received 3 and 5 h of time in bed for seven nights demonstrated highly significant negative slopes, about 0.75 and 0.50 mm/s per day, respectively. Latency to pupil constriction shows similarly ordered effects across groups, with a significant positive slope in the 3-h group.

In restricted sleep conditions of 3 h per night over 1 week, decreases in saccadic velocity correlated

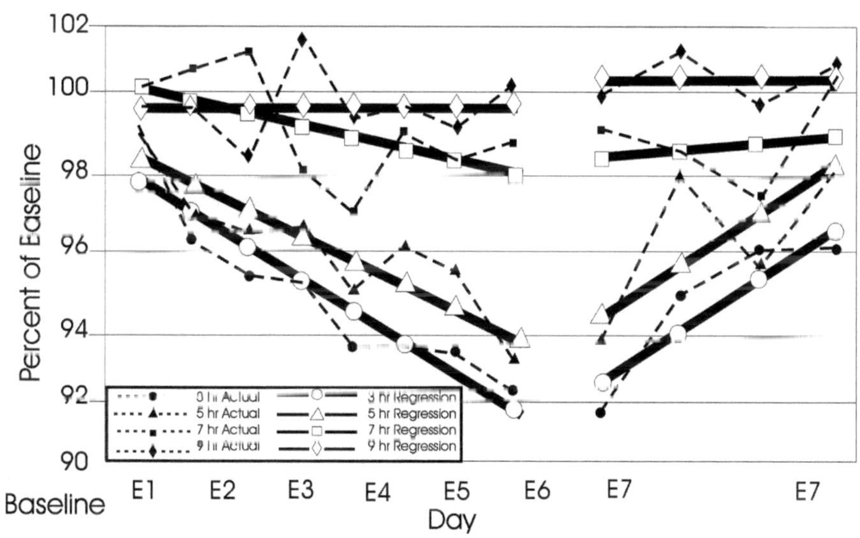

Fig. 7.8 Changes in group mean saccadic velocity with four doses of sleep (3, 5, 7, and 9 h) over a 7-night experimental period a 3-night recovery period (Russo, Thomas et al. 2003)

highly with increases in simulator driving accidents. Additionally, latency to pupil constriction increases were correlated with driving accident increases in the 3-h group. Rowland et al. (2005) found similarly high correlations with a study of continuous total sleep deprivation between saccadic velocity, simulator driving accidents, latency to pupil constriction, and accidents.

Of interest in the Rowland et al. (2005) study was the result that only one night of recovery sleep after two nights of total sleep deprivation returned saccadic velocity and constriction latency to baseline, while in the chronic partial sleep deprivation study, 3 days of recovery sleep did not yield return to baseline of the same measures. Those findings suggest that the brain, vis-a-vis oculomotor function, may have been reacting to chronic partial sleep deprivation with an adaptation response mechanism that required substantially more time from which to recover than an accommodation response from brief total sleep deprivation.

Final Thoughts

Sleep research represents a relatively new form of scientific exploration. In this chapter, we have attempted to demonstrate the intricate relationship between traumatic brain injuries and sleep disorders. Physicians can gain valuable insight into their patient's current neurological disorders by asking questions about sleep patterns and examining polysomnographical data. Moreover, behavioral or pharmacological interventions aimed at treating sleep may improve neurologic outcomes and long-term quality of life measurements. Continued research into this budding field will prove fruitful for all parties involved.

References

Aldrich MS. Sleep medicine. New York, NY: Oxford University Press; 1999.

Balachandran D, Ewing S, Murray BJ, Lebeau L, Mullington JM. Human host response during chronic partial sleep deprivation. Sleep. 2002;25:A106–7.

Balkin T. Effects of sleep schedules on commercial motor vehicle driver performance. Washington, DC: U.S. Dept. of Transportation, Federal Motor Carrier Safety Administration; 2000.

Balkin TJ, Bliese PD, et al. Comparative utility of instruments for monitoring sleepiness-related performance decrements in the operational environment. J Sleep Res. 2004;13(3):219–27.

Belenky G, Wesensten NJ, et al. Patterns of performance degradation and restoration during sleep restriction and subsequent recovery: a sleep dose–response study. J Sleep Res. 2003;12(1):1–12.

Brown ID, Tickner AH, et al. Effect of prolonged driving on overtaking criteria. Ergonomics. 1970;13(2):239–42.

Buysse DJ, Reynolds 3rd CF, et al. The Pittsburgh Sleep Quality Index: a new instrument for psychiatric practice and research. Psychiatry Res. 1989;28(2):193–213.

Carskadon MA, Dement WC, et al. Guidelines for the multiple sleep latency test (MSLT): a standard measure of sleepiness. Sleep. 1986;9(4):519–24.

Cohen M, Oksenberg A, et al. Temporally related changes of sleep complaints in traumatic brain injured patients. J Neurosurg Psychiatry. 1992;55(4):313–15.

Cuff P, Russo M, Stetz M, Stetz T. The prevalence of sleep/wake disturbances in mild traumatic brain injury. J Neuro Sci. 2009;285:S272.

Eriksson KS, Sergeeva OA, et al. Orexins/hypocretins and aminergic systems. Acta Physiol (Oxf). 2010;198(3): 263–75.

Gangwisch JE, Malaspina D, et al. Inadequate sleep as a risk factor for obesity: analyses of the NHANES I. Sleep. 2005;28(10):1289–96.

George B, et al. Night sleep disorders during recovery of severe head injuries. Neurochirurgie. 1981;27:35–38.

Hoddes E, Zarcone V, et al. Quantification of sleepiness: a new approach. Psychophysiology. 1973;10(4):431–6.

Horne JA, Pettitt AN. High incentive effects on vigilance performance during 72 hours of total sleep deprivation. Acta Psychol (Amst). 1985;58(2):123–39.

Johns MW. A new method for measuring daytime sleepiness: the Epworth sleepiness scale. Sleep. 1991;14(6): 540–5.

Mendelson WB. Hynotic medications: Mechanisms of action and pharmacologic effects principles and practice of sleep medicine. Philadelpha, Saunders CO., 2005.

Minors D, Waterhouse J, et al. Effect of sleep loss on core temperature when movement is controlled. Ergonomics. 1999;42(4):647–56.

Mitler MM, Gujavarty KS, et al. Maintenance of wakefulness test: a polysomnographic technique for evaluation treatment efficacy in patients with excessive somnolence. Electroencephalogr Clin Neurophysiol. 1982;53(6):658–61.

Moldofsky H. Sleep and the immune system. Int J Immunopharmacol. 1995;17(8):649–54.

Montano N, Cogliati C, et al. One night sleep deprivation alters primarily cardiac sympathovagal balance. Sleep. 2005;28:A134.

Ohayon MM. Epidemiology of insomnia: what we know and what we still need to learn. Sleep Med Rev. 2002;6(2):97–111.

Orff HJ, Ayalon L, et al. Traumatic brain injury and sleep disturbance: a review of current research. J Head Trauma Rehabil. 2009;24(3):155–65.

Orthmann JL, Rogers NL, et al. Changes in plasma growth hormone levels following chronic sleep restriction. Sleep. 2001;24:A248–149.

Pagel JF. Excessive daytime sleepiness. Am Fam Physician. 2009;79(5):391–6.

Ron S, Algom D, et al. Time-related changes in the distribution of sleep stages in brain injured patients. Electroencephalogr Clin Neurophysiol. 1980;48(4):432–41.

Rowland LM, Thomas ML, et al. Oculomotor responses during partial and total sleep deprivation. Aviat Space Environ Med. 2005;76(7 Suppl):C104–13.

Russo M, Stetz M, et al. Excessive daytime sleepiness in mild traumatic brain injury patients (mTBI). Sleep. 2009;32:A311.

Russo M, Thomas M, et al. Oculomotor impairment during chronic partial sleep deprivation. Clin Neurophysiol. 2003;114(4):723–36.

Russo MB, Kendall AP, et al. Visual perception, psychomotor performance, and complex motor performance during an overnight air refueling simulated flight. Aviat Space Environ Med. 2005;76(7 suppl): C92–103.

Russo MB, Sing H, et al. Visual neglect: occurrence and patterns in pilots in a simulated overnight flight. Aviat Space Environ Med. 2004;75(4):323–32.

Spiegel K, Leproult R, et al. Adaptation of the 24-h growth hormone profile to a state of sleep debt. Am J Physiol Regul Integr Comp Physiol. 2000;279(3): R874–83.

Spiegel K, Sheridan JF, et al. Effect of sleep deprivation on response to immunization. JAMA. 2002;288(12): 1471–2.

Spiegel K, Tasali E, et al. Brief communication: Sleep curtailment in healthy young men is associated with decreased leptin levels, elevated ghrelin levels, and increased hunger and appetite. Ann Intern Med. 2004;141(11):846–50.

Taheri S, Lin L, et al. Short sleep duration is associated with reduced leptin, elevated ghrelin, and increased body mass index. PLoS Med. 2004;1(3):e62.

Thomas M, Sing H, et al. Neural basis of alertness and cognitive performance impairments during sleepiness. I. Effects of 24 h of sleep deprivation on waking human regional brain activity. J Sleep Res. 2000;9(4): 335–52.

Thomas M, Thorne D, et al. The relationship between driving accidents and microsleep during cumulative partial sleep deprivation. J Sleep Res. 1998;7 suppl 2:275.

Thomas ML, Sing H, et al. Neural basis of alertness and cognitive performance impairments during sleepiness II Effects of 48–72 hours of sleep deprivation on waking human regional brain activity. Thalamus Relat Syst. 2003;2(3):199–229.

Thorne D, Thomas M, et al. Accident rate, attention and performance in a driving simulator during 64 hours of progressive sleep deprivation. J Sleep Res. 1997;26 Suppl 1:634.

Thorne D, Thomas M, et al. Driving-simulator accident rates before, during, and after one week of restricted night sleep. Sleep. 1998;21 Suppl 3:235.

Thorpy MJ, Westbrook PR, et al. The clinical use of the Multiple Sleep Latency Test. The Standards of Practice Committee of the American Sleep Disorders Association. Sleep. 1992;15(3):268–76.

Welsh A, Thomas M, et al. Effect of 64 hours of sleep deprivation on accidents and sleep events during a driving simulator. Sleep. 1998;21 suppl 3:234.

Zeitzer JM, Friedman L, et al. Insomnia in the context of traumatic brain injury. J Rehabil Res Dev. 2009;46(6): 827–36.

Vestibular Consequences of mTBI

8

Michael E. Hoffer, Kim Gottshall, and Erik S. Viirre

Abstract

Damage to vestibular function is a common and under-recognized consequence of mild Traumatic Brain Injury. Untreated vestibular disorders can lead to vertigo, imbalance, and slow improvement after mTBI. Fortunately, diagnosis and management of vestibular dysfunction, if made routine, can be quickly and successfully carried out. Common conditions, including Benign Positional Vertigo, can be detected by history and verified and treated by bedside testing. Simple medical management and, crucially, directed physical therapy can greatly improve the condition of most patients. In this chapter, an algorithmic approach is presented to assist in the diagnosis and management of vestibular system problems after head injury.

Keywords

Vestibular • Vertigo • Balance • Dizziness • Benign positional vertigo • Migraine • Spatial disorientation

Introduction

The vestibular organs are crucial for motion sensation and maintenance of balance. Imbedded in the temporal bones, they are well protected, and yet ultimately are vulnerable to concussive shock from abrupt force applied to the head through blunt trauma or overpressure from explosive blasts. A variety of injuries can occur to the vestibular organ with traumatic brain injury (TBI), both acute and chronic. Dysfunction of the vestibular organs results in continuous or intermittent vertigo and reduction of balance, including increasing the risk of falls. In addition, injury can occur in a number of places in

M.E. Hoffer, M.D., F.A.C.S.
Department of Otolaryngology, Naval Medical Center, San Diego, CA, USA

K. Gottshall, Ph.D.
Physical Therapy Department, Naval Medical Center San Diego, San Diego, CA, USA

Department of Neurosciences, School of Medicine, University of California-San Diego, San Diego, CA, USA

E.S. Viirre, M.D., Ph.D. (✉)
Department of Neurosciences, School of Medicine, University of California-San Diego, San Diego, CA, USA

Naval Health Research Center, San Diego, CA, USA
e-mail: eviirre@ucsd.edu

J.W. Tsao (ed.), *Traumatic Brain Injury: A Clinician's Guide to Diagnosis, Management, and Rehabilitation*, DOI 10.1007/978-0-387-87887-4_8, © Springer Science+Business Media, LLC 2012

the central vestibular pathway which can also cause impairment in balance function and equilibrium.

It is our opinion that vestibular dysfunction is often unrecognized after TBI due to the attention paid to primary injuries to the scalp, skull, and brain. Rapid recognition of the possibility of vestibular disorders after TBI should lead to screening for these problems and their prompt treatment. The great advantage of such screening and recognition is that appropriate treatment can often be immediately rendered. For example, lack of recognition of the presence of benign positional vertigo (BPV), one consequence of TBI, can mean that as head injury patients try to mobilize, they are struck with terrible vertigo. This vertigo can result in falls and drastic exacerbation of patients' other symptoms, such as headache and memory loss. The patient is, thus, bedridden or mobility impaired for a long period, even months. Fortunately, a simple treatment, the Canalith Repositioning Maneuver (Helminski et al. 2010) can immediately cure BPV and hugely improve mobilization and even mental status. Other vestibular disorders can also be detected and managed expeditiously to improve recovery. For example, a study of blast-injured subjects in Operation Iraqi Freedom demonstrated improvement if their blast-triggered migraine-related vertigo was diagnosed and treated (Hoffer et al. 2010).

For the purposes of this chapter, we confine our discussion to mild traumatic brain injury (mTBI). mTBI is the most common disorder seen in the current wars in Southwest Asia and is increasingly becoming a more important topic due to the number of sports-related episodes of concussion, a form of mTBI (Hoffer et al. 2010; McCrory et al. 2009). The symptoms of mTBI can be myriad, but one of the most common is dizziness. Assessment for vestibular disorders should be part of the standard clinical doctrine for acute and chronic management of head-injured patients. In this chapter, we review this assessment from an anatomic and physiologic point of view and for the appropriate clinical approach. We briefly outline treatment approaches to the various disorders.

Vestibular Anatomy and Physiology

The vestibular organs are simply accelerometers that provide information to the brain about the motion of the head. Inside the utricle and the macula are the otolith organs. The otoliths are calcium carbonate crystals fixed in a gelatinous matrix that rests on hair cells. The otoliths are detectors of linear acceleration, either motion in a straight line or slow tilting of the head relative to gravity. In contrast, the semicircular canals (SCCs) are rotational or angular accelerometers. They are hollow and fluid filled. Inertia of fluid in the canals as the head turns results in the deviation of the cupula, the acceleration sensor in each canal. Signals from the hair cells in the otoliths and the SCCs are transmitted along the auditory nerve, in parallel with the signals from the cochlea that encode sound stimuli. In the brainstem, vestibular signals are combined and are modulated and adapted by cerebellar circuits. Disruption of the otoliths, SCCs, auditory nerves, and brainstem circuits are all potential sites of dysfunction of the vestibular system. Active disturbance of these systems results in vertigo and damage to the systems means loss of acceleration information to the brain and loss of balance. Understanding the pathophysiology, loss of function, and neural adaptation of the vestibular system is key to the management of TBI-induced disorders.

mTBI from Blunt Versus Explosive Blast Trauma

In this discussion, we examine two types of mTBI. We first look at mTBI secondary to blunt head injury (closed head injury); then, we examine the vestibular disorders associated with mTBI seen after an explosive blast.

Blunt head injury is by far the most common cause of mTBI in the civilian world and is receiving increased attention due to sports-related etiologies, commonly termed "concussion." Such sports-related injuries can occur in high-profile professional athletes as well as the young soccer prodigy playing at the local park on Saturday

Table 8.1 Vestibular disorders after closed head injury

Entity	History	Physical exam	Vestibular tests
Positional vertigo (PTBPV)	Positional vertigo	Nystagmus on Dix–Hallpike test or modified Dix–Hallpike test	No other abnormalities
Exertional dizziness (PTEID)	Dizziness during and right after exercise	Abnormalities in challenged gait testing	No other abnormalities
Migraine-associated dizziness (PTMAD)	Episodic vertigo with periods of unsteadiness	Abnormalities in challenged gait testing	VOR gain, phase, or symmetry abnormalities
	Headaches	+/– Abnormalities on head impulse testing	High-frequency VOR abnormalities
		Normal static posture tests	Normal posturography
Spatial disorientation (PTSpD)	Constant feeling of unsteadiness worsened by standing but still present when sitting or lying down	Abnormalities on standard gait tests	VOR gain, phase, or symmetry abnormalities High-frequency VOR abnormalities
		+/– Abnormalities on head impulse testing	Abnormal posturography
	Drifting to one side while walking Shifting weight when standing still	Abnormalities on static posture tests	Central findings on rotation chair testing

morning. Work in our laboratory over the last several years has allowed us to characterize the vestibular disorders seen after closed head injury (Hoffer et al. 2004, 2009). Table 8.1 shows the characteristics of the four classes of balance disorders seen after blunt trauma. Post-traumatic benign positional vertigo (PTBPV) is identical to idiopathic BPV. It is characterized by short episodes of vertigo that occur when changing head or body position (rolling over in bed, looking up, etc.) (Gordon et al. 2002). The episodes last only a few seconds. PTBPV is discussed in more detail below. Post-traumatic exercise-induced dizziness (PTEID) is dizziness that occurs after the completion of physical activity. These individuals complain of unsteadiness or feeling off balance after they finish exercise. They do not generally complain of vertigo. The third class of dizziness seen is post-traumatic migraine-associated dizziness (PTMAD). In this classification, which has received increasing attention over the last several years, individuals complain of a variety of transient types of dizziness. Individuals can have vertigo, unsteadiness, or visual abnormalities. The episodes are intermittent and can last from seconds to hours. Most individuals have more than one type of dizziness episode. In this disorder, migraine headache (either coincident with or distinct from the dizziness) is one of the hallmark symptoms. PTMAD is discussed in more detail below. The final class of dizziness seen after blunt head trauma is post-traumatic spatial disorientation (PTSpD). In this symptom, complex individuals complain of unsteadiness when standing still or moving quickly. They also have unsteadiness on uneven surfaces or when walking in poor light conditions. Like the migraine-associated dizziness patients, this group of individuals may have headaches, but unlike that group headaches are rarely one of the dominant symptoms. The hallmark of this condition is the need to use light touch when standing still to avoid from wobbling. We have been able to describe the frequency of these disorders and this data is shown in Fig. 8.1. It should be noted that the frequency of PTBPV is likely underestimated in this group since many of these individuals may have resolved the BPV prior to presenting to our clinic.

While blast-related mTBI may seem less relevant, it is becoming an increasingly important etiology of mTBI. Well over 80% of all war injuries are blast-related mTBI in isolation. In the civilian world, air bags, compressors, pneumatic tools, and a number of other job site risks have resulted in a sharp rise in the number of blast-related mTBI cases. Dizziness is the number one

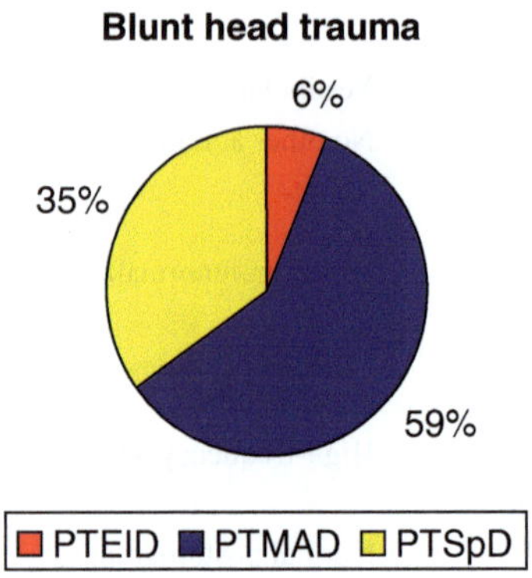

Fig. 8.1 Comparisons of dizziness: blunt head trauma

symptom of blast-related mTBI (Hoffer et al. 2010). Blast-induced mTBI differs from blunt mTBI in a number of ways (Hoffer et al. 2009). The classes of dizziness are in agreement with this finding. Table 8.2 shows the classes of dizziness seen after blast-induced mTBI. The post-blast BPV (PBBPV) is identical to the PTBPV with transient positional-induced vertigo episodes. On the other hand, the post-blast exertional dizziness (PBED) which was formerly termed post-blast exercise-induced dizziness is dramatically different from the PTEID in that post-blast individuals get unsteady upon starting to exercise (rather than at the completion of the episode). The symptoms of unsteadiness and disequilibrium as well as headaches are the same, but the temporal relationship of these symptoms to exercise is much different and, hence, more troubling to the patient. The final two classes, post-blast dizziness and post-blast dizziness with vertigo (PBD and PBDV), are characterized by the following two symptoms—constant unsteadiness which is made worse by more challenging balance environments (uneven surfaces, poor light conditions, moving quickly, etc.) and constant headaches which fluctuate in severity. The presence of additional episodic vertigo separates the two disorders. The relative frequency of these dizziness types is shown in Fig. 8.2. Unlike after blunt head injury, the frequency of PBBPV, while likely slightly higher than zero, is very small. The classification systems have proved helpful in a variety of ways. They can be understood and are essential to guide treatment and rehabilitation. They also provide prognostic details which help in patient management. Equally important is that they provide a diagnosis for patients who too often have been told that the dizziness is "something they got from the head injury" and "give it time—it will go away."

Table 8.2 Balance disorders seen after blast exposure

Entity	History	Physical exam	Vestibular tests
Positional vertigo (PBBPV)	Positional vertigo	Nystagmus on Dix–Hallpike test or modified Dix–Hallpike test	No other abnormalities
Exertional dizziness (PBED)	Dizziness during exercise	Abnormalities in challenged gait test	No other abnormalities
Blast-induced disequilibrium (PBD)	Constant feeling of unsteadiness when standing and walking worse with challenging environments Constant headache	Abnormalities in challenged gait Abnormalities in tandem Romberg Abnormalities with quick head motion	Abnormal posturography Abnormal target acquisition, dynamic visual acuity, and gaze stabilization +/– VOR gain, phase, or symmetry abnormalities
Blast-induced disequilibrium with vertigo (PBDV)	Constant feeling of unsteadiness when standing and walking worse with challenging environments Constant headache Episodic vertigo	Abnormalities in challenged gait Abnormalities in tandem Romberg Abnormalities with quick head motion	Abnormal posturography Abnormal target acquisition, dynamic visual acuity, and gaze stabilization VOR gain, phase, or symmetry abnormalities

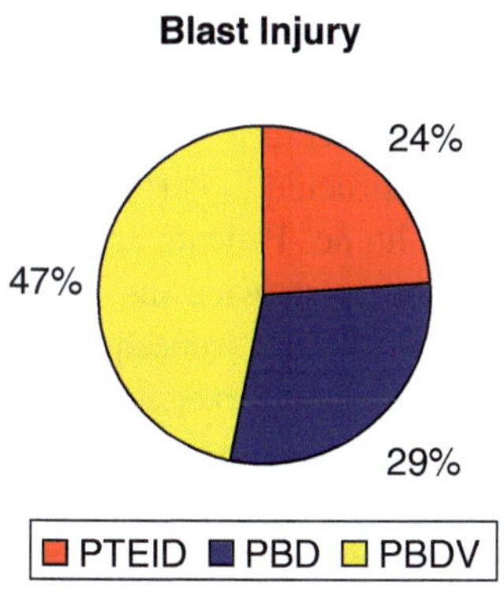

Fig. 8.2 Comparisons of dizziness: blast injury

Post-traumatic Benign Positional Vertigo

BPV is the most common condition causing vertigo. BPV is simply the result of calcium carbonate crystals broken loose from the otolith organ ending up in the SCCs. Clinicians involved in the diagnosis or treatment of patients that present with vertigo or imbalance should know how to elicit a history of BPV and carry out the Dix–Hallpike test for the diagnosis. The Canalith-Repositioning maneuver (CRM, or as it is commonly known, the Epley Maneuver) is a simple, safe procedure that can immediately cure BPV. If one is familiar with the diagnosis of BPV, the CRM is a powerful addition to one's clinical armamentarium. A full description of the Dix–Hallpike test and the CRM is given in Viirre (Viirre et al. 2005). In summary, one looks for a history of brief vertigo attacks that are provoked by head movements; rolling over in bed, bending over, or reaching up. The vertigo lasts for seconds and should stop as the patient lies still. Note that motion sickness and imbalance from a spell of vertigo can last for minutes or hours after the actual vertigo episode. The Dix–Hallpike test is carried out with a patient on an examining bench. While being held securely by the examiner, the patient's head is turned 45° to the right or left. The patient is then thrust backward rapidly. Onset of a vertigo sensation accompanied by torsional nystagmus (a clockwise or anticlockwise rotation of the eyes as the patient looks straight ahead) is diagnostic. The CRM is a simple continuation of movements once a positive Dix–Hallpike test is elicited. With the head extended back so it is below the horizontal plane, a sequence of turns of the head and body will remove the offending calcium carbonate crystals from the SCC.

Post-traumatic Migraine-Associated Dizziness

Migraine is one of the most common genetic disorders, present in approximately one in six women and one in ten men. Migraine is a disease complex of which headache is the most common symptom. Migraine aura is well recognized and its presence is diagnostic of migraine, and almost half of migraineurs have dizziness and vertigo episodes (Vuković et al. 2007). The high incidence of migraine in the general population suggests that a high percentage of people with TBI will have concomitant migraine, even if they were not symptomatic prior to their injury. The post-traumatic headache, dizziness, cognitive difficulties, and symptoms not localized to the head may well be present in TBI patients as the result of the onset of migraine headaches.

Migraine headache is diagnosed by using the International Headache Society criteria for headache (International Headache Society Classification). There are no diagnostic tests for migraine-related dizziness, but vertigo in a patient who meets the migraine headache criteria, must have migraine considered in the differential diagnosis. Because of the variable penetrance of the condition, review for a family history of recurrent headaches, dizziness, and/or motion sensitivity may be fruitful, even if a formal diagnosis of migraine is not reported in the family.

Treatment of migraine can be effectively carried out by lifestyle and medical management. In TBI patients, particular attention must be paid to provision of adequate regular sleep, regular meals, and a well-designed activity program (see below). Medical management includes use of calcium channel blockers (Verapamil), and possible use of beta blockers (Inderal) and carbonic anhydrase inhibitors (Topirimate). Topirimate, in particular, has been studied in the TBI dizziness population and has been found to be effective not only for the dizziness and vertigo, but also for headache control in patients (Gode et al. 2010).

Treatment

The vestibular physical therapy rehabilitation strategy employs specific exercises designed to decrease dizziness, increase balance function, and increase general activity levels. Exercises to decrease dizziness focus on exposure to specific stimuli for habituation or attenuation of the dizziness response in the brain. Balance retraining involves exercises designed to improve organization of sensory information for balance control and coordination of muscle responses. General activity exercise involves a daily aerobic exercise program of progressive walking, cycling, or swimming (Gottshall and Hoffer 2010; Teggi et al. 2009).

A vestibular physical therapy (VPT) program for mTBI patients consists of exercise procedures that target the vestibulo-ocular reflex (VOR), cervico-ocular reflex (COR), depth perception (DP), somatosensory retraining (SS), dynamic gait, and aerobic function (Gottshall and Hoffer 2010; Teggi et al. 2009). The VOR, COR, and DP exercises are graded in difficulty, based on velocity of head and object motion, and progression of body positioning from sitting to standing to walking. The SS exercises are graded in difficulty by narrowing the base of support, making the surface uneven, or changing the surface from firm to soft. Large-amplitude head and trunk movements are also employed to increase somatosensory input. These exercises included the Proprioceptive Neuromuscular Facilitation (PNF) techniques of slow reversal head and neck patterns, modified chopping and lifting for head and trunk in progression from supine, to sitting, and to standing postures, and total body mass rolling activities. Varied walking exercises are graded in difficulty by changing direction, performing with the eyes closed, increasing speed of ambulation, walking on soft surfaces, or navigating stairs. An aerobic home exercise program progressively increases the time, speed, or distance that the patient can tolerate. All patients are encouraged to work at their maximum tolerance while performing the VPT and are instructed to perform the exercises twice daily at home. Patients are monitored by the physical therapist twice the first week, and once a week for the subsequent 7 weeks. Compliance to the home exercise program is surveyed by the physical therapist during patient visits.

An objective assessment is performed for all mTBI patients by the vestibular physical therapist. A functional test battery consisting of an impulse head thrust test, Fukuda step test, Romberg test, tandem Romberg test, and Dynamic Gait Index (DGI) is administered to each patient (Herman et al. 2009). In addition, the Dizziness Handicapped Index (DHI) (Jacobson and Newman 1990) and the Activities-Specific Balance Confidence (ABC) Scale (Powell and Myers 1995) surveys are administered. The above measurements are obtained pre-treatment, during treatment, and post-treatment (6–8 weeks after beginning treatment). Subjective patient reports of degree and length of imbalance perception are documented throughout treatment. The length of time required for patients to return to work after the initiation of physical therapy is monitored.

As we have noted, vestibular complaints are the most frequent sequelae of blast-induced mTBI (Helminski et al. 2010). VPT has been established as the most important treatment modality for this group of patients. Nevertheless, there is little work objectively documenting the impact of VPT on this group of patients. Studies have been completed in the past examining clinical measures like the Glasgow Coma Scale (GCS) on overall recovery pattern after TBI, but outcome measures specifically aimed at examining the adequacy of vestibular tests to track vestibular recovery have been lacking (Sandhaug et al. 2010). Scherer and Schubert reinforced the need for best practices in vestibular assessment for formulation of appropriate VPT treatment strategies (Scherer and Schubert 2009). Now, the application of vestibular testing and rehabilitation in this patient population is needed to provide information on objective outcome measures (Scherer and

Schubert 2009). VPT is most effective when applied in a customized fashion, tailored to individual patient deficits and needs. While we and others have developed VPT procedures that are applied in "best practices" for blast-induced mTBI vestibular patients (Hoffer et al. 2009), these therapies must be customized for the patient entry level of function and expectation level of recovery. Knowledge of the patient's disability and diagnosis is critical to building the foundation for return to activity, work, or participation in sports. There has been documentation on the reliability of CDP as a diagnostic tool and on the reliability of the DGI as a diagnostic tool (Herman et al. 2009; Gottshall et al. 2003; Mishra et al. 2009; Nashner and Peters 1990), but those studies have not looked at the head injury population which tends to have a different type of vestibular profile than those tested in previous studies. The head injury population is also a younger population than the previous studies represent. Similarly, over the past 5 years, there are several studies (Whitney et al. 2009; Goebel et al. 2006; Badaracco et al. 2007; Pritcher et al. 2008) examining the GST as an outcome measure correlated with postural stability. In these studies, the patient groups were small and again the populations were far different from head-injured blast patients, in terms of vestibular dysfunction and age. What might be considered normal for an older vestibular patient (post-stroke, etc.) would still be wholly unacceptable in a young military population intent on returning to active duty. Our study represents a demonstration of a suite of vestibular tests successfully utilized to judge outcomes in patients with both blunt and blast-induced mTBI with vestibular disorders in the active duty military. Vestibular clinical centers will establish their own normative values for tests on patients of similar age and activity level. The standard results of these tests can be used to determine return-to-duty/work status as well as return-to-physical activity status. While the entire suite of tests provides valuable information, our data indicates that the vertical GST is the most sensitive outcome predictor for a young, military population. This likely indicates that recovery of vestibular function is frequency and velocity dependent. This observation agrees with the work of Paige (Paige 1989) in which linearity and symmetry of the VOR were examined.

Management of TBI-Related Dizziness: An Algorithm

Based on the disorders described above, we have derived a simple algorithm to aid in the management of dizziness post-TBI. In Fig. 8.3, branch points are based on historical or physical findings. Diagnostic categories are indicated in separate shaded boxes. The simplest, and perhaps the most important, item is the first: the Dix–Hallpike test. The test should be done on all patients with any complaint of dizziness. This simple procedure and its readily observable sign of torsional nystagmus is the definitive test of BPV, and leads to the definitive treatment, the canalith repositioning maneuver. Once BPV has been tested for and treated, further complaints of dizziness depend on whether the injury is blunt or blast related.

On the blunt trauma-related arm of disorders, PTEID is defined by dizziness *after* exercise and is treated with appropriate VPT. If there are interspersed episodes of headaches, PTMAD should be suspected. A combination of traditional migraine prophylaxis pharmaceuticals and VPT is most effective. Finally, in the blunt trauma-related arm, if there is persistent unsteadiness during low-effort walking or even during standing, PTSpD is present, and it requires a differently configured program of VPT.

After blast-related trauma, there may be dizziness (PBED) at the onset of exercise. VPT is effective here. Post-blast, there may be a complaint of constant dizziness. PBD may be reduced with migraine medications. If there are interspersed episodes of vertigo, then PBD + Vertigo is present and in addition to migraine prophylaxis, diuretics such as hydrochlorothiazide or acetazolamide can be effective in reducing the vertigo episodes. As can be seen, a knowledgeable physical therapist is essential for management of this group of patients as well as a diagnostician familiar with the acute post-trauma categories.

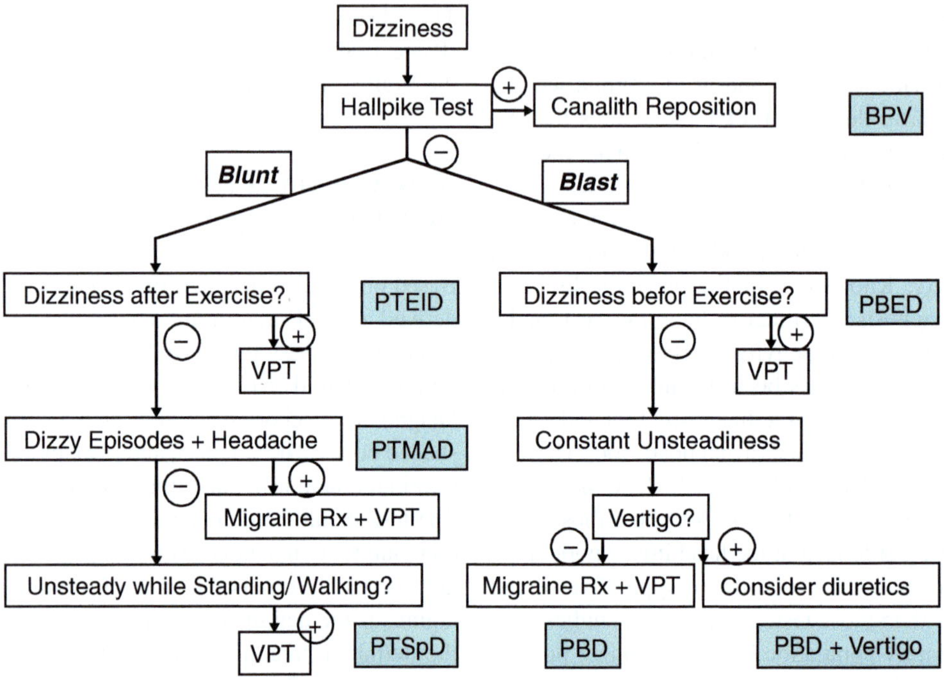

Fig. 8.3 Algorithm for management of TBI-related dizziness

Advanced Concepts in Vestibular Consequences of TBI

Blunt and blast mTBI have been demonstrated to result in a variety of medical conditions and syndromes. These vary from simple in diagnosis and management, such as BPV, to the more complex, such as PTSpD. Fortunately, observers can be readily trained to recognize these various conditions and initiate management. Since dizziness is the leading complaint post-TBI, deployment of formalized protocols and training programs should be implemented in both military and civilian environments such as football, where mTBI is frequent. Medical personnel should be trained to recognize and treat such conditions as migraine-related TBI syndromes.

Despite recent work in the area, there is still a great deal of research with respect to mTBI that is needed. Critical among these are deploying known countermeasures for mTBI, determining the pathophysiology of mTBI so that even more specific countermeasures can be developed, studying the effects of multiple blasts and head impacts, and developing diagnostic and therapeutic tools that are mobile, rugged, and easy to use.

References

Badaracco C, Labini FS, Meli A, Angelis ED, Tufarelli D. Vestibular rehabilitation outcomes in chronic vertiginous patients through computerized dynamic visual acuity and Gaze stabilization test. Otol Neurotol. 2007;28:809–13.

Gode S, Celebisoy N, Kirazli T, Akyuz A, Bilgen C, Karapolat H, Sirin H, Gokcay F. Clinical assessment of topiramate therapy in patients with migrainous vertigo. Headache. 2010;50(1):77–84.

Goebel JA, Tungsiripat N, Sinks B, Carmody J. Gaze stabilization test: a new clinical test of unilateral vestibular dysfunction. Otol Neurotol. 2006;28:68–73.

Gordon CR, Joffe V, Levite R, Gadoth N. Traumatic benign paroxysmal positional vertigo: diagnosis and treatment. Harefuah. 2002;141(11):944–7.

Gottshall KR, Hoffer ME. Tracking recovery of vestibular function in individuals with blast-induced head trauma using vestibular-visual-cognitive interaction tests. J Neurol Phys Ther. 2010;34(2):94–7.

Gottshall KR, Drake A, Gray N, McDonald E, Hoffer ME. Objective vestibular tests as outcome measures in head injury patients. Laryngoscope. 2003;113:1736–50.

Helminski JO, Zee DS, Janssen I, Hain TC. Effectiveness of particle repositioning maneuvers in the treatment of benign paroxysmal positional vertigo: a systematic review. Phys Ther. 2010;90(5):663–78.

Herman T, Inbar-Borovsky N, Brozgol M, Giladi N, Hausdorff JM. The Dynamic Gait Index in healthy older adults: the role of stair climbing, fear of falling and gender. Gait Posture. 2009;29(2):237–41.

Hoffer ME, Gottshall KR, Moore RJ, Balough BJ, Wester DC. Characterizing and treating dizziness after mild head trauma. Otol Neurotol. 2004;25(2):135–8.

Hoffer ME, Donaldson C, Gottshall KR, Balaban C, Balough BJ. Blunt and blast head trauma: different entities. Int Tinnitus J. 2009;15(2):115–8.

Hoffer ME, Balaban C, Gottshall KR, Balough BJ, Maddox MR, Penta JR. Blast exposure: vestibular consequences and associated characteristics. Otol Neurotol. 2010;31(2):232–6.

International Headache Society Classification: ICHD-II. http://ihsclassification.org/en/02_klassifikation/.

Jacobson GP, Newman CW. The development of Dizziness Handicap Inventory. Arch Otolaryngol Head Neck Surg. 1990;116:424–7.

McCrory P, Meeuwisse W, Johnston K, Dvorak J, Aubry M, Molloy M, Cantu R. Consensus statement on concussion in sport – the third international conference on concussion in sport held in Zurich, November 2008. Phys Sportsmed. 2009;37(2):141–59. Review.

Mishra A, Davis S, Speers R, Shepard NT. Head shake computerized dynamic posturography in peripheral vestibular lesions. Am J Audiol. 2009;18(1):53–9.

Nashner LM, Peters JF. Dynamic posturography in the diagnosis and management of dizziness and balance disorders. Neurol Clin. 1990;8(2):331–49.

Paige GD. Nonlinearity and asymmetry in the human vestibuloocular reflex. Acta Otolaryngol. 1989;108:1–8.

Powell LE, Myers AM. The Activities-specific Balance Confidence (ABC) scale. J Gerontol A Biol Sci Med Sci. 1995;50(1):M28–34.

Pritcher MR, Whitney SL, Marchetti GF, Furman JM. The influence of age and vestibular disorders on gaze stabilization: a pilot study. Otol Neurotol. 2008;29:982–8.

Sandhaug M, Andelic N, Vatne A, Seiler S, Mygland A. Functional level during sub-acute rehabilitation after traumatic brain injury: course and predictors of outcome. Brain Inj. 2010;24:740–7.

Scherer MR, Schubert MC. Traumatic brain injury and vestibular pathology as a comorbidity after blast exposure. Phys Ther. 2009;89(9):1–13.

Teggi R, Caldirola D, Fabiano B, Recanati P, Bussi M. Rehabilitation after acute vestibular disorders. J Laryngol Otol. 2009;123(4):397–402.

Viirre ES, Purcell I, Baloh RW. How i do it. The Dix-Hallpike test and the canalith repositioning maneuver. Laryngoscope. 2005;115(1):184–7.

Vuković V, Plavec D, Galinović I, Lovrencić-Huzjan A, Budisić M, Demarin V. Prevalence of vertigo, dizziness, and migrainous vertigo in patients with migraine. Headache. 2007;47(10):1427–35.

Whitney SL, Marchetti GF, Pritcher M, Furman JM. Gaze stabilization and gait performance in vestibular dysfunction. Gait Posture. 2009;29(2):194–8.

Post-traumatic Headache

9

Jay C. Erickson and Brett J. Theeler

Abstract

Headaches are a common symptom following traumatic head injury. Post-traumatic headaches often resolve in the first few months after injury, but chronic headaches may persist for years in some cases. The characteristics of post-traumatic headaches are heterogeneous and frequently resemble primary headache disorders. Classifying the phenotype of post-traumatic headache helps guide treatment. A comprehensive diagnostic and therapeutic approach is required to successfully address the headaches as well the comorbid conditions that can perpetuate the headache syndrome. A combination of pharmacologic and non-pharmacologic interventions may be necessary to achieve a favorable outcome.

Keywords

Post-traumatic headache • Migraine • Concussion • Brain trauma • Pain • Headache prophylactic medication • Headache abortive medication

Introduction

Headache is among the most common symptoms following traumatic brain injury. Headaches frequently develop as part of the acute post-traumatic syndrome and may continue to occur for months or years after the injury. Post-traumatic headaches (PTHAs) contribute to disability, lost productivity, healthcare costs, and decreased quality of life among TBI patients. Understanding headache diagnosis and headache management are, therefore, essential skills for clinicians who care for TBI patients. This chapter discusses the classification, epidemiology, clinical features, and diagnosis of PTHAs and provides a framework for formulating an effective treatment plan.

Definitions

Headaches are classified as either primary or secondary headache disorders (Headache Classification Subcommittee of the International

J.C. Erickson, M.D. (✉)
Neurology Service, Madigan Army Medical Center, Tacoma, WA, USA
e-mail: Jay.Erickson@us.army.mil

B.J. Theeler, Ph.D.
187th Medical Battalion, Fort Sam Houston, TX, USA

J.W. Tsao (ed.), *Traumatic Brain Injury: A Clinician's Guide to Diagnosis, Management, and Rehabilitation*, DOI 10.1007/978-0-387-87887-4_9, © Springer Science+Business Media, LLC 2012

Table 9.1 Diagnostic criteria for acute and chronic post-traumatic headaches (Headache Classification Subcommittee of the International Headache Society 2004)

5.1.1 *Acute post-traumatic headache attributed to moderate or severe head injury*
(A) Headache, no typical characteristics known, fulfilling criteria C and D
(B) Head trauma with at least one of the following:
1. Loss of consciousness for >30 min
2. Glasgow Coma Scale (GCS) < 13
3. Post-traumatic amnesia for >48 h
4. Imaging demonstration of a traumatic brain lesion
(C) Headache develops within 7 days after head trauma or after regaining consciousness
(D) One of the following:
1. Headache resolves within 3 months after head trauma
2. Headache persists, but 3 months have not yet passed since head trauma
5.1.2 *Acute post-traumatic headache attributed to mild head injury*
(A) Headache, no typical characteristics known, fulfilling criteria C and D
(B) Head trauma with all of the following:
1. Either no loss of consciousness, or loss of consciousness <30 min
2. GCS ≥ 13
3. Symptoms and/or signs diagnostic of concussion
(C) Headache develops within 7 days after head trauma
(D) One of the following:
1. Headache resolves within 3 months after head trauma
2. Headache persists, but 3 months have not yet passed since head trauma
5.2.1 *Chronic post-traumatic headache attributed to moderate or severe head injury*
(A) Headache, no typical characteristics known, fulfilling criteria C and D
(B) Head trauma with at least one of the following:
1. Loss of consciousness for >30 min
2. GCS < 13
3. Post-traumatic amnesia for >48 h
4. Imaging demonstration of a traumatic brain lesion
(C) Headache develops within 7 days after head trauma or after regaining consciousness
(D) Headache persists for >3 months after head trauma
5.2.2 *Chronic post-traumatic headache attributed to mild head injury*
(A) Headache, no typical characteristics known, fulfilling criteria C and D
(B) Head trauma with all of the following:
1. Either no loss of consciousness, or loss of consciousness <30 min
2. GCS ≥ 13
3. Symptoms and/or signs diagnostic of concussion
(C) Headache develops within 7 days after head trauma
(D) Headache persists for >3 months after head trauma

Headache Society 2004). Primary headaches are not caused by an identifiable underlying illness, injury, or exposure. Examples include tension-type headache and migraine. In contrast, secondary headaches are attributable to a specific inciting event, exposure, or condition such as traumatic, infectious, neoplastic, inflammatory, systemic, or toxic processes. PTHAs are classified as secondary headaches because they are caused by head or neck trauma. PTHAs are among the most common types of secondary headache disorders.

The diagnostic criteria for different types of PTHAs are summarized in Table 9.1. According to the International Classification of Headache Disorders, 2nd Edition (ICHD-2), headaches attributed to head or neck trauma include seven different secondary headache syndromes: acute PTHA, chronic PTHA, acute and chronic headache attributed to whiplash injury, headache attributed to traumatic intracranial hematoma, post-craniotomy headache, and headache attributed to other head or neck trauma (Headache Classification Subcommittee of the International Headache Society 2004). Acute PTHAs begin within 7 days of head trauma and are further classified according to the severity of head trauma (Headache Classification Subcommittee of the International Headache Society 2004). PTHAs that persist beyond 3 months after the inciting head trauma are classified as chronic PTHAs (Headache Classification Subcommittee of the International Headache Society 2004). The criteria for acute and chronic headache attributed to whiplash injury are similar but imply a traumatic mechanism with acceleration/deceleration of the neck associated with neck pain at the time of injury (Headache Classification Subcommittee of the International Headache Society 2004).

The current criteria for classifying PTHAs have been criticized as they are based solely on the time from the traumatic event and the severity of the head trauma, but do not include any description of the head or neck pain (Lenaerts 2008; Formisano et al. 2009; Evans 2004). Additionally, requiring the onset of headache within 7 days after injury may not adequately ascribe a post-traumatic etiology in some cases. An increased time period up to 6 months has been recommended by some experts (Evans 2004). Moreover, the 3-month latency period distinguishing between acute and chronic PTHA is arbitrary and based upon observational studies rather than biologic mechanisms (Lenaerts 2008; Formisano et al. 2009; Evans 2004).

When a preexisting primary headache disorder, such as migraine, is made worse by head trauma, it can be classified as either a migraine or as both a migraine and a PTHA as per the clinician's judgement (Headache Classification Subcommittee of the International Headache Society 2004). Marked worsening of the primary headache disorder in close temporal relation to trauma and development of different headache features after trauma, including ineffectiveness of medications that had previously been effective, are some factors that support adding a diagnosis of PTHA in patients with preexisting primary headache disorders.

Epidemiology

Every year in the USA, an estimated 1.8 million individuals develop acute PTHA and 400,000 individuals develop chronic PTHA (Lenaerts et al. 2004). The incidence of acute headache following mild traumatic head injury ranges from 31 to 96% (Lenaerts et al. 2004; Packard 1999; Solomon 2005; Faux and Sheedy 2008; Stovner et al. 2009). Headaches occur after moderate to severe traumatic head injury in 4.3 to 37% of patients (Yamaguchi 1992; Couch and Bearss 2001; Walker et al. 2005). PTHAs tend to decline over time, occurring in 31–96% of patients in the first month after trauma, 32–78% at 2–3 months after trauma, 8–35% at 1 year, and 20% at 3–4 years (Lenaerts et al. 2004; Packard 1999; Solomon 2005; Faux and Sheedy 2008; Stovner et al. 2009; Packard and Ham 1993). A review of 1,670 patients from 12 studies revealed that 58% of patients with traumatic brain injury had chronic headaches, though this study did not distinguish between PTHA, primary headaches, and non-traumatic causes of secondary headaches (Nampiaparampil 2008).

The epidemiology of headache after a whiplash injury is less well defined. An estimated 1–6% of individuals have chronic whiplash symptoms (Solomon 2005; Freeman et al. 1999). Headaches occur immediately after whiplash injury in 49–82% of patients and chronic symptoms lasting a year or longer occur in 8–82% of patients (Solomon 2005; Balla and Karnaghan 1987; Schrader et al. 2006; Sterner et al. 2001; Vanderploeg et al. 2009). According to the current classification system, headaches that develop beyond 7 days after whip lash injury are not classified as a PTHA (Headache Classification Subcommittee of the International Headache Society 2004).

There is an inverse relationship between the severity of head injury and the incidence of PTHA. Headaches tend to occur more frequently, and are more likely to persist, after mild head injury compared to moderate or severe head injury (Solomon 2005; Yamaguchi 1992; Couch and Bearss 2001). Of 377 patients with severe head trauma, only 4–23% had headaches a year later (Formisano et al. 2009). Further, the rate of headache after very severe TBI (GCS less than or equal to 8, coma duration 15–60 days) was 4.3% compared to 23.4% in patients with severe TBI (GCS less than or equal to 8, coma duration 3–14 days) in this study (Formisano et al. 2009). The presence of an abnormal CT scan of the brain and a prolonged period of amnesia, both suggesting a more severe head injury, are associated with fewer reported headaches (Yamaguchi 1992). Other symptoms of the post-concussion syndrome also occur more often after mild head injury (Vanderploeg et al. 2009). The reasons for this apparent clinical paradox are uncertain.

The incidence of acute PTHAs in children is 30–80%, a rate similar to that seen in adult populations (Wilson and Krolczyk 2006; Kirk et al. 2008). PTHAs tend to resolve in the majority of children within a year (Kirk et al. 2008; Moscato et al. 2005). Chronic PTHAs have a prevalence of only 3.2–6.8% among children after head injury (Kirk et al. 2008; Moscato et al. 2005).

There is significant disparity in the prevalence of PTHAs in different countries which may relate to social, ethnic, and cultural factors. In Lithuania, for example, only 4% of individuals reported PTHAs that continued for more than 1 month after a concussion (Mickeviciene et al. 2002). The lower prevalence of PTHA in certain countries may be explained by different cultural and social expectations of post-traumatic symptoms as well as lower rates of litigation in those countries (Solomon 2005; Packard 1992).

Military combatants are at risk for PTHAs due to head or neck trauma sustained during military service (Evans 2008). Ten to twenty-five percent of the US Army soldiers returning from Iraq or Afghanistan have a head or neck injury (Hoge et al. 2008; Okie 2005). In a study of 978 returning US Army soldiers who had a concussion while deployed to a combat theater, the prevalence of any type of headache was 98% and the prevalence of PTHA was 37% (Theeler et al. 2009).

Several risk factors for developing a chronic PTHA have been identified. Female sex is a risk factor (Jensen and Nielsen 1990). Lower educational level and low socioeconomic status have been suggested as risk factors for chronic PTHA, but evidence supporting these assertions is contradictory (Packard 1999; Faux and Sheedy 2008; Stovner et al. 2009). Although a causal relationship has not been proven, psychiatric symptoms such as depression, anxiety, anger, and personality change are increased in patients with PTHA and may be important contributors to the development of chronic PTHA and increased headache-related disability (Tatrow et al. 2003a; Keshavan et al. 1981). Prior headache history appears to be an important predictor of chronic PTHA (Faux and Sheedy 2008; Stovner et al. 2009; Jensen and Nielsen 1990). As mentioned previously, the risk of chronic PTHA is inversely related to the injury severity with a higher incidence of headache after mild head injuries compared to more severe head injuries (Formisano et al. 2009; Solomon 2005; Yamaguchi 1992; Couch and Bearss 2001). Shorter duration of post-traumatic amnesia as a marker of head injury severity is also associated with an increased risk of chronic PTHA (Yamaguchi 1992).

Pathophysiology

There are multiple pain-sensitive anatomic structures of the head and neck which are capable of causing head pain. The trigeminal nerve is the major pathway for transmitting nociceptive stimuli for the head (Fig. 9.1). The trigeminal nerve contains nociceptive afferents from the anterior scalp, anterior cranium, face, mouth, teeth, temporomandibular joints, sinuses, cranial blood vessels, and meninges. Injury to any of these structures can cause head pain. The greater and lesser occipital nerves, which arise from the C2 and C3 cervical spinal roots, convey nociceptive stimuli from the posterior head and scalp (Fig. 9.1). Painful stimuli from structures of the cervical spine are conveyed largely by the cervical nerve roots. The central processes of trigeminal pain neurons and cervical pain neurons converge

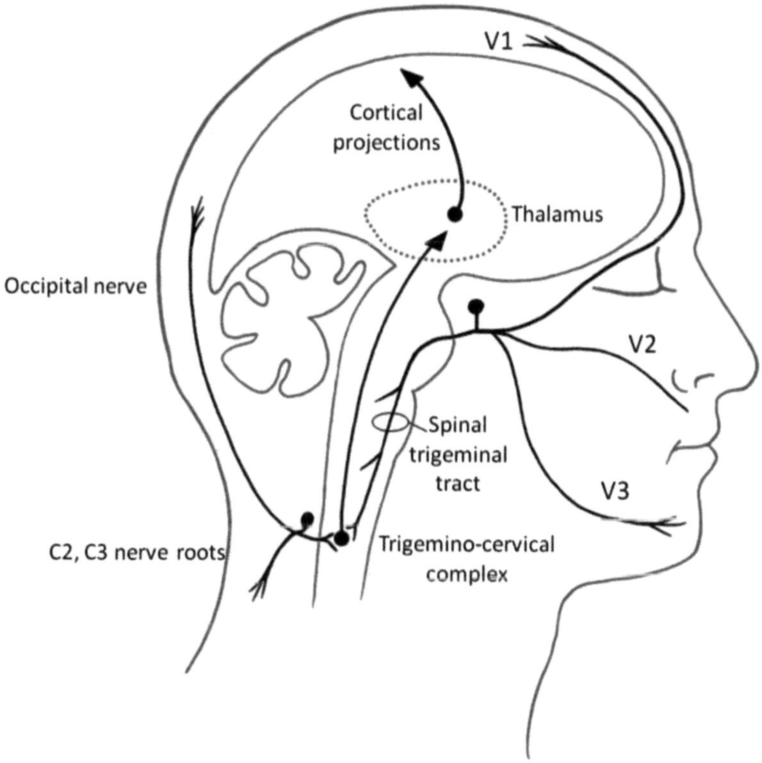

Fig. 9.1 Major neuroanatomic pathways conveying pain from the head and neck

within the central nervous system in the upper cervical spinal cord. The convergence of these two anatomic pain pathways is known as the trigeminocervical complex (Bartsch and Goadsby 2003). Some second-order neurons in this region receive inputs from both cervical and trigeminal pain afferents. Thus, peripheral activation of one pain system (trigeminal or cervical) can produce central activation of the other system. The trigeminocervical complex helps explain why injury of neck structures can cause head pain. It also helps explain why activation of the trigeminal pain pathway can produce pain in the posterior head and neck.

Headaches following concussion or mild head injury are rarely associated with an identifiable underlying structural injury (Hughes et al. 2004). A number of potential pathophysiologic mechanisms may contribute to the development of PTHAs even in the absence of identifiable structural injury. Head trauma can trigger a cascade of neurochemical and neurocellular events in both the central and peripheral nervous systems that may activate nociceptive systems, though the precise mechanisms have not been elucidated (Lenaerts et al. 2004; Packard 1999; Giza and Hovda 2001). PTHAs, especially those possessing migraine-like features, may share the same pathophysiology as migraines, including central sensitization, altered neurotransmitter signaling, altered cortical excitability, release of neuropeptides from trigeminal nerve terminals, and cerebral vasoreactivity (Packard and Ham 1997). There is evidence that trauma can trigger migraine headaches in previously asymptomatic individuals (Weiss et al. 1991). Patients with post-traumatic migraines may have a latent genetic predisposition to migraine that clinically manifests after mild head trauma.

Irritation, activation, or compression of the occipital nerves, trigeminal nerve, or other peripheral nerves of the head may be a source of headache after trauma. This can result in neuralgic pain in the distribution of the involved nerve. Traumatic injury to muscular, skeletal, and ligamentous structures of the cervical spine can also cause pain to be referred to the head (Bogduk 2004). It is uncertain if injury to central neural pathways in the brain stem or cerebral cortex is a significant contributor to the genesis of PTHA. Theoretically, damage to central anti-nociceptive systems or activation of central pro-nociceptive systems could contribute to head pain.

The multiple mechanisms of head pain described above are not exclusive of one another. A patient may have multiple mechanisms acting in concert. Therefore, identifying all potential sources of head pain in each patient is important for developing a successful therapeutic plan.

Clinical Features

PTHAs are highly heterogeneous, both clinically and mechanistically, and many different headache types have been reported after head trauma (Haas 1996). PTHAs do not possess any unique clinical symptoms that clearly distinguish them from non-traumatic headache disorders, other than having the onset in close temporal relationship to head or neck trauma.

In civilian populations, approximately 72% of headaches attributed to head trauma are bilateral in location (Lew et al. 2006). A frontal location has been reported in 50%, followed by holocephalic (18%), hemicranial (13%), and bitemporal (10%) (Lew et al. 2006). Eighty-three percent of PTHAs are non-throbbing. The pain may be described as either dull or sharp (Walker et al. 2005; Lew et al. 2006). Seventy-one percent of PTHAs are aggravated by physical activity or exertion and over 60% are mild to moderate in severity (Lew et al. 2006). Sensitivity to light and sound occurs in 35 and 29% of patients, respectively (Lew et al. 2006). Nausea occurs in 16–31% while vomiting occurs in 12–14% of patients with PTHAs (Lew et al. 2006).

Headaches after whiplash injury are located in the occipital region in 46% of patients. Generalized head pain or non-occipital locations occur in 54% of cases (Evans 2004). One study found that head pain associated with whiplash injury was rarely severe (Schrader et al. 2006). Other features that may be seen in post-whiplash headaches include aggravation of symptoms by exertion or activity, photophobia, and phonophobia (Schrader et al. 2006; Lew et al. 2006).

Headaches developing after head trauma often possess the same characteristics as primary headache disorders (Lew et al. 2006; Haas 1996; Baandrup and Jensen 2005). Between 70 and 96% of headaches attributed to head trauma would otherwise meet ICHD-2 criteria for a primary headache disorder at some time following head injury (Lew et al. 2006; Haas 1996). PTHAs most commonly resemble tension-type headache or migraine headache (Haas 1996; Baandrup and Jensen 2005). This is clinically relevant because treatments for PTHAs are selected based on the primary headache disorders that they resemble. For example, PTHAs resembling migraines are treated with therapies known to be effective for migraine. Thus, it is useful for clinicians to classify PTHAs according to well-recognized headache types or syndromes. The major subgroups of headaches after trauma include tension-type headache, migraine, trigeminal autonomic cephalagias, cranial neuralgias, cervicogenic headaches, and medication-overuse headache. Each of these is briefly described in the following paragraphs and outlined in Table 9.2.

Approximately 33% of PTHAs resemble tension-type headaches with a wide range of 6–85% seen in different studies (Evans 2004; Walker et al. 2005; Lew et al. 2006). Tension-type headache is typically bilateral and of mild or moderate severity. The pain quality is pressing or tightening in nature and not aggravated by routine physical activity. Tension-type headache may be accompanied by either light or sound sensitivity, but not nausea (Headache Classification Subcommittee of the International Headache Society 2004).

Approximately 28–60% of PTHAs resemble migraine (Walker et al. 2005; Theeler et al. 2009; Lew et al. 2006; Haas 1996). Migraine headaches are the most common form of PTHA after military-related mild head trauma (Theeler et al. 2009). Migraine characteristics include head pain

Table 9.2 Features of common types of headache syndromes after head trauma

Headache type	Laterality	Duration	Severity	Quality	Other symptoms	Comments
Migraine	Unilateral, asymmetric, or bilateral	4–72 h	Moderate or severe	Often throbbing or pulsatile	Nausea or vomiting Photophonosensitivity Aura Avoidance of physical activity	Patient may lie down in a dark, quiet place
Tension type	Bilateral	30 min to several hours	Mild or moderate	Steady, squeezing	No nausea May have either light or sound sensitivity	Patient can usually function. OTCs often helpful
Occipital neuralgia	Unilateral	Continuous and/or brief episodes	Variable	Steady and/or "shooting"	Parasthesias in distribution of occipital nerve	Palpation over the occipital nerve reproduces pain
Cervicogenic	Unilateral or bilateral	Variable	Mild or moderate	Usually dull, steady, or "aching"	Neck pain, soreness, and/or stiffness HA triggered by neck movements or postures	Cervical muscle tenderness and/or spasm
Medication-overuse HA	Bilateral	Continuous	Mild or moderate	Usually steady	May have additional headaches characteristic of the underlying, original headache disorder that resulted in overuse	Use of analgesics >15 days/month. Headache often occurs after the analgesic has "worn off"

that is moderate or severe, unilateral or asymmetric, throbbing or pulsatile in quality, aggravated by or causes avoidance of routine physical activity, and accompanied by either nausea and vomiting or both light and sound sensitivity (Headache Classification Subcommittee of the International Headache Society 2004). The headache attacks last several hours to several days without treatment. Aura, a transient focal neurologic symptom that is most often visual in nature and precedes or accompanies the headache, occurs in a minority of patients with migraine and is not required for a headache to be considered a migraine. The term "post-traumatic migraine" is often used to describe PTHAs that would otherwise meet diagnostic criteria for migraine, although it is not listed as a diagnosis in ICHD-2. Post-traumatic migraines may not be distinguishable from idiopathic migraine by clinical features or responsiveness to treatment (Weiss et al. 1991).

Head trauma can precipitate the development of trigeminal autonomic cephalalgias, but these are relatively rare presentations of PTHAs (Evans 2004). Trigeminal autonomic cephalalgias manifest as unilateral headache accompanied by prominent autonomic manifestations, such as conjuctival injection, lacrimation, ptosis, mioisis, eyelid edema, rhinorrhea, or facial sweating abnormalities (Headache Classification Subcommittee of the International Headache Society 2004). Specific subtypes of trigeminal autonomic cephalalgias include cluster headache, paroxysmal hemicrania, hemicrania continua, and SUNCT (short-lasting, unilateral, neuralgiform headache attacks with conjunctival injection and tearing) (Headache Classification Subcommittee of the International Headache Society 2004).

Cranial neuralgias can result from head trauma (Evans 2004; Lenaerts et al. 2004; Packard 1999). Occipital neuralgia is probably the most common neuralgiform disorder following head or neck injury and typically presents with persistent, moderate, unilateral head pain with episodes of brief, severe, lancinating pain radiating from the occipital area to the side of the head. Trigeminal neuralgia and neuralgias involving the terminal branches of the trigeminal nerve, such as supraorbital neuralgia and infra-orbital neuralgia, can also occur after head trauma. Compression, stretching, or other forms of injury to these peripheral nerves, their branches, or their central connections can cause pain in the distribution of the affected nerve. The pain is typically stabbing, jabbing, or lancinating. There may be severe brief paroxysms of pain that are superimposed on persistent, less severe pain in the distribution of the nerve. There is usually tenderness over the nerve, and there may be sensory impairment in the distribution of the nerve as well.

Cervicogenic headaches occur when pain is generated or referred from a source in the cervical spine, such as cervical discs, facet joints, or myofascial structures (Bogduk 2004). Patients with this category of headaches usually have persistent or intermittent neck discomfort as part of their presentation. There may be neck or occipital tenderness with or without trigger points. Headaches may be triggered by certain neck movements or positions. Cervicogenic headache is often located in the occipital area or posterior head region but may also affect anterior head regions. The head pain can be unilateral or bilateral.

Medication-overuse headache, sometimes called analgesic rebound headache, is an important contributor to chronic headaches following head trauma. Nineteen to forty-two percent of patients with PTHAs develop this secondary headache disorder (Haas 1996; Baandrup and Jensen 2005). Medication-overuse headache develops in susceptible patients when frequent use of acute analgesic medication is continued over a prolonged period of time. Analgesic overuse is defined as use of acute analgesics 15 or more days per month for more than 3 months (Headache Classification Subcommittee of the International Headache Society 2004). Medication-overuse headache is typically bilateral, mild to moderate, and non-throbbing. It occurs at least 15 days per month and often occurs daily. The headache usually begins several hours after consuming the offending analgesic. The patient becomes trapped in a cycle of escalating headaches and increasing medication use. The diagnosis is confirmed when headaches improve after cessation of the overused analgesic. Typically, the headaches worsen for 1 or 2 weeks after analgesic cessation and then gradually improve over the next 4–6 weeks. Medication-overuse headache can occur with any type of pain medication, though combination medications containing one or more simple analgesics coupled with opioids, caffeine, or butalbital have the highest risk (Dodick and Freitag 2006).

Differential Diagnosis

The vast majority of patients with PTHAs after mild head trauma do not have an underlying, life-threatening condition. However, the clinician must ask the following question: "Are the headaches a harbinger of a serious underlying disorder that would significantly alter prognosis or require specific treatment?" Table 9.3 lists causes of headaches after head trauma. It is beyond the scope of this chapter to describe each of these disorders in detail. Clinicians who routinely evaluate patients after head trauma should be familiar with the key features of these disorders in order to avoid delays in diagnosis.

There are a number of "danger signs" that should alert the clinician to the possibility of a potentially serious medical condition causing headaches. Danger signs include altered mental status, focal neurologic symptoms or deficits, progressively worsening headache pattern, intractable headache, thunderclap headaches (rapid-onset headaches with maximal pain at the onset), headaches induced by position, valsalva, or exertion, systemic or constitutional symptoms, as well as new headache after 50 years of age (Silberstein 2000). Headaches with atypical features can also be a sign of an underlying abnormality. Unfortunately, headaches fully resembling primary headaches can occur in patients with serious underlying medical conditions.

Clinical Evaluation

The major goals of the clinical evaluation are to exclude serious underlying etiologies, establish an accurate headache diagnosis, determine the impact of the headaches on the individual, and identify important comorbid conditions which may be perpetuating or exacerbating the headaches. This information is essential to formulating an effective therapeutic plan.

Table 9.3 Causes of headache after trauma

Dangerous causes of headache:
• Cerebral vein or sinus thrombosis
• Subdural or epidural hematoma
• Intracerebral hemorrhage
• Subarachnoid hemorrhage
• Low or high intracranial pressure
• Hydrocephalus
• Carotid or vertebral artery dissection
• Cavernous-carotid fistula
• Cerebral aneurysm
• Skull fracture
• Cervical vertebra fracture
• Cervical disc protrusion
Primary headache disorders:
• Migraine
• Tension-type headache
• Cluster headache
• Others
Neuralgiform headaches:
• Occipital neuralgia
• Supraorbital or infraorbital neuralgia
• Trigeminal neuralgia
• Scalp laceration-associated neuralgia
Cervicogenic headaches:
• Cervical myofascial pain
• Cervical ligament strain
• Cervical disc protrusion
• C2–C3 facet joint dysfunction
Other causes:
• Medication-overuse (rebound) headache
• Medication side effect
• Sinus injury
• TMJ disorders
• Post-craniotomy headache
• Ocular pain (various causes)
• Chemical meningitis
• Headache due to a non-traumatic cause
• Headache due to a psychiatric condition
• Somatization
• Malingering

History

The history obtained from the patient is the most important part of the clinical evaluation. A detailed description of the headache should be obtained, including onset, location, quality,

Table 9.4 Clinical evaluation of subacute and chronic headaches after head trauma

History:
• Severity and mechanism of trauma
• Detailed description of headache(s) prior to and since head trauma
– Onset
– Location
– Severity
– Duration
– Frequency
– Quality
– Triggers
– Associated symptoms
– Functional impact
– Change in pattern over time
• Current and past headache therapies
– Doses
– Duration of treatment
– Side effects
– Response to treatment
• Other neurologic symptoms during or between headaches
• Past and current medical problems
• Social history including caffeine use and current stressors including legal issues
• Family history of headaches
Physical exam:
• Vital signs
• Complete neurologic exam
• Head and neck exam
– Range of motion
– Cervical muscle spasm
– Trigger points
– Cephalic or ocular bruits
Screening instruments:
• Headache Impact Test (HIT-6)
• Migraine Disability Assessment Scale (MIDAS)
• PTSD checklist
• Beck Depression Inventory or PHQ-9
• Neurobehavioral Symptom Inventory
• Pittsburgh Sleep Quality Index
Imaging:
• Review any prior imaging
• Obtain imaging if "danger sign" (see text)
• Use clinical judgment if no danger signs are present
– Brain MRI ± MR angiogram
– C-spine MRI ± MR angiogram

frequency, severity, duration, associated symptoms, triggers, functional impact, and changes in pattern over time. The specific characteristics of PTHAs can be used to classify them into categories that have treatment implications. We find it useful to categorize PTHAs into those resembling migraine, tension-type headaches, cervicogenic headache, neuralgiform headache, or probable medication-overuse headache as described in the Clinical Features section of this chapter. An individual patient may have more than one type of headache, so it is important to obtain a detailed description of each headache type. It is also important to ask about headaches that existed prior to the traumatic injury and whether there has been a marked change in the pattern of preexisting headaches.

Patients should be asked about the occurrence of focal neurologic symptoms, either during or between headache attacks, as well as other "red flags" (see previous section). Post-traumatic migraines may be accompanied by an aura which typically manifests as transient visual disturbance. Other focal neurologic symptoms in patients with a history of head trauma should not be attributed to a migraine aura without first excluding other causes.

The clinician must ascertain all current and previously attempted headache therapies, including medications and non-pharmacologic treatments. The dose, effectiveness, tolerability, side effects, and duration of each therapy should be determined. This information is essential for determining whether a specific therapy has received an adequate trial and for identifying the presence of medication-overuse headache. Common pitfalls in headache treatment include prescribing nonoptimal doses, failing to treat with prophylactic agents for a sufficient period of time, and continuing to prescribe medications causing medication-overuse headache. Understanding the clinical response a patient had to specific medications can also have diagnostic utility. For example, headaches that are rapidly relieved by a triptan medication are very likely to be migraines.

A number of standardized instruments can aid in the evaluation of patients with PTHAs. As previously mentioned, visual or verbal analog pain scales are useful for grading pain severity and tracking changes in pain over time. An instrument to measure headache-associated disability is highly recommended in order to better understand how the headaches are impacting the function of the patient. The Headache Impact Test-6 (HIT-6) and the Migraine Disability Assessment Scale (MIDAS) are two widely used disability scales, although neither one has been specifically validated in patients with PTHA (Kosinksi et al. 2003; Stewart et al. 2001).

Patients with PTHAs often have concurrent medical and psychological conditions that can perpetuate or exacerbate headaches. Such conditions include insomnia, other sleep disorders, post-traumatic stress disorder (PTSD), depression, and chronic non-headache pain disorders (Packard 1992; Packard 2008; Silver et al. 2009; Glaesser et al. 2004). These conditions should be screened for during the clinical evaluation. Standardized instruments can aid in detecting and monitoring comorbid conditions. Useful instruments include the PTSD symptom checklist, Beck depression inventory, and Pittsburgh Sleep Quality Index (Blanchard et al. 1996; Beck et al. 1996; Buysse et al. 1989).

Physical Exam

Patients with headaches should undergo a careful neurologic examination, including vital signs and evaluation of mental status, cranial nerves, motor function, sensation, coordination, gait, and reflexes. The vast majority of patients with headaches after mild head injury will not have focal or lateralizing motor, sensory, or reflex abnormalities. It is important to examine the optic discs for papilledema, the pupils for anisocoria, the eyelids for ptosis, and the eyes for chemosis, proptosis, or orbital edema. Careful palpation for cranial, occipital, and cervical trigger points should be performed.

Imaging

All patients with moderate or severe traumatic brain injury, and many patients with concussion or mild head trauma, should undergo a head CT during the acute evaluation. Head CT is recommended in the acute period for patients who lost consciousness even if the neurologic exam is normal (Inamasu et al. 2000; Borczuk 1995; American Academy of Neurology Practice Parameter 1997). When patients present with subacute or chronic headaches following mild head trauma, the clinician must decide whether neuroimaging is needed to exclude a potential underlying contributory abnormality. Head CT or MRI has been recommended in patients whose headaches worsen or persist longer than 1 week after concussion (American Academy of Neurology Practice Parameter 1997). However, the yields of head CT and standard brain MRI are low in patients with a history of mild head trauma (Hughes et al. 2004). Specific signs that suggest the need for neuroimaging in non-acute headache patients include abnormal neurologic examination findings, progressively worsening headache pattern, and headaches induced by position or valsalva (Silberstein 2000). Headaches that fail to respond to an appropriate trial of therapy or possess atypical features not conforming to common headache phenotypes are additional indications for imaging.

Brain MRI is more sensitive than CT and is the imaging study of choice in the subacute setting. MR or CT angiogram should be utilized in patients in whom arterial dissection, aneurysm, vasospasm, or carotid-cavernous fistula are considerations. MR or CT venogram should be performed in patients with possible cerebral vein thrombosis, a condition which can be triggered by trauma and has variable manifestations including headache, signs of elevated intracranial pressure, focal seizures, and/or focal neurologic symptoms. Cervical spine MRI may be utilized in patients with suspected cervicogenic headaches to assess for structural abnormalities, such as herniated discs or cervical nerve root impingement.

Other Diagnostic Studies

Lumbar puncture is rarely needed in the evaluation of PTHA. However, measuring the opening pressure is an important diagnostic tool for excluding low or high CSF pressure in selected cases. Patients with low CSF pressure headaches due to a dural tear, which can be caused by mild trauma, have head pain triggered by moving into an upright posture and relieved by lying back down. CSF analysis may also be used to exclude infectious or inflammatory etiologies of headache in selected cases.

Treatment

The treatment of PTHAs can be both challenging and rewarding. To date, there have been no randomized, controlled clinical trials evaluating the efficacy of any therapies for PTHAs. No treatments have been developed specifically for PTHA nor are there any FDA-approved medications with this indication. Therefore, treatments that are known to be effective for primary headache disorders, such as migraine or tension-type headache, are typically employed.

Our approach to treating PTHAs is outlined in Fig. 9.2. A systematic and rational approach to treatment is recommended. The major goals of treatment are to abort headache attacks, decrease headache frequency, and reduce disability. Classification of the headache type is an important step in developing an individualized treatment plan. As discussed in the following sections and outlined in Fig. 9.2, a wide variety of pharmacologic and non-pharmacologic therapies can be utilized to optimize the outcome of different subtypes of PTHA.

Abortive Medications

Abortive headache treatments provide acute relief of individual attacks of headache. The goal is to achieve complete relief or nearly complete relief of head pain as rapidly as possible so that the patient can resume normal activities. A practical goal is to achieve headache relief within 2 h of the onset.

Nonsteroidal anti-inflammatory drugs (NSAIDs) are a good first choice for most types of PTHAs (Fig. 9.2). NSAIDs are effective for

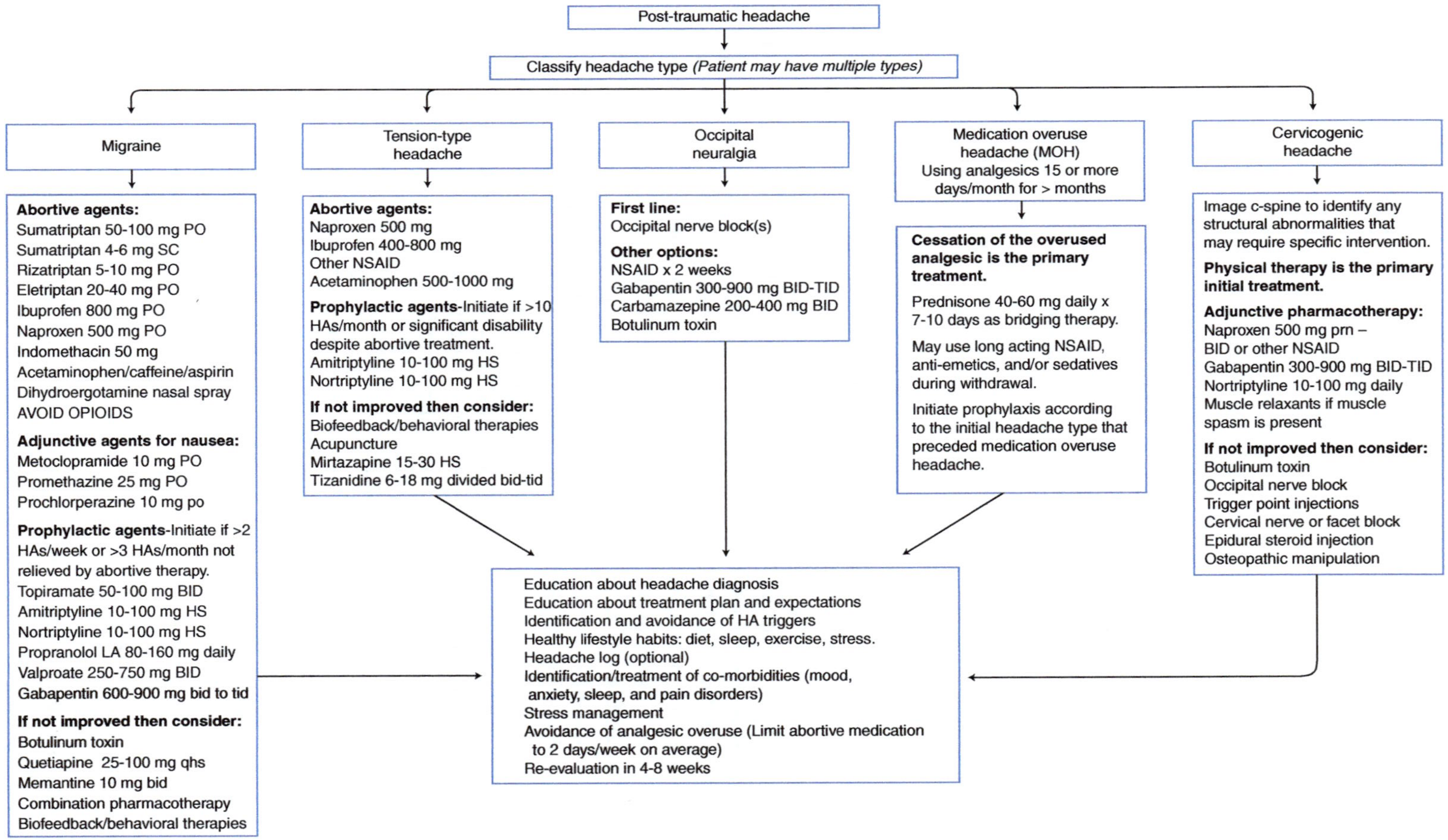

Fig. 9.2 Treatment algorithm (according to headache subtypes)

migraine, tension-type headache, and cervicogenic headache (Silberstein 2000; Evers et al. 2009; Bogduk and Govind 2009; Lenaerts 2009). The specific NSAID agent is not especially important, though naproxen and ibuprofen are the most widely used. Ketorolac injection may be helpful for those who cannot take, or do not respond to, oral medications.

The triptan class of medications should be tried in patients with migraine-type PTHAs that fail to respond adequately to NSAIDs (Fig. 9.2). Triptans are serotonin receptor agonists that are selectively effective for migraine pain and are FDA approved for the treatment of acute migraine. Uncontrolled studies suggest that these agents are effective for aborting attacks of PTHA (Lew et al. 2006). There are more than half a dozen triptan agents on the market and there are several different routes of administration. Oral triptan agents are effective for the majority of patients with migraine. Patients who have rapid-onset headaches or who develop severe nausea or vomiting early in the headache attack may benefit from a nasal or subcutaneous route of administration. Triptans have an excellent safety record, though should be used with caution in patients with vascular risk factors and should be avoided in patients with uncontrolled hypertensions because of their vasoconstriction properties. Patients who experience nausea or vomiting during acute migraine attacks should be prescribed an antiemetic agent, such as metoclopramide or promethazine (Fig. 9.2). Triptan agents may be given in combination with an NSAID for enhanced effectiveness.

There are a variety of combination analgesic products that are marketed for acute treatment of headaches. Such products include Fioricet, Fiorinal, Midrin, and Excedrin. These products may be helpful for patients with infrequent attacks of mild–moderate migraine headache. Excedrin has evidence supporting its effectiveness in migraine, but the other agents have not been rigorously tested (Silberstein 2000). Anecdotally, these agents do not seem to be highly effective for chronic PTHAs and often lead to overuse and dependence. Fioricet and Fiorinal contain butalbital, a barbiturate, which can cause sedation and dependence. Midrin also has sedating properties. Many of these products contain acetaminophen which can reach hepatotoxic levels if the patient uses multiple doses or takes other acetaminophen-containing products. All of these products are relatively short acting and many patients require repeated doses. These properties may contribute to the risk of developing rebound headache with these agents. Patients using these medications must, therefore, be educated about their potentially addictive properties and the risk of developing medication-overuse headache. We do not consider these products first-line treatments for PTHAs and avoid using them in patients who have two or more headaches per week because of the risk of developing rebound headaches.

Opioid medications are generally not highly effective for most headache types and should not be used as first-line headache abortive agents (Silberstein 2000; Borczuk 1995). Opioids should be avoided as much as possible in patients with chronic PTHAs as opioid use is associated with a greater risk of developing chronic daily headache. Opioids, however, are sometimes needed as rescue therapy for severe, intractable headache attacks not responding to multiple first-line abortive agents.

Treatment of medication-overuse headache requires cessation of the causative analgesic agent (Fig. 9.2) (Dodick and Silberstein 2008). Sudden cessation of the offending agent can usually be accomplished, although patients taking large amounts of butalbital-containing products should be tapered gradually to prevent drug-withdrawal seizures. Likewise, patients on large doses of opioids may need to be tapered down or monitored to prevent severe withdrawal symptoms. Cessation of analgesic medication inevitably results in worsening daily headaches for about 2 weeks followed by a gradual improvement back to an episodic headache pattern within 6 weeks. Patients must understand that withdrawal headaches are expected for at least 2 weeks and must be fully committed to the treatment plan. A 7-day course of prednisone 40–60 mg daily may be used to minimize withdrawal headaches (Pageler et al. 2008). A long-acting triptan (naratriptan or frovatriptan) or long-acting NSAID (naproxen or meloxicam) may be used sparingly for severe exacerbations (Dodick and Silberstein 2008). Sleep-inducing medication, antiemetics, and adequate hydration may be helpful during the withdrawal period.

Headache Prevention Medications

Patients who experience frequent headaches may benefit from daily use of headache prophylactic medication. Because most patients with PTHAs experience spontaneous resolution in the first few weeks after injury, many practitioners do not initiate prophylactic therapy until some period of time has passed. It remains to be determined whether initiation of headache prophylactic therapy in the first few days or weeks after injury mitigates acute PTHAs or decreases the likelihood of developing chronic PTHAs. At this time, there is insufficient evidence to guide the decision as to when after the injury headache prophylaxis should be started. However, most practitioners would agree that patients who continue to experience frequent headache more than 2 months after the injury are appropriate candidates for prophylactic therapy.

In general, patients who experience two or more moderate–severe headache attacks per week or 3 or more days of impaired activities per month, over a period of several months, despite use of abortive medications are good candidates for headache prophylactic medication (Silberstein 2000). A practical treatment goal of prophylactic medication is a 50% or greater reduction in headache attack frequency. Prophylactic medications require a minimum of 4 weeks to take effect. They should be started at a low dose to minimize side effects and gradually increased over weeks or even months until the frequency of headaches decreases, side effects develop, or the highest target dose is reached. Patience on the part of both the patient and provider is critical. Switching prophylactic agents prematurely, without first titrating up the dose or treating for a minimum of 6 weeks, is a common mistake that should be avoided.

There are no randomized, controlled trials of prophylactic medications for PTHAs. Agents known to be effective for primary headache disorders are used to treat patients with PTHAs. Uncontrolled studies provide limited support for using amitriptyline, propranolol, or valproate for prophylaxis of chronic PTHAs (Bogduk 2004; Lew et al. 2006; Packard 2000; Tyler et al. 1980). Selection of the prophylactic agent is based primarily on the specific headache type (Fig. 9.2).

Amitriptyline, propranolol, topiramate, and valproate have strong evidence of efficacy as prophylaxis for migraine headaches and the latter three agents are FDA approved for migraine prevention (Silberstein 2000; Evers et al. 2009). Other medications that can be useful for migraine prevention include nortriptyline, gabapentin, and calcium channel blockers (Silberstein 2000; Evers et al. 2009). In clinical practice, if PTHAs have migraine features (i.e., post-traumatic migraine), then a prophylactic agent known to be effective for migraine should be tried (Fig. 9.2). Selection of a migraine prophylactic agent is influenced by the patient's comorbid conditions. One should try to avoid prophylactic agents that will aggravate comorbid conditions and select an agent that may benefit one or more comorbid conditions. Propranolol, or another beta blocker, is a good choice for patients with post-traumatic migraine who also have hypertension or essential tremor. Topiramate is optimal for patients with migraine with comorbid obesity or epilepsy. Valproate is appropriate for post-traumatic migraines in the setting of comorbid bipolar disorder or epilepsy, but must be used with caution owing to its teratogenicity, risk of hepatotoxicity, and propensity for promoting weight gain.

Tricyclic antidepressants, such as amitriptyline or nortriptyline, are appropriate first-line agents for prophylaxis of PTHAs resembling tension-type headaches (Lenaerts 2009). TCAs have evidence for efficacy in tension-type headache, though are unproven for PTHAs. Muscle relaxants have no proven benefit for tension-type headache but are sometimes prescribed. Other prophylactic agents that may be helpful for tension-type headache are tizanidine, mirtazapine, and topiramate.

Post-traumatic neuralgiform headaches, such as occipital neuralgia or trigeminal neuralgia, may benefit from an anticonvulsant. Carbamazepine is the most established agent for trigeminal neuralgia (Gronseth et al. 2008). Oxcarbazepine is also effective for trigeminal neuralgia (Gronseth et al. 2008). Gabapentin can be used to treat occipital neuralgia (Fig. 9.2). Lamotrigine is another option for neuralgiform headaches. It is well tolerated and has minimal adverse cognitive side effects, but must be slowly titrated up to minimize the risk of a serious mucocutaneous reaction.

Non-pharmacologic Therapies

A variety of non-pharmacologic interventions may be helpful in treating PTHAs. Such treatments include behavioral therapies, physical modalities, and injection procedures. There are no randomized, controlled trials evaluating the effectiveness of any of these approaches for PTHAs, but there is evidence supporting their use in other headache disorders. Most non-pharmacologic techniques have minimal to no adverse effects and may be used as an adjunct to pharmacologic treatments.

All patients with PTHAs should receive education about their diagnosis and treatment plan. Patients with acute PTHAs should be reassured that their headaches are likely to improve over time. Patients with chronic PTHAs should be informed that there are numerous therapies that may alleviate headaches but it may take multiple trials to optimize treatment. Patients should be given clear instructions about the goals and proper uses of any prescribed medications. Establishing realistic expectations and enlisting the active participation of the patient will improve compliance.

Lifestyle modification is a simple, yet often overlooked, technique. Patients should be encouraged to establish healthy meal, sleep, and exercise patterns. Patients may identify specific triggers for their headaches which can be avoided. Caffeine overuse, smoking, and alcohol use can contribute to headaches. A headache log may help identify potential triggers in some cases.

Several uncontrolled studies of relaxation therapy and biofeedback have shown favorable results in PTHA (Gurr and Coetzer 2005; Tatrow et al. 2003b). These techniques seem to be especially helpful for patients with PTHAs who have significant muscle tightness, anxiety, or insomnia. The efficacy of these techniques for migraine headache is well established (Silberstein 2000).

Physical modalities, such as physical therapy, osteopathic manipulation therapy, acupuncture, and massage, have not been evaluated for PTHA. These techniques may be useful as adjuncts to medical therapy, particularly in patients with suspected cervical sources of pain (Fig. 9.2). Physical therapy is an important initial step in treating post-traumatic cervicogenic headache.

Procedures

Occipital nerve blocks, performed by injection of local anesthetic with or without steroid, can be helpful for treating a variety of headache types, most notably occipital neuralgia (Tobin and Flitman 2009). One case series showed an 80% response rate of post-traumatic occipital neuralgia following nerve blockade (Hecht 2004). Occipital nerve blocks can also help alleviate cervicogenic headache and migraine headaches (Tobin and Flitman 2009).

Other techniques that may be considered are botulinum toxin injections or trigger point injections of craniocervical muscles. These approaches are well suited for patients with cervical myofascial pain and muscle tenderness as prominent features (Bogduk 2004; Bogduk and Govind 2009; Freund and Schwartz 2001). The efficacy of these treatments for PTHA has not been systematically studied. The efficacy of botulinum toxin injections for tension-type headache and migraine is also uncertain. Nonetheless, there is considerable anecdotal reports and clinical experience with these approaches. Headaches secondary to C2–C3 facet joint dysfunction can be treated with facet joint blocks or cervical medial branch blocks (Bogduk 2004; Bogduk and Govind 2009).

Occipital neurolysis, occipital nerve decompression surgery, and implantation of occipital nerve stimulators are potentially useful treatments for refractory headaches. Studies are needed to validate the usefulness of these more invasive techniques before they can be routinely recommended for use in PTHA.

Treatment of Comorbid Conditions

Treating headaches in isolation, without taking into account comorbid conditions, can contribute to treatment failure. Identifying and treating concurrent conditions are important steps in optimizing the headache care plan. Comorbid conditions may limit treatment options or provide therapeutic opportunities. One should avoid headache treatments that may exacerbate comorbid conditions and select headache treatments that benefit one or more comorbid conditions. Conditions comorbid with PTHA that may influence selection of headache prophylactic medication include concurrent primary headache disorders, sleep disorders, epilepsy, hypertension, alcohol abuse, depression, anxiety, PTSD, obesity, analgesic overuse, postamputation limb pain, and other chronic pain disorders. Patients with psychological or psychiatric conditions should be evaluated and treated for these conditions, ideally by a mental health professional.

Summary

PTHAs are a heterogeneous syndrome that can be challenging and rewarding to treat. PTHAs are currently defined as headaches, with any features, that begin within 7 days of a traumatic head or neck injury. Such headaches often resolve in the first few months after injury, but chronic headaches can persist for years. A comprehensive diagnostic and therapeutic approach is needed to establish an individualized treatment plan that addresses all of the potential underlying causes of head pain as well as comorbid conditions that can perpetuate the headache syndrome. PTHAs often resemble primary headache disorders and are treated in a similar manner. Classifying the phenotype of PTHA helps guide treatment. A combination of pharmacologic and nonpharmacologic interventions may be necessary to achieve a favorable outcome. Studies are needed to identify the biological mechanisms that generate PTHAs and to determine the most effective therapies.

References

American Academy of Neurology Practice Parameter. The management of concussion in sports. Neurology. 1997;48:581–5.

Baandrup L, Jensen R. Chronic post-traumatic headache—a clinical analysis in relation to the international headache classification 2nd edition. Cephalalgia. 2005;25(2):132–8.

Balla J, Karnaghan J. Whiplash headache. Clin Exp Neurol. 1987;23:179–82.

Bartsch T, Goadsby PJ. The trigeminocervical complex and migraine: current concepts and synthesis. Curr Pain Headache Rep. 2003;7(5):371–6.

Beck AT, Steer RA, Ball R, Ranieri W. Comparison of beck depression inventories. J Pers Assess. 1996;67(3):588–97.

Blanchard EB, Jones-Alexander J, Buckley TC, Forneris CA. Psychometric properties of the PTSD checklist. Behav Res Ther. 1996;34(8):669–73.

Bogduk N. The neck and headaches. Neurol Clin. 2004;22(1):151–71.

Bogduk N, Govind J. Cervicogenic headache:an assessment of the evidence on clinical diagnosis, invasive tests, and treatment. Lancet Neurol. 2009;8(10): 959–68.

Borczuk P. Predictors of intracranial injury in patients with mild head trauma. Ann Emerg Med. 1995;25: 731–6.

Buysse DJ, Reynolds III CF, Monk TH, Berman SR, Kupfer DJ. The Pittsburgh Sleep Quality Index: a new instrument for psychiatric practice and research. Psychiatry Res. 1989;28(2):193–213.

Couch JR, Bearss C. Chronic daily headache in the post-traumatic syndrome: relation to extent of head injury. Headache. 2001;41(6):559–64.

Dodick D, Freitag F. Evidence-based understanding of medication-overuse headache: clinical implications. Headache. 2006;46 suppl 4:S202–11.

Dodick DW, Silberstein SD. How clinicians can detect, prevent, and treat medication overuse headache. Cephalalgia. 2008;28(11):1207–17.

Evans RW. Post-traumatic headaches. Neurol Clin. 2004;22(1):237–49. viii.

Evans RW. Expert opinion: posttraumatic headaches among United States soldiers injured in Afghanistan and Iraq. Headache. 2008;48(8):1216–25.

Evers S, Afra J, Frese A, Goadsby PJ, Linde M, May A, Sandor PS, European Federation of Neurological Societies. EFNS guideline on the drug treatment of migraine- revised report of an EFNS task force. Eur J Neurol. 2009;16(9):968–81.

Faux S, Sheedy J. A prospective controlled study in the prevalence of posttraumatic headache following mild traumatic brain injury. Pain Med. 2008;9(8):1001–11.

Formisano R, Bivona U, Catani S, D'Ippolito M, Buzzi MG. Post-traumatic headache: facts and doubts. J Headache Pain. 2009;10:145–52.

Freeman MD, Croft AC, Rossignol AM, Weaver DS, Reiser M. A review and methodologic critique of the literature refuting whiplash syndrome. Spine (Phila Pa 1976). 1999;24(1):86–96.

Freund B, Schwartz M. Treatment of chronic cervical-associated headache with botulinum toxin a: a pilot study. Headache. 2001;40(3):231–6.

Giza CC, Hovda DA. The neurometabolic cascade of concussion. J Athletic Train. 2001;36(3):228–35.

Glaesser J, Neuner F, Lütgehetmann R, Schmidt R, Elbert T. Posttraumatic stress disorder in patients with traumatic brain injury. BMC Psychiatry. 2004;4:5–11.

Gronseth G, CruccuAlksne J, Argoff C, Brainin M, Burchiel K, Nurmikko T, Zakrzewska JM. Practice parameter: the diagnostic evaluation and treatment of trigeminal neuralgia (an evidence-based review): report of the Quality Standards Subcommittee of the American Academy of Neurology and the European Federation of Neurological Societies. Neurology. 2008;71(15):1183–90.

Gurr B, Coetzer BR. The effectiveness of cognitive-behavioral therapy for post-traumatic headaches. Brain Inj. 2005;19(7):481–91.

Haas DC. Chronic post-traumatic headaches classified and compared with natural headaches. Cephalalgia. 1996;16(7):486–93.

Headache Classification Subcommittee of the International Headache Society. The international classification of headache disorders: 2nd edition. Cephalalgia. 2004;24 suppl 1:9–160.

Hecht JS. Occipital nerve blocks in postconcussive headaches: a retrospective review and report of ten patients. J Head Trauma Rehabil. 2004;19(1):58–71.

Hoge CW, McGurk D, Thomas JL, Cox AL, Engel CC, Castro CA. Mild traumatic brain injury in U.S. Soldiers returning from Iraq. N Engl J Med. 2008;358(5):453–63.

Hughes DG, Jackson A, Mason DL, Berry E, Hollis S, Yates DW. Abnormalities on magnetic resonance imaging seen acutely following mild traumatic brain injury: correlation with neuropsychological tests and delayed recovery. Neuroradiology. 2004;46:550–8.

Inamasu J, Shingo H, Katsunori A, Sadao S, Takeshi K, Naoki A. CT scans essential after posttraumatic loss of consciousness. Am J Emerg Med. 2000;18:810–1.

Jensen OK, Nielsen FF. The influence of sex and pre-traumatic headache on the incidence and severity of headache after head injury. Cephalalgia. 1990;10:285–93.

Keshavan MS, Channabasavanna SM, Reddy GN. Post-traumatic psychiatric disturbances: Patterns and predictors of outcome. Br J Psychiatry. 1981;1981(138):157–60.

Kirk C, Nagiub G, Abu-Arafeh I. Chronic post-traumatic headache after head injury in children and adolescents. Dev Med Child Neurol. 2008;50(6):422–5.

Kosinksi M, Bayliss MS, Bjorner JB, Ware JE, Garber WH, Batenhorst A, Cady R, Dahlof CG, Dowson A, Tepper S. A six-item short-form survey for measuring headache impact: the HIT-6. Qual Life Res. 2003;12(8):963–74.

Lenaerts ME. Post-traumatic headache: from classification challenges to biological underpinnings. Cephalalgia. 2008;28 suppl 1:12–5.

Lenaerts ME. Pharmacotherapy of tension-type headache (TTH). Expert Opin Pharmacother. 2009;10(8):1261–71.

Lenaerts ME, Couch JR, Couch JR. Posttraumatic headache. Curr Treat Options Neurol. 2004;6(6):507–17.

Lew HL, Lin PH, Fuh JL, Wang SJ, Clark DJ, Walker WC. Characteristics and treatment of headache after traumatic brain injury: a focused review. Am J Phys Med Rehabil. 2006;85(7):619–27.

Mickeviciene D, Shrader H, Nestvold K, Surkiene D, Kunickas R, Stover LJ, Sand T. A controlled historical cohort study on the post-concussion syndrome. Eur J Neurol. 2002;9(6):581–7.

Moscato D, Peracchi MI, Mazzotta G, Savi L, Battistella PA. Post-traumatic headache from moderate head injury. J Headache Pain. 2005;6(4):284–6.

Nampiaparampil DE. Prevalence of chronic pain after traumatic brain injury: a systematic review. JAMA. 2008;300(6):711–9.

Okie S. Traumatic brain injury in the war zone. N Engl J Med. 2005;352:2043–7.

Packard RC. Post-traumatic headache:permanency and relationship to legal settlement. Headache. 1992;32:496–500.

Packard RC. Epidemiology and pathogenesis of posttraumatic headache. J Head Trauma Rehabil. 1999;14(1):9–21.

Packard RC. Treatment of chronic daily posttraumatic headache with divalproex sodium. Headache. 2000;40:736–9.

Packard RC. Chronic post-traumatic headache: associations with mild traumatic brain injury, concussion, and post-concussive disorder. Curr Pain Headache Rep. 2008;12:67–73.

Packard RC, Ham LP. Posttraumatic headache: determining chronicity. Headache. 1993;33:133–4.

Packard RC, Ham LP. Pathogenesis of posttraumatic headache and migraine: a common headache pathway? Headache. 1997;37:142–52.

Pageler L, Katsarava Z, Diener HC, Limmroth V. Prednisone vs. placebo in withdrawal therapy following medication overuse headache. Cephalalgia. 2008;28(2):152–6.

Schrader H, Stovner LJ, Obelieniene D, Surkiene D, Mickeviciene D, Bovim G, Sand T. Examination of the diagnostic validity of headache attributed to whiplash injury: a controlled, prospective study. Eur J Neurol. 2006;13(11):1226–32.

Silberstein SD. Practice parameter: evidence-based guidelines for migraine headache: report of the quality standards committee of the American Academy of Neurology. Neurology. 2000;55:754–62.

Silver JM, McAllister TW, Arciniegas DB. Depression and cognitive complaints following mild traumatic brain injury. Am J Psychiatry. 2009;166:653–61.

Solomon S. Chronic post-traumatic neck and head pain. Headache. 2005;45(1):53–67.

Sterner Y, Toolanen G, Knibestöl M, Gerdle B, Hildingsson C. Prospective study of trigeminal sensibility after whiplash trauma. J Spinal Disord. 2001;14(6):479–86.

Stewart WF, Lipton RB, Dowson AJ, Sawyer J. Development and testing of the Migraine Disability Assessment (MIDAS) Questionnaire to assess headache-related disability. Neurology. 2001;56(6 suppl 1):S20–8.

Stovner LJ, Schrader H, Mickeviciene D, Surkiene D, Sand T. Headache after concussion. Eur J Neurol. 2009;16(1):112–20.

Tatrow K, Blanchard EB, Hickling EJ, Silverman DJ. Posttraumatic headache: biopsychosocial comparisons with multiple control groups. Headache. 2003a;43(7):755–66.

Tatrow K, Blanchard EB, Silverman DJ. Post-traumatic headache: an exploratory treatment study. Appl Psychophysiol Biofeedback. 2003b;28(4):267078.

Theeler BJ, Flynn F, Erickson JC. Post-traumatic headaches after mild head injury in U.S. soldiers returning from Iraq or Afghanistan. Neurology. 2009;72(11 suppl 3):A496–97.

Tobin J, Flitman S. Occipital nerve blocks: when and what to inject? Headache. 2009;49(10):1521–33.

Tyler GS, McNeely HE, Dick ML. Treatment of post traumatic headache with amitriptyline. Headache. 1980;20(4):213–6.

Vanderploeg R, Vanderploeg R, Belanger HG, Curtiss G. Mild traumatic brain injury and post traumatic stress disorder and their associations with health symptoms. Arch Phys Med Rehabil. 2009;90:1084–93.

Walker WC, Seel RT, Curtiss G, Warden DL. Headache after moderate and severe traumatic brain injury: a longitudinal analysis. Arch Phys Med Rehabil. 2005;86(9):1793–800.

Weiss HD, Stern BJ, Goldberg J. Post-traumatic migraine: chronic migraine precipitated by minor head or neck trauma. Headache. 1991;31(7):451–6.

Wilson MC, Krolczyk SJ. Pediatric post-traumatic headache. Curr Pain Headache Rep. 2006;10(5):387–90.

Yamaguchi M. Incidence of headache and severity of head injury. Headache. 1992;32(9):427–31.

Seizures After TBI

10

John Betjemann and Karen Parko

Abstract

Representing approximately 5% of epilepsy in the civilian population and up to 50% in certain military populations, post-traumatic epilepsy (PTE) warrants both increased clinical attention and research considerations. In this chapter, we discuss the important definitions when considering post-traumatic epilepsy including the timing of post-traumatic seizures and the severity of head injuries. We also review the epidemiology and risk factors for in both the civilian population and the military, as these groups vary significantly. In addition, we elucidate potential pathophysiologic mechanisms underlying PTE and consider its role as a model for epileptogenesis in current and future research. Our clinical discussion focuses on the timing of post-traumatic seizures, the utility of diagnostic testing, the evidence for treatment of PTE and ultimately outcomes. We highlight the relevant studies in each section and underscore the theme that more research is certainly needed.

Keywords

Epilepsy • Traumatic brain injury • Post-traumatic epilepsy • Seizure • Anticonvulsant • Epidemiology • Antiepileptic drugs • Post-traumatic seizures • Epileptogenesis

J. Betjemann, M.D.
Department of Clinical Neurology, University of California at San Francisco, San Francisco, CA, USA

K. Parko, M.D. (✉)
Department of Clinical Neurology, University of California at San Francisco, San Francisco, CA, USA

VA Epilepsy Centers of Excellence, San Francisco VA Medical Center, San Francisco, CA, USA
e-mail: Karen.Parko@va.gov

Introduction

Since ancient times, traumatic brain injury (TBI) has been associated with the development of epilepsy. In *"Injuries of the Head,"* Hippocrates (460–357 B.C.) recognized that a wound to the left temporal region could cause convulsions of the right side of the body (Caveness et al. 1979). Physicians of the same era also came to recognize these post-traumatic seizures as a poor

J.W. Tsao (ed.), *Traumatic Brain Injury: A Clinician's Guide to Diagnosis, Management, and Rehabilitation*, DOI 10.1007/978-0-387-87887-4_10, © Springer Science+Business Media, LLC 2012

prognostic sign. More detailed descriptions of traumatic brain injuries resulting in seizures can be found during the Renaissance. However, post-traumatic epilepsy (PTE) remained largely under-appreciated until the late nineteenth century. For instance, in a series of 67 patients described by French physician Leuret in 1843, epilepsy was believed to arise from a head injury in just one case while "fear" was the most common etiology, responsible for 35 cases (Lowenstein 2009).

Epilepsies are divided into either primary or secondary based on their etiology. Primary epilepsies are idiopathic and likely represent genetic syndromes. Secondary epilepsies are acquired from a brain insult (trauma, infections, tumors, strokes). Accounting for 5% of all epilepsy in the general population and 20% of acquired, or symptomatic epilepsy, TBI is now widely recognized as an important etiologic consideration in the epilepsy population (Hauser et al. 1991). Moreover, in certain military populations, the probability of developing PTE can exceed 50%. Although PTE has become more readily recognized and studied, it has proven extremely difficult to treat both medically and surgically. PTE is also beginning to serve as a model for epileptogenesis in an effort to identify novel biomarkers and target truly antiepileptogenic therapies.

In this chapter we:

1. Review the varied definitions as they pertain to classifying post-traumatic seizures and severity of brain injuries.
2. Discuss the epidemiology and risk factors for PTE in both general and military populations.
3. Explore the pathophysiology of PTE.
4. Examine the types of seizures in PTE and the timing of the onset of seizures.
5. Review potential diagnostic tools.
6. Detail what is known regarding the treatment of post-traumatic seizures and epilepsy.
7. Look at the impact of PTE on outcomes.
8. Conclude with an update on PTE as a model of epileptogenesis, animal models, biomarkers, and novel therapeutic strategies.

Definitions

PTE is a heterogeneous condition, and one of the major challenges in studying PTE and interpreting existing data is recognizing the various definitions that are employed. Most investigators have made the distinction between PTE, or recurrent unprovoked seizures following TBI, and seizures immediately following a head injury. As such, the following definitions are widely accepted:

- *Immediate seizures*: occurring less than 24 h after injury.
- *Early seizures*: occurring between 24 h and 7 days after injury.
- *Late seizures*: occurring more than 7 days after injury.

Immediate and early seizures are believed to be the result of acute injury and do not constitute epilepsy while recurrent late seizures define PTE.

The other main set of definitions to consider involves rating the severity of head injury. The most widely accepted definitions characterize head injuries into the following three severities:

- *Mild*: Glasgow Coma Scale (GCS) 13–15, alteration in consciousness ≤24 h, loss of consciousness <30 min, post-traumatic amnesia ≤24 h, and negative cerebral imaging.
- *Moderate*: GCS 9–12, alteration in consciousness >24 h, loss of consciousness between 30 min and 24 h, post-traumatic amnesia between 24 h and 7 days, and either positive or negative cerebral imaging.
- *Severe*: GCS 3–8, alteration in consciousness >24 h, loss of consciousness ≥24 h, post-traumatic amnesia ≥7 days, and usually positive cerebral imaging.

Within these definitions, positive cerebral imaging is mainly defined as the presence of a skull fracture, cerebral contusion, or intracranial hemorrhage of any type.

While the main focus of this book is mild TBI, unfortunately very little is known about mild TBI and the development of PTE. This may be a manifestation of mild TBI patients not coming to medical attention. In addition, within the military there existed a stigma against reporting mild head injuries. This chapter highlights each instance in which studies have addressed mild TBI; however, we also spend considerable time discussing moderate and severe TBI.

Epidemiology and Risk Factors

When evaluating the overall risk for developing epilepsy following common brain injuries, severe TBI confers a relative risk of 29 times that of the general population, placing it behind only brain tumors and subarachnoid hemorrhage (Herman 2002). In general, risk factors with a relative risk greater than 10 are believed to have a strong causal relationship while those between 4 and 10 have a probable causal relationship (Herman 2002). Figure 10.1, adapted from Dr. Susan Herman's 2002 article in *Neurology* summarizes these relative risks and clearly illustrates the strong relationship between the severity of head injury and the risk of developing PTE.

Despite the fact that PTE accounts for a significant portion of all epilepsy, there have been relatively few studies examining the incidence of PTE in the civilian population. Once again, these studies are quite heterogeneous in both their definitions and methodology. For the purposes of this discussion, we separate these studies by the population examined (i.e., population-based versus patients admitted to a facility). For each we consider their definition of head injuries, incidence of early and/or late seizures, and their respective risk factors.

Population-Based Studies

Annegers et al. (1980) published a large population-based study following a cohort of 2,747 civilians in Rochester, Minnesota, over a total of 28,176 person-years. There were 1,640 mild head injuries defined as either unconsciousness or post-traumatic amnesia for less than 30 min without evidence of a skull fracture. The 912 moderate head injuries were defined by skull fractures or loss of consciousness or post-traumatic amnesia for more than 30 min. Severe head injuries, of which there were 195, had at least one of the following features: brain contusion (diagnosed by abnormal neurologic exam or by observation during surgery), intracranial hematoma, or more than 24 h of either unconsciousness or post-traumatic

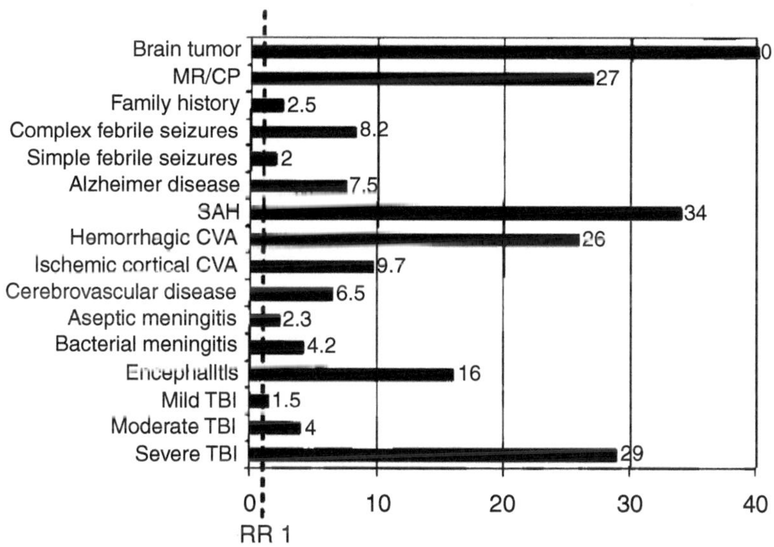

Fig. 10.1 Relative risk for unprovoked seizures after common brain injuries. The dotted vertical line represents the general population risk for unprovoked seizures. MR/CP = mental retardation/cerebral palsy; SAH = subarachnoid hemorrhage; CVA = cerebrovascular accident; TBI = traumatic brain injury. (adapted from Herman 2002)

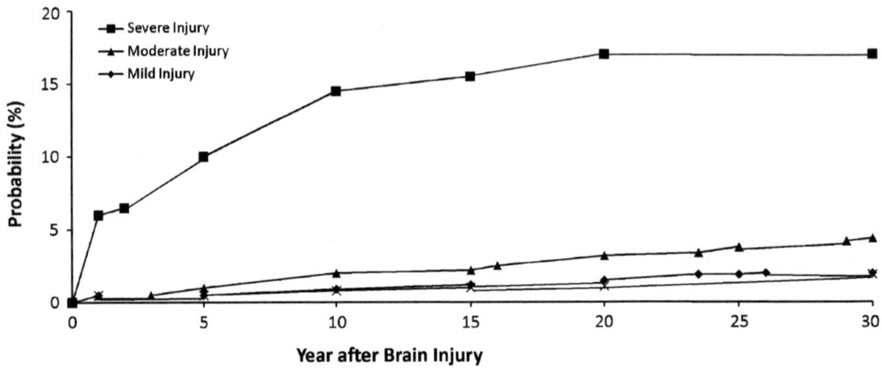

Fig. 10.2 Cumulative probability of unprovoked seizures in 4541 patients with traumatic brain injuries according to the severity of the injury and the incidence of seizures in the general population. The cumulative incidence in the population was derived from incidence rates, with the use of the density method to convert the rate to risk estimates. The asterisks indicate the incidence in the general population at specific points in time (adapted from Annegers 1998)

amnesia. Early seizures were defined as occurring "while still suffering from the direct effects of the head injury," up to 2 weeks after injury. Early seizures were observed in 2.1% with the main risk factors being age <15 years and severe head injury. Late, unprovoked seizures occurred in 1.9% with the main risk factors being severe head injury and the presence of early seizures. Broken down by severity, the risk of PTE within 1 year of severe TBI was 7.1% and 11.5% within 5 years. For moderate head injuries, the risks were 0.7% and 1.6%, respectively and for mild head injuries, 0.1% and 0.6%, respectively. As such, the authors concluded that the risk of PTE following a mild head injury was no greater than the risk experienced by the general population.

Utilizing the same definitions as the previous study, Annegers et al. published a second population-based study in 1998. This cohort was comprised of 4,541 children and adults living in Olmsted County, Minnesota and was followed for 53,222 person-years. Figure 10.2 depicts the cumulative probability of seizures based on severity of injury compared to the general population. They found a significantly elevated risk of PTE among severe and moderate head injuries as evidenced by the following standardized incidence ratios: 17.0 (CI, 12.3–23.6), 2.9 (1.9–4.1), and 1.5 (1–2.2) for severe, moderate and mild head injuries, respectively. When looking specifically at mild head injuries, the increased risk of seizures abated after 5 years, after which the risk of epilepsy was no greater than the risk incurred by the general population. When considering severe head injuries, they noted a significantly increased risk of seizures more than 10 years after injury. Finally, employing a multivariate model of analysis the authors demonstrated an increased risk of late seizures, or PTE, with severe injury, brain contusion or hematoma, loss of consciousness or post-traumatic amnesia for >24 h and an age of 65 years or older.

Studies of Hospitalized Patients

A somewhat more heterogeneous group of studies exists examining the incidence of seizures in TBI patients admitted to the hospital or a TBI rehabilitation center. Not surprisingly, the rate of early and late post-traumatic seizures is higher in these studies compared to the population-based studies.

- Briefly, one study followed 896 consecutive patients admitted to the hospital and calculated incidences of 4.2% and 10.2% for early and late seizures, respectively (Jennett and

Lewin 1960). Of note, late epilepsy was defined as “one or more late fits,” and prophylactic phenobarbitone was prescribed for patients who were deemed likely to develop epilepsy. Early seizures were more likely in patients with >24 h of post-traumatic amnesia, depressed skull fracture, and intracranial hematoma. The risk of late seizures was increased by intracranial hematoma alone and a combination of depressed skull fracture and >24 h of post-traumatic amnesia.

- A second study followed 137 consecutive head injury patients admitted to the hospital for a median of 12 months (Angeleri et al. 1999). The incidence of late seizures was 13.1% and the risk of PTE was increased by low GCS (3–8), the presence of a single lesion on CT (particularly temporal or frontal), the presence of early seizures (defined as occurring within 4 weeks of injury), and the development of a focal EEG abnormality 1 month after injury.
- Englander et al. (2003) investigated the rate of PTE among 647 TBI patients admitted to one of four trauma centers. The study preselected for moderate and severe head injuries by including only those patients with a positive CT scan within 7 days of injury or a best GCS score of ≤10 in the first 24 h post-injury. Late post-traumatic seizures, defined as occurring more than 1 week after injury, occurred in 10.2% of the population. Of note, many of the patients were initially treated with prophylactic phenytoin; however, to remain in the study phenytoin had to be discontinued by week 4. The investigators found an increased risk of seizures associated with multiple or bilateral contusions, dural penetration, the need for multiple intracranial surgeries, subdural hematoma requiring evacuation, and midline shift greater than 5 mm. Interestingly, the investigators found that the probability of unprovoked seizures at 2 years was related to the number of cerebral contusions with approximately 25% probability for patients with multiple contusions, 8% for a single contusion, and 6% for no contusions.
- One final study evaluated the incidence of early (<1 week after injury) and late post-traumatic seizures (>1 week) in 490 consecutive patients admitted to a rehabilitation program for post-injury problems in education and employment (Asikainen et al. 1999). Based on this patient population, the study involved mainly those with moderate to severe TBI, though patients with the most severe injuries were also excluded, as they were unlikely to be admitted to the rehabilitation facility. Early post-traumatic seizures were seen in 16.3% of all patients and were significantly more likely in patients under age 8. PTE was observed in 25.3% and those with early seizures or depressed skull fractures had a statistically significant increased risk.

The findings of these studies as well as two pediatric studies are well summarized in Table 10.1 adapted from Garga and Lowenstein (2006).

The Military Experience

Much of what is known about TBI and the development of PTE stems from studies of combat veterans from World War I to present day conflicts. With rates as high as 53%, the general risk of PTE in the traumatic brain injured military population is substantially higher than in the civilian population. This increased risk has been associated with a higher proportion of severe traumatic brain injuries, particularly those involving dural penetration. Over time and conflicts, the rate of incidence of PTE following missile injuries has remained remarkably consistent (Table 10.2). As seen in civilian studies, the rate of development of PTE is highest in the first year following injury across all injury severities. That said, the incidence of epilepsy within 5 years of injury ranges from 22 to 43% and is approximately 50% by 10 years, evidence that a significant number of veterans develop epilepsy many years after injury (Lowenstein 2009).

The Vietnam Head Injury Study (VHIS) has provided some of the most extensive longitudinal

Table 10.1 Incidence of early and late post-traumatic seizures in civilian populations

Study	Feature	*N*	Early seizure (%)	Risk factors	Late seizure (%)	Risk factors
Jennett and Lewin (1960)	Admitted	896	4.2	PTS >24 h, age <5 years, skull fracture, intracranial hemorrhage	10.2	Early seizure, PTA >24 h, depressed skull fracture, intracranial hematoma
Annegers et al. (1980)	Population admitted,	2,747	2.1	Age <15 years, severe injury	1.9	Severe injury, early seizure
Desai et al. (1983)	pediatric	702	4.1	Age <16 years, focal neuro deficits, LOC/PTA >30 min, skull fracture, intracranial hematoma	N/A	N/A
Annegers et al. (1998)	Population	4,541	2.6	Not evaluated	2.1	Severe injury, brain contusion, subdural hematoma, LOC/PTA >24 h
Hahn et al. (1988)	Admitted, pediatric	937	9.8	GCS 3–8, diffuse cerebral edema, acute subdural hematoma	N/A	N/A
Angeleri et al. (1999)	Admitted	137	8		13.1	GCS 3–8, early seizures, single brain CT lesions, EEG focus
Asikainen et al. (1999)	TBI Rehab Center	490	16.3	Age <8 years	25.3	Early seizures, depressed skull fracture
Englander et al. (2003)	Admitted with CT findings or GCS 3–10	647	3	N/A	10.2	Multiple or bilateral cortical contusions, dural penetration, multiple intracranial operations, midline shift >5 mm, evacuated SDH

PTA post-traumatic amnesia, *LOC* loss of consciousness, *GCS* Glasgow coma scale, *TBI* traumatic brain injury, *SDH* subdural hematoma

Table 10.2 Post-traumatic epilepsy following craniocerebral missile wounds in armed conflicts during the twentieth century (adapted from Salazar et al., 1999)

			Post-traumatic epilepsy (%)	
Conflict	Author(s), year	No. of patients	5 years	10–15+ years
WWI	Credner, 1930	1,990	38	50
WWI	Ascroft, 1941	317	35	–
WWI	Caviness, 1966	82	–	50
WWII	Russell & Whitty, 1952	820	43	–
WWII	Walker & Erculei, 1969	739	34	–
Korean War	Caveness et al., 1962	211	36	–
Korean War	Taylor & Kretschmann, 1971	474	–	50
Vietnam War	Caveness et al. 1979	1,135	34	–
Vietnam War	Salazar et al. 1985, 1987	520	34	51
Iran–Iraq	Aarabi, 1990	489	32	–
Lebanon	Brandvold et al., 1990	46	22	–

data regarding the development of PTE. Of the 421 Vietnam veterans with penetrating head injury, 53% had PTE 15 years after injury (Salazar et al. 1985). Moreover, the risk of developing PTE within 1 year of injury was nearly 580 times that of the general age-matched population. Ten to fifteen years later, the risk of developing PTE in this population was still 25 times higher than the general population. Recently, phase 3 of the VHIS was published. This portion of the study evaluated 199 of the original VHIS veterans and demonstrated the prevalence of seizures to be 43.7% 30–35 years after injury, similar to the prevalence found in phase 2, 20 years earlier (Raymont et al. 2010). In addition, 12.6% experienced very late onset of PTE with their first seizure occurring more than 14 years after injury.

Naturally, the data from prior wars are cause for serious concern over the injuries and their possible life-long consequences for current service men and women in the Middle East conflicts. TBI has been dubbed the "signature injury" of these conflicts because of the nature of injuries sustained from explosives such as improvised explosive devices. Nearly 22% of the wounded soldiers evaluated at Landstuhl Regional Medical Center in Germany have sustained injuries to the head, face, or neck (Okie 2005). Experts believe this number can serve as a rough estimate of the incidence of TBI in the current conflicts and in fact likely underestimates the true percentage. By comparison, in the Vietnam War only 12–14% of all combat casualties had sustained a head injury (Okie 2005). In addition, the mortality rate for Vietnam soldiers who sustained head injuries approached 75%, whereas many more of our current soldiers are surviving their injuries because of faster access to improved medical care and better body armor. As a result, we are likely to see a significant number of soldiers returning from the Middle East conflicts with TBI and potentially PTE.

Pathophysiology

As mentioned previously, early post-traumatic seizures do not constitute PTE and are felt to be an epiphenomenon of the underlying brain injury or a marker for the severity of injury (Herman 2002). Accordingly, early and late seizures should be considered separately and are believed to have different pathologic mechanisms. This concept is further supported by the ability to suppress early seizures with antiepileptics without significantly altering the incidence of PTE. The exact pathophysiologic mechanisms underlying PTE are not completely understood and continue to be investigated. Evidence suggests a multifactorial process including contributions from blood–brain barrier changes, parenchymal hemorrhage, release of excitotoxins, and free radical damage (Herman 2002). More specifically, the pathophysiology varies according to the type of injury. Closed head injuries cause edema, diffuse axonal injury, and ischemia resulting in the release of toxic mediators (Agrawal et al. 2006). Penetrating injuries lead to the formation of epileptogenic focal cortical scars. Evidence also exists linking hemorrhagic infarction to the formation of an epileptic focus through ferrous deposits and a resulting cascade that culminates in cell death (Agrawal et al. 2006).

Types of Seizures and Timing of Seizures

Seizure types observed in PTE have been examined in a few studies, but ultimately no consistent themes have emerged. Approximately two-thirds of patients with PTE will experience either generalized seizures or focal onset seizures with secondary generalization, while others will have only focal seizures (Agrawal et al. 2006). Specifically, Haltiner et al. (1997) observed 60 patients with moderate to severe TBI and found that 31 had generalized seizures, 20 had focal onset seizures, and 9 had focal onset seizures with secondary generalization. Similar percentages were noted by Englander et al. (2003) in the study of patients admitted to trauma centers. In the more recently published phase 3 of the VHIS trial, the most common clinical seizure type experienced were focal onset seizures with alteration of consciousness (formerly called complex partial seizures).

The presentation of PTE varies widely. Most studies indicate that the risk of developing PTE is highest in the first 1–2 years post-injury. Data from the VHIS revealed that while 57% of PTE developed within 1 year of injury, over 18% experienced their first seizure more than 5 years after injury, and 7% experienced their first seizure 10 or more years after injury (Salazar et al. 1985). Others have demonstrated 80% of PTE presenting in the first year with up to 90% by 18 months (Englander et al. 2003). From the large population-based study of civilians in Olmsted County, Minnesota, it became clear that following a mild TBI the risk of developing PTE remained elevated for only 5 years, while the risk remained increased for 10 years in moderate TBI and for at least 20 years in the severe TBI population (Annegers et al. 1998). Exactly how long the risk remains elevated is unclear and the data mentioned earlier from phase 3 of the VHIS demonstrated new cases of PTE some 30–35 years after injury. While it seems certain that the risk of developing PTE many years after injury persists, it becomes difficult to accurately estimate this risk as people develop other independent risk factors for epilepsy as they age (i.e., stroke or dementia).

Diagnostic Testing

Even today, diagnostic testing to predict the development of PTE is quite limited and often adds little to the clinical evaluation and careful consideration of the previously discussed risk factors. In a large EEG study, over 1,000 EEGs were reviewed from 722 patients (Jennett and van de Sande 1975). Many of these patients would have been classified as having suffered a severe TBI and in fact the rate of PTE in this population was 43%. These records were compared to a control series of EEGs from all TBI patients at another hospital, many of whom sustained mild traumatic brain injuries. The investigators found no significant difference in the rate of EEG abnormalities between 510 patients with PTE and 391 without, regardless of the time since injury. In addition, they found that 20% of patients with PTE had at least one normal EEG within the first 3 months post-injury. As such, the authors ultimately concluded that EEG added little to the clinical evaluation in terms of predicting the development of PTE.

Brain imaging can demonstrate evidence of prior traumatic injury and can, therefore, be helpful in predicting the development of PTE; however, imaging may also be normal, as is typically the case in mild TBI. A prospective study from India included 381 consecutive patients admitted for mild head injury, GCS 13–15 (Thiruppathy and Muthukumar 2004). Thirty-eight percent were found to have positive findings on CT scan and these abnormal scans were predicted by low GCS admission score (13–14), abnormal neurologic exam and fractures detected on skull x-rays. Accordingly, the decision to image a patient should be based on clinical presentation. At this point in time imaging is not recommended for most patients with mild TBI and is not helpful in predicting risk of PTE in this population.

For more severe head injuries, both CT and MRI findings can be correlated to the occurrence of PTE. Perhaps the earliest study to investigate CT scans' ability to predict PTE investigated 233 patients admitted for head trauma from 1977 to 1978 (D'Alessandro et al. 1982). Head injuries were divided into two groups; severe, which was characterized by loss of consciousness greater than 24 h, focal neurologic signs, early seizures, depressed skull fracture, intracranial hematoma, or brain contusion, or mild-moderate which encompassed all other injuries. Eleven patients (5%) developed PTE, all of whom fell into the severe TBI category. In this particular study, only patients with radiographic evidence of a focal cerebral lesion developed PTE, and the risk seemed particularly elevated with the combination of intracerebral hemorrhage coupled with extracerebral hematoma. Data from the VHIS demonstrated a significant relationship between total brain volume loss as measured on CT scan 15 years after injury and the development of PTE (Salazar et al. 1985). In addition, independent of brain volume loss, location of injury (i.e., resulting in hemiparesis, aphasia, visual field loss, or organic mental disorder) also conferred a higher risk of PTE. As mentioned earlier, more recent studies have also underscored the importance of abnormal CT scans in predicting PTE (Angeleri et al. 1999; Englander et al. 2003).

Studies have also examined the utility of MRI in predicting PTE. Angeleri et al. (1999) compared MRIs from 137 patients with TBI. In particular they were interested in the presence of hemosiderin 1 year after injury. While there was no difference in the percentage of patients with "isolated hemosiderin zones," the group with PTE was significantly more likely to have focal gliotic hemosiderin lesions in their cortex, again underscoring the importance of lesion location. In a study from India in 2003, Kumar et al. employed Magnetization Transfer (MT) MRI to predict PTE. MT imaging, a novel MRI sequence, had previously been utilized for more accurate detection of diffuse axonal injury and perilesional gliosis in neurocysticercosis-related seizures (Kumar et al. 2003). They found that MT abnormalities extending beyond the lesion seen on standard T2 imaging predicted a higher rate of PTE and that, while hemosiderin alone did not confer a higher risk of PTE, gliotic scar surrounding hemosiderin did. Significant research regarding neuroimaging in TBI is ongoing and will hopefully soon be able to more accurately stratify an individual's risk of developing PTE.

Treatment

Numerous trials have been undertaken to evaluate the potential for medications to be truly antiepileptogenic and prevent the development of PTE. While most of the trial designs were similar, there was some variability in time to treatment following injury, length of follow-up, and monitoring of compliance. In addition, most trial designs included a period of monitoring after the medication had been stopped to see if the drug was truly antiepileptogenic or whether it was merely suppressing seizures (Temkin 2009).

The largest study to date was a randomized, double-blind, placebo-controlled study evaluating the effectiveness of phenytoin in preventing PTE in 404 patients with severe TBI (Temkin et al. 1990). Patients were randomized to either phenytoin or placebo, and treatment was initiated within 24 h. The patients were treated for 1 year, during which time serum drug levels were monitored to ensure compliance. Treatment was discontinued after 1 year and the patients were followed for a second year to assess potential antiepileptogenic effects of early treatment. The investigators found that treatment with phenytoin significantly reduced the number of early seizures (those occurring in the first week after injury). In the phenytoin group 3.6% had early seizures versus 14.2% assigned to placebo (risk ratio 0.27, CI 0.12–0.62). Between day 8 and the end of the first year of treatment, 21.5% in the phenytoin group and 15.7% in the placebo group experienced late seizures. By the end of the second year, the rates were 27.5% and 21.1% in the phenytoin and placebo arms, respectively. A small, similarly designed study also found no difference in the rate of PTE in children given phenytoin versus placebo (Young et al. 1983).

Multiple other studies have investigated the potential antiepileptogenic effects of some of the older anticonvulsants in either monotherapy or combination therapy. Data from studies of phenobarbital monotherapy and phenytoin combined with phenobarbital were inconclusive because of small sample sizes resulting in wide confidence intervals (Temkin 2009). One study of carbamazepine monotherapy demonstrated a significant reduction in early seizures but no effect on late seizures (Temkin 2009). A single study compared valproate to phenytoin for the treatment of early seizures and the prevention of late seizures (Temkin et al. 1999). There was no significant difference in the rate of early seizures between the valproate and phenytoin treatment groups and valproate had no significant effect on the rate of late seizures. These treatment trials are well summarized in Fig. 10.3 adapted from Temkin *Epilepsia* 2009.

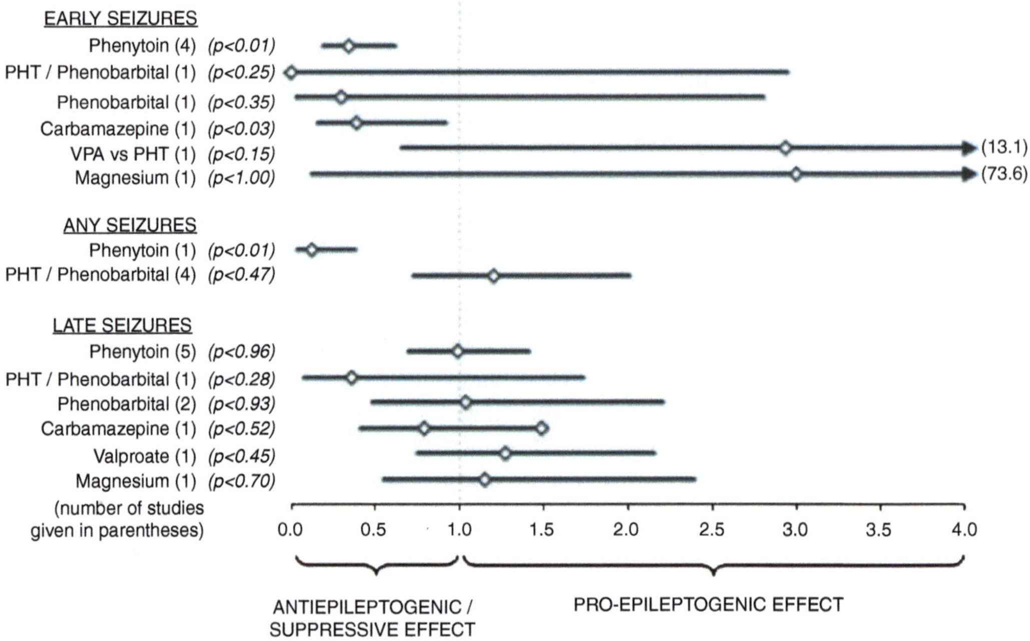

Fig. 10.3 Meta-analysis results for seizure prevention after traumatic brain injury. The relative risk for each drug and time frame is marked by a diamond on a line that indicates the 95% confidence interval for that relative risk. A relative risk of 1, representing no treatment effect, is marked by the dashed vertical line (adapted from Temkin 2009)

In 2003, the American Academy of Neurology released a practice parameter discussing the use of antiepileptics for prophylaxis in severe TBI (Chang and Lowenstein 2003). They concluded that phenytoin prophylaxis was effective in decreasing the risk of early (within 1 week of injury) post-traumatic seizures. In addition, it was felt that antiepileptic prophylaxis was likely not effective in decreasing the risk of late post-traumatic seizures. Of note, the newer antiepileptics have not been studied, and certainly trials evaluating their effectiveness in treating and preventing PTE are warranted.

While little has been reported on the subject, surgical therapy may be an option for patients with PTE and should be considered. Traumatic brain injuries rarely result in the development of mesial temporal sclerosis; however, lesionectomies or resective surgeries of an identified epileptic focus are possible. In addition, a vagal nerve stimulator may be considered in patients with frequent seizures. Thus, referral to a comprehensive epilepsy center is warranted, especially in medically refractory cases of PTE.

Outcomes

Remission rates for PTE range from 25 to 40% meaning that a large number of patients will remain on antiepileptics for their lifetime (Frey 2003). It stands to reason that people with frequent seizures during the first year after injury will continue to have frequent seizures and have a smaller chance of remission. Thus, outcomes are affected not only by the injury and PTE, but also by the treatments used to suppress seizures, and medical and surgical therapies are not without significant side effects.

A study of World War II veterans with penetrating head injuries demonstrated that while head injury alone did not shorten life expectancy, head injury coupled with PTE did significantly shorten life expectancy (Corkin et al. 1984). Others found that the presence of PTE correlated with a lower level of overall general function as measured by the Glasgow Outcome Scale in mainly moderate to severe TBI rehabilitation patients (Asikainen et al. 1999). In the same study the authors found no difference in the rate of independent employment between TBI patients with and without PTE, with approximately one third being unable to work in each group.

Epileptogenesis

Epileptogenesis involves the process whereby the normal, nonepileptic brain transforms into one that generates spontaneous, recurrent, and unprovoked seizures (Jensen 2009). TBI provides one of the clearest models of epileptogenesis in that an inciting injury results in the development of post-traumatic seizures. One key feature of this process that has been identified through observation as well as through animal models is the presence of a latent period between the injury and the onset of seizures. As previously discussed, this latent period is quite variable and can last for years in humans. Researchers have focused on this period of time to identify the various changes that occur in the brain during epileptogenesis and view it as a critical time period to target truly antiepileptogenic therapies.

The cascade of changes that occur following a TBI are quite complex. Some early changes involve gene induction and neurotransmitter modifications as well as modifications of ion channel and transporter proteins (Jensen 2009). Within a few days after injury there is evidence of neuronal death and inflammation. The later changes include axonal sprouting and dendritic modifications, such as mossy fiber sprouting—in essence the formation of abnormal excitatory connections (Prince et al. 2009). Some models of epileptogenesis have demonstrated structural alterations in interneurons leading to less effective GABAergic inhibitory neurotransmission (Prince et al. 2009).

In an effort to better understand the various processes that define epileptogenesis, researchers have attempted to create animal models of TBI and PTE. Naturally, this is fraught with difficulties as brain injury is a very heterogeneous disorder that differs from person to person in terms of the location of injury, mechanism of injury, and extent of injury. While multiple animal models exist, only the rat lateral fluid-percussion model has been reported to consistently result in late spontaneous seizures (Pitkanen et al. 2009). Briefly, this model involves craniectomy followed by direct impact to the epidural space in the form of a liquid pulse transmitted via a saline-filled cylinder (Pitkanen et al. 2009). The severity of injury can be controlled by the weight and height of a pendulum that strikes the cylinder and creates the liquid pulse. This mode of injury mimics human TBI well in that it causes direct cortical injury as well as deep white matter damage. From this model, researchers have begun to study diagnostic and predictive technologies, including imaging and electrophysiologic techniques. In addition, they have begun to study novel therapies such as medications that block glutamate receptors or calcium channels, caspase inhibitors, antiapoptotic agents, and stem cell transplantation (Jensen 2009). Despite some successes, none of these treatment strategies have been translated to human trials (Jensen 2009).

References

Aarabi B. Surgical outcome in 435 patients who sustained missilehead wounds during the Iran-Iraq War. Neurosurgery. 1990;27:692–695; discussion 695.

Agrawal A, Timothy J, Pandit L, Manju M. Post-traumatic epilepsy: an overview. Clin Neurol Neurosurg. 2006;108:433–9.

Angeleri F, Majkowski J, Cacchio G, Sobieszek S, D'Acunto S, Gesuita R, Bachleda A, Polonara G, Krolicki L, Signorino M, Salvolini U. Posttraumatic epilepsy risk factors: one-year prospective study after head injury. Epilepsia. 1999;40:1222–30.

Annegers J, Grabow J, Groover R, Laws E, Elveback L, Kurland L. Seizures after head trauma: a population stuffy. Neurology. 1980;30:683–9.

Annegers JF, Hauser WA, Coan SP, Rocca WA. A population-based study of seizures after traumatic brain injuries. N Engl J Med. 1998;338:20–4.

Asikainen I, Kaste M, Sarna S. Early and late posttraumatic seizure in traumatic brain injury rehabilitation patients: brain injury factors causing late seizures and influence of seizures on long-term outcome. Epilepsia. 1999;40:584–9.

Ascroft P. Traumatic epilepsy after gunshot wounds at the head. Br Med J. 1941;1:739–744.

Brandvold B, Levi L, Feinsod M, George ED. Penetrating craniocerebral injuries in the Israeli involvement in the Lebanese conflict, 1982–1985. Analysis of a less aggressive surgical approach. J Neurosurg. 1990; 72:15–21.

Caveness WF, Meirowsky AM, Rish BL, Mohr JP, Kistler JP, Dillon JD, Weiss GH. The nature of posttraumatic epilepsy. J Neurosurg. 1979;50:545–53.

Caveness WF, Walker AE, Ascroft PB. Incidence of posttraumatic epilepsy in Korean veterans as compared with those from World War I and World War II. J Neurosurg. 1962;19:122–129.

Caviness V. Epilepsy and craniocerebral injury in warfare. In Caveness W, Walker A (Eds) Head Injury: Conference Proceedings. JB Lippincott, Philadelphia, PA. 1966;220–234.

Credner L. Klinische und soziale auswirkungen von hirnsschdigungen. Z. Gesamte Neurollogie et Psychiatrie. 1930;126:721–757.

Chang BS, Lowenstein DH. Quality standards subcommittee of the American academy of neurology. Practice parameter: antiepileptic drug prophylaxis in severe traumatic brain injury: report of the quality standards subcommittee of the American academy of neurology. Neurology. 2003;60(1):10–6.

Corkin S, Sullivan EV, Carr FA. Prognostic factors for life expectancy after penetrating head injury. Arch Neurol. 1984;41(9):975–7.

D'Alessandro R, Tinuper P, Ferrara R, Cortelli P, Pazzaglia P, Sabattini L, Frank G, Lugaresi E. CT scan prediction of late post-traumatic epilepsy. J Neurol Neurosurg Psychiatry. 1982;45:1153–5.

Desai BT, Whitman S, Coonley-Hoganson R, Coleman TE, Gabriel G, Dell J. Seizures and civilian head injuries. Epilepsia. 1983;24:289–96.

Englander J, Bushnik T, Duong TT, Cifu DX, Zafonte R, Wright J, Hughes R, Bergman W. Analyzing risk factors for late post-traumatic seizures: a prospective, multicenter investigation. Arch Phys Med Rehabil. 2003;84:365–73.

Frey LC. Epidemiology of posttraumatic epilepsy: a critical review. Epilepsia. 2003;44 suppl 10:11–7.

Garga N, Lowenstein DH. Posttraumatic epilepsy: a major problem in desperate need of major advances. Epilepsy Current. 2006;6:1–5.

Hahn YS, Fuchs S, Flannery AM, Barthel MJ, McLone DG. Factors influencing posttraumatic seizures in children. Neurosurgery. 1988;22:864–7.

Haltiner AM, Temkin NR, Dikmen SS. Risk of seizure recurrence after the first late posttraumatic seizure. Arch Phys Med Rehabil. 1997;78:835–40.

Hauser WA, Annegers JF, Kurland LT. Prevalence of epilepsy in Rochester, Minnesota, 1940–1980. Epilepsia. 1991;31:429–45.

Herman ST. Epilepsy after brain insult: targeting epileptogenesis. Neurology. 2002;59 Suppl 5:S21–6.

Jennett WB, Lewin W. Traumatic epilepsy after closed head injuries. J Neurol Neurosurg Psychiatry. 1960;23:295–301.

Jennett B, van de Sande J. EEG prediction of post-traumatic epilepsy. Epilepsia. 1975;16:251–6.

Jensen FE. Posttraumatic epilepsy: treatable epileptogenesis. Epilepsia. 2009;50 Suppl 2:1–3.

Kumar R, Gupta RK, Husain M, Vatsal DK, Chawla S, Rathore RKS, Pradhan S. Magnetization transfer MR imaging in patients with posttraumatic epilepsy. Am J Neuroradiol. 2003;23:218–24.

Lowenstein DH. Epilepsy after head injury: an overview. Epilepsia. 2009;50 Suppl 2:4–9.

Okie S. Traumatic brain injury in the war zone. N Engl J Med. 2005;352:2043–7.

Pitkanen A, Immonen RJ, Grohn OHJ, Kharatishvili I. From traumatic brain injury to posttraumatic epilepsy: what animal models tell us about the process and treatment options. Epilepsia. 2009;50 Suppl 2:21–9.

Prince DA, Parada I, Scalise K, Graber K, Jin X, Shen F. Epilepsy following cortical injury: cellular and molecular mechanisms as targets for potential prophylaxis. Epilepsia. 2009;50 Suppl 2:30–40.

Raymont V, Salazar AM, Lipsky R, Goldman D, Tasick G, Grafman J. Correlates of posttraumatic epilepsy 35 years following combat brain injury. Neurology. 2010;75:224–9.

Russell W, Whitty C. Studies in traumatic epilepsy. Part 1 (Factors influencing the incidence of epilepsy after brain wounds). J Neurol Neurosurg Psychiatry. 1952;15:93–98.

Salazar AM, Jabbari B, Vance SC, Grafman J, Amin D, Dillon JD. Epilepsy after penetrating head injury. I. Clinical correlates: a report of the Vietnam Head Injury Study. Neurology. 1985;35:1406–14.

Salazar A, Aarabi B, Levi L, Feinsod M. Posttraumatic epilepsy following craniocerebral missile wounds in recent armed conflicts. In Aarabi B, Kaufman HH, Dagi TF, George ED, Levy ML. (Eds) Missile Wounds of the Head and Neck. Vol. 2, Thieme, Park Ridge, IL. 1999;281–292.

Salazar A, Grafman J, Jabbari B, Vance SC, Amin D. Epilepsy and cognitive loss after penetrating head injury. In Wolf P, Dam W, Janz M et al. (Eds) Advances in Epileptology. Raven Press, New York. 1987;627–631.

Taylor ASJ, Kretschmann C. Posttraumatic Symptoms in Head Injured Veterans of the Korean Campaign. National Institute of Neurological Disorders and Stroke, Bethesda, MD. (1971).

Temkin NR. Preventing and treating posttraumatic seizures: the human experience. Epilepsia. 2009;50 Suppl 2:10–3.

Temkin NR, Dikmen SS, Anderson GD, Wilensky AJ, Holmes MD, Cohen W, Newell DW, Nelson P, Awan A, Winn HR. Valproate therapy for prevention of posttraumatic seizures: a randomized trial. J Neurosurg. 1999;91:593–600.

Temkin NR, Dikmen SS, Wilensky AJ, Keihm J, Chabal S, Winn HR. A randomized, double-blind study of phenytoin for the prevention of post-traumatic seizures. N Engl J Med. 1990;323:497–502.

Thiruppathy SP, Muthukumar N. Mild head injury: revisited. Acta Neurochir (Wein). 2004;146(10):1075–83.

Walker E, Erculei F. Head Injured Med. Charles C Thomas, Springfield, IL. (1969).

Young B, Rapp RP, Norton JA, Haack D, Tibbs PA, Bean JR. Failure of prophylactically administered phenytoin to prevent late post-traumatic seizures. J Neurosurg. 1983;58:236–41.

Endocrine Disturbances Following TBI

11

Victoria Tepe and Arthur Guerrero

Abstract

TBI-related neuroendocrine abnormalities can occur across all injury severity levels as the result of compression, swelling, necrosis, hemorrhage, lacerations, strain, shear, or vascular damage to hypothalamic-pituitary brain structures. The prevalence of TBI-related hormonal dysfunction may be as high as 40%. Almost without exception, civilian researchers agree that there is a need to screen TBI patients for neuroendocrine abnormalities in the acute, post-acute, or recovery phases of TBI. In the military setting, there is a need to better understand how comorbidities such as PTSD might interact with TBI-related hormonal dysfunction and to distinguish the endocrine effects of mild TBI in particular.

Keywords

Hormone(s) • Hormone replacement therapy (HRT) • Hypopituitarism • Hypothalamus/hypothalamic • Neuroendocrine (dysfunction, abnormality) • Pituitary (insufficiency, dysfunction, screening) • Hypothalamic-pituitary-adrenal (HPA) axis

V. Tepe, Ph.D. (✉)
Contractor, Defense Centers of Excellence for Psychological Health and Traumatic Brain Injury, Arlington, VA, USA

Survivability/Vulnerability Information Analysis Center, Booz Allen Hamilton, Dayton, OH, USA
e-mail: Tepe_Victoria@bah.com

A. Guerrero, M.D.
Endocrinology and Metabolism Service, Department of Medicine, Tripler Army Medical Center, Honolulu, HI, USA

Abbreviations

ACTH	Adrenocorticotropic hormone
ADH	Antidiuretic hormone (vasopressin)
BINT	Blast-induced neurotrauma
BMI	Body mass index
bTBI	Blast-induced TBI
CT	Computed tomography
FSH	Follicle stimulating hormone fatigue
GCS	Glasgow Coma Scale
GH	Growth hormone
GHD	Growth hormone deficiency

J.W. Tsao (ed.), *Traumatic Brain Injury: A Clinician's Guide to Diagnosis, Management, and Rehabilitation*,
DOI 10.1007/978-0-387-87887-4_11,

HPA	Hypothalamic–pituitary axis
HRT	Hormone replacement therapy
ICP	Intracranial pressure
LH	Luteinizing hormone
mTBI	Mild traumatic brain injury
PTHP	Post-traumatic hypopituitarism
PTSD	Post-traumatic stress disorder
T4	Free thyroxine
TBI	Traumatic brain injury
TSH	Thyroid stimulating hormone

Introduction

Traumatic brain injury (TBI) is defined as the result of external force, which may include the head being struck by or striking an object (blunt impact), foreign body penetration of the brain, brain acceleration/deceleration movement, or forces from an external event such as a blast or explosion (see Taber et al. 2006). The large majority (75–90%) of civilian TBIs are classified as mild TBI (mTBI).

TBI is a significant public health concern, as each year some 1.7 million or more Americans sustain non-fatal brain injury (CDC 2006; Rutland-Brown et al. 2006). In the civilian sector, these injuries are usually the result of motor vehicle accidents (50%), falls (30%), or violence (20%). TBIs are most common among individuals 15–24 years of age, very young children (less than 5 years of age), and people 75 years of age and above. An estimated 2% of Americans currently live with TBI-related disability and related costs (Thurman et al. 1999). TBIs represent nearly one-third of all injury-related deaths in the USA annually, and are the leading cause of death and disability among young adults.

In the military setting, TBI is a known risk faced by personnel in combat and in the course of specific high-risk military activities (e.g., parachuting; see Ivins et al. 2003). This is a significant concern for the US military, even when TBI is diagnosed as mild. In addition to a dramatically increased risk for medical discharge due to moderate or severe TBI, military personnel with mTBI are more likely to be discharged for behavioral causes, including alcoholism, drug use, and criminal conviction (Ommaya et al. 1996). As the individual and operational costs of these injuries become increasingly obvious, so does the need for state-of-the-art medical care, treatment, and recovery services. It is especially important that military TBI be accurately and effectively diagnosed with the clearest possible medical understanding and recognition of potential physiological, psychological, and behavioral sequelae and comorbidities.

The purpose of this chapter is to document recent findings with respect to TBI-related neuroendocrine abnormalities and to relate these findings as specifically as possible to the military medical setting, where it may be especially difficult to differentiate symptoms of TBI, endocrine dysfunction, and combat-related stress reactions. To the extent the available literature allows, we also consider what is known about neuroendocrine abnormalities, which extend across all severities of TBI, with respect to specific psychiatric comorbidities including post-traumatic stress disorder (PTSD) and depression. Finally, we offer conclusions with respect to prevalence, screening, and knowledge gaps that require additional research.

Endocrine Sequelae of TBI

Until fairly recently, evidence for TBI-related neuroendocrine dysfunction was limited primarily to anecdotal reports, case studies, and autopsy findings (see Edwards and Clark 1986). The first report of TBI-related pituitary insufficiency appeared as a case study published nearly 100 years ago (Cyran 1918, as cited in Bondanelli et al. 2005). Although subsequent published autopsy series observed injuries to hypothalamic and/or pituitary structures in 26–86% of fatal head trauma (Ceballos 1966; Crompton 1971; Daniel et al. 1959; Kornblum and Fisher 1969), they involved only patients who died as the result of their injuries. Thus, it was unknown to what extent such injuries occurred among patients who sustained relatively less severe brain trauma. In 1942, a review of the literature available at the time included 595 cases of pituitary insufficiency, finding just four of them related specifically to brain injury (Escamilla and Lisser 1942). Thus, it was generally believed that although TBI-related pituitary dysfunction was possible, it was probably also rare.

This perspective changed dramatically with the publication of a case series review of more than 300 patients who were shown to have suffered pituitary dysfunction resulting from TBI (Benvenga et al. 2000). Among these patients, hormonal abnormalities were frequent due to pituitary dysfunction. Additional findings indicated that such abnormalities might occur even in cases of mild head trauma and that they could persist for years after initial injury.

More recent data have shown that endocrine dysfunction can be found to occur in as many as 40% of all TBI patients, due to TBI-related damage of hypothalamic–pituitary brain structures (Ghigo et al. 2005; Krahulik et al. 2009; Tanriverdi et al. 2010). As will be discussed later, pituitary abnormalities are seen across all severities of TBI, and no specific finding is predictive of which hormonal abnormalities will occur. Although resulting hormonal abnormalities are common, symptoms are easily overlooked or mistaken for other TBI-related sequelae. Left undiagnosed and untreated, neuroendocrine disorders can impair rehabilitation and lead to long-term medical and psychological problems.

Mechanisms of Neuroendocrine Dysfunction

Located at the base of the brain, the hypothalamus and pituitary gland are vulnerable to TBI-related trauma in general. Hormonal dysfunction can result from primary or secondary lesions to the hypothalamus, the pituitary, or the pituitary stalk. Hypothalamic and pituitary lesions can be caused by TBI-related vascular damage, strain and/or shear on white matter between structures, compression, swelling, necrosis, hemorrhage, or laceration (Crompton 1971; Edwards and Clark 1986; Kelly et al. 2000; Rothman et al. 2007; Yuan and Wade 1991). The anterior pituitary gland, in particular, is a common site of TBI-related injury and subsequent hormonal dysfunction. Located in the lateral regions of the pituitary gland, somatotrophic and gonadotrophic cells are thought to be more vulnerable due to their location and fragile blood supply. Distributed more centrally, corticotrophic and thyrotrophic cells may be somewhat less vulnerable (Benvenga et al. 2000).

The hypothalamus secretes and releases hormones that stimulate or suppress the production of hormones in the anterior pituitary gland. Anterior pituitary hormones—adrenocorticotropic hormone (ACTH), thyroid stimulating hormone (TSH), luteinizing hormone/follicle stimulating hormone (LH/FSH), growth hormone (GH), and prolactin—stimulate the release of product substances from other target glands and organs throughout the body (Fig. 11.1). The posterior pituitary, also known as the neurohypophysis, is a collection of direct neuronal projections from the hypothalamus; it receives two hormones—oxytocin and vasopressin—directly from the hypothalamus.

The term hypopituitarism refers to abnormally reduced secretion of any one or more pituitary hormones.[1] Some studies have suggested that the most common hormonal effect of TBI-related hypopituitarism is growth hormone deficiency (GHD) resulting from somatotrophic cell death due to impaired blood and oxygen supply (Ghigo et al. 2005; Kelly et al. 2000). The least commonly observed abnormality is TSH deficiency (Thompson 2007). The case series review published by Benvenga and colleagues in 2000 observed TBI-related hypopituitarism leading to

[1]The term *panhypopituitarism* is used when most or all pituitary hormones are affected. The term *pituitary dysfunction* is used to describe any abnormality in the hypothalamic–pituitary–end organ axis.

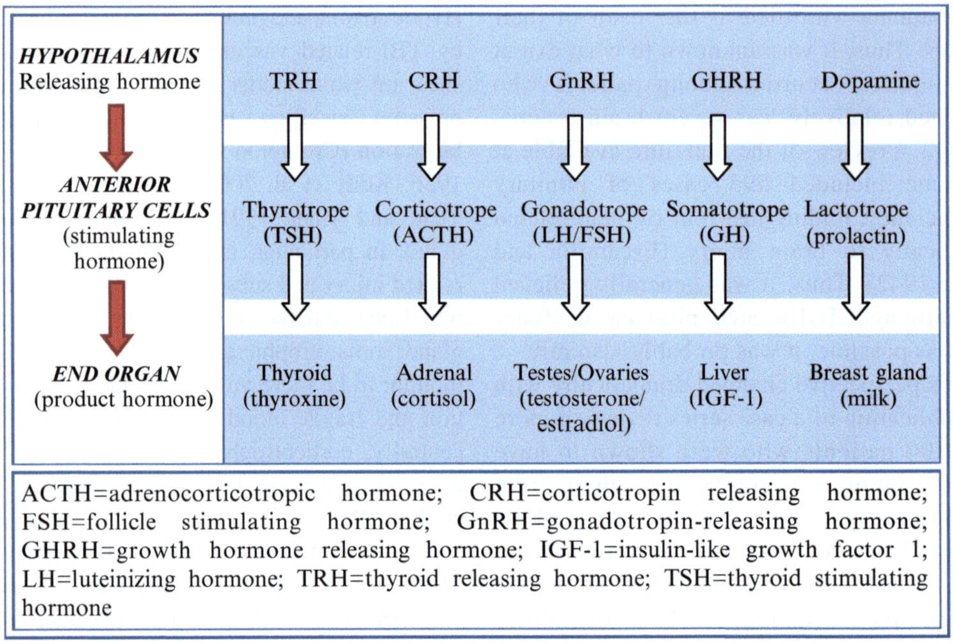

Fig. 11.1 The hypothalamus secretes hormones, which mediate production of anterior pituitary hormones, which stimulate release of product hormones from target organs

deficiencies in gonadotropin, ACTH, TSH, and GH, as well as abnormally high levels of prolactin (hyperprolactinemia).

Over the last 10 years, other studies have identified one or more of these same hormonal abnormalities at varying frequencies in TBI patients. Table 11.1 presents an overview of specific hormonal abnormalities reported to occur in the acute and/or chronic phases of TBI. Rothman et al. (2007) offer an informative review of the clinical spectrum of TBI-related neuroendocrine deficits and their respective underlying mechanisms.

Prevalence and Symptoms of Neuroendocrine Dysfunction

In general, research reported over the most recent decade has shown that the incidence of neuroendocrine disorders consequent to TBI may be as high as 40%, and that at least 20–30% of adult TBI patients will likely develop a disorder of at least one endocrine function (Ghigo et al. 2005; Krahulik et al. 2009). Most disorders emerge within the first year post-injury. Some are transient, while others may persist for months or years. Post-traumatic hypopituitarism (PTHP) has been linked to adverse outcomes in both the acute and chronic stages of TBI (Behan et al. 2008; Bondanelli et al. 2007; Cohan et al. 2005; Klose and Feldt-Rasmussen 2008), but early diagnosis and treatment can improve the outcome (Krahulik et al. 2009). Left untreated, neuroendocrine disorders can cause neurological deficits, complicate treatment, and lead to mental illness (Bavisetty et al. 2008; Dikmen et al. 2004; Hellawell et al. 1999).

Despite its evident prevalence, PTHP probably goes unrecognized and untreated in many or even most cases due to misattribution of symptoms and lack of screening for pituitary dysfunction. Hormonal deficiencies align with a variety of initial symptoms which, depending on other health status or injury factors, may or may not be immediately obvious as due to pituitary dysfunction. Numerous authors have called attention to the need for routine screening of all TBI patients in the acute and/or post-acute phases of TBI (Bavisetty et al. 2008; Berg et al. 2009;

Table 11.1 Overview of hormonal abnormalities associated with TBI

Abnormality	Hormone(s)	Onset	Reference(s)
Adrenal insufficiency (anterior pituitary)	↓ ACTH-cortisol	<3 months	Agha et al. (2005), Cohan et al. (2005), Kleindienst et al. (2009)
		≥3 months	Agha et al. (2004), Aimaretti et al. (2004, 2005), Herrmann et al. (2006), Kelly et al. (2000), Kleindienst et al. (2009), Klose et al. (2007), Leal-Cerro et al. (2005), Lieberman et al. (2001), Popovic et al. (2004), Schneider et al. (2006), Tanriverdi et al. (2006)
Diabetes insipidus (posterior pituitary)	↓Vasopressin (ADH)	<3 months	Agha et al. (2005), Boughey et al. (2004), Krahulik et al. (2009)
Growth hormone deficiency (anterior pituitary)	↓ GH IGF-1	<3 months	Agha et al. (2005), Kleindienst et al. (2009), Tanriverdi et al. (2006)
		≥3 months	Agha et al. (2004), Aimaretti et al. (2004, 2005), Bavisetty et al. (2008), Bondanelli et al. (2004), Herrmann et al. (2006), Kelly et al. (2000), Kleindienst et al. (2009), Klose et al. (2007), Leal-Cerro et al. (2005), Lieberman et al. (2001), Popovic et al. (2004), Schneider et al. (2006), Tanriverdi et al. (2006)
Hyperprolactinemia (anterior pituitary)	↑ Prolactin	<3 months	Agha et al. (2005), Tanriverdi et al. (2006)
		≥3 months	Agha et al. (2004), Aimaretti et al. (2004, 2005), Bondanelli et al. (2004), Klose et al. (2007), Lieberman et al. (2001), Popovic et al. (2004), Schneider et al. (2006), Tanriverdi et al. (2006)
Hypogonadism (anterior pituitary)	↓Gonadotropin LH/FSH Testosterone/estradiol	<3 months	Agha et al. (2005), Cernak et al. (1999), Kleindienst et al. (2009), Tanriverdi et al. (2006)
		≥3 months	Agha et al. (2004), Aimaretti et al. (2004, 2005), Bavisetty et al. (2008), Bondanelli et al. (2004), Herrmann et al. (2006), Kelly et al. (2000), Klose et al. (2007), Leal-Cerro et al. (2005), Lieberman et al. (2001), Popovic et al. (2004), Schneider et al. (2006), Tanriverdi et al. (2006)
Hypothyroidism (anterior pituitary)	↓ TSH ↓ T4	<3 months	Cernak et al. (1999), Kleindienst et al. (2009), Tanriverdi et al. (2006)
		≥3 months	Aimaretti et al. (2004, 2005), Bondanelli et al. (2004), Herrmann et al. (2006), Kelly et al. (2000), Klose et al. (2007), Leal-Cerro et al. (2005), Lieberman et al. (2001), Popovic et al. (2004), Schneider et al. (2006), Tanriverdi et al. (2006)

Bushnik et al. 2007; Krahulik et al. 2009; Powner et al. 2006; Powner and Boccalandro 2008; Raverot et al. 2009; Sesmilo et al. 2007; Thompson 2007; Yollin et al. 2007). In 2005, an international panel of neuroendocrinologists and rehabilitation physicians released a consensus statement recommending that prospective and retrospective screening of pituitary function be performed for all patients with moderate-to-severe TBI (Ghigo et al. 2005). The panel found that pituitary screening is essential for these patients, and emphasized that baseline screening should be routine in particular for TBI patients who are hospitalized for at least 1 day due to their injuries. Because PTHP can occur regardless of TBI severity level, pituitary screening may also be warranted for mTBI patients (Guerrero and Alfonso 2010; Tanriverdi et al. 2010; Thompson 2007).

Hormonal deficiencies align with a variety of initial symptoms which, depending on other health status or injury factors, may or may not be immediately obvious as due to pituitary dysfunction. Differential diagnosis is less difficult when hormonal deficiencies persist and lead to increasingly distinct physical symptoms (see Schneider et al. 2005). Chronic GHD in adults leads to reduced muscle mass and increased body fat around the waist. ACTH deficiency may cause secondary adrenal insufficiency which can be life threatening; this may present initially as weight loss, anemia, hypoglycemia, and hyponatremia (low sodium levels). Symptoms of chronic TSH deficiency include fatigue, constipation, weight gain, hair loss, low blood pressure, and reduced heart rate. Gonadotropin (LH/FSH) deficiencies may lead to a loss of libido, infertility, and increased risk of osteoporosis. Men with LH deficiency may develop anemia, loss of body hair, and muscle mass. Women with FSH deficiency may experience amenorrhea. Vasopressin (ADH) deficiency is observed as diabetes insipidus, which manifests as excessive dilute urine production, dehydration, extreme thirst, and dangerously high sodium blood levels in patients with limited access to water. Symptoms of ADH/vasopressin deficiency can be masked by ACTH deficiency (Prabhakar and Shalet 2006).

Overview of Military TBI

In a recent study of soldiers deployed to Iraq, clinician-confirmed TBI history (primarily mTBI) was identified in more than one of every five (22.8%) soldiers from a Brigade Combat Team (Terrio et al. 2009). This is consistent with the finding that 22% of soldiers wounded in Iraq and Afghanistan have sustained injuries to the head, face, or neck (Okie 2005). Other studies have found that as many as 28% of military personnel have sustained at least mTBI while deployed to conflicts in Iraq and Afghanistan (Warden 2006). In cooperation with the Armed Forces Health Surveillance Center, the Defense and Veterans Brain Injury Center (DVBIC) tracks and analyzes the incidence of military TBI based on actual medical diagnoses of TBI within the US armed forces (Table 11.2). Their findings show a steady increase in diagnosed TBI on an annual basis since 2005; military TBI incident diagnoses have more than doubled over the last 5 years, an increase perhaps influenced by a growing awareness of brain injury in military settings. The large majority (78–83%) of these injuries are diagnosed as mTBIs.

Most TBIs sustained by US troops during combat in Iraq and Afghanistan are closed-head injuries due to explosion/blast from improvised explosive devices (IEDs) (Galarneau et al. 2008; Warden 2006). One study observed that even among 1,303 military patients with explosive injury only to the lower extremities, more than half (665) also had neurological symptoms consistent with TBI (Cernak et al. 1999). Although the precise pathophysiological effects of blast injury to the brain are not yet fully understood, recent clinical and experimental findings have shown that blast injuries can and do cause brain damage associated with biochemical changes and cognitive impairment (Cernak et al. 2001). Rapid pressure shifts from explosive blast can cause concussion, contusion, and cerebral infarct due to the formation of air emboli in blood vessels (Ling et al. 2009; Mayorga 1997). At Walter Reed Army Medical Center, admitted patients who have been exposed to blast are now routinely

Table 11.2 Military TBI incident diagnoses by year (2000–2010) within the US armed forces

Calendar year	2000	2001	2002	2003	2004	2005	2006	2007	2008	2009	2010 (Q1)	Total
TBI incident diagnoses	10,963	11,830	12,469	12,886	13,271	12,025	16,873	23,002	28,557	27,862	7,604	178,876

DVBIC source data updated as of May 20, 2010, available at http://www.dvbic.org/TBI-Numbers.aspx

evaluated for brain injury. In recent years, some 59% of these patients have been diagnosed with TBI (Warden 2006).

Diagnostic Challenges

Possible neuropsychiatric sequelae and/or co-occurring symptoms associated with mTBI include a variety of cognitive deficits (e.g., memory and attention impairment), mood disorder (e.g., depression, anxiety), apathy, changes in behavior, sleep disturbances, chronic pain, and headache (Jorge and Starkstein 2005; Kreutzer et al. 2001; Nampiaparampil 2008; Rao and Lyketsos 2000; Riggio and Wong 2009). These effects have been observed and reported among military patients with TBI. Terrio and colleagues (2009) found that soldiers with TBI were more likely also to report post-injury and post-deployment somatic and/or neuropsychiatric symptoms. In a study of US Navy and Marine Corps Combat Trauma Registry (CTR) data, Galarneau et al. (2008) observed higher morbidity and medical utilization among patients with severe TBIs, and more mental conditions among patients with milder TBI.

Subtle long-term effects of mTBI on attention and memory can emerge gradually and persist for months or years after original injury (Bohnen et al. 1992; Bohnen and Jolles 1992; Ponsford et al. 2000; Trudeau et al. 1998; Vanderploeg et al. 2005). Long after initial injury, such symptoms may be attributed to other life or combat-related stressors, other medical circumstances, or psychological conditions. Otherwise healthy individuals are often able to adapt, compensate, and manage subjectively subtle changes in cognition, mood, and energy. If judgment itself is impaired, the brain-injured person may be among the last to recognize the possible seriousness of his or her own symptoms.

Neurological and psychiatric comorbidity further complicates the diagnostic and treatment challenges of military TBI and mTBI. Pituitary dysfunction is often associated with signs and symptoms common to other maladies and sequelae of TBI, including post-concussion syndrome (Hofman et al. 2002; Ryan and Warden 2003), stress (Bryant 2008), or PTSD (Kim et al. 2007). These might include fatigue, insomnia, impaired cognition and memory loss, difficulty concentrating, emotional, and mood disturbance, and a sense of social isolation (Bay and Xie 2009; Belmont et al. 2006; Bushnik et al. 2007; Carroll et al. 1998; Deijen et al. 1996; Rosen et al. 1994). Thus, when TBI occurs in combination with psychiatric injury or disorder, it can be especially difficult to establish a clear basis for the evaluation and treatment of symptoms or changes in mood, cognition, and behavior.

There is a known association between TBI and anxiety disorders, particularly PTSD (Hiott and Labbate 2002), and patients with TBI are at greater risk of developing psychiatric disorders such as depression and PTSD (Bryant and Harvey 1998; Kim et al. 2007). Military patients in particular may present with symptoms that meet the diagnostic criteria for both. This is not surprising, given that the frontal and temporal brain areas implicated for involvement in PTSD are also especially vulnerable to TBI (see Kennedy et al. 2007). Areas of neuroanatomical overlap include the orbitofrontal cortex, the dorsolateral prefrontal cortex, the hippocampus, and tracts which connect the amygdala and the medial prefrontal cortex (see also Stein and McAllister 2009).

It is not known precisely to what extent TBI-related neuropsychiatric and behavioral sequelae may be the clinically observable results of hormonal dysfunction. PTSD has also been linked to altered stress-related responses in the hypothalamic–pituitary–adrenal (HPA) axis[2] (Davidson et al. 2004; McFarlane et al. 1997).

Although the basis for pituitary dysfunction may differ—for example, as the result of direct

[2] Normally in response to stress, the hypothalamus releases corticotrophin-releasing hormone (CRH) which in turns signals the pituitary gland to release adrenocorticotropic hormone (ACTH). This signals the adrenal gland to release cortisol, which facilitates physiological adaptation to stress. However, this function appears to be disrupted by chronic stress and/or trauma exposure. PTSD has been associated with high CRH levels and low ACTH and cortisol levels observable within 1–2 h after trauma exposure.

damage or loss of receptor cells vs. increased cell numbers and sensitivity—altered pituitary function leads ultimately to many of the same clinically observable symptoms. Thus, it may be difficult to ascertain psychological vs. biological causality based on clinical symptoms alone. Unless TBI patients are screened for pituitary dysfunction, it may be difficult to correctly establish and treat the basis of these complaints. Left untreated, hormonal abnormalities can adversely affect patient outcome (Della Corte et al. 1998; Hackl et al. 1991) and may complicate or worsen other TBI-related physical and psychological sequelae (Bavisetty et al. 2008; Kleindienst et al. 2009). Hormonal deficiencies might also play a role in psychosocial problems that are often associated with TBI and sometimes hamper rehabilitation (Dijkers 2004; Dikmen et al. 1995; Morton and Wehman 1995; Schneider et al. 2005).

Review of the Literature

The overarching intent of this chapter is to address the question of whether/how neuroendocrine abnormalities might complicate or confound the diagnosis and treatment of TBI. Several authors have observed that findings regarding endocrine abnormalities can differ depending on what criteria are applied to define hormonal deficiency, and on what assessment methods are used to ascertain hormonal functional status (e.g., Guerrero and Alfonso 2010). Specifically, there is evidence to suggest that hypopituitarism may be overlooked by basal testing alone, suggesting a need for inclusion of additional dynamic (stimulation) tests to more precisely assess hormonal function (Bernard et al. 2006; Faust et al. 2008; Kokshoorn et al. 2010;Schneider et al. 2008a). Commentary offered by Sesmilo et al. (2007) provides an informative overview of considerations for evaluative testing.

More than a dozen review papers have been published on the topic of neuroendocrine disorder consequent to TBI (Table 11.3). These works consider the problem of TBI-related hypothalamic–pituitary dysfunction in depth, and all conclude that pituitary hormonal deficiency is a frequent, serious, and largely unrecognized result of TBI. Hormonal deficiencies can arise in either the acute or chronic phase of TBI, and in general point to the need for routine or improved diagnostic screening procedures to identify and manage hormonal abnormalities by replacement therapy as appropriate. It is also widely recognized that the early symptoms of pituitary dysfunction often mimic other TBI symptoms, sequelae, and comorbidities, including depression, anxiety, post-concussion syndrome, and PTSD.

Although methodological differences have led to variant incidences reported in clinical studies, key and consistent findings of recent literature reviews affirm that the prevalence of TBI-related hypopituitarism is far greater than previously believed. It seems that while TBI-related hypopituitarism usually presents as an isolated deficiency of just one hormone, 10–15% of TBI patients suffer multiple hormonal deficiencies. In the acute phase of TBI, gonadal hormone deficits are very common, affecting as many as 80% of patients (Bondanelli et al. 2005; Ghigo et al. 2005;. Hyperprolactinemia has been reported to occur in more than half of TBI patients (Agha et al. 2004, 2005; Dimopoulou et al. 2004; Klose et al. 2007). The incidence of other acute hormone abnormalities is estimated as GH 18%, adrenal 15–16%, thyroid 10–30%, and vasopressin as high as 40% (Behan et al. 2008; Rothman et al. 2007). Diabetes insipidus can occur in the acute phase of TBI, but is uncommon and is usually transient.

Recent reviews also demonstrate a general consensus that hypopituitarism occurs in 25–40% of patients in the post-acute phase (>3 months) of TBI (Agha et al. 2007; Behan et al. 2008; Bondanelli et al. 2005; Ghigo et al. 2005). Post-traumatic pituitary deficiencies can develop well into TBI recovery, with one cohort study reporting dysfunction out to 5 years (Bondanelli et al. 2004). In the majority of studies, the most commonly observed post-acute isolated abnormality is GH deficiency, which affects 15–30% of TBI patients and may be severe in as many as 12–15% (Popovic et al. 2005; Urban et al. 2005). The timeframe and extent of recovery from post-acute

Table 11.3 Literature reviews (2005–2010)

Author(s), Journal	Title	Findings
Agha et al. (2007), British J Neurosurg, 21, 210–16	Hypopituitarism following traumatic brain injury (TBI)	Addresses the need to identify and manage TBI-related hormone deficiencies to reduce morbidity, aid recovery, and avoid long-term complications of pituitary failure
Behan et al. (2008), J Neurol Neurosurg Psychiatry, 79, 753–59	Neuroendocrine disorders after traumatic brain injury	Observes post-traumatic hypopituitarism (PTHP) associated with adverse outcome in acute and chronic phases after TBI. Addresses the need to identify and manage TBI-related hormone deficiencies to optimize recovery, improve quality of life, and avoid long-term adverse consequences
Bondanelli et al. (2005), Eur J Endocrinol, 152, 679–91	Hypopituitarism after traumatic brain injury	Emphasizes the need for accurate evaluation, long-term follow-up, and adequate replacement therapy
Ghigo et al. (2005), Brain Inj, 19, 711–24	Consensus guidelines on screening for hypopituitarism following traumatic brain injury	Recommends systematic screening of pituitary function for all patients with moderate-to-severe TBI at risk of developing pituitary deficits. Suggests patients will benefit and rehabilitation may be enhanced by appropriate hormonal replacement therapy
Guerrero and Alfonso (2010), Mil Med, 175, 574–80	Traumatic brain injury-related hypopituitarism: a review and recommendations for screening combat veterans	Extends recommendations for screening and treatment of combat veterans based on findings from the civilian research literature Observes that additional studies will be required to determine whether there is a need to modify these recommendations based on unique needs of the military patient population
Kennedy et al. (2007), J Rehabil Res Dev, 44, 895–920	Post-traumatic stress disorder and post-traumatic stress disorder-like symptoms and mild traumatic brain injury	Addresses TBI-related genetic, structural, endocrine, and neurochemical changes similar to those noted in the pathophysiology of PTSD. Observes that some of these changes may enhance the biological risk of PTSD or PTSD-like syndrome in TBI patients
Klose and Feldt-Rasmussen (2008), Pituitary, 11, 255–61	Does the type and severity of brain injury predict hypothalamo–pituitary dysfunction?	Observes that it has not yet been possible to identify early hormone alterations useful to the prediction of long-term PTHP. Finds outcome studies have indicated that PTHP is of clinical significance, which may justify introduction of neuroendocrine screening in TBI
Popovic et al. (2005), J Endocrinol Invest, 28, 61–4	Hypopituitarism following traumatic brain injury (TBI): call for attention	Addresses psychometric evaluation and neurocognitive testing as measures needed to support hormonal replacement. Addresses preliminary studies which show that subjects treated with GH experience significant improvements in concentration, memory, depression, anxiety, and fatigue
Powner et al. (2006), Neurocrit Care, 5, 61–70	Endocrine failure after traumatic brain injury in adults	Urges greater awareness of hypopituitarism as a possible complication of TBI. Encourages appropriate testing

(continued)

Table 11.3 (continued)

Author(s), Journal	Title	Findings
Powner and Boccalandro (2008), Curr Opin Crit Care, 14, 163–66	Adrenal insufficiency following traumatic brain injury in adults	Addresses adrenal gland failure or the inability to produce adrenocorticotropin and other pituitary hormones as a possible consequent of TBI. Recommends all patients sustaining severe traumatic brain injury should be tested for endocrine failure (adrenal, thyroid, and growth hormone) 3 months after injury
Riggio and Wong (2009), Mt Sinai J Med, 76, 163–72	Neurobehavioral sequelae of traumatic brain injury	Recommends evaluation of post-traumatic brain injury patients with neurobehavioral sequelae to include carefully structured history and physical exam with emphasis on neurological and psychiatric function. Adjunctive evaluations tailored to the context of the individual patient with neuroimaging, neurophysiological, and neuropsychiatric testing
Rothman et al. (2007), J Neuropsychiatry Clin Neurosci, 19, 363–72	The neuroendocrine effects of traumatic brain injury	Reviews the clinical spectrum of neuroendocrine deficits after TBI and their underlying mechanisms. Future studies of the effects of hormonal replacement on recovery are recommended
Schneider et al. (2005), J Neurotrauma, 22, 937–46	Anterior pituitary hormone abnormalities following traumatic brain injury	Observes that post-traumatic anterior pituitary dysfunction may aggravate symptoms of brain injury. Cautions that when undiagnosed, anterior pituitary dysfunction may lead to potentially fatal endocrine crises
Schneider et al. (2007), JAMA, 298, 1429–38	Hypothalamopituitary dysfunction following traumatic brain injury and aneurysmal subarachnoid hemorrhage: a systematic review	Found the prevalence of hypopituitarism was greater in patients with severe compared with those with mild or moderate traumatic brain injury. Early neuroendocrine abnormalities were transient in some patients while, less commonly, hypopituitarism evolved over time in others. Patients with PTHP showed an impaired quality of life and an adverse metabolic profile
Tanriverdi et al. (2010), Pituitary, 13, 146–53	Pituitary function in subjects with mild traumatic brain injury: a review of literature and proposal of a screening strategy	Finds that patients with mTBI are also vulnerable to pituitary dysfunction. Recommends screening mTBI patients who are hospitalized for at least 24 h, who have abnormal initial CTs, or who develop signs/symptoms of hypopituitarism post-TBI
Urban et al. (2005), Brain Inj, 19, 349–58	Anterior hypopituitarism following traumatic brain injury	Emphasizes anterior pituitary hormonal function assessment is crucial. Observes that hormone replacement therapy could allow treatment and correction of underlying causes of TBI sequelae

hormonal deficiencies varies widely (Rothman et al. 2007).

Based on the available recent literature, there is no conclusive evidence of a direct relationship between hypopituitarism and recovery (vs. fatality) from TBI. However, it is important to recognize that studies are typically forced to exclude very severely injured patients who die quickly as a result of their injuries or who are disabled to the extent that they cannot be tested as research subjects. The high incidence of hypothalamic–pituitary lesions observed on autopsy suggests that there may be a link between damage to these structures and TBI outcome. In fact, TBI-related hypopituitarism has been linked to adverse health outcome in acute and post-acute stages of TBI (Agha et al. 2007; Behan et al. 2008; Klose et al. 2007). Potentially severe sequelae include ischemic heart disease and shortened life span (Urban et al. 2005) as well as a number of other medical issues that can develop in relation to specific hormonal abnormalities when they are left untreated (Bondanelli et al. 2005; Kelly et al. 2000). Additional possible effects of PTHP include reduced quality of life (Cuneo et al. 1992; Schneider et al. 2007) and impaired rehabilitation (Urban et al. 2005).

In general, the risk of hypopituitarism is relatively higher for patients who have sustained more severe brain injuries (Bondanelli et al. 2005; Klose and Feldt-Rasmussen 2008; Popovic et al. 2005; Schneider et al. 2007). However, patients with mTBI also face a substantial risk of developing pituitary deficiencies (Tanriverdi et al. 2010). No specific findings have yet been reported to suggest a link between the severity level of TBI and specific types of hormonal abnormalities. Nor are there any findings to suggest that hypopituitarism might be any more or less likely for specific mechanisms of injury or injury location (Ghigo et al. 2005). However, among patients who sustain more severe TBIs, endocrine abnormalities are observed most often in cases that involve basal skull fractures, hypothalamic edema, diffuse axonal injuries, increased intracranial pressure (ICP), hyponatremia and/or hypotension, prolonged unresponsiveness, and/or extended stay in intensive care (Schneider et al. 2007).

Twenty-two clinical research studies have been published in recent years (Table 11.4). Six of these studies were prospective (acute/post-acute to 1- to 3-year post-injury) investigations of TBI-related neuroendocrine dysfunctional prevalence and/or risk factors (Bushnik et al. 2007; Kleindienst et al. 2009; Klose et al. 2007; Krahulik et al. 2009; Schneider et al. 2008b; Tanriverdi et al. 2007b). Ten studies were retrospective investigations involving assessments within the first 12 months post-TBI (Bavisetty et al. 2008; Bondanelli et al. 2007; Leon-Carrion et al. 2007) or at least 1-year post-TBI (Faust et al. 2008; Klose et al. 2007; Pavlovic et al. 2009; Stojanovic et al. 2008; Tanriverdi et al. 2008; Yollin et al. 2007). Mossberg et al. (2008) assessed post-TBI aerobic capacity in relation to GH deficiency in the "post-acute" recovery phase, unspecified. Two studies were based on retrospective review of data from TBI patients' charts (Schneider et al. 2008a; Wachter et al. 2009). Four studies investigated the prevalence of neuroendocrine abnormalities found during the acute phase of TBI, within 24–48 h of injury (Berg et al. 2009; Llompart-Pou et al. 2008; Tanriverdi et al. 2007a; van der Eerden et al. 2010).

Of the 22 studies shown in Table 11.4, 13 included mild, moderate, and severe TBI patient cohorts[3] (Bavisetty et al. 2008; Kleindienst et al. 2007; Klose et al. 2007; Krahulik et al. 2009; Mossberg et al. 2008; Schneider et al. 2008b; Tanriverdi et al. 2007a, b, 2008; van der Eerden et al. 2010; Wachter et al. 2009; Yollin et al. 2007). Five studies included only moderate and severe TBI patients (Berg et al. 2009; Bondanelli et al. 2007; Llompart-Pou et al. 2008; Pavlovic et al. 2009; Stojanovic et al. 2008), and one included severe TBI patients only (Leon-Carrion et al. 2007). Three studies did not specify patient TBI severity levels (Bushnik et al. 2007; Faust et al. 2008; Schneider et al. 2008a).

Generally consistent with the findings of earlier studies, findings from the majority of very recent clinical studies indicate overall incidence of TBI-related pituitary dysfunction at 20–40% (Bavisetty et al. 2008; Berg et al. 2009; Bondanelli et al. 2007; Krahulik et al. 2009; Llompart-Pou et al. 2008; Pavlovic et al. 2009; Schneider et al. 2008a; Tanriverdi et al. 2007a; Wachter et al. 2009; Yollin et al. 2007). Lower overall incidences (1–15%) were reported in two studies that employed dynamic hormone tests (e.g., insulin tolerance test, ACTH-stimulation test) at 13 months post-injury (Klose et al. 2007) and in an emergency department-based cohort under

[3]TBI severity levels are usually defined by Glascow Coma Scale (GSC) scores; mild = 13–15; moderate = 9–12; severe = <9.

Table 11.4 Clinical studies (2007–2010)

Author(s), Journal	Title	TBI patient sample (GCS severity level)	PD × TBI severity (GCS)	Findings
Bavisetty et al. (2008), Neurosurgery, 62, 1080–94	Chronic hypopituitarism after traumatic brain injury: risk assessment and relationship to outcome	$N=70$ Mild Moderate Severe	NS	Patients tested 6–9 months post-injury. Incidence of major hormonal deficiency was 21%, including GH deficiency or insufficiency (16%) and hypogonadism (11%). Patients with major deficiencies had more abnormal acute CT findings, greater BMI, worse disability rating scores, greater rates of depression, and worse quality of life scores in the energy and fatigue, emotional well-being, and general health domains. Major deficiencies were associated with diffuse brain swelling, intracerebral hemorrhage, and multiple contusions
Berg et al. (2009), Exp Clin Endocrinol Diabetes. EPub ahead of print	Prevalence of anterior pituitary dysfunction in patients following traumatic brain injury in a German multi-centre screening program	$N=246$ Moderate Severe	NS	Studied prevalence of anterior pituitary dysfunction across five German endocrine centers. 246 patients underwent baseline endocrine tests. Incidence of impaired pituitary function was found in 21%, predominantly secondary hypogonadism and hypothyreosis
Bondanelli et al. (2007), J Neurotrauma, 24, 1687–98	Anterior pituitary function may predict functional and cognitive outcome in patients with traumatic brain injury undergoing rehabilitation	$N=72$ Moderate (10) Severe (62)	NS	Evaluated relationship between pituitary function and TBI outcome in 72 patients with moderate and severe TBIs undergoing rehabilitation at 6–12 months post-injury. Incidence of overall pituitary dysfunction was 31%; anterior hypopituitarism incidence was 26%. GCS and GH peak were strong predictors of outcome, indicating a negative influence of pituitary dysfunction and a positive influence of normal GH secretion on recovery during post-TBI rehabilitation
Bushnik et al. (2007), Brain Inj, 21, 559–66	Fatigue after TBI: association with neuroendocrine abnormalities	$N=64$ nr	nr	Prospective study evaluated association between neuroendocrine findings and fatigue in TBI patients 1-year post-injury. Incidence of pituitary abnormalities was 90%. Fatigue scores were elevated compared to published control data. Higher GH levels were associated with higher scores, in contradiction to expectation of a relationship between GH deficiency and fatigue

Faust et al. (2008), Endocr Abstr, 16, P433	Unusual pattern of pituitary insufficiencies following traumatic brain injury evaluated by insulin tolerance test	$N=90$ nr	nr	Patients studied at 12 months post-TBI. In addition to standard basal endocrine measures, patients were administered the insulin tolerance test (ITT). Overall prevalence of pituitary insufficiency was 52%, with ACTH (39%) being the most common, followed by GH (12%). Authors conclude that ITT is safe diagnostic tool that revealed an unusual pattern with ACTH as predominant deficiency
Kleindienst et al. (2007), Endocr Abstr, 13, P231	A prospective longitudinal study of anterior pituitary dysfunction following traumatic brain injury	$N=71$ Mild Moderate Severe	Persistent GH deficiency correlated with TBI severity ($p=0.036$)	Prospective study to identify predictors of late endocrine insufficiency. Pituitary function was assessed in acute, post-acute, and 24–36 months. Hypopituitarism was detectable in 70% of patients initially and 50% late after TBI. Age, BMI, initial GCS, and mechanical ventilation were correlated with persistent GH deficiency
Klose et al. (2007), Clin Endocrinol, 67, 193–201	Prevalence and predictive factors of post-traumatic hypopituitarism	$N=104$ Mild (44) Moderate (20) Severe (40)	Increased risk of hypopituitarism after severe TBI (vs. mTBI, $p=0{\cdot}004$)	Cross-sectional cohort study of hospitalized patients evaluated 13 months post-injury showed hypopituitarism incidence of 15% with GH most frequently affected. Pituitary insufficiency risk was elevated in severe (vs. mild) TBI and in patients with increased ICP. Obesity was noted as possible confound for pituitary dysfunction
Klose et al. (2007), Clin Endocrinol, 67, 598–606	Acute and long-term pituitary insufficiency in traumatic brain injury: a prospective single-centre study	$N=46$ Mild (22) Moderate (9) Severe (15)	Hypopituitarism more frequently associated with severe TBI (vs. mTBI, $p=0{\cdot}02$)	12-Month prospective study of prevalence and hormone alterations. Incidence of hormone alterations was 76% in the acute TBI phase, with thyroid and gonadal hormone alterations most common. Acute alterations did not predict long-term hypopituitarism. Post-acute incidence was 13%, with GH deficiency most common. Long-term hypopituitarism was frequent only in severe TBI patients
Krahulik et al. (2009), J Neurosurg, Epub ahead of print	Dysfunction of hypothalamic hypophysial axis after traumatic brain injury in adults	$N=89$ Mild Moderate Severe	nr	Prospective study to determine incidence and risk factors for endocrine dysfunction. Patients were evaluated at time of injury and 3, 6, and 12 months post-injury. Primary hormonal dysfunction was found in 21%; major deficits included GH, hypogonadism, and diabetes insipidus. MRIs demonstrated empty sella syndrome in patients with major hormonal deficits. Brain swelling and cranial base fracture were identified as risk factors

(continued)

Table 11.4 (continued)

Author(s), Journal	Title	TBI patient sample (GCS severity level)	PD × TBI severity (GCS)	Findings
Leon-Carrion et al. (2007), Brain Inj, 21, 871–75	Cognitive deterioration due to GH deficiency in patients with traumatic brain injury: a preliminary report	$N=22$ Severe	N/A	Between-group study examined hormonal deficit vs. TBI influence on cognitive and behavioral disorders in 22 severe TBI patients, 11 of whom had isolated GH deficiency. Evaluation at 6 months post-TBI found greater cognitive deficits (attention, executive function, memory, and emotion) among GH-deficient patients
Llompart-Pou et al. (2008), Neurocritical Care, 9, 230–36	Acute hypothalamic–pituitary–adrenal response in traumatic brain injury with and without extracerebral trauma	$N=165$ Moderate Severe	nr	Evaluated impact of systemic injury (extracerebral trauma, ECT) on HPA axis response. Adrenal insufficiency was found at 24–48 h post-injury in 24% of patients, with increased risk in patients with low plasma ACTH and patients with hemorrhagic shock. Patients with and without ECT had comparable acute HPA response. Adrenal insufficiency did not affect outcome
Mossberg et al. (2008), J Clin Endocrinol Metab, 93, 2581–87	Aerobic capacity and growth hormone deficiency after traumatic brain injury	$N=35$ Mild (5) Moderate Severe	N/A	Study of post-acute recovery phase to assess aerobic capacity in relation to GH deficiency. TBI patients overall had below normal aerobic capacity, but with higher peak oxygen consumption in TBI patients with normal GH vs. insufficient and deficient GH. GH abnormality presents possible increased risk for secondary cardiorespiratory disability
Pavlovic et al. (2009), Eur J Neurol, Epub ahead of print	Chronic cognitive sequelae after traumatic brain injury are not related to growth hormone deficiency in adults	$N=60$ Moderate Severe	NS	Retrospective cross-sectional study of endocrine and cognitive function at least 1-year post-injury. GH deficiency or insufficiency was found in 33% of patients independent of trauma severity and age at trauma. There were no significant differences in neuropsychological tests between patients having TBI with GH deficiency, insufficiency, or normal secretion
Schneider et al. (2008b), Clin Endocrinol, 68, 206–12	Predictors of anterior pituitary insufficiency after traumatic brain injury	$N=78$ Mild Moderate Severe	NS	Assessed clinical and radiological risk factors for PTHP; assessments performed at 3 and 12 months post-TBI. Results identified diffuse axonal injury, basal skull fracture, and older age as major risk factors for TBI-related hypopituitarism

Schneider et al. (2008a), Endocr Abstr, 16, OC1.1	Structured assessment of neuroendocrine dysfunction following traumatic brain injury and aneurysmal subarachnoid hemorrhage in 921 patients: the German Interdisciplinary Database	$N=594$ nr	nr	Data were gathered from a national registry of TBI and SAH patients with endocrine assessments to assess 921 patients. In patients with only basal pituitary assessments, ACTH, and GH impairments were found in 44% of TBI patients. Prevalence of hypopituitarism was greater (52%) among patients with at least one stimulation test. This suggests that hypopituitarism may be overlooked if only basal values are gathered
Stojanovic et al. (2008), Endocr Abstr, 16, P396	The effects of growth hormone deficiency following moderate and severe traumatic brain injury on cognitive functions	$N=61$ Moderate Severe	nr	Examined neurobehavioral functions in patients with TBI-related GH deficiency at least 1 year after TBI. GH-deficient patients had lower cognitive test scores than GH normal patients on executive cognitive function measures
Tanriverdi et al. (2007a), Brain Inj, 21, 433–39	Pituitary functions in the acute phase of traumatic brain injury: Are they related to severity of the injury or mortality?	$N=104$ Mild (49) Moderate (24) Severe (31)	Basal cortisol and testosterone (males) positively correlated, prolactin negatively correlated with TBI severity (severe vs. mild or moderate TBI, $p<0.05$)	Studied pituitary functions within 24 h of TBI to identify relationships between pituitary hormones, TBI severity, and mortality. Post-TBI mortality (20) was unrelated to basal pituitary hormone levels. Age and TBI severity were related to mortality. Pituitary deficiencies included TSH (4%), gonadotropin (40%), ACTH (9%), and GH (20%). Basal hormone cortisol, prolactin, and testosterone were related to TBI severity
Tanriverdi et al. (2007b), Clin Endocrinol, 1–7	Three year prospective investigation of anterior pituitary function after traumatic brain injury: a pilot study	$N=30$ Mild (19) Moderate (6) Severe (5)	NS	Three-year prospective follow-up of anterior pituitary function. GH deficiency was the most common dysfunction, improving over time in 54% of patients with mild or moderate TBI. Among patients with ACTH deficiency at 1 year, 83% recovered after 3 years. Severe TBI patients showed ACTH and GH deficiencies persisting to the third year
Tanriverdi et al. (2008), Eur J Endocrinol, 159, 7–13	Antipituitary antibodies after traumatic brain injury: is head trauma-induced pituitary dysfunction associated with autoimmunity?	$N=29$ Mild (18) Moderate (6) Severe (5)	nr	Study of TBI patients at 3-year follow-up evaluation of antipituitary antibodies (APAs) and pituitary function, compared against normal control subjects. APAs were detected in 45% of TBI patients, with none found in normal controls. There was a significant relationship between APA positivity and TBI-related hypopituitarism. APA was also associated with low GH response. Autoimmunity may contribute to the development of TBI-induced hypopituitarism

(continued)

Table 11.4 (continued)

Author(s), Journal	Title	TBI patient sample (GCS severity level)	PD × TBI severity (GCS)	Findings
van der Eerden et al. (2010), Eur J Endocrinol, 162, 19	Should anterior pituitary function be tested during follow-up of all patients presenting at the emergency department because of traumatic brain injury?	*N* = 107 Mild (77) Moderate Severe	nr	Assessed prevalence of pituitary dysfunction in an emergency department-based cohort screened for anterior pituitary insufficiency using strict endocrinological diagnostic criteria. Abnormalities were found in 14% of patients, with more extensive evaluation finding dysfunction in one patient only
Wachter et al. (2009), J Clin Neurosci, 16, 202–8	Pituitary insufficiency after traumatic brain injury	*N* = 55 Mild (17) Severe (34) Unknown (3)	nr	Retrospective study of patient charts to investigate relationship between hypopituitarism, neuropsychological changes, and CT findings. Pituitary insufficiency prevalence was 25%. Neuropsychological complaints were present in 67%, associated with intracerebral hemorrhagic lesions but not with pituitary insufficiency
Yollin et al. (2007), Endocr Abstr, 14, P545	Is there an endocrine explanation for persistent neuropsychological disabilities long after traumatic brain injury (TBI)?	*N* = 50 Mild (10) Moderate (2) Severe (38)	nr	Studied prevalence of pituitary dysfunction in patients with TBIs and neuropsychological disabilities at least 1-year post-TBI. Findings included 46% patients showing at least one anterior pituitary deficiency (TSH (12%), ACTH (20%), GH (40–45%)). Hypopituitarism unrelated to GCS, initial CTs, GOS, self-sufficiency, or return to work. High risk for deficiencies justifies pituitary exploration long after TBI

TBI severity classification varied across studies; for the majority, a post-resuscitative Glasgow Coma Scale (GCS) score of 3–8 corresponded to severe, 9–12 corresponded to moderate, and 13–15 corresponded to mTBI

Notes: *GCS* Glasgow Coma Scale, *nr* not reported, *NS* not significant, *PD* pituitary dysfunction strict endocrinological screening and diagnostic criteria (van der Eerden et al. 2010). Notably higher rates of pituitary hormonal deficiency were reported in three studies which observed incidence as high as 70–76% in the acute phase and 50–52% in the post-acute phase of TBI (Faust et al. 2008; Kleindienst et al. 2007; Klose et al. 2007). Bushnik et al. (2007) reported pituitary abnormalities in 90% of patients studied for TBI-related fatigue 1-year post-injury. Variations in the reported prevalence of hypopituitarism are not unusual, likely due to differences in diagnostic criteria, assessment techniques, and clinical confounds in various patient cohorts (see review by Kokshoorn et al. 2010). For example, although several studies of hormonal abnormalities in acute TBI have reported evidence that gonadal and/or thyroid deficiencies are the most common (40–76%) (Berg et al. 2009; Klose et al. 2007; Tanriverdi et al. 2007a), Schneider et al. (2008a) found that ACTH and GH deficiencies were most common in a large review of TBI patients who had received at least one hormone simulation test.

Studies involving TBI patients assessed 3 months to 3 years after original injury showed GH deficiency to be most frequent abnormality, with reported incidence ranging from 12 to 63% (Bavisetty et al. 2008; Bondanelli et al. 2007; Klose et al. 2007; Krahulik et al. 2009; Tanriverdi et al. 2007b; Yollin et al. 2007). Hypogonadism was also noted among 10–26% or more of post-acute patients in some studies (Bavisetty et al. 2008; Bondanelli et al. 2007; Krahulik et al. 2009). Faust et al. (2008) found ACTH to be the most common deficiency among patients who were tested with baseline endocrine measures as well as the insulin tolerance test. Notably, Tanriverdi et al. (2007b) observed that although GH and ACTH deficiencies improved over time in 54% and 83% of TBI patients, respectively, these deficiencies persisted to the third year of follow-up among individuals with severe TBIs.

Several investigators have addressed possible specific relationships between GH and/or ACTH deficiencies and other injury or health factors of interest. GH deficiency may be associated with reduced aerobic capacity and increased risk for secondary cardiorespiratory disability (Mossberg et al. 2008). However, Bushnik et al. (2007) found an unexpected positive correlation between GH levels and fatigue in TBI patients. Possible predictor variables for persistent GH deficiency are consistent with those for TBI-related hypopituitarism generally, including age, body mass index (BMI), obesity, initial GCS, and mechanical ventilation (Kleindienst et al. 2007; Schneider et al. 2008b). Llompart-Pou et al. (2008) observed an increased risk for adrenal insufficiency in patients with hemorrhagic shock, but found no increased risk among patients with extracerebral trauma. A recent study by Tanriverdi et al. (2008) suggests that autoimmunity may contribute to the development of TBI-related hypopituitarism, finding antipituitary antibodies in 45% of TBI patients (vs. none in normal controls) and an association between antipituitary antibodies and low GH response in particular.

It is not yet clear whether or to what extent TBI-related GH deficiency might affect neuropsychological function. There is some evidence that TBI patients who are GH deficient may show greater cognitive deficits (attention, executive function, memory, and emotion) (Leon-Carrion et al. 2007; Stojanovic et al. 2008). However, other studies have failed to find any clear relationship between pituitary dysfunction and neuropsychological measures of cognitive function (Pavlovic et al. 2009; Wachter et al. 2009; Yollin et al. 2007).

Consistent with conclusions drawn by prior reviews, the most recent research literature indicates general agreement that although patients who sustain mTBI are at risk for developing TBI-related pituitary abnormalities, moderate-to-severe (vs. mild) TBI probably presents a relatively greater risk for TBI-related hormonal sequelae (Klose et al. 2007; Krahulik et al. 2009; Tanriverdi et al. 2007a), and deficiencies are more likely to persist for months or years in patients with severe TBI (Klose et al. 2007; Tanriverdi et al. 2007b). However, fewer than half of the clinical studies we reviewed sought or reported significant differences associated with TBI severity. Just three of these studies reported statistically significant effects of initial GCS score on pituitary function beyond the early acute injury phase (Kleindienst et al. 2007; Klose et al. 2007). As a whole, the recent body of literature provides no clear basis by which to conclude that specific hormonal abnormalities are more or less often associated with specific levels of TBI severity (GCS scores), injury locations, or mechanisms of injury.

Schneider and colleagues (2008b) identified specific risk factors for TBI-related pituitary abnormalities to include diffuse axonal injury, basal skull fracture, and older age. Pituitary abnormalities have also been linked to abnormal acute CT findings, greater BMI (Bavisetty et al. 2008), increased ICP (Klose et al. 2007), and empty sella syndrome[4] (Krahulik et al. 2009). Bavisetty et al. (2008) observed that although initial GCS scores were not predictive of TBI-related hypopituitarism, TBI patients with major hormonal deficiencies 6–9 months post-injury had more severe brain injuries based on their CT findings ($p<0.014$). Specifically, this effect was associated with CT findings of diffuse brain swelling, evacuated intracerebral hemorrhage, or multiple contusions (see also Wachter et al. 2009). Krahulik et al. (2009) observed brain swelling and cranial base fracture as significant risk factors for TBI-related hormonal deficits, and Klose et al. (2007) reported that TBI-related pituitary deficiencies were associated with increased ICP. However, other studies in this series also considered specific aspects of TBI and found no significant predictive injury characteristics (Bondanelli et al. 2007; Klose et al. 2007; Pavlovic et al. 2009).

Finally, two recent studies showed relationships between hypopituitarism and TBI recovery and outcome. Bondanelli et al. (2007) evaluated the relationship between pituitary function and TBI outcome in patients undergoing rehabilitation after moderate or severe TBI, finding a negative influence of pituitary dysfunction (GH deficiency) on cognitive and functional recovery during rehabilitation. Bavisetty et al. (2008) found that TBI patients with major pituitary deficiencies had worse disability rating scores, higher rates of depression, and worse quality of life scores in the energy, fatigue, emotional well-being, and general health domain measures taken 6–9 months post-injury.

[4]Empty sella syndrome involves the sella turcica, which is the bony structure that surrounds the pituitary gland. This structure may appear empty on imaging studies due to shrinkage or flattening of the pituitary, which may occur as the result of direct damage or injury-related fluid compression.

Conclusions and Recommendations

A fast-growing body of evidence suggests that neuroendocrine dysfunction is a common consequence of TBI, and further that if left untreated, it has the potential to compromise patient health, recovery, and outcome. Current evidence strongly supports routine acute and post-acute screening for pituitary hormonal abnormalities in TBI patients generally, and especially among moderate-to-severe TBI patients in whom endocrine disruption might be expected to have the greatest immediate or long-term health impact. Among those who have suffered severe TBI, pituitary hormonal deficits may persist for months or years post-injury.

Based upon the findings of the current review and those published previously, it is reasonable to conclude that neuroendocrine abnormalities can be expected to occur in 20–40% of TBI patients. Although there seems to be emerging agreement that more severe TBIs present relatively greater risk for neuroendocrine dysfunction, relatively few studies have observed statistically significant differences to support this conclusion based upon GCS severity assessment scores. Just 4 of the 22 clinical studies here reviewed observed statistically significant effects of TBI severity based on initial patient GCS scores (Kleindienst et al. 2007; Klose et al. 2007; Tanriverdi et al. 2007a). Six studies analyzed for TBI severity effects and found none (Bavisetty et al. 2008; Berg et al. 2009; Bondanelli et al. 2007; Pavlovic et al. 2009; Schneider et al. 2008b; Tanriverdi et al. 2007b). Several earlier studies also reported finding no association between initial TBI severity level and the occurrence of hypopituitarism (Agha et al. 2004; Aimaretti et al. 2004; Lieberman et al. 2001;

Schneider et al. 2006). Moreover, it is apparent that patients with mTBI are at risk for TBI-related hypopituitarism (Tanriverdi et al. 2010).

This raises the possibility that current TBI severity criteria and related assessment tools fail to capture potentially significant aspects or parameters of injury that could signal an elevated risk to hypothalamic–pituitary structures in particular. There is a need for additional research to determine what, if any injury-related factors, circumstances, imaging studies, or other clinical measures might reliably support early risk assessment for primary or secondary hypothalamic–pituitary involvement irrespective of diagnosed TBI severity level based on GCS scores. To date, the identification of such factors has been limited primarily to severe injury scenarios involving diffuse axonal damage, basal skull fracture, hypotensive or hypoxic insult, and increased ICP. Age, BMI, and obesity have been identified as general risk factors. The literature also provides no clear and consistent evidence linking hormonal effects to specific brain injury location or mechanism of injury, to include blast-related TBI as found in the combat military population. This further suggests the need to identify and capture other injury-related parameters that may represent the potential for injury to hypothalamic–pituitary structures in particular.

Gonadal (LH/FSH; 80%) deficiencies are most commonly observed in relation to the acute phase of TBI. It is not clear whether this number may be exaggerated by the so-called "eugonadal sick syndrome"[5] or by exposure to opiates after injury, with subsequent resolution in the post-acute phase. Hyperprolactemia has also been observed to occur in more than half of acute patients. Although transient diabetes insipidus in the acute phase of TBI is uncommon (<4%), it may occur less severely as partial deficiency in as many as 26% of TBI patients (Agha et al. 2005; Tsagarakis et al. 2005) and may in some cases persist well beyond the first few months post-TBI (Agha et al. 2005; Krahulik et al. 2009). Thyroid abnormalities (TSH; 10–30%) have been reported, but may be confounded by euthyroid sick syndrome,[6] which accounts for a significantly lower prevalence in the chronic phase. GH (18%) and ACTH (15%) deficiencies may also occur in the acute phase of TBI. In the post-acute and chronic phases of TBI, somatotrophic (GH) and corticotropic (ACTH) deficiencies are reported frequently, affecting 15–20% of TBI patients. However, additional research is needed to more precisely identify the relative prevalence of isolated TBI-related hormonal abnormalities with respect to their relevant risk factors, etiology, time course, and relationships to other variables that may influence patient treatment and outcome.

Findings from the available research literature do not yet support clear expectations as to how TBI-related hormonal abnormalities might alter the early clinical presentation of patients with TBI. Additional research is needed to ascertain the time course of TBI-related hormonal disruption, the onset of which likely varies by relationship to primary or secondary injury factors. Whether or not the signs and symptoms of hormonal impairments are clinically observable might also depend to a large extent on the context, severity, and circumstances of original injury. Subsequent to initial assessment, hormonal sequelae can be easily mistaken for or masked by similar symptoms associated with post-concussion syndrome or psychiatric comorbidity. Subtle symptoms may be missed entirely. These diagnostic challenges reinforce the importance of basal and stimulation tests as needed to rule out or diagnose hormonal deficiencies

[5]Since the 1970s, transient hypogonadism has been described in acute illness. The degree of hypothalamic–pituitary–gonadal axis suppression is related to the severity of illness in critical care patients. It has been proposed that there is both primary and secondary hypogonadism; however, the mechanism is poorly understood. There is no established role for treatment.

[6]Assessment of thyroid function in patients with nonthyroidal illness is difficult, especially in the critically ill. Many such patients have low serum concentrations of both thyroxine (T4) and triiodothyronine (T3) and their serum thyrotropin (TSH) concentration also may be low. Proposed mechanisms include an alteration in thyroid binding proteins, and decreased 5′-monodeiodination activity which reduces T4 to T3 conversion. Thyroid function returns to normal after convalescence. Treatment is generally held unless there is other evidence to suggest a hypothyroid state.

that might otherwise be obscured by co-occurring physical, cognitive, and psychosocial changes consequent to TBI.

Almost without exception, civilian researchers in this area agree that there is a need to screen TBI patients for neuroendocrine abnormalities common in the acute, post-acute, or recovery phases of TBI. The most conservative recommendation is that all TBI patients who need hospitalization for at least 24 h should be screened for pituitary abnormalities, and that this should include mTBI patients who have CT abnormality or who develop signs and symptoms suggestive of hypopituitarism at any time post-TBI (Tanriverdi et al. 2010).

Although no clear consensus has yet developed concerning what specific tests are both optimal and cost-effective, in the acute phase of TBI it is especially important to evaluate rapidly (typically by basal cortisol level) to determine if there is adrenal insufficiency, which is a potentially life-threatening condition. Thyroid baseline testing is also warranted in the acute phase, prior to hospital discharge, though results should be interpreted with caution because thyroid function tests can be altered in any acute illness.

Following the acute phase, Tanriverdi et al. (2010) recommend that all pituitary hormonal axes should again be evaluated at 3–6 months post-injury and then followed for 3 years of surveillance. However, full implementation of these guidelines is generally restricted to endocrinologists able to perform dynamic hormonal testing. Another recent review reiterates the recommendation to have a low threshold for screening for pituitary dysfunction in combat veterans following any severity TBI and proposes readily available screening tests with indications for referral to an endocrinologist (Guerrero and Alfonso 2010). In addition, future research would be helpful to ascertain the potential benefits of routine screening and early intervention on long-term TBI recovery and rehabilitation.

Where TBI-related hormonal abnormalities are identified, the question is raised how and when to intervene therapeutically. Potentially beneficial effects of hormone replacement therapy (HRT) on cognitive, mood, and physical function have been documented in other patient populations (Azad et al. 2003; Bhasin et al. 1997; Carroll et al. 1998; Maruff and Falleti 2005). More recently, HRT has been demonstrated in TBI patients with GH deficiencies, with findings to suggest that GH treatment may exert a positive effect on patient quality of life (Kreitschmann-Andermahr et al. 2008; Yollin et al. 2008). The benefits of GH replacement are well-established in patients where GH deficiency is clear and persistent (Monson 2003); however, GH therapy has been shown to increase mortality in critically ill adults (Ruokonen and Takala 2002; Takala et al. 1999). Additional prospective, randomized studies are needed to determine whether and when HRT is appropriate in treating the unique considerations of TBI-related hormonal deficiencies that may be borderline, ambiguous, transient, or complicated by other clinical symptoms. Studies are also needed to determine how HRT affects long-term aspects of TBI such as recovery and rehabilitation.

Not yet addressed by the research literature is the question of why some patients may recover from TBI-induced hormonal abnormalities more quickly than others, and/or without intervention. Although it seems unlikely that recovery is strictly a function of original TBI severity level, additional research is needed to profile endocrinological risk and recovery. Conflicting findings also call attention to the need for more studies of how and to what extent TBI-related pituitary hormonal deficiencies may be expected to influence neurobehavioral and cognitive function.

Considerations for Military TBI

Largely unique to the realm of military medicine is the problem of blast-induced neurotrauma (BINT), or blast-induced TBI (bTBI), which now accounts for majority of TBIs sustained by US military personnel engaged in current conflicts in Iraq and Afghanistan (Galarneau et al. 2008; Warden 2006). More than two-thirds of all US military casualties since the beginning of conflicts in Iraq and Afghanistan have been due to explosive weapons (Defense Manpower Data Center 2010) and more than half of US troops who are injured by explosive blast are also diagnosed with TBI. Although the precise pathophysiology of BINT itself is not yet fully understood, the basic mechanisms of explosive injuries are well-summarized in a recently published review by Cernak and Noble-Haeusslein (2010). Blast-related pressure shifts can cause concussion, contusion, vasospasm, edema, metabolic changes, cerebral infarct, and neurological symptoms consistent with TBI (Cernak and Noble-Haeusslein 2010; Ling et al. 2009). Blast effects can also cause brain damage associated with biochemical changes and cognitive deficit (Cernak et al. 2001). Studies based on experimental animal models suggest that TBI and BINT share many possible primary and secondary effects in common, including elevated ICP, diffuse axonal injury, metabolic and physiological disturbances, and cognitive sequelae (Armonda et al. 2006; Belanger et al. 2009; Ling et al. 2009). However, other studies suggest that changes associated with BINT may differ from non-blast-related TBI in terms of their timing and frequency (Ling et al. 2009). Further experimental and clinical studies are needed to determine whether and how BINT might influence hypothalamic–pituitary function. Implementation of routine pituitary screening in military patients with BINT could provide essential information not otherwise generally available in civilian medical settings, and studies are underway.

Another key challenge in the context of military TBI is the need to differentiate between TBI and PTSD when symptoms overlap. Kennedy et al. (2007) provide a comprehensive review of the literature on PTSD and PTSD-like symptoms concurrent with mTBI. Brain regions implicated in PTSD are also vulnerable to TBI, including the orbitofrontal and dorsolateral prefrontal cortices, the hippocampus, and tracts connecting the amygdala and medial prefrontal cortex. Moreover, PTSD itself has been linked to altered HPA axis function, manifesting as elevated hypothalamic corticotrophin-releasing hormone and reduced cortisol levels within hours of exposure to trauma (Davidson et al. 2004; McFarlane et al. 1997). In PTSD, this is due primarily to increased sensitivity and numbers of glucocorticoid receptors, which in turn creates an increase in negative feedback to the pituitary. However, these alterations are associated with symptoms that can be difficult to distinguish from those of TBI-related pituitary dysfunction. Co-occurring symptoms of TBI and PTSD include cognitive deficits (memory, attention) mood disorder, apathy, sleep disturbance, chronic pain, and headache. Particularly in the case of mTBI, it may be very difficult to determine whether persistent neuropsychiatric symptoms are due to neurological vs. psychological disorder. In fact, comorbidity is common and military personnel often present with symptoms that meet the diagnostic criteria for both TBI and PTSD. Effective treatment and rehabilitation requires accurate diagnosis, particularly for mTBI which may be missed and is usually not initially visible on imaging studies. A better understanding of the biological interface between TBI and PTSD may be facilitated by studies that focus specifically on endocrine effects of mTBI in particular.

Depression and chronic stress also involve changes which manifest as HPA alterations. In depression and chronic stress, the number of glucocorticoid receptors is reduced. Three recent studies point to chronic and perceived stress and hypocortisolemia (low blood cortisol level) as potentially significant contributors to post TBI fatigue and depression (Bay and Donders 2008; Bay and Xie 2009; Bay et al. 2009).

The literature does not yet support conclusions about how TBI patients who also suffer from psychiatric comorbidities or chronic stress might present differently from those who do not, or how the presence or absence of TBI-related neuroendocrine dysfunction might interact. The greater need may be in determining how to diagnose any or all of these maladies correctly in the face of multiple common symptoms, as is a challenge frequently encountered in military medical settings.

Recommendations

Several knowledge gaps exist, calling attention to the need for a better understanding of when to expect and how to distinguish TBI-related hormonal abnormalities from other maladies. Specifically, additional clinical studies involving civilian and/or military TBI populations are needed to address specific research objectives as follows:

- Identify specific risk and recovery factors for TBI-related neuroendocrine dysfunction.
- Document the costs vs. benefits of routine endocrine screening on TBI recovery and rehabilitation outcome.
- Specify relationships between TBI-related hormonal deficiencies and behavioral, cognitive functional, and mood disorders.
- Ascertain the time course of TBI-related hormonal abnormalities.

We also identified three additional research objectives as being especially important to the improved understanding and treatment of neuroendocrine abnormalities specifically in the context of military TBI:

- Determine the prevalence of BINT-related neuroendocrine abnormalities.

  Additional research is needed to determine whether and how BINT may influence hypothalamic–pituitary function. Implementation of routine pituitary screening in military patients with BINT can provide essential information not otherwise generally available in civilian medical settings.
- Identify risk factors and prevalence of neuroendocrine sequelae of mTBI.

  An improved understanding of the biological interface between TBI and PTSD may be facilitated by research to specifically address endocrine sequelae of mTBI. Symptoms of hormonal dysfunction may be identical to those associated with psychiatric disorder and cognitive, mood, and behavioral changes sometimes associated with post-concussion syndrome. Additional research in this area may inform etiology and support differential diagnosis.
- Assess outcome effects of HRT.

  Clinical research involving civilian subjects suggests that HRT may be effective as intervention for TBI-related neuroendocrine dysfunction, especially in the case of GHD. There is a need for careful review and evaluation of HRT with respect to its possible usefulness and considerations unique to the military medical context.

The military medical setting offers valuable opportunities to address risk and injury factors that are largely unique to military and veteran populations, yet potentially very informative to medical science in general. Likewise, findings drawn from civilian patient populations can and should inform military medical science and practice. TBIs are unfortunately common in both realms, underscoring the need for additional research to improve diagnosis, treatment, and recovery.

References

Agha A, Phillips J, O'Kelly P, et al. The natural history of post-traumatic hypopituitarism: implications for assessment and treatment. Am J Med. 2005;118:1416.

Agha A, Phillips J, Thompson CJ. Hypopituitarism following traumatic brain injury (TBI). Br J Neurosurg. 2007;21:210–6.

Agha A, Rogers B, Mylotte D, et al. Neuroendocrine dysfunction in the acute phase of traumatic brain injury. Clin Endocrinol. 2004;60:584–91.

Agha A, Sherlock M, Phillips J, et al. The natural history of post-traumatic neurohypophysial dysfunction. Eur J Endocrinol. 2005;152:371–7.

Aimaretti G, Ambrosio MR, Di Somma C, et al. Traumatic brain injury and subarachnoid haemorrhage are conditions at high risk for hypopituitarism: screening study at 3 months after the brain injury. Clin Endocrinol. 2004;61:320–6.

Aimaretti G, Ambrosio MR, Di Somma C, et al. Residual pituitary function after brain injury-induced hypopituitarism: a prospective 12-month study. J Clin Endocrinol Metab. 2005;90:6085–92.

American Academy of Neurology. Practice parameter: the management of concussion in sports (summary statement). Report of the Quality Standards Subcommittee. Neurology. 1997;48:581–5.

Armonda RA, Bell RS, Vo AH, et al. Wartime traumatic cerebral vasospasm: recent review of combat casualties. Neurosurgery. 2006;59:1215–25.

Azad N, Pitale S, Barnes WE, et al. Testosterone treatment enhances regional brain perfusion in hypogonadal men. J Clin Endocrinol Metab. 2003;88:306–8.

Bavisetty S, Bavisetty S, McArthur DL, et al. Chronic hypopituitarism after traumatic brain injury: risk assessment and relationship to outcome. Neurosurgery. 2008;62:1080–94.

Bay E, Donders J. Risk factors for depressive symptoms after mild-to-moderate traumatic brain injury. Brain Inj. 2008;22:233–41.

Bay E, Xie Y. Psychological and biological correlates of fatigue after mild-to-moderate traumatic brain injury. West J Nurs Res. 2009;31:731–47.

Bay E, Sikorski A, Gao F. Functional status, chronic stress, and cortisol response after mild-to-moderate traumatic brain injury. Biol Res Nurs. 2009;10:213–25.

Behan LA, Phillips J, Thompson CJ, Agha A. Neuroendocrine disorders after traumatic brain injury. J Neurol Neurosurg Psychiatry. 2008;79:753–9.

Belanger HG, Kretzmer T, Yoash-Gantz R, et al. Cognitive sequelae of blast-related versus other mechanisms of brain trauma. J Int Neuropsychol Soc. 2009;15:1–8.

Belmont A, Agar N, Hugeron C, et al. Fatigue and traumatic brain injury. Ann Readapt Med Phys. 2006;49: 370–4.

Benvenga S, Campenni A, Ruggeri RM, Trimarchi F. Hypopituitarism secondary to head trauma. J Clin Endocrinol Metab. 2000;85:1353–61.

Berg C, Oeffner A, Schumm-Draeger PM, et al. Prevalence of anterior pituitary dysfunction in patients following traumatic brain injury in a German multi-centre screening program. Exp Clin Endocrinol Diabete. 2009. EPub ahead of print. http://www.ncbi.nlm.nih.gov/pubmed/19691014. Accessed 18 Jan 2010.

Bernard F, Outtrim J, Menon DK, Matta BF. Incidence of adrenal insufficiency after severe traumatic brain injury varies according to definition used: clinical implications. Br J Anaesth. 2006;96:72–6.

Bhasin S, Storer TW, Berman N, et al. Testosterone replacement increases fat-free mass and muscle size in hypogonadal men. J Clin Endocrinol Metab. 1997;82: 407–13.

Bohnen N, Jolles J. Neurobehavioral aspects of postconcussive symptoms after mild head injury. J Nerv Ment Dis. 1992;180:683–92.

Bohnen N, Jolles J, Twijnstra A. Neuropsychological deficits in patients with persistent symptoms six months after mild head injury. Neurosurgery. 1992;30:692–6.

Bondanelli M, Ambrosio MR, Zatelli MC, et al. Hypopituitarism after traumatic brain injury. Eur J Endocrinol. 2005;152:679–91.

Bondanelli M, Ambrosio MR, Cavazzini L, et al. Anterior pituitary function may predict functional and cognitive outcome in patients with traumatic brain injury undergoing rehabilitation. J Neurotrauma. 2007;24: 1687–97.

Bondanelli M, De Marinis L, Ambrosio MR, et al. Occurrence of pituitary dysfunction following traumatic brain injury. J Neurotrauma. 2004;21:685–96.

Boughey JC, Yost MJ, Bynoe RP. Diabetes insipidus in the head-injured patient. Am Surg. 2004;70:500–3.

Bryant RA. Disentangling mild traumatic brain injury and stress reactions. N Engl J Med. 2008;358:525–6.

Bryant RA, Harvey AG. Relationship between acute stress disorder ad posttraumatic stress disorder following mild traumatic brain injury. Am J Psychiatry. 1998;155: 625–9.

Bushnik T, Englander J, Katznelson L. Fatigue after TBI: association with neuroendocrine abnormalities. Brain Inj. 2007;21:559–66.

Carroll PV, Christ ER, Bengtsson B-A. Growth hormone deficiency in adulthood and the effects of growth hormone replacement: a review. J Clin Endocrinol Metab. 1998;83:382–95.

Cassidy JD, Carroll LJ, Peloso PM, et al. Incidence, risk factors and prevention of mild traumatic brain injury: results of the WHO Collaborating Centre Task Force on Mild Traumatic Brain Injury. J Rehabil Med. 2004;36:28–60.

Ceballos R. Pituitary changes in head trauma: analysis of 102 consecutive cases of head injury. Ala J Med Sci. 1966;3:185–98.

Centers for Disease Control and Prevention. Traumatic Brain Injury in the United States: emergency department visits, hospitalizations, and deaths. Prepared by Division of Injury Response, National Center for Injury Prevention and Control, Centers for Disease Control and Prevention, U.S. Department of Health and Human Services; 2006.

Cernak I, Noble-Haeusslein LJ. Traumatic brain injury: an overview of pathobiology with emphasis on military populations. J Cereb Blood Flow Metab. 2010;30(2): 255–66.

Cernak I, Savic J, Ignjatovic D. Blast injury from explosive munitions. J Trauma. 1999;47:96–103.

Cernak I, Wang Z, Jiang J, Bian X, Savic J. Ultrastructural and functional characteristics of blast injury-induced neurotrauma. J Trauma. 2001;50:695–706.

Cohan P, Wang C, McArthur DL, et al. Acute secondary adrenal insufficiency after traumatic brain injury: a prospective study. Crit Care Med. 2005;33:2358–66.

Correa R, Mena I, Sidney Z, et al. Neuro-functional and endocrine findings in patients with post-traumatic stress disorder. Alasbimn J. 2009; 11, Article No. AJ44 -1.

Crompton MR. Hypothalamic lesions following closed head injury. Brain. 1971;94:165–72.

Cuneo RC, Salomon F, McGauley GA, et al. The growth hormone deficiency syndrome in adults. Clin Endocrinol. 1992;37:387–97.

Cyran E. Hypophysenschädigung durch Schädelbasisfraktur. Dtsch Med Wschr. 1918;44:1261.

Daniel PM, Prichard MML, Treip CS. Traumatic infarction of the anterior lobe of the pituitary gland. Lancet. 1959;2:927–30.

Davidson JR, Stein DJ, Shalev AY, Yehuda R. Posttraumatic stress disorder: acquisition, recognition, course and treatment. J Neuropsychiatry Clin Neurosci. 2004;16: 135–47.

Defense Manpower Data Center. Global war on terrorism: casualties by reason. 2010. Retrieved on 22 Jan

2010 from http://siadapp.dmdc.osd.mil/personnel/CASUALTY/gwot_reason.pdf.

Deijen JB, De Boer H, Blok GJ, Van der Veen EA. Cognitive impairments and mood disturbances in growth hormone deficient men. Psychoneuroendocrinology. 1996;21:313–22.

Della Corte F, Mancini A, Valle D, et al. Provocative hypothalamopituitary axis tests in severe head injury: correlation with severity and prognosis. Crit Care Med. 1998;26:1419–26.

Dijkers MP. Quality of life after traumatic brain injury: a review of research approaches and findings. Arch Phys Med Rehabil. 2004;85:21–35.

Dikmen SS, Bombardier CH, Machamer JE, Fann JR, Temkin NR. Natural history of depression in traumatic brain injury. Arch Phys Med Rehabil. 2004;85:1457–64.

Dikmen SS, Ross BL, Machamer JE, Temkin NR. One year psychosocial outcome in head injury. J Int Neuropsychol Soc. 1995;1:67–77.

Dimopoulou I, Tsagarakis S, Theodorakopoulou M, et al. Endocrine abnormalities in critical care patients with moderate-to-severe head trauma: incidence, pattern and predisposing factors. Intensive Care Med. 2004;30:1051–7.

Edwards OM, Clark JD. Post-traumatic hypopituitarism. Six cases and a review of the literature. Medicine. 1986;65:281–90.

Escamilla RF, Lisser H. Simmonds' disease: a clinical study with review of the literature. J Clin Endocrinol. 1942;2:65–96.

Faust M, Wille J, Schumann C, et al. Unusual pattern of pituitary insufficiencies following traumatic brain injury evaluated by insulin tolerance test. Endocr Abstr. 2008;16:P433.

Galarneau MR, Woodruff SI, Dye JL, et al. Traumatic brain injury during Operation Iraqi Freedom: findings from the United States Navy-Marine Corps Combat Trauma Registry. J Neurosurg. 2008;108:950–7.

Ghigo E, Masel B, Aimaretti G, et al. Consensus guidelines on screening for hypopituitarism following traumatic brain injury. Brain Inj. 2005;19:711–24.

Guerrero AF, Alfonso A. Traumatic brain injury-related hypopituitarism: a review and recommendations for screening combat veterans. Mil Med. 2010;175:574–80.

Hackl JM, Gottardis M, Wieser C, et al. Endocrine abnormalities in severe traumatic brain injury—a cue to prognosis in severe craniocerebral trauma? Intensive Care Med. 1991;17:25–9.

Hellawell DJ, Taylor RT, Pentland B. Cognitive and psychosocial outcome following moderate or severe traumatic brain injury. Brain Inj. 1999;13:489–504.

Herrmann BL, Rahder J, Kahlke S, et al. Hypopituitarism following severe traumatic brain injury. Exp Clin Endocinol Diabetes. 2006;114:316–21.

Hiott DW, Labbate L. Anxiety disorders associated with traumatic brain injuries. NeuroRehabilitation. 2002;17:345–55.

Hofman PAM, Verhey FRJ, Wilmink JT, et al. Brain lesions in patients visiting a memory clinic with postconcussional sequelae after mild to moderate brain injury. J Neuropsychiatry Clin Neurosci. 2002;14:176–84.

Ivins BJ, Schwab K, Warden D, et al. Traumatic brain injury in U.S. Army paratroopers: prevalence and character. J Trauma. 2003;55:617–21.

Jorge RE, Starkstein S. Pathophysiologic aspects of major depression following traumatic brain injury. J Head Trauma Rehabil. 2005;20:475–87.

Kelly DF, Gaw Gonzalo IT, Cohan P, et al. Hypopituitarism following traumatic brain injury and aneurysmal subarachnoid hemorrhage: a preliminary report. J Neurosurg. 2000;93:743–52.

Kennedy JE, Jaffee MS, Leskin GA, et al. Posttraumatic stress disorder and posttraumatic stress disorder-like symptoms and mild traumatic brain injury. J Rehabil Res Dev. 2007;44:895–920.

Kim E, Lauterbach EC, Reeve A, Arciniegas DB, et al. Neuropsychiatric complications of traumatic brain injury: a critical review of the literature (a report by the ANPA Committee on Research). J Neuropsychiatry Clin Neurosci. 2007;19:106–27.

Kleindienst A, Brabant G, Bock C, et al. Neuroendocrine function following traumatic brain injury and subsequent intensive care treatment: a prospective longitudinal evaluation. J Neurotrauma. 2009;26:1–2.

Kleindienst A, Weigel D, Bock C, et al. A prospective longitudinal study of anterior pituitary dysfunction following traumatic brain injury. Endocr Abstr. 2007;13:P231.

Klose M, Feldt-Rasmussen U. Does the type and severity of brain injury predict hypothalamo-pituitary dysfunction? Does post-traumatic hypopituitarism predict worse outcome? Pituitary. 2008;11:255–61.

Klose M, Juul A, Struck J, et al. Acute and long-term pituitary insufficiency in traumatic brain injury: a prospective single-centre study. Clin Endocrinol. 2007;67:598–606.

Kokshoorn NE, Wassemaar MJ, Biermasz NR, et al. Hypopituitarism following traumatic brain injury: prevalence is affected by the use of different dynamic tests and different normal values. Eur J Endocrinol. 2010;162:11–8.

Kornblum RN, Fisher RS. Pituitary lesions in craniocerebral injuries. Arch Pathol. 1969;88:242–8.

Krahulik D, Zapletalova J, Frysak Z, Vaverka M. Dysfunction of hypothalamic-hypophysial axis after traumatic brain injury in adults. J Neurosurg. 2009. EPub ahead of print. http://www.ncbi.nlm.nih.gov/pubmed/19929195. Accessed 15 Jan 2010.

Kreitschmann-Andermahr I, Poll EM, Reineke A, et al. Growth hormone deficient patients after traumatic brain injury – baseline characteristics and benefits after growth hormone replacement. An analysis of the German KIMS database. Growth Horm IGF Res. 2008;18:472–8.

Kreutzer JS, Seel RT, Gourley E. The prevalence and symptom rates of depression after traumatic brain injury: a comprehensive examination. Brain Inj. 2001;15:561–2.

Leal-Cerro A, Flores JM, Rincon M, et al. Prevalence of hypopituitarism and growth hormone deficiency in adults long-term after severe traumatic brain injury. Clin Endocrinol. 2005;62:525–32.

Leon-Carrion J, Leal-Cerro A, Cabezas M, et al. Cognitive deterioration due to GH deficiency in patients with traumatic brain injury: a preliminary report. Brain Inj. 2007;21:871–5.

Lieberman SA, Oberoi AL, Gilkinson CR, et al. Prevalence of neuroendocrine dysfunction in patients recovering from traumatic brain injury. J Clin Endocrinol Metab. 2001;86:2752–6.

Ling G, Bandak F, Armonda R, et al. Explosive blast neurotrauma. J Neurotrauma. 2009;26:815–25.

Llompart-Pou JA, Raurich JM, Perez-Barcena J, et al. Acute hypothalamic-pituitary-adrenal response in traumatic brain injury with and without extracerebral trauma. Neurocrit Care. 2008;9:230–6.

Maruff P, Falleti M. Cognitive function in growth hormone deficiency and growth hormone replacement. Horm Res. 2005;64 Suppl 3:100–8.

Mayorga MA. The pathology of primary blast overpressure injury. Toxicology. 1997;121:17–28.

McFarlane AC, Atchison M, Yehuda R. The acute stress response following motor vehicle accidents and its relations to PTSD. Ann N Y Acad Sci. 1997;821: 437–41.

Monson JP. Long-term experience with GH replacement therapy: efficacy and safety. Eur J Endocrinol. 2003;148 Suppl 2:S9–14.

Morton MV, Wehman P. Psychosocial and emotional sequelae of individuals with traumatic brain injury: a literature review and recommendations. Brain Inj. 1995;9:81–92.

Mossberg KA, Masel BE, Gilkison CR, Urban RJ. Aerobic capacity and growth hormone deficiency after traumatic brain injury. J Clin Endocrinol Metab. 2008;93:2581–7.

Nampiaparampil DE. Prevalence of chronic pain after traumatic brain injury: a systematic review. J Am Med Assoc. 2008;300:711–9.

Okie S. Traumatic brain injury in the war zone. N Engl J Med. 2005;352:2043–7.

Ommaya AK, Salazar AM, Dannenberg AL, et al. Outcome after traumatic brain injury in the U.S. military medical system. J Trauma. 1996;41:972–5.

Pavlovic D, Pekic S, Stojanovic M, et al. Chronic cognitive sequelae after traumatic brain injury are not related to growth hormone deficiency in adults. Eur J Neurol. 2009. Epub ahead of print. http://www3.interscience.wiley.com/journal/123228501/abstract. Accessed 20 Jan 2010.

Ponsford J, Willmott C, Rothwell A, et al. Factors influencing outcome following mild traumatic brain injury in adults. J Int Neuropsychol Soc. 2000;6: 568–79.

Popovic V, Oekic C, Oavlovic D, et al. Hypopituitarism as a consequence of traumatic brain injury (TBI) and its possible relation with cognitive disabilities and mental distress. J Endocrinol Invest. 2004;27:1048–54.

Popovic V, Aimaretti G, Casanueva FF, Ghigo E. Hypopituitarism following traumatic brain injury (TBI): call for attention. J Endocrinol Invest. 2005;28: 61–4.

Powner DJ, Boccalandro C. Adrenal insufficiency following traumatic brain injury in adults. Curr Opin Crit Care. 2008;14:163–6.

Powner DJ, Boccalandro C, Alp MS, Vollmer DG. Endocrine failure after traumatic brain injury in adults. Neurocrit Care. 2006;5:61–70.

Prabhakar VKB, Shalet SM. Aetiology, diagnosis, and management of hypopituitarism in adult life. Postgrad Med J. 2006;82:259–66.

Rao V, Lyketsos C. Neuropsychiatric sequelae of traumatic brain injury. Psychosomatics. 2000;41: 95–103.

Raverot G, et al. Preliminary results of French collaborative evaluation (DEPHY-TC) in patients with suspected pituitary abnormalities after traumatic brain injury and subarachnoid hemorrhage. ENDO 2009, abstract. 2009. P3-625.

Riggio S, Wong M. Neurobehavioral sequelae of traumatic brain injury. Mt Sinai J Med. 2009;76:163–72.

Rosen T, Wiren L, Wilhelmsen L, et al. Decreased psychological well-being in adult patients with growth hormone deficiency. Clin Endocrinol. 1994;40:111–6.

Rothman MS, Arciniegas DB, Filley CM, et al. The neuroendocrine effects of traumatic brain injury. J Neuropsychiatry Clin Neurosci. 2007;19:363–72.

Ruokonen E, Takala J. Dangers of growth hormone therapy in critically ill patients. Curr Opin Clin Nutr Metab Care. 2002;5:199–209.

Rutland-Brown W, Langlois JA, Thomas KE, Yongli L. Incidence of traumatic brain injury in the United States, 2003. J Head Trauma Rehabil. 2006;21:544–8.

Ryan LM, Warden DL. Post concussion syndrome. Int Rev Psychiatry. 2003;15:310–6.

Schneider HJ, Kreitschmann-Andermahr I, Ghigo E, et al. Hypothalamopituitary dysfunction following traumatic brain injury and aneurismal subarachnoid hemorrhage: a systematic review. JAMA. 2007;298: 1429–38.

Schneider HJ, Schneider M, Saller B, et al. Prevalence of anterior pituitary insufficiency 3 and 12 months after traumatic brain injury. Eur J Endocrinol. 2006;154: 259–65.

Schneider HJ, Schneider M, Tuschy U, et al. Structured assessment of neuroendocrine dysfunction following traumatic brain injury and aneurysmal subarachnoid hemorrhage in 921 patients: the German Interdisciplinary Database. Endocr Abstr. 2008a;16:OC1.1.

Schneider M, Schneider HJ, Stalla GK. Anterior pituitary hormone abnormalities following traumatic brain injury. J Neurotrauma. 2005;22:937–46.

Schneider M, Schneider HJ, Yassouridis A, et al. Predictors of anterior pituitary insufficiency after traumatic brain injury. Clin Endocrinol. 2008b;68:206–12.

Sesmilo G, Halperin I, Puig-Domingo M. Endocrine evaluation of patients after brain injury: what else is needed to define specific clinical recommendations? Hormones. 2007;6:132–7.

Stein MB, McAllister TW. Exploring the convergence of posttraumatic stress disorder and mild traumatic brain injury. Am J Psychiatry. 2009. EPub ahead of print. http://ajp.psychiatryonline.org/cgi/content/abstract/appi.ajp.2009.08101604v1. Accessed 13 Jan 2010.

Stojanovic M, Pekic S, Pavlovic D, et al. The effects of growth hormone deficiency following moderate and severe traumatic brain injury on cognitive functions. Endocr Abstr. 2008;16:P396.

Taber KH, Warden DL, Hurley RA. Blast-related traumatic brain injury: what is known? J Neuropsychiatry Clin Neurosci. 2006;18:141–5.

Takala J, Ruokonen E, Webster NR, et al. Increased mortality associated with growth hormone treatment in critically ill adults. N Engl J Med. 1999;341: 785–92.

Tanriverdi F, DeBellis A, Bizzarro A, et al. Antipituitary antibodies after traumatic brain injury: is head trauma-induced pituitary dysfunction associated with autoimmunity? Eur J Endocrinol. 2008;159:7–13.

Tanriverdi F, Senyurek H, Unluhizarci K, et al. High risk of hypopituitarism after traumatic brain injury: a prospective investigation of anterior pituitary function in the acute phase and 12 months after trauma. J Clin Endocrinol Metab. 2006;91:2105–11.

Tanriverdi F, Unluhizarci K, Kelestimur F. Pituitary function in subjects with mild traumatic brain injury: a review of literature and proposal of a screening strategy. Pituitary. 2010;13:146–53.

Tanriverdi F, Ulutabanca H, Unluhizarci K, et al. Pituitary functions in the acute phase of traumatic brain injury: are they related to severity of the injury or mortality? Brain Inj. 2007a;21:433–9.

Tanriverdi F, Ulutabanca H, Unluhizarci K, et al. Three years prospective investigation of anterior pituitary function after traumatic brain injury: a pilot study. Clin Endocrinol. 2007b. 1–7.

Terrio H, Brenner LA, Ivins BJ, et al. Traumatic brain injury screening: preliminary findings in a U.S. Army Brigade Combat Team. J Head Trauma Rehabil. 2009;24:14–23.

Thompson C. Traumatic brain injury-induced hypopituitarism: whom and when to test. Endocr Abstr. 2007; 14:S1.1.

Thurman DJ, Alverson C, Dunn KA, et al. Traumatic brain injury in the United States: a public health perspective. J Head Trauma Rehabil. 1999;14:602–15.

Trudeau DL, Anderson J, Hansen LM, et al. Findings of mild traumatic brain injury in combat veterans with PTSD and a history of blast concussion. J Neuropsychiatry Clin Neurosci. 1998;10:308–13.

Tsagarakis S, Tzanela M, Dimopoulou I. Diabetes insipidus, secondary hypoadrenalism and hypothyroidism after traumatic brain injury: clinical implications. Pituitary. 2005;8:251–4.

Urban RJ, Harris P, Masel B. Anterior hypopituitarism following traumatic brain injury. Brain Inj. 2005;19: 349–58.

van Den Berghe G. Novel insights into the neuroendocrinology of critical illness. Eur J Endocrinol. 2000;143: 1–13.

van der Eerden A, Twicker M, Sweep F, et al. Should anterior pituitary function be tested during follow-up of all patients presenting at the emergency department because of traumatic brain injury? Eur J Endocrinol. 2010;162:19.

Vanderploeg RD, Curtiss G, Belanger HG. Long-term neuropsychological outcomes following mild traumatic brain injury. J Int Neuropsychol Soc. 2005; 11:228–36.

Wachter D, Gundling K, Oertel MF, et al. Pituitary insufficiency after traumatic brain injury. J Clin Neurosci. 2009;16:202–8.

Warden D. Military TBI during the Iraq and Afghanistan wars. J Head Trauma Rehabil. 2006;21:398–402.

Yollin E, Kozlowski O, Fontaine P, et al. Effects of 6 months growth hormone treatment in GH deficient patients (GHD) long after traumatic brain injury (TBI). Endocr Abstr. 2008;16:P403.

Yollin E, Kozlowski O, Soudan B, et al. Is there an endocrine explanation for persistent neuropsychological disabilities long after traumatic brain injury (TBI)? Endocr Abstr. 2007;14:P545.

Yuan X-Q, Wade CE. Neuroendocrine abnormalities in patients with traumatic brain injury. Front Neuroendocrinol. 1991;12:209–30.

12 Confronting Mild TBI and Co-occurring Post-traumatic Stress Disorder Symptoms in Combat Deployed Service Members

Justin S. Campbell, Jeffrey H. Greenberg, and Jennifer M. Weil

Abstract

Traumatic Brain Injury (TBI) and Post-traumatic Stress Disorder (post-traumatic stress disorder) have been called the signature injuries of the wars in Iraq and Afghanistan. While post-traumatic stress disorder is frequently associated with exposure to traumatic events such as combat, surviving head injuries is a novel phenomenon likely associated with improved protective headgear, adept field medical attention, and the ability to expeditiously evacuate injured persons to upper echelon care facilities as indicated. Frequently, disorders (psychological and physical) are viewed discretely in spite of a mounting evidence base that suggests that these and similar injuries tend to co-occur. This chapter explores TBI and post-traumatic stress disorder in a historical context, identifies available assessment and treatment modalities, highlights a global approach to case conceptualization, and suggests research lines to address the key questions about developing simultaneous assessment and treatment models for the co-occurrence of TBI and post-traumatic stress disorder as well as other potentially confounding injuries.

Keywords

Traumatic brain injury • Post-traumatic stress disorder • Co-occurring disorders • Military health care • Veteran's health care • Assessment • Treatment • Case conceptualization

Introduction

To date, many thousands of service members have been deployed to Iraq and Afghanistan—Operation Iraqi Freedom (OIF) and Operation Enduring Freedom (OEF). These conflicts have placed military personnel at high risk for experiencing traumatic events that may affect coping capacities as well as injuries by blasts, vehicle crashes, and other war-related dangers. Epidemiological studies

J.S. Campbell, Ph.D.
U.S. Navy Space and Naval Warfare Systems Pacific, San Diego, CA, USA

J.H. Greenberg, Ph.D. (✉)
Altarum Institute, Washington, DC, USA
e-mail: Jgreenberg16@hotmail.com

J.M. Weil, Ph.D.
Deployment Health Clinical Center, Defense Centers of Excellence for Psychological Health and Traumatic Brain Injury, Arlington, VA, USA

J.W. Tsao (ed.), *Traumatic Brain Injury: A Clinician's Guide to Diagnosis, Management, and Rehabilitation*,
DOI 10.1007/978-0-387-87887-4_12,

examining the incidence of post-traumatic stress disorder (post-traumatic stress disorder) and traumatic brain injury (TBI) among service members have suggested high rates of both psychological and medical conditions as compared to civilian populations (Hoge et al. 2004). Yet, few studies have examined the prevalence of post-traumatic stress disorder co-occurring with TBI, and many scientists and clinicians argue whether or not a person who has experienced impaired consciousness associated with a mild TBI (mTBI), otherwise termed "concussion," can develop post-traumatic stress disorder (Bryant 2001). Given that effective treatments are predicated on understanding the mechanisms and experiential processes that mediate a disorder, it is vital to disentangle the relationship between these conditions. The current chapter reviews the evidence of post-traumatic stress disorder and TBI among service member populations, discusses the potential that these two conditions may co-occur, presents valid and reliable screening/assessment tools that mental health professionals can use to assess post-traumatic stress disorder and TBI, highlights the latest empirical treatments for both disorders, and provides recommendations for future directions in understanding the interaction between post-traumatic stress disorder and TBI.

Diagnostic Definitions

What Is post-traumatic stress disorder?

post-traumatic stress disorder is a clinical disorder that may result after a person experiences a traumatic event. According to the Diagnostic and Statistical Manual-Fourth Edition-Text Revised (DSM-IV-TR) American Psychiatric Association (APA, 1994), a person may be diagnosed with post-traumatic stress disorder if the following five criterion sets are met. First, the individual must have experienced a real or imaged event that is physically threatening to himself or herself or others and invokes intense fear, helplessness, or horror. Second, the person reports symptoms related to reexperiencing the traumatic event, such as disturbing memories, thoughts, and/or nightmares. These reexperiencing symptoms are often triggered by reminders (e.g., watching the news, being in a crowd, attending a memorial service). Third, the person actively attempts to avoid thoughts, feelings, and/or reminders of the trauma. Avoidance attempts may include isolating self from social support and social activities or using maladaptive coping strategies to manage feelings of anxiety, such as substance abuse. Fourth, the person describes symptoms of hyperarousal such as sleep disturbances (e.g., initial insomnia, frequent waking throughout the night, and early morning rising), hypervigilance (e.g., excessive and unnecessary guarding or watchful behavior), and exaggerated startle response (feeling jumpy when hearing a sound or other reminder of the event). Finally, a person reports that these symptoms have persisted for at least 1 month post exposure to the traumatic event. Persons diagnosed with post-traumatic stress disorder experience impairment in social, occupational, or other areas of functioning. Impairment for less than 3 months is considered acute, whereas symptoms that last longer than 3 months are considered chronic (APA 1994). post-traumatic stress disorder can have a "delayed onset" which is defined as at least 6 months post stress exposure. Prior to 1 month of symptoms, individuals who meet criteria for post-traumatic stress disorder may be diagnosed with Acute Stress Disorder (ASD). If symptoms are present after 1 month, the diagnosis is changed to post-traumatic stress disorder. Table 12.1 summarizes symptoms for criterions B–D.

What Is TBI?

The Defense and Veterans Brain Injury Center (DVBIC) defines a TBI as a blow or a jolt to the head or a penetrating head injury that disrupts the function of the brain. Not all blows or jolts to the head result in a TBI. The severity of such an injury may range from "mild"—a brief change in mental status with or without loss of consciousness (LOC)—to "severe," an extended period of unconsciousness or amnesia after the injury. The terms "concussion" and "mild TBI" are interchangeable

Table 12.1 Criterion B–D symptoms for post-traumatic stress disorder from the DSM-IV-TR

Criterion	Symptoms	# of symptoms required for diagnosis
B (Reexperiencing symptoms)	1. Recurrent and intrusive recollections of the event including images, thoughts, or perceptions 2. Recurrent distressing dreams of the event 3. Acting or feeling as if the traumatic event were recurring 4. Intense psychological distress at exposure to internal or external cues that symbolize or resemble an aspect of the traumatic event 5. Physiological reactivity on exposure to internal or external cues that symbolize or resemble an aspect of the traumatic event	One or more
C (Avoidance symptoms)	1. Efforts to avoid thoughts, feelings, or conversations associated with the trauma 2. Efforts to avoid activities, places, or people that arouse recollections of the trauma 3. Inability to recall an important aspect of the trauma 4. Markedly diminished interest or participation in significant activities 5. Feeling of detachment or estrangement from others 6. Restricted range of affect 7. Sense of foreshortened future	Three or more
D (Hypervigilance symptoms)	1. Difficulty falling or staying asleep 2. Irritability or outbursts of anger 3. Difficulty concentrating 4. Hypervigilance 5. Exaggerated startle response	Two or more

Table 12.2 Symptoms of TBI

TBI category	Associated symptoms
Mild	• May remain conscious or may experience a loss of consciousness for a few seconds or minutes • Headache • Confusion • Lightheadedness • Dizziness • Blurred vision or tired eyes • Ringing in the ears • Bad taste in the mouth • Fatigue or lethargy • Change in sleep patterns • Behavioral or mood changes • Trouble with memory, concentration, attention, or thinking
Moderate/severe	• Same symptoms as above • Headache that gets worse or does not go away • Repeated vomiting or nausea • Convulsions or seizures • An inability to awaken from sleep • Dilation of one or both pupils of the eyes • Slurred speech • Weakness or numbness in the extremities • Loss of coordination • Increased confusion, restlessness, or agitation

(DVBIC 2010). Symptoms of a TBI are typically categorized as mild, moderate, severe, or penetrating, depending on the severity of symptoms. Table 12.2 provides symptom descriptions used when diagnosing TBI.

Are post-traumatic stress disorder and TBI Similar?

The nosology for post-traumatic stress disorder and TBI overlaps in the areas of sleep disturbance, behavior and mood changes, and problems with concentration, attention, memories, and thinking. Even more challenging from a diagnostic perspective is that many of the symptoms of TBI may yield maladaptive avoidance behaviors, such as strategies to avoid activities, places, and individuals. These avoidance behaviors are common for individuals meeting post-traumatic stress disorder diagnostic criteria.

Prevalence Estimates

Post-traumatic Stress Disorder

Data from the National Comorbidity Study-Replication, an epidemiological study examining lifetime prevalence of various psychiatric disorders among the US population, indicated that 3% of study participants met the criteria for post-traumatic stress disorder during the past year (Kessler et al. 2005a), whereas 8.7% of study participants met the criteria for post-traumatic stress disorder during their lifetime (Kessler et al. 2005b).

Epidemiological data examining service members' pre-deployment have suggested that rates of post-traumatic stress disorder are similar (5%) to those of civilian populations (Hoge et al. 2004). However, when examining service members at post-deployment, data has indicated that post-traumatic stress disorder is common, with approximately 9–12% of OIF and 5–6% OEF meeting the diagnostic criteria. This includes data from the Millennium Cohort Study, a large sample study of deployed combat veterans (Hoge et al. 2004; Hoge et al. 2006; Smith et al. 2008). Other studies support these findings (Vasterling et al. 2006; Adamson et al. 2008) and report data that many deployed service members are experiencing symptoms of post-traumatic stress disorder.

Limitations to the latter prevalence estimates for OIF/OEF populations should be noted, including that these data are based on self-report surveys (screening instruments) rather than clinical assessment tools to diagnose post-traumatic stress disorder. Despite these limitations, the base rate for post-traumatic stress disorder among deployed military service members exceeds the rates of both non-deployed service members and civilian populations and warrants the need for appropriate screening, assessment, and effective treatment for this population.

Traumatic Brain Injury

Approximately 5.8 million people (3%) in the general US population suffer with chronic disability due to head injury (Kim et al. 2007). The Centers for Disease Control (CDC) and prevention reports that 1.7 million people are treated and released with a TBI, 27,500 are hospitalized, and 52,000 individuals die annually from TBI (CDC 2010). While these numbers are daunting, they likely represent an underrepresentation of the number of individuals who experience a TBI annually as many people who suffer a head injury never seek medical care. In the civilian population, the leading causes are falls (28%), motor vehicle accidents (20%), struck by or against events (19%), and assaults (11%) (CDC 2010). In combat situations, TBI is typically associated with improvised explosive devices (IEDs) and other forms of blast exposure and may be caused by penetrating foreign objects and rapid acceleration/deceleration of the brain within the skull, all of which can result in brain contusions involving shearing and tearing of nerve fibers (DVBIC 2010). Additionally, overpressurization in the brain due to close proximity blast waves emanating from IED and rocket/mortar explosions are thought to produce harmful biochemical alterations in the brain (Kennedy et al. 2007) and diffuse injury to connective, integrative white matter tracts (Stein and McAllister 2009).

The majority of combat duty in OIF and OEF has been sustained by the US Army and Marine Corps personnel. Therefore, it can be hypothesized that these service members may have the highest incidence of TBI in the military. In a large cross-sectional survey of the US Army Soldiers (N=2,525) examining the prevalence of mTBI, data revealed that approximately 15% of soldiers met the mTBI criteria (Hoge et al. 2008). mTBI was defined as an affirmative response to any one of the three questions indicating LOC or being "knocked out," "being dazed, confused, or seeing stars," or "not remembering the injury." Findings also revealed that soldiers with mTBI experienced more intense combat, and blast injury (singular as well as multiple exposures), and were more likely to be hospitalized for their injuries than soldiers who did not sustain a head injury (Hoge et al. 2008). Findings from other studies are consistent, suggesting that estimates for mTBI range from 7 to 30% (Schneiderman et al. 2008; Ramchand et al. 2008; Kennedy et al. 2007; Vasterling et al. 2006). These rates exceed the rates for post-traumatic stress disorder, suggesting that brain injuries do not always result in post-traumatic stress disorder.

Co-occurring post-traumatic stress disorder and TBI

Some scientists argue that it is unlikely for individuals to develop post-traumatic stress disorder if a head injury is sustained. Why? There is a theoretical premise which asserts that post-traumatic stress disorder symptoms are a fear-conditioned memory of the traumatic event (Resick 2001). Consequently, if a person sustains a head injury that results in an LOC, the ability to encode memories should be disrupted and thus the person is incapable of forming a fear-conditioned memory (Sbordone and Liter 1995). Throughout the past decade, research has challenged this perspective, suggesting that a person may have both post-traumatic stress disorder and TBI (Bryant 2001).

Bryant and Harvey conducted a series of studies investigating the relationship between post-traumatic stress disorder and TBI (Bryant and Harvey 1998; Harvey and Bryant 2000; see also Bryant 2001; Harvey et al. 2003) among civilian populations. For example, in a study examining 79 automobile accident victims who were admitted to a trauma hospital during a 10-month period, 13.9% met the criteria for post-traumatic stress disorder at 1 month after sustaining the trauma and 24% met the criteria for post-traumatic stress disorder at 6 months (Bryant and Harvey 1998). Even more disturbing, at 2 years post assessment, 22% of the 79 participants met the criteria for post-traumatic stress disorder (Harvey and Bryant 2000). In another study, conducted by Bombardier et al. (2006) evaluating post-traumatic stress disorder in 125 patients from a trauma hospital who sustained definite TBI (excluding uncomplicated mTBI as well as several other medical-social history factors that might complicate diagnosis), 11.3% met the criteria for post-traumatic stress disorder at 6 months following the trauma. The most common sources of trauma in this sample were motor vehicle accident (49%), falls (32%), assault (7%), and others (12%). In contrast, Glasser et al. (2004) investigated post-traumatic stress disorder in 46 patients with TBI in a neurological rehabilitation clinic. Patients who maintained consciousness (n=15) were compared to patients who lost consciousness (n=31) during the trauma. Individuals who lost consciousness were less likely to develop post-traumatic stress disorder (3.2%) than those who retained consciousness (26.7%).

Research among military populations has suggested that post-traumatic stress disorder commonly co-occurs with TBI (Hoge et al., 2008). For example, in a study by Hoge et al. (2008), examining 2,525 US Army infantry soldiers 3–4 months after returning from deployment, post-deployment rates of post-traumatic stress disorder were highest for those with mTBI with associated LOC (range: 4.3–43.9%), followed by mTBI with altered mental status (range: 10.7–27.3%). Those with non-TBI-related injuries had a 16.2% post-traumatic stress disorder prevalence. For those in the sample with no injuries,

9.1% screened positive for post-traumatic stress disorder. LOC rivaled even combat exposure in a hierarchical logistic regression model predicting post-traumatic stress disorder with numerous risk variables. Additional multivariate modeling found that an LOC was a significant predictor, but mediated by post-traumatic stress disorder and depression (no longer significant when those variables were entered into the model). This last finding suggests that mTBI is most correlated to poor deployment health outcomes when co-occurring with post-traumatic stress disorder and depression. In contrast, data from the Adamson et al. (2008) national phone survey of 1,965 soldiers post deployment (Schell and Marshall 2008) reported a weighted percentage of comorbidity at just 1%, despite finding that 13.8% of the sample screened positive for probable post-traumatic stress disorder and 19.5% screened positive for probable TBI. Limitations to these studies and the vast differences in estimates include the various methodologies applied to determine TBI status and severity, as well as a reliance upon self-reports rather than clinician-confirmed examinations. It is also important to consider that exposure to combat experiences that increase the risk for blast exposure varies greatly by service and type of occupational specialty of service members deployed to OIF/OEF assignments. For instance, combat maneuver units such as those surveyed by Hoge et al. (2008) are more likely to patrol "outside the wire" and come into contact with IEDs and rocket attacks compared to service members assessed in broad population surveys (Schell and Marshall 2008; Schneiderman et al. 2008).

Despite the diversity of methods employed in the study of co-occurring post-traumatic stress disorder and TBI and estimates of prevalence, all of these studies suggest that it is possible for an individual to present with concurrent symptoms of post-traumatic stress disorder and TBI. Bryant (2001) posits four possible explanations. First, despite an LOC for the TBI event itself, the pain, anxiety, and suffering surrounding the event may form the genesis of a traumatic memory. Second, when it is impossible to create conscious declarative memories for a TBI event, unconsciously coded implicit memories for the event may still result in traumatic memories despite impaired consciousness. Third, individuals may modify or create memories of otherwise fragmented TBI-related experiences. Lastly, neurological trauma associated with TBI may also interact with the neurological systems that mediate the expression of post-traumatic stress disorder.

Bryant's potential explanations for post-traumatic stress disorder/TBI comorbidity are plausible for military populations; however, it should be noted that in civilian populations the co-occurrence of post-traumatic stress disorder and TBI is more likely to result from a single incident, such as an automobile accident or an assault (Langlois et al. 2006), whereas in combat-deployed military personnel, there may be numerous traumatic incidents over the course of a deployment which both meet the criterion A for post-traumatic stress disorder and result in LOC (Kennedy et al. 2007). Service members who present with co-occurring post-traumatic stress disorder and TBI symptoms likely represent a complex patient history involving multiple exposures to traumatic experiences or repeat stressors and injuries over the course of several months and multiple combat deployments.

Clinical Management

Post-traumatic Stress Disorder

The APA (APA 2004) recommends that individuals at risk for post-traumatic stress disorder should be screened for recent/remote trauma exposure and for those individuals who are positive a diagnostic assessment should be conducted. Diagnostic assessment should include a complete evaluation that assesses the symptoms of post-traumatic stress disorder, including dissociative, reexperiencing, avoidance/numbing, and hyperarousal symptom clusters and their temporal sequence relative to the trauma (i.e., before versus after 1 month from the traumatic event). The guidelines for persons diagnosed with post-traumatic stress disorder suggest that interventions and activities that ensure physical and psychological safety, required medical care, and self-care resources should and made available. Examples of psychiatric management goals which are consistent with the APA guidelines include establishing a therapeutic alliance, ongoing assessment of safety and psychiatric status, ongoing assessment of comorbid disorders and treatment response, and increasing the patient's capacity to cope with the psychosocial effects of trauma. The practice guideline also identifies effective treatments for the symptoms of post-traumatic stress disorder, such as psychopharmacology, psychotherapy, psychoeducation, and other supportive measures. Combinations of these treatment approaches may offer benefits; however, it should be noted that research related to treatment combinations is not currently available. Subsequent sections of this chapter highlight screening, assessment, and treatment tools that are widely used with combat-related post-traumatic stress disorder populations and are consistent with the APA treatment guidelines.

Screening and Assessment for Military Populations

Several valid and reliable screening and assessment instruments have been tested with military populations. These instruments are described below and are frequently used in both research and clinical settings.

Screening Tools: post-traumatic stress disorder Checklist

The post-traumatic stress disorder checklist (PCL) which is frequently used in epidemiological research to examine trends and rates of post-traumatic stress disorder is available in three versions: civilian, military, and trauma specific. The PCL is a 17-item self-report measure that assesses each of the 17 post-traumatic stress disorder symptoms. Using a 5-item Likert scale, the PCL asks individuals to estimate symptom severity. Scoring criteria for the 17-item screener is based upon a 1–5 point criteria with a score of 1 representing "not at all" and a score of 5 representing "extremely." The cutoff score for this instrument is 50. Numerous studies have indicated that the PCL is a valid and reliable screening instrument (Ruggierro et al. 2003; Lang et al. 2003).

Primary Care post-traumatic stress disorder Screener

This four-item screen (Prins and Ouimette 2004) has been studied in Veterans Affairs hospital general medical clinic patients, and appears to have strong sensitivity (0.78) and specificity (0.87) at the optimal cutoff score of 3 versus the Clinician-Administered post-traumatic stress disorder Scale (CAPS—see description below). This self-report screening tool uses yes/no response options with scores ranging from 0 (all questions marked "no") to 4 (all questions marked "yes").

Mississippi Scale for Combat-Related post-traumatic stress disorder

This 35-item self-report measure assesses post-traumatic stress disorder symptoms as well as associated features (i.e., substance abuse, suicidality, depression). Using a 5-point Likert scale, individuals are asked to identify symptom severity. Scores can range from 35 to 175 (Keane et al. 1988 Feb).

The post-traumatic stress disorder scales discussed above are brief, easy to use, administer, and score. Although these screening tools should not be substituted for a thorough clinical interview, providers treating large numbers of service members at risk for an exposure to a traumatic event may find these tools useful in situations of limited time and/or resources. For patients that screen positive for post-traumatic stress disorder, follow-up assessment tools should be used to determine if the patient meets diagnostic criteria. Two assessments frequently used for military populations are described below.

Assessment Tools: CAPS

The CAPS is the gold standard post-traumatic stress disorder structured clinical interview. This 30-item assessment measure corresponds to the DSM-IV criteria for post-traumatic stress disorder and is used to make current (past month) or lifetime diagnosis of post-traumatic stress disorder. Items assess the 17 symptoms of post-traumatic stress disorder, the impact of symptoms on social and occupational functioning, and the improvement in symptoms since previous administrations. The CAPS should be administered by trained clinicians, researchers, or paraprofessionals. A symptom is counted as present if it has a frequency of 1 and severity of 2 (Blake et al. 1995).

The Keane post-traumatic stress disorder Scale

Used by clinicians and researchers, the Keane post-traumatic stress disorder scale which is derived from the Minnesota Multiphasic Personality Inventory-2 (MMPI-2) has been found to be a useful indicator of post-traumatic stress disorder (Lyons and Keane 1992). This 46-item scale uses the same norms based on the MMPI-2 standardization of 1,138 males and 1,462 females sampled from the general population. A useful feature of the Keane post-traumatic stress disorder scale is that it may be difficult for a patient to fake "bad" due to the difficulty in identifying specific items on this scale from the hundreds of items on the lengthy MMPI-2. Further, the MMPI-2 contains validity scales explicitly designed to detect invalid responding.

post-traumatic stress disorder Treatment Models

Several treatment models have been studied and found to be effective with military populations. The following sections describe these models.

1. *Exposure and behavioral therapy.* In a large-scale review of randomized, controlled trials for the treatment of post-traumatic stress disorder, the National Academies of Science (2007) concluded that the only therapeutic modality with sufficient evidence to warrant a recommendation was exposure therapy. This is based upon the principles of Classical Conditioning (Pavlov 1927) which asserts that a person who is exposed to stimuli that, through biologically and/or cognitive pairing with life-threatening situations, will develop conditioned fear and startle responses. The goal of exposure treatments is to facilitate habituation when stimuli are present through the use of safe and supportive environments. Habituation in the presence of conditioned stimuli will ultimately decrease fear or startle responses. Exposure as a treatment can be applied either gradually or rapidly (i.e., a technique known as flooding [Foa and Chambless 1978]) to help patients habituate to their traumatic experiences. Prolonged Exposure (PE) therapy for post-traumatic stress disorder consists of nine to twelve 90-min sessions that include psychoeducation, imaginal exposure (i.e., a detailed recounting of the trauma that should elicit affective responses), and in vivo exposure (i.e., continual and progressive first-hand exposure to stimuli that elicit affective response) (Foa et al. 2007). For those treating combat-related post-traumatic stress disorder, exposure therapy may emphasize habituation to reminders of the trauma rather than actual traumatic events themselves, hence the recent application of modalities such as virtual reality (Reger and Gahm 2008). A key goal of PE is the reduction of the patient's avoidant behaviors in the face of feared situations and stimuli, a critical step towards reducing relative distress surrounding traumatic experiences and helping patients to return to full functioning (Foa and Kozak 1986).
2. *Cognitive processing therapy (CPT).* CPT, originally developed for female sexual assault survivors, has been frequently applied to veteran populations. The CPT model uses an exposure approach that directs the patient to write about the traumatic event. These narratives are generally fraught with "stuck points." Stuck points are cognitive distortions (inaccurate beliefs or thoughts) that impact the patient's perception of the trauma, thereby facilitating continued avoidance, distress, and affective arousal when exposed to cues associated with the trauma. The goal of CPT is not to eliminate cognitions of the trauma, but rather to teach the patient how to live *with* the trauma. Living with the trauma could mean learning to trust when appropriate, openly grieving a loss, or understanding that justice is an ideal rather than a guarantee. Narrative writing should continue as long as stuck points or inaccuracies persist. Patient encounters require that the patients repeatedly read aloud their accounts of the trauma to facilitate habituation to the traumatic event. To evaluate progress, the PCL or another symptom-driven

screen/assessment should be repeatedly administered. Initially, the patients should show evidence of elevated PCL scores due to distress experienced while encountering the traumatic event; however, with time and continual exposure, PCL scores should decrease to subthreshold clinical levels along with the distress associated with reliving the trauma. At the conclusion of treatment, patients should (a) be able to grieve accurately, (b) assign responsibility, (c) understand that they were unable to control the trauma from happening, (d) accept that they must live with the trauma rather than perseverating on the cognition that wishes the trauma had never happened, and (e) concurrently experience significantly decreased distress and an ability to reengage in their lives despite the occurrence of the trauma(s).

3. *Cognitive behavioral therapy (CBT).* At the theoretical core of CBT therapies is the classic Beck model of Cognitive Therapy. Beck's model was originally designed to address depression (1979) and emphasizes the relationship among cognition, emotions, and behaviors. Specifically, cognitive-based models help the patient identify erroneous thoughts and belief systems that cause distress in individuals and are intricately associated with feelings and patterns of behavior. Since the model's genesis, CBT has been used for many psychiatric disorders including post-traumatic stress disorder and substance abuse. Clinicians working with military populations may have challenges using a CBT approach, particularly for post-traumatic stress disorder. For example, military populations are trained to be "on guard," and watch for potential signs of danger in the environment. This hypervigilance is protective in a combat situation, yet in a civilian situation this same thought processing and behavioral response may be interpersonally inhibiting and socially problematic. For persons who may be redeployed to combat, challenging these thoughts may be unrealistic as hypervigilance is often a necessary attribute in the combat zone.

4. *Psychopharmacology for post-traumatic stress disorder.* Psycho-pharmacological approaches to the treatment of post-traumatic stress disorder are another treatment used in the management of post-traumatic stress disorder symptoms. Despite research to support the use of psychopharmacological treatments, it should be noted that neither the National Academies of Science report or the APA practice guideline (1994) endorses any one particular psychopharmacological approach for the treatment of post-traumatic stress disorder. Typically, selective serotonin reuptake inhibitors (SSRIs) such as Prozac (Fluoxetine) are used as a first line of treatment for patients meeting the diagnostic criteria for post-traumatic stress disorder (Davidson et al. 1991; Lineberry et al. 2006). Other psychopharmacological treatments used to treat post-traumatic stress disorder are tricyclic antidepressants, monoamine oxidase inhibitors (MAOIs), the neurological agent carbamazepine, beta blockers, clonidine, and lithium and benzodiazepines such as valium or klonopin (Davidson et al. 1991).

   Aside from symptom management, the drug propanalol, a beta adrenergic blocker, has been studied to determine its impact in blocking the encoding of traumatic memories that are thought by some to be a primary causal agent of post-traumatic stress disorder (Pitman et al. 2002). Additionally, GABA agonist hypnotics such as Ambien (Zolpidem) are being studied to determine their impact in reducing many of the sleep-related problems associated with post-traumatic stress disorder (Bobo et al. 2007).

   Other pharmacological options that may be used to address post-traumatic stress disorder-associated sleep problems, atypical antipsychotics such as Abilify (Aripiprazol), Zyprexa (Olanzapine), Seroquel (Quetiapine), and Risperdal (Risperidone), may help impact and improve sleep function (Lineberry et al. 2006). The alpha-1 adrenergic antagonist Prazosin, typically prescribed for hypertension, has recently received a great deal of attention because of studies linking it with reduced nightmares in veterans suffering from post-traumatic stress disorder (Peskind et al. 2003; Maher et al. 2006; Raskind et al. 2006).

5. *Emerging psychotherapeutic approaches.* While not yet extensively studied for treatment

of post-traumatic stress disorder, Hayes et al.'s Acceptance and Commitment Therapy (ACT) may be a promising intervention. In contrast to CBT, the ACT model helps patients to identify and work towards goals, rather than focusing on modifying thoughts, feelings, and behaviors (Hayes et al. 1999). In this model, the patient is able to reduce avoidance behaviors and increase value-based living. The five principles of ACT are as follows:

1. Develop an understanding that trying to avoid emotional pain will not work. Pain and distress are normal parts of life.
2. Understand that trying to control the problem is itself a source of distress.
3. Develop the ability to separate one's self from one's thoughts.
4. Stop the struggle with one's own thoughts.
5. Commit to action.

Aside from ACT, a growing movement within the field of post-traumatic stress disorder therapy is the use of integrative medical treatments, an approach known collectively as complementary and alternative medicine (CAM). Of the CAM approaches, acupuncture is receiving some attention as a promising approach for post-traumatic stress disorder. For example, in a randomized, controlled study conducted by Holifield et al. (2007), findings suggested that patients receiving acupuncture in conjunction with CBT showed a substantial reduction in post-traumatic stress disorder symptoms compared to participants who received CBT alone and a wait-list control group. Other CAM modalities being studied for the treatment of post-traumatic stress disorder include exercise therapy, massage therapy, relaxation and mindfulness techniques, and yoga. These modalities teach skills that can be readily incorporated into a healthy lifestyle, and, most importantly, appear to have little risk of doing harm. On the periphery of CAM techniques are spiritual counseling, music and art therapy, Qi Gong, Tai Chi, and Reiki. Despite the objectively benign nature of these alternative practices, practitioners are nonetheless urged to proceed with caution with respect to the application of all the approaches described in the alternative approaches section given the paucity of empirical evidence examining their efficacy and propensity for doing further harm.

Traumatic Brain Injury

During the past decade, institutions such as the CDC, Department of Defense (DoD), and Congress have been establishing workgroups to identify guidelines for the screening, assessment, and treatment of mTBI. Presently, the DoD has developed a clinical practice guideline for theater management of TBI which includes an assessment and treatment algorithm.

Screening and Assessment: Head injury symptomatology in combat zones, especially those associated with exposure to blasts from IEDs, is likely to copresent with gross physical trauma to the entire body, making head injury assessment a secondary or tertiary consideration to more vital diagnostic and treatment endeavors. Therefore, when patients sustain blast injuries or enter treatment in an unconscious state for unknown reasons, care should be taken to ensure that these patients are screened for cognitive impairment once an assessment of their post-head injury cognitive function is appropriate. Although there are a number of assessment models designed to identify individuals meeting the diagnostic criteria for TBI, few service members undergo screening for cognitive impairment. Why? Lack of resources and knowledge in both the caregivers and the patients limits both screening and assessment endeavors. However, once a person has been flagged for an assessment to investigate the impact of head trauma, there are a number of assessment modalities that may be used (Schwab et al. 2007).

Glasgow Coma Scale

Primary assessment of acute head injury can be accomplished through the Glasgow Coma Scale (GCS) (Teasdale and Jennett 1974). The GCS measures three factors of neurological functioning: eye opening, motor response, and verbal response. Scores range from 1 to 6 with total scale scores ranging from 3 to 18. While there are other factors associated with assessing a TBI such as CT scans (e.g., imaging) and length of LOC, the GCS is considered a gold standard model for rapidly assessing neurological functioning and is most useful for prognosticating clinical outcomes in moderate to severe TBI.

Military Acute Concussion Evaluation

A tool that can be utilized by first responders, derived from the Sideline Assessment of Concussion (SAC) frequently used on college and professional football players, is the Military Acute Concussion Evaluation (MACE) (DVBIC 2006). The MACE can be administered in approximately 10 min and comprises three main sections: history, screening neurological examination, and cognitive evaluation. The history section asks the provider to obtain a description of the incident, cause of the injury, determining the presence or absence of a helmet, investigation of anterograde and retrograde amnesia, and LOC. The neurological examination assesses ocular (papillary response and eye tracking), verbal (speech fluency and word finding), and motor (pronator drift and gait and coordination) functions. The cognitive portion includes an assessment of orientation to various factors of time, immediate memory, brief neurological screening, recalling digits backwards, and a delayed recall of the items on the immediate memory word list. The MACE can be scored to produce three outcomes: (a) no concussion, (b) concussion with LOC, (c) or concussion with no LOC (DVBIC 2006). A diagnosis of concussion can be made from the history section alone. *Repeatable Battery for the Assessment of Neuropsychological Status (RBANS).* Use of repeatable assessment batteries such as the RBANS (Randolph 1998) is another assessment model. This assessment tool measures a variety of neuropsychological and neurocognitive performance constructs identifying the current status. The multiple forms available from the RBANS lend the instrument to longitudinal evaluation of patient progress (Randolph 1998).

Pre-deployment Neuropsychological Assessment

In response to the high incidence of combat-related TBI, the DoD Assistant Secretary of Defense for Health Affairs (ASD-HA) released a directive that all service members shall have a neurocognitive evaluation prior to deployment. While a number of different automated neurocognitive instruments are available, the ASD-HA directed that the Automated Neuropsychological Assessment Metrics (ANAM) would be used by all branches of the armed services until a thorough comparison of multiple neurocognitive tools could be completed. The ANAM, also known as ANAM4, is a battery of tests which have been normed for service member populations. The current ANAM4 TBI battery measures the following domains: simple reaction time, code substitution (learning), procedural reaction time, mathematical processing, matching to sample, code substitution (delayed). Additionally, the battery includes a demographics page, TBI questionnaire, sleepiness scale, and mood scale. This instrument is a relative of the initial ANAM, a battery of neuropsychological tests developed by the DoD for research purposes over the past 30 years.

Treatment of Traumatic Brain Injury: The treatment model for mTBI in military settings is fairly straightforward, starting with rest and sustenance in the initial aftermath of the incident. Medications that inhibit blood clotting should be avoided as diffuse bleeding throughout the brain remains a possibility. Close observation during the initial stages of the trauma is warranted in case symptoms worsen (e.g., reports of a worsening headache). Pharmacological interventions have been employed to address a number of the symptoms of TBI, such as using Triptan agents to treat headache (Lane and Arciniegas 2002). For mTBI symptoms that do not remit, a number of treatment models are being explored. For example, Hyperbaric Oxygen Therapy (HBOT) is being evaluated by the DoD as part of a clinical trial (Golden et al. 2002).

Assessment of TBI with the Potential for Comorbid post-traumatic stress disorder: TBI, because of its propensity for acute life-threatening conditions, takes priority upon intake. For those suffering with moderate or severe TBI or a penetrating head wound, practitioners in combat hospitals will likely emphasize only life-saving care prior to medical evacuation of the patient to a higher, more definitive level of care. For those suffering from mTBI, the real issue at hand is whether or not the patients are seen by medical staff in conjunction with their injury. For those who are adequately healthy and conscious, and seen in close proximity to their injury, assessments such as the MACE can be conducted. In many cases, the patients may not seek out medical care and misinterpret or ignore the initial symptoms of mTBI or concussion. When these patients finally are evaluated, perhaps in a mandatory screening prior to departing the combat zone or due to complaints for other injuries, a more thorough neurocognitive screening, such as the RBANS, can be conducted. Given the traumatic nature of many instances that result in TBI in the combat zone, it is reasonable to screen for the presence of ASD—the precursor to post-traumatic stress disorder—during the course of the assessment. A positive screen for ASD warrants a future evaluation for post-traumatic stress disorder if symptoms do not remit. ASD may be identified using standard screening instruments designed for post-traumatic stress disorder; however, it is important to remember that temporal factors delineate ASD from post-traumatic stress disorder. In addition, the amount of time in which one experiences post-traumatic stress disorder may further confound the diagnosis. Alternative clinical disorders in the mood, anxiety, and substance abuse families may be present as well as social and other behavioral problems. Many individuals will have some type of psychological response to a traumatic event; however, the majority does not proceed to experiencing acute or chronic post-traumatic stress disorder. Evaluation based upon clinical decision making and case conceptualization are warranted as individuals experiencing early traumatic stress symptoms may present with variable responses dependent on their coping or recovery pathway.

Granacher (2008) has been one of the few to offer a detailed strategy for assessment of TBI patients thought to also be at risk for post-traumatic stress disorder. With respect to assessment, Grenacher notes that "comprehensive neuropsychiatric assessment is the most important single tool with which to determine whether a patient with post-traumatic stress disorder has co-morbid TBI." This model includes the following: (a) review records of TBI event, (b) detailed neuropsychiatric history, (c) mental status and neurological examination, (d) brain imaging with MRI, (e) standard neurocognitive assessment, (f) standard behavioral assessments, and (g) laboratory testing. Obviously, some of these recommendations are impractical for clinicians working in deployed environments (e.g., MRI, laboratory testing, and, depending upon the availability of neuropsychologists or neuropsychiatrists, the standard neurocogntive assessment).

Treatment Models for TBI with Comorbid post-traumatic stress disorder: The Institute of Medicine (IOM) report on the evidence related to the treatment of post-traumatic stress disorder forcefully states: "The scientific evidence on treatment modalities for post-traumatic stress disorder does not reach the level of certainty that would be desired for such a common and serious condition among Veterans" (IOM 2007). Given that the identification of efficacious treatment for post-traumatic stress disorder alone is in such a state, it should come as no surprise that the literature has little to offer with respect to evidence-based treatments for comorbid TBI and post-traumatic stress disorder.

Prior to the start of the wars in Iraq and Afghanistan, Bryant (2001) noted that there is no approach currently applied that can differentiate between the overlapping symptoms in TBI and post-traumatic stress disorder. In fact, many clinicians overlook one condition for the sake of an unduly warranted focus on the other condition. Bryant (2001) also argued that best practices in post-traumatic stress disorder therapy may need to be modified if TBI is suspected. In particular, LOC or other encoding problems may preclude therapies that rely on recall of the traumatic event such as imaginal exposure. Further, deficits in attention may make cognitive therapies challenging and require use of strategies and techniques (cue cards, written reminders) that mitigate TBI-induced problems with sustained attention and memory. Finally, Bryant advocated early cognitive therapy after the identification of TBI as a means to prevent the development of cognitions that cause individuals to inaccurately attribute TBI-induced symptoms to some sort of psychological disturbance.

Posttraumatic Stress Disorder Assessment and Treatment Model

Event	Assessment	Treatment	Clinical Outcomes
A criterion A event such as a shooting, crime or exposure to disaster. The individual experiences fear or horror, although freezing may also be a common response. Impairment and symptoms are noted in several criterion areas. These areas are re-experiencing the event through thoughts or dreams, avoidance of stimuli that are reminders of the event, physiological arousal such as sleep difficulties, hypervigilance and exaggerated startle response, the symptoms last greater than a month and result in clinically significant distress in multiple areas of functioning.	Assessment for Posttraumatic Stress-Disorder includes multiple steps: Initial use of screeners such as the Posttraumatic Stress Disorder Checklist (PCL) or the Mississippi Scale for Posttraumatic Stress Disorder identify symptoms consistent with a diagnosis of Posttraumatic Stress Disorder. A diagnosis of Posttraumatic Stress Disorder should include use of the Clinician Administered Posttraumatic Stress Disorder Scale (CAPS). The CAPS is the gold standard clinical assessment measuring the DSM-IV criteria for Posttraumatic Stress Disorder. Further models such as the Minnesota Multiphasic Personality Inventory –II (MMPI-II) Posttraumatic Stress Disorder Keane Scale (PK) have been significantly correlated with the diagnosis of Posttraumatic Stress Disorder. The MMPI-II contains scales to identify invalid answering.	While a number of models have been identified to address Posttraumatic Stress Disorder, the literature generally supports the use of exposure-based treatment models. These models include Prolonged Exposure Therapy (PET) and Cognitive Processing Therapy (CPT). Psychopharmacological agents such as selective serotonin reuptake inhibitors (SSRI) have been identified as appropriate treatments. Additionally, Ambien and Prazosin have been identified as useful models for sleep disturbance and nightmare reduction respectively. Further models such as Acceptance and Commitment Therapy (ACT) and Complementary and Alternative Medicine (CAM) may yield promising treatments.	Successful treatment is correlated with improvement in functioning across multiple domains. Often individuals with Posttraumatic Stress Disorder hope that treatment will conclude with them feeling as though the trauma had never happened. This treatment goal is rarely realized. Treatment models that are successful reduce avoidance of feared stimuli, reduce re-experiencing of the event, reduce hyperarousal and bio-physiological reactivity. As a result anxiety and distress are reduced. Successful treatment results in individuals able to engage in their lives and experience significantly reduced distress. It should be noted that relapses, especially around anniversaries or strong reminders of the event may occur and result in a renewed need for treatment.

Fig. 12.1 post-traumatic stress disorder assessment and treatment model

TBI Assessment and Treatment Model

Event	Assessment	Treatment	Clinical Outcomes
TBI may be caused by multiple types of impacts or insults to the head. In the civilian population, TBI is most frequently associated with motor vehicle accidents, falls and assaults. In the military population, currently blast exposure is the most frequent cause of TBI. Other causes of injury are motor vehicle accidents and bullet/shrapnel wounds.	Assessment for TBI includes multiple steps: While most TBI cases are mild in nature and full recovery is expected within hours to days, moderate, severe or penetrating TBI may also be present. Initial screening for a TBI should be completed using the Military Acute Concussion Evaluation (MACE). A positive diagnosis can be made from the history section of the MACE. Further evaluation can be made using an automated neuropsychological test assessing cognitive performance across multiple domains. Follow up assessment can include use of the Repeatable Battery for the Assessment of Neuropsychological Status (RBANS).	Treatment for TBI is a fairly straightforward endeavor. Generally, recovery is assisted by rest and access to a quiet environment as well as pain medication that does not impact clotting. Individuals who continue to experience problems secondary to TBI including: pain, balance, agitation, cognitive impairment and memory problems may be offered alternative treatment models. These models include use of the triptan medications for pain, hyperbaric oxygen treatment and cognitive rehabilitation. Further treatment models continue to be explored.	The majority of individuals with TBI are expected to make a full recovery within hours to days of the injury. Further recovery may take several weeks to months; however expectation of recovery is critical to a positive recovery curve. Full recovery is associated with return to function akin to function before the injury. Research continues to examine TBI, looking at questions such as the impacts of multiple TBI.

Fig. 12.1 (continued)

In a subsequent review paper developed by McMillan et al. (2003), the authors advocate for the use of CBT for the treatment of post-traumatic stress disorder following TBI citing four case studies and one quasi-experimental design that demonstrated efficacy for the approach. The authors state: "CBT may be of particular value to people with cognitive disability because it is structured, educative, and interactive."

Adjunctive problem-focused methods and services commonly offered to individuals suffering from TBI alone might also prove useful for individuals presenting with both post-traumatic stress disorder and TBI. Examples are patient/caregiver education, self-care and independent living skills training, referral to supported housing services, family skills training, social skills training, vocational rehabilitation, case management, religious/spiritual advisement, and substance abuse treatment (Kennedy et al. 2007).

Some pharmacotherapy interventions may target co-occurring symptoms of TBI and post-traumatic stress disorder. Shared symptoms of irritability, flash anger, and violent outbursts can be addressed with anticonvulsants (e.g., carbamazepine, gabapentin, valproate). Insomnia can be treated with the atypical antipsychotic Quetiapine (Kennedy et al. 2007). However, Kennedy and colleagues were quick to point out that individuals suffering from TBI may be more sensitive to both side and primary effects of medications, and therefore the introduction of pharmacotherapy to any patient with TBI should be made with lower starting doses and close observation while gradually increasing the dosage to therapeutic levels. The authors also note a paucity of literature examining the utility of combined pharmacotherapy and psychotherapy for the treatment of concurrent TBI/post-traumatic stress disorder.

Taber and Hurley (2009) advocate for use of therapeutic interventions that involve rescripting or reprocessing approaches for individuals suffering concurrently from post-traumatic stress disorder and TBI. These approaches focus less on the traumatic event, which for sufferers of TBI can be helpful in cases of LOC or amnesia for the traumatic event; instead the focus is directed at reducing self-directed attributions of shame, guilt, and anger.

Summary and Recommendations

Lew et al. (2008) noted the following: "No empirically validated therapies exist to treat comorbid post-traumatic stress disorder, depression, and post-concussive disorders, which may be confounded by self-medicated alcohol/substance misuse, abuse, or dependence." It is proposed that clinicians who expect to work with individuals experiencing comorbid post-traumatic stress disorder and TBI may have to follow a model that specifically addresses the uniqueness of their patients (case conceptualization) while customizing a treatment that draws from both treatment literatures and is tailored to the unique symptom presentation of the patient (Fig. 12.1).

This chapter was designed to give mental health providers who work with veterans or recent combat deployers, and especially those providers working in austere environments, with a starting point for developing their own approach to the assessment and treatment of comorbid post-traumatic stress disorder and TBI. The discussion of prevalence rates indicates that post-traumatic stress disorder will present a challenge to almost any provider who works with a population that has endured multiple combat tours of duty. With respect to TBI, first responders and emergency trauma providers are almost certain to encounter cases of severe, moderate, and mild TBI; however, providers outside of casualty collection points are more likely to experience a heavier post-traumatic stress disorder than TBI caseload. For those presenting with TBI symptoms due to combat, providers should know that their patient has likely already met one of the criteria for post-traumatic stress disorder and may score high on Cluster D hyperarousal symptoms that emphasize some degree of cognitive impairment and sleep problems that logically follow some forms of TBI. Likewise, when a patient presents with elevated Cluster D symptoms on post-traumatic stress disorder assessments, the provider may give serious consideration to pursuing additional assessment to investigate the presence of TBI. In either case, professional clinical judgment buttressed by empirical evaluation of symptom patterns is warranted.

In closing, we strongly recommend that mental health practitioners who work with combat-deployed service members become familiar with and follow the guidelines for the treatment of patients with ASD and post-traumatic stress disorder (APA 2004). These guidelines are quite relevant for individuals at risk for TBI, as the guidelines emphasize the collection of a thorough history of traumatic events and evaluation for potential comorbid conditions. For those service members who (a) screen high for post-traumatic stress disorder using self-reported screening instruments, (b) are known to have a previous diagnosis of post-traumatic stress disorder, or (c) present with symptoms strongly indicative of post-traumatic stress disorder, an additional screen for a history of blast exposure or head injury requires few additional resources. Similarly, when combat-exposed service members report primarily with complaints of symptoms related to blast exposure or other head injuries, administration of a short post-traumatic stress disorder screening instrument, such as the PCL, has little risk with potentially important benefits. In this latter scenario, the provider may have to administer the screening instrument orally if the symptoms make self-report problematic. In either case, short screening questions aimed at determining a history of head trauma, combined with short, self-reported post-traumatic stress disorder screens, provide a logical, low-cost, low-risk means for determining which service members receive more thorough screening such as that prescribed by the APA.

References

Adamson DM, Burnam MA, Burns RM, Caldarone LB, Cox RA, D'Amico E, Diaz C, Eibner C, Fisher G, Helmus TC, Jaycox LH, Karney BR, Kilmer B, Marshall GN, Martin LT, Meredith LS, Metscher KN, Osilla KC, Pacula RL, Ramchand R, Ringel JS, Schell TL, Sollinger JM, Tanielian T, Vaiana Kayla ME, Williams M, Michael Yochelson MR. Invisible wounds of war: psychological and cognitive injuries, their consequences, and services to assist recovery. Santa Monica, CA: Rand Corporation; 2008.

American Psychiatric Association. Diagnostic and Statistical manual of mental disorders. 4th ed. Washington, DC: Author; 1994.

American Psychiatric Association (APA). Practice guideline for the treatment of patients with acute stress disorder and posttraumatic stress disorder, Vol. Nov. Arlington, VA: American Psychiatric Association; 2004. p. 57.

Beck AT. Cognitive therapy and the emotional disorders. New York, NY: Penguin Books; 1979.

Blake DD, Weathers FW, Nagy LM, Kaloupek DG, Gusman FD, Charney DS, Keane TM. The development of a clinician-administered posttraumatic stress disorder scale. J Traumatic Stress. 1995;8(1):75–90. Review.

Bobo WV, Warner CH, Warner CM. The management of post traumatic stress disorder (posttraumatic stress disorder) in the primary care setting. Southern Med J. 2007;100(8):797–802.

Bombardier CH, Fann JR, Temkin N, Esselman PC, Pelzer E, Keough M, Dikmen S. Posttraumatic stress disorder symptoms during the first six months after traumatic brain injury. J Neuropsychiatry Clin Neurosci. 2006;18:501–8.

Bryant RA. Posttraumatic stress disorder and traumatic brain injury: can they co-exist? Clin Psychol Rev. 2001;21:931–48.

Bryant RA, Harvey AG. Relationship between acute stress disorder and posttraumatic stress disorder following mild traumatic brain injury. Am J Psychiatry. 1998;155:625–9.

Centers for Disease Control and Prevention. Facts about traumatic brain injury; 2010.

Davidson J, Roth S, Newman E. Flouxetine in posttraumatic stress disorder. J Traumatic Stress. 1991;4(3):419–23.

Defense and Veterans Brain Injury Center; 2010.

Defense and Veterans Brain Injury Center. Military Acute Concussion Examination; 2006.

Foa EB, Chambless DL. Habituation of subjective anxiety during flooding in imagery. Beh Res Ther. 1978;16(6):391–9.

Foa EB, Hembree EA, Rothbaum BO. Prolonged exposure therapy for posttraumatic stress disorder: emotional processing of traumatic experiences: therapists guide. Oxford: Oxford University Press; 2007.

Foa EB, Kozak MJ. Emotional processing of fear: exposure to corrective information. Psychol Bull. 1986;99:20–35.

Glasser J, Neuner F, Lutgehetmann R, Schmidt R, Elbert T. Posttraumatic stress disorder in patients with traumatic brain injury. BMC Psychiatry 2004;4:5. http://www.biomedcentral.com/1471-244X/4/5.

Golden ZL, Neubauer R, Golden CJ, Greene L, Marsh J, Mleko A. Improvement in cerebral metabolism in chronic brain injury after hyperbaric oxygen therapy. Int J Neurosci. 2002;112(2):119–31.

Granacher Jr RP. Commentary: applications of functional neuroimaging to civil litigation of mild traumatic brain injury. J Am Acad Psychiatry Law. 2008;36(3):323–8.

Harvey AG, Bryant RA. Two-year prospective evaluation of the relationship between acute stress disorder and posttraumatic stress disorder following mild traumatic brain injury. Am J Psychiatry. 2000;157:626–8.

Harvey AG, Brewin CR, Jones C, Kopelman MD. Coexistence of posttraumatic stress disorder and traumatic brain injury: towards a resolution of the paradox. J Int Neuropsychol Soc. 2003;9:663–76.

Hayes SC, Strosahl KD, Wilson KG. An experiential approach to behavior change: acceptance and commitment therapy. New York, NY: Guilford Press; 1999.

Hoge CW, Castro CA, Messer SC, McGurk D, Cotting DI, Koffman RL. Combat duty in Iraq and Afghanistan, mental health problems, and barriers to care. N Engl J Med. 2004;351:13–22.

Hoge CW, Auchterlonie JL, Milliken CS. Mental health problems, use of mental health services, and attrition from military service after returning from deployment to Iraq or Afghanistan. J Am Med Assoc. 2006;295: 1023–32.

Hoge CW, McGurk D, Thomas JL, Cox AL, Engel CC, Castro CA. Mild traumatic brain injury in US soldiers returning from Iraq. The New England Journal of Medicine. 2008;358:453–63.

Holifield M, Sinclair-Lian N, Warner TD, HammerSchlag R. Acupuncture for posttraumatic stress disorder: a randomized controlled pilot trial. J Nerv Mental Dis. 2007;195(6):504–13.

Keane TM, Caddell JM, Taylor KL. Mississippi scale for combat-related posttraumatic stress disorder: three studies in reliability and validity. J Consult Clin Psychol. 1988;56(1):85–90.

Kennedy JE, Jaffee MS, Leskin GA, Stokes JW, Leal FO, Fitzpatrick PJ. Posttraumatic stress disorder and posttraumatic stress disorder-like symptoms and mild traumatic brain injury. J Rehabil Res Dev. 2007;44: 895–920.

Kessler RC, Chiu WT, Demler O, Walters EE. Prevalence, severity, and comorbidity of 12-Month DSM-IV disorders in the National Comorbidity Survey Replication. Arch Gen Psychiatry. 2005a;62:617–27.

Kessler RC, Berguland P, Demler O, Jin R, Walters EE. Lifetime prevalence and age-of-onset distributions of DSM-IV disorders in the National Comorbidity Survey Replication. Arch Gen Psychiatry. 2005b;2:593–602.

Kim E, Lauterback EC, Reeve A, Arciniegas DB, Coburn KL, Mendez MF, Rummans TA, Coffey EC. Neuropsychiatric complications of traumatic brain injury: a critical review of the literature (a report by the ANPA Committee on Research). J Neuospychiatry Clin Neurosci. 2007;19:106–27.

Lane JC, Arciniegas DB. Post traumatic headache. Current treatment options. Neurology. 2002;4(1):89–104.

Lang AJ, Laffaye C, Satz LE, Dresselhaus TR, Stein MB. Sensitivity and specificity of the posttraumatic stress disorder checklist in detecting posttraumatic stress disorder in female veterans in primary care. J Trauma Stress. 2003;16(3):257–64.

Langlois JA, Rutland-Brown W, Wald MM. The epidemiology and impact of traumatic brain injury: a brief overview. J Head Trauma Rehabil. 2006;21:375–8.

Lew HL, Vanderploeg RD, Moore DF, Schwab K, Friedman L, Yesavage J, Keane TM, Warden DL, Sigford BJ. Overlap of mild TBI and mental health conditions in returning OIF/OEF service members and veterans. J Rehabil Res Dev. 2008;45(3):xi–xvi.

Lineberry TW, Ramaswamy S, Bostwick JM, Rundell JR. Traumatized troops: how to treat combat related posttraumatic stress disorder. J Fam Pract. 2006;5(5):39–52.

Lyons JA, Keane TM. Keene posttraumatic stress disorder scale: MMPI and MMPI-2 update. J Traumatic Stress. 1992;5(1):111–17.

Maher MJ, Rego SA, Asnis GM. Sleep disturbances in patients with posttraumatic stress disorder: epidemiology, impact and approaches to management. CNS Drugs. 2006;20(7):567–90.

McMillan TW, Williams WH, Bryant R. Posttraumatic stress disorder and traumatic brain injury: a review of causal mechanisms, assessment, and treatment. Neuropsychol Rehabil. 2003;13(1–2):149–64.

National Academies of Science, Institute of Medicine. Treatment of posttraumatic stress disorder: an assessment of the evidence. Washington, DC: National Academies Press; 2007.

Pavlov IP. Conditioned reflexes: an investigation of the physiological activity of the cerebral cortex. York University; 1927. http://psychclassics.asu.edu/Pavlov/.

Prins A, Ouimette P. Corrigendum. The Primary Care posttraumatic stress disorder screen (PC-posttraumatic stress disorder): development and operating characteristics. Primary Care Psychiatry. 2004;4:151.

Ramchand R, Karney B, Osilla K, Burns R, Calderone L. Prevalence of posttraumatic stress disorder, Depression, and TBI among returning service members. In: Tanielian T, Jaycox L, editors. Invisible wounds of war: psychological and cognitive injuries, their consequences, and services to assist recovery. Santa Monica, CA: Rand Corporation; 2008. p. 35–82.

Peskind ER, Bonner LT, Hoff DJ, Raskind MA. Prazosin reduces trauma-related nightmares in older men with chronic posttraumatic stress disorder. J Geriatr Psychiatry Neurol. 2003;16(3):165–71.

Pitman RK, Sanders KM, Zusman RM, Healy AR, Cheema F, Lasko NB, Cahill L, Orr SP. Pilot study of secondary prevention of posttraumatic stress disorder with propranolol. Biol Psychiatry. 2002;51(2):189–92.

Randolph, C. (1998). Repeatable Battery for the Assessment of Neuropsychological Status: Manual. PsychCorp

Raskind MA, Peskind ER, Hoff DJ, Hart KL, Holmes HA, Warren D, Shofer J, O'Connell J, Taylor F, Gross C, Rohde K, McFall M. A parallel group placebo controlled study of prazosin for trauma nightmares and sleep disturbance in combat veterans with posttraumatic stress disorder. Biol Psychiatry. 2006;61(8):928–34.

Reger GM, Gahm GA. Virtual reality exposure therapy for active duty soldiers. J Clin Psychol. 2008;64: 940–6.

Resick PA. Stress and trauma. Philadelphia, PA: Taylor and Frances Group; 2001.

Ruggierro KJ, Del Ben K, Scotti J, Rabalais AE. Psychometric properties of the posttraumatic stress disorder Checklist-Civilian Version. J Traumatic Stress. 2003;16(5):495–502.

Sbordone RJ, Liter JC. Mild traumatic brain injury does not produce posttraumatic stress disorder. Brain Inj. 1995;9:405–12.

Schell TL, Marshall GN. Survey of individuals previously deployed to OEF/OIF. In: Tanielian T, Jaycox L, editors. Invisible wounds of war: psychological and cognitive injuries, their consequences, and services to assist rec*overy*. Santa Monica, CA: Rand Corporation; 2008. p. 87–113.

Schneiderman AI, Braver ER, Kang HK. Understanding sequelae of injury mechanisms and mild traumatic brain injury incurred during the conflicts in Iraq and Afghanistan: Persistent postconcussive symptoms and posttraumatic stress disorder. Am J Epidemiol. 2008;167:1446–52.

Schwab KA, Ivins B, Cramer G, Johnson W, Sluss-Tiller M, Kiley K, Lux W, Warden D. Screening for traumatic brain injury in troops returning from deployment in Afghanistan and Iraq: initial investigation of the usefulness of a short screening tool for traumatic brain injury. J Head Trauma. 2007;22: 377–89.

Smith TC, Ryan MA, Wingard DL, Slymen DJ, Sallis JF, Kritz-Silverstein D. New onset and persistent symptoms of posttraumatic stress disorder self reported after deployment and combat exposure: prospective population based US military cohort study. Br Med J. 2008;335(7640):336–71.

Stein MB, McAllister TW. Exploring the convergence of posttraumatic stress disorder and mild-traumatic brain injury. Am J Psychiatry. 2009;166(768–776).

Taber KH, Hurley RA. posttraumatic stress disorder and combat-related injuries: functional neuroanatomy. J Neuropsychiatry Clin Neurosci. 2009;21:1–4.

Teasdale G, Jennett B. Assessment of coma and impaired consciousness. A practical scale Lancet. 1974; 2(7872):81–4.

Vasterling JJ, Proctor SP, Amoroso P, Kane R, Heeren T, White RF. Neuropsychological outcomes of army personnel following deployment to the Iraq war. J Am Med Assoc. 2006;296:519–29.

Behavioral and Psychiatric Comorbidities of TBI

13

Robert L. Collins, Nicholas J. Pastorek, Andra T. Tharp, and Thomas A. Kent

Abstract

Traumatic brain injury (TBI) is associated with a variety of behavioral consequences, including symptoms of depression, anxiety, aggression, and impulse control and overlaps with many of the symptoms of post-traumatic stress and post-traumatic stress disorder. There are many challenges to researchers and clinicians, including heterogeneity of the injury, distinguishing premorbid characteristics from the consequences of the TBI, lack of specificity in diagnostic criteria, and the absence of systematic therapeutic trials. In this chapter, we present an overview of the literature on psychiatric and behavioral consequences of TBI, highlighting those studies that investigate the incidence of these conditions, contribution of premorbid functioning to subsequent symptoms, and characteristics of mild TBI (frequently referred to as concussion) that provide clues to distinguishing it from other psychiatric comorbidities. Our analysis of the available literature suggests that in some, but not all cases, TBI may diminish inhibitory

Robert L. Collins, Nicholas J. Pastorek, and Andra L. Teten contributed equally to this work.

R.L. Collins, Ph.D., A.B.P.P. • T.A. Kent, M.D. (✉)
Neurology Care Line, Michael E. DeBakey VA Medical Center, Houston, TX, USA

Department of Neurology, Baylor College of Medicine, Houston, TX, USA
e-mail: robert.collins3@va.gov; tkent@bcm.edu

N.J. Pastorek, Ph.D., A.B.P.P.
Rehabilitation Care Line, Michael E. DeBakey VA Medical Center, Houston, TX, USA

Department of Psychiatry and Behavioral Sciences, Baylor College of Medicine, Houston, TX, USA
e-mail: nicholas.pastorek@va.gov

A.T. Tharp, Ph.D.
Menninger, Department of Psychiatry and Behavioral Sciences, Baylor College of Medicine, Houston, TX, USA
e-mail: atharp@cdc.gov

J.W. Tsao (ed.), *Traumatic Brain Injury: A Clinician's Guide to Diagnosis, Management, and Rehabilitation*,
DOI 10.1007/978-0-387-87887-4_13,

control over certain behaviors while in others, there may be an exacerbation of clinical expression of psychiatric symptoms. Treatment needs to consider whether there is a unique sensitivity to adverse events in patients who have suffered a TBI and prospective trials should be encouraged.

Keywords
Impulsive aggression • Post-concussion syndrome • Suicide • Post-traumatic stress disorder • Depression • Traumatic brain injury • Military • Veteran • Aggression

Introduction

An estimated 1.7 million Americans sustain a traumatic brain injury (TBI) each year (Faul et al. 2010) and over 5.3 million (2% of the US population) are currently living with a disability from TBI that requires assistance in activities of daily living (Brain Injury Association of America 2009). Men are 1.5 times more likely to sustain a TBI than women, and military activities increase the risk of TBI (Schwab et al. 2007). Approximately 35.2% of TBIs are caused by falls, 17.3% by motor vehicle accidents, 16.5% by being struck by something or striking one's head against something, and 10% by assaults (Faul et al. 2010). Among military personnel serving in a warzone, explosive blasts are the leading cause of TBI (Champion et al. 2009). TBI is associated with a variety of subsequent neurological disorders, including epilepsy, Alzheimer's disease, and Parkinson's disease (National Institute of Neurological Disorders and Stroke 2002). TBI has also been associated with a number of psychiatric and behavioral effects, including the development of mood and anxiety disorders, aggressive behavior, and post-traumatic stress (PTS) and post-traumatic stress disorder (PTSD).

TBI Psychiatric and Behavioral Comorbidities

Development of mood and anxiety disorders has been reported following TBI with anxiety and depression occurring most frequently in mild TBI (mTBI) (described below). Variation in the frequency of these disorders has been reported across studies. Some research suggests that depressive symptoms are more frequent than those associated with anxiety (Deb and Crownshaw 2004) though depression may be more likely to remit (Hibbard et al. 1998). An estimated 6–77% (as reported in Horner et al. 2008) of those with TBI report post-injury depression, although Levin et al. (2001) found that the prevalence of depression following TBI (17%) did not differ from that experienced following general trauma (6%). The wide range of prevalence estimates is believed to result from variation across studies in injury severity, method of diagnosis (for TBI and depression), and other methodological issues (Horner et al. 2008). The problem is further complicated by an overlap in symptoms between TBI and depression (e.g., sleep disturbance). Prevalence of anxiety after TBI has been reported as high as 70%, but a meta-analysis found the prevalence of anxiety disorders following TBI to be 29%, with 23% for mTBI (Moore et al. 2006). Levin et al. (2001) found that the prevalence of depression following TBI did not differ for mild (18%) and moderate (11%) TBI. Variation also occurs based on anxiety disorder (Deb and Crownshaw 2004; Fann et al. 1995). Substantial comorbidity may occur (Moore et al. 2006); for example, Hibbard et al. (1998) found that 44% of their sample with TBI reported two or more Axis I disorders an average of 8 years following injury. Among 1,560 adults who completed telephone interviews 1 year following TBI, approximately 40% reported clinically significant symptoms of mood or anxiety disorders (Horner et al. 2008). Most work with the development of anxiety disorders involves PTSD, which is described in detail below.

The examination of co-occurring depression and TBI has been complicated by a variety of methodological factors, including variation across studies in sample characteristics, severity and definition of TBI and depression, and assessment instrument (Horner et al. 2008). Studies examining risk factors for depression after TBI have yielded mixed results (for discussion, see Levin et al. 2001; Rosenthal et al. 1998; Moldover et al. 2004); for example, some have found that older age (Levin et al. 2005) and female gender (Glenn et al. 2001) significantly predict post-injury depression, whereas others have reported that these were not significant predictors (Mooney et al. 2005; Seel et al. 2003; Hibbard et al. 2004; Rapoport et al. 2003). Although it is unclear what proportion of individuals with TBI have mood and anxiety disorders prior to their injury, in general, 6.7% of individuals over the age of 18 in the USA experience major depression and 18% experience an anxiety disorder each year (Kessler et al. 2005). With the exception of suicide-related TBI, it is unclear if psychiatric disorders pose a risk for TBI, though some studies have found that premorbid psychiatric disorders, such as alcohol abuse, anxiety, and depression, increase the risk of post-injury depression or anxiety (Horner et al. 2008; Hibbard et al. 1998; Jorge and Robinson 2002; Moldover et al. 2004). Depression following TBI has been associated with poorer cognitive functioning (Chamelian et al. 2006; Keiski et al. 2006) and poorer psychosocial functioning (Draper et al. 2007; Hibbard et al. 2004) than reported by those without depression. It has also been associated with a failure to recover as expected following TBI (Mooney et al. 2005).

That said, the etiology of these deficits is unclear; negative outcomes such as poor psychosocial functioning have been hypothesized to be the cause (Bay et al. 2008) and the consequence (Draper et al. 2007) of depression. It is also possible that for some individuals, depression following TBI may reflect an organic etiology (Levin et al. 2005) associated with the neurological issues associated with TBI; for example, lesions in the regions such as the left dorsofrontal cortex, left basal ganglia, or right posterior hemisphere have distinguished depressed and nondepressed patients with TBI (Rosenthal et al. 1998). Differentiating a diagnosis of depression from other issues following TBI is complicated (Jorge and Robinson 2002), as psychiatric symptoms following TBI, such as irritability and anger, are common to PTSD, depression, aggression, and some neuroanatomical lesions. It is also counterintuitive that symptoms of depression and anxiety are more common among those with mild than those with more severe injuries, though lack of awareness associated with severe TBI has been hypothesized as a possible explanation (Moldover et al. 2004). Taken together, this research suggests that the development of psychiatric issues following TBI may represent the developmental concept of *equifinality*, in which the same outcome (e.g., depression) may result from disparate causes and circumstances, such as premorbid dysfunction, poor psychosocial functioning after TBI, or nature and anatomic location of TBI.

Just as depression and other psychiatric conditions are associated with an increased risk of suicide in soldiers returning from combat deployments (Pietrzak et al. 2009; Tanielian and Jaycox 2008), a history of combat-related TBI must also be considered when assessing suicide risk of returning soldiers and veterans. In their review of the relation between TBI and suicidality, Simpson and Tate (2007) conclude that those recovering from TBI have a three- to fourfold increased risk of committing suicide relative to the general population, and that this increase appears to remain constant at least through the first 15 years post-injury. A recent Danish population-based study including nearly 150,000 subjects examined the relation between TBI severity and suicide risk (Teasdale and Engberg 2001). While those with severe TBI, as defined by the presence of cerebral contusions or intracranial hemorrhages, demonstrated the highest risk of suicide (i.e., 4.1 times increased risk) relative to the general population, those classified with a concussion still demonstrated an increased risk of suicide (i.e., three times increased risk). It has been suggested, however, that the increased rates of suicide for mTBI are likely related to post-injury and/or concomitant psychosocial factors, whereas suicidality following severe TBI is likely related to the injury and subsequent sequelae (Simpson and Tate 2007). Given that the vast majority of combat-related TBIs from the current wars in Iraq and Afghanistan are classified as mild (Tanielian and Jaycox 2008), the relation between TBI severity and suicidality must be carefully considered in order to fully appreciate the potential implications for health management of returning military personnel and veterans. Although causal attribution cannot be drawn from correlational studies, the possibility that such an association exists between combat-related concussion and suicide has extremely important implications for mental health screening and suicide prevention efforts given the relatively high incidence of history of concussion in returning military personnel (estimated to be between 5 and 20% of service members in deployed units [Tanielian and Jaycox 2008]). Future attempts to further explicate the complex relation between concussion and suicide must take into account the various shared risk factors between TBI and suicidality (e.g., young age, male gender, substance abuse, aggression/impulsivity) to determine the extent to which concussion uniquely contributes to suicide risk (Wasserman et al. 2008).

Aggressive behavior following TBI complicates rehabilitation (Nott et al. 2006), is a concern for caregivers (Johnson and Balleny 1996), and has been associated with lower psychosocial functioning 10 years following injury (Draper et al. 2007). The prevalence of aggression following TBI differs based on definition/severity of TBI, definition and assessment of aggression, reporting period, reporter (self, caregiver, staff), sample, and timing of assessment. Aggression following TBI may be expressed as agitation (Kim 2002; Nott 2006), intimate partner violence (Arango-Lasprilla et al. 2008; Marsh and Martinovich 2006), suicide attempts (Oquendo 2004), sexual violence or sexual disinhibition (DelBello 1999; Kelly et al. 2008), verbal aggression (Dyer et al. 2006), or physical aggression (Alderman 2007). As in the general population, verbal aggression typically is more frequent than physical aggression (Kelly et al. 2008; Dyer et al. 2006). The frequency of aggression following TBI has ranged from 11 to 96% based on the form of violence and the assessment instrument used (as reported in Tateno et al. 2003). Using the Overt Aggressive Scale (OAS, Yudofsky et al. 1986), Tateno et al. (2003) found that 33.7% of patients with TBI compared to 11.5% of patients without TBI reported aggressive acts in the 6 months following their injury. The frequency also varies based on the sample, severity of TBI, and duration of time since injury, with more agitation and aggression reported soon after the injury (Nott et al. 2006). For example, using the Overt Aggression Scale—Modified for Neurorehabilitation (OAS-MNR, Alderman et al. 1997), Alderman (2007) reported 5,548 episodes of aggression perpetrated by 108 patients with severe neurological damage over 14 days on an inpatient unit. The authors noted that the episodes were triggered by staff prompts or erupted with no apparent provocation. Using the OAS, Baguley et al. (2006) reported that rates of aggression among patients with moderate to severe TBI fluctuated over the 5 years following injury, but that at any given time approximately 25% of patients with TBI were expressing "severe" aggression. Johnson and Balleny (1996) reported that among individuals who survived severe TBI and were followed for 3 years, 55% of those whose injury occurred more than 18 months ago compared to 13% of those whose injury occurred less than 18 months ago had verbal or physical aggression as reported by family members; however, severity of behavioral problems (aggression and other problems) was not significantly correlated with the severity of head injury. Using the Buss Perry Aggression Scale (BPAQ, Buss and Perry 1992), Dyer et al. (2006) compared a sample of participants with TBI to those with spinal cord injury (SCI), and those without injury on measures of anger, aggression, and impulsivity 10 years following injury. Participants with TBI (severity not specified) reported more impulsivity, anger, and verbal aggression than those with SCI. When caregiver's reports were used, participants with TBI were also rated as more verbally aggressive than those with SCI. TBI has also been associated with anger and aggression among forensic samples. Slaughter et al. (2003) randomly selected 69 inmates of a county jail of whom 87% (67% mild, 33% moderate/severe) reported a lifetime history of TBI and 36% (80% mild, 20% moderate/severe TBI) reported a TBI in the past year. Based on the Brief Anger and Aggression Questionnaire (BAAQ, Maiuro et al. 1987), more extreme anger and aggression were reported by those with TBI than those without. Similarly, using the index offense of record, Brewer-Smyth et al. (2004) found that women incarcerated for a violent crime had more traumatic brain injuries with loss of consciousness in their lifetimes than those incarcerated for a nonviolent crime; however, only one participant convicted of a violent crime reported severe brain injury.

TBI and aggression has been examined among military samples; Vietnam veterans with TBI from penetrating brain wounds reported more aggression and violence than those without TBI (Grafman et al. 1996). At the time this chapter was written, the association between TBI and aggression had not been examined systematically among military personnel serving in Operation Enduring Freedom and Operation Iraqi Freedom, but the consequences of TBI are a concern given the proliferation of improvised explosive devices (IEDs) used in these conflicts. Among the personnel serving in Iraq, it is estimated that approximately 11% meet the criteria for mild TBI through surveys (MHAT V 2008). In a similar vein among a sample of 2,525 Army infantry soldiers serving in Iraq, Hoge et al. (2008) reported that 4.9% reported loss of consciousness and 10.3% reported altered mental status. Although survey data provides clues about the possible scope of the problem, survey reports of TBI symptoms and criteria are not necessarily confirmed by a clinical assessment and, therefore, may not accurately estimate prevalence.

Aggression following TBI often co-occurs with other post-injury psychiatric and psychosocial issues, such as anger (Dyer et al. 2006), hostility (Oquedo et al. 2004), impulsivity (Dyer et al. 2006), depression (Baguley et al. 2006), PTS, PTSD (Bryant 2001), and substance abuse (Draper et al. 2007). Though premorbid factors such as alcohol use may influence the presence (TBI vs. no TBI, Oquedo et al. 2004) and etiology (i.e., whether due to violent or nonviolent causes, Schopp et al. 2006) of TBI, these factors seem to be less predictive of post-injury aggression than the other post-injury psychosocial issues. For example, in a 5-year follow-up study, age and depressive symptoms, as rated with the Beck Depression Inventory (Beck 1988), were the only factors that predicted aggression at 6-, 24-, and 60-month follow-up (Baguley et al. 2006). The disorders and symptoms co-occurring with aggression following TBI are similar to those in non-TBI samples: Anger and hostility have been associated with PTSD (Orth and Wieland 2006) and irritability and aggressive outbursts have been observed among depressed patients (Haller and Kruk 2006). Impulsivity and substance use, specifically alcohol use, have been associated with a variety of violent acts, and are thought to be associated via shared biological substrates or altered social information processing (Hoaken and Steward 2003; Moeller et al. 2001). The comorbidity may also be an artifact of the diagnostic criteria for Axis I and Axis II disorders, which may include irritability, anger, impulsivity, and aggression (APA 2000). Given these similarities, it is unclear what distinguishes TBI aggression from that observed among non-injured individuals and consequently what novel aspects for TBI-aggression treatment would need to be considered. Because TBI involves lesions to the brain, usually in the frontal lobes, it is possible that specific executive function deficits experienced by individuals with TBI and aggression may provide clues to understanding the phenomenology and treatment of this behavioral problem. Group differences on executive deficits have been examined among individuals with TBI based on the etiology of their injury (violent vs. nonviolent), with results suggesting that premorbid factors, and not the nature of injury, influence the outcome following TBI (Machamer et al. 2003; Schopp et al. 2006). In a study of sex differences in executive functions among individuals with TBI, women outperformed men on neuropsychological assessments, but premorbid factors and factors related to the injury were most predictive of neuropsychological functioning among men and women (Niemeier et al. 2007). When comparing men with and without TBI who were receiving court-ordered treatment for intimate partner violence, men with TBI had poorer executive functioning and lower post-injury IQ than the non-TBI batterers (March and Martinovich 2006). Underscoring the importance of considering premorbid differences, these studies do not yet definitively establish how executive functions may be associated with aggression post-TBI.

Among aggressive individuals without TBI, studies of executive deficits have primarily involved examining neuropsychological differences between those with impulsive versus premeditated subtypes of aggressive behavior. Impulsive aggression is characterized as a hair-trigger response to a threat with a behavioral loss of control, and premeditated aggression is a planned act usually carried out for a specific purpose or goal (Barratt et al. 1991; Barratt et al. 1997b; Stanford et al. 2003). The neuropsychological correlates of impulsive aggression include specific language and executive function deficits, particularly verbal performance that involves more complex analyses (Villemarette-Pittman et al. 2003; Miller et al. 2008). Trauma survivors with impulsive aggression also evidenced alexithymia, which is an inability to recognize and articulate one's emotional experience, suggesting that verbal deficits may also be associated with emotional awareness deficits (Teten et al. 2008). The pattern of executive function deficits and other characteristics, such as similar neuroanatomical lesions (Greve et al. 2002), lack of self-awareness (Dyer et al. 2006), and language difficulties (Wood et al. 2006), suggests that post-TBI aggression is likely to be the impulsive subtype of aggression. Moreover, impulsive aggression is overrepresented among veterans with PTSD such that in one study over 70% of male veterans with PTSD compared to 29% of those without PTSD reported impulsive aggression (Teten et al. 2010). The frequent co-occurrence of PTSD and TBI (described below) may provide further evidence that post-TBI aggression is primarily impulsive aggression. Characterizing this problematic behavior would provide a framework for conceptualizing aggressive behaviors co-occurring with TBI and introduce novel approaches to treatment, such as anticonvulsants (Stanford et al. 2005) and cognitive behavioral therapy (McCloskey et al. 2008).

Orbitofrontal regions have been associated with alterations in behavior including impulse control since reports of the prototypical patient with frontal injury (Damasio et al. 1994; Stein and Moeller 2005). Studies specifically of impulsive aggression among individuals with TBI suggest associations with lesions of the ventromedial prefrontal cortex (Greve et al. 2002) using neuropsychological testing sensitive to this region (e.g., Revised Strategy Application Test). One difficulty in generalizing subtypes of aggression and their relationship to neuroanatomical underpinnings from the extensive literature on aggression in TBI is that impulsivity and impulsive aggression are often equated, whereas, at least in highly impulsive individuals with antisocial behavior, the degree of impulsivity does not itself distinguish those with predatory vs. impulsive aggression, but the existence of language impairments and parietal electrophysiological processing differences did distinguish them (Barratt et al. 1997a). This research suggests that impulsivity alone is not sufficient to cause an individual to become impulsively aggressive and it is likely that additional deficits that may be associated with TBI are important to this condition. Initial work in long-term survivors of severe TBI with impulsive aggression did not demonstrate these specific neuropsychological abnormalities, suggesting that there may be alternative pathways to impulsive aggression (Greve et al. 2001). However, in this study, premorbid functioning was associated with impulsive aggression, suggesting that it may be difficult retrospectively to delineate the specific contribution of the TBI to the behaviors of interest.

The Relationship Between Mild TBI and PTSD

There is considerable interest in the potential relationship between mTBI and PTSD given the context in which both occur during military deployment. To better understand this issue, a background on mTBI is provided with an emphasis on those characteristics that complicate the separation of the consequences of mTBI from PTSD.

Epidemiology and Classification of mTBI with a Focus on Symptoms

Approximately 70–90% of head injuries are classified as mild in nature (Kraus and Nourjah 1988; Sosin et al. 1996). Incidence rates of mTBI in the civilian population, however, are widely considered to be underestimated since approximately 25% of individuals suffering an mTBI do not seek medical attention (Centers for Disease Control and Prevention 2003). As with moderate to severe TBI, the rate of mTBI is greatest in males and young adults and the most common mechanisms include motor vehicle accidents and falls (Cassidy et al. 2004). Similar to the civilian population, the majority of military TBIs are mild. In fact, the incidence of mTBI in contemporary warfare may be on the rise due to the prevalent use of explosive munitions (i.e., IEDs and mines). In one study, 22.8% of soldiers returning from the Iraq War were noted to have a history of at least one mTBI during deployment, most of which were mild in nature (Terrio et al. 2009). It is estimated that by 2008 as many as 300,000 soldiers had suffered an mTBI in the wars in Iraq and Afghanistan (Tanielian and Jaycox 2008), although this may be an inflated estimate based on the lack of validity of the diagnostic criteria used to derive the approximation (Hoge et al. 2009). These issues are important to address as the definitions and context affect our understanding of the psychological and psychiatric effects of TBI.

Characterization of the personal and economic impact of mTBI is complicated by the lack of uniformity in the definition (Centers for Disease Control and Prevention 2003). The diagnosis of mTBI is based on the assessment of acute injury severity characteristics immediately following an injury to the head resulting from blunt trauma and/or acceleration or deceleration forces. Most contemporary mTBI classification schemes require a period of impaired consciousness (including loss of consciousness), memory dysfunction for a period of time surrounding the injury (i.e., retrograde or post-traumatic amnesia), or neurological or physiological dysfunction (e.g., seizures, lethargy, and vomiting) proximal to the time of injury. A consensus group associated with the American Congress of Rehabilitation Medicine (ACRM) defined mTBI as any one of the following: any period of loss of consciousness, any loss of memory for events before or after the accident, any alteration in mental state at the time of the accident, or any focal neurological deficits that may or may not be transient (ACRM 1993). Historically, this was an important departure from previously held notions that an observed loss of consciousness was required to establish a history of mTBI (Ruff 2005), although it should be noted that other diagnostic systems may require a loss of consciousness to establish a history of mTBI (Diagnostic and Statistical Manual of Mental Disorders-IV-TR 2000). In order to create a clearer boundary between those with mild versus those with moderate to severe TBI, the ACRM consensus group suggested that those with mTBI experience a loss of consciousness of no greater than 30 min, experience a post-traumatic amnesia of no greater than 24 h, and should have a Glasgow Coma Scale (GCS) score of 13 or greater within 30 min after their injury. The ACRM definition of mTBI has gained traction in the research and clinical community over the last 15 years and has been adapted by other health agencies (Centers for Disease Control and Prevention 2003).

Various subclassifications of mTBI have been also proposed which take into account the length of loss of consciousness or altered mental status as in the case of sports-related concussion (American Academy of Neurology 1997) or the presence or absence of positive neuroimaging findings (Levin et al. 1987). The American Academy of Neurology classification system specifies three grades of concussion: Grade 1 being defined by transient confusion, no loss of consciousness, and concussion symptoms or mental status abnormalities that resolve in less than 15 min; Grade 2 being defined by transient confusion, no loss of consciousness, and concussion symptoms or mental status abnormalities lasting more than 15 min; and Grade 3 being defined by any loss of consciousness. In the context of sports, the American Academy of Neurology recommends that only those players experiencing a Grade 1 concussion who demonstrate a normal sideline assessment (while at rest and with exertion) should return to play the same day. Players with persisting symptoms after a Grade 1 concussion and those with Grade 2 or 3 concussions should not return to play on the same day. In order to determine readiness to return to play and overall neurologic status after a concussion, the American Academy of Neurology also advocates for repeated observation and assessment over the course of recovery (American Academy of Neurology 1997).

Although general consensus has been reached regarding the diagnostic criteria for mTBI, several shortcomings of the diagnostic system have been identified. Without direct observation from trained bystanders or emergency medical technicians, there is no way to verify that the minimal criteria for mTBI were present at the time of the injury (i.e., brief period of altered mental status). Despite the apparent fallibility of relying on retrospective, self-reported changes in mental status to establish a history of mTBI, this is considered standard practice in diagnosing mTBI (Alexander 1995; Ruff 2005) and has been recommended by the Centers for Disease Control in cases of nonmedically attended TBI (Centers for Disease Control and Prevention 2003). Additionally, alcohol and recreational drugs present at the time of injury or therapeutic drugs administered in the immediate post-injury period can cause alterations in consciousness and perturbations in autobiographic memory, all of which can be mistaken for injury-related alterations in mental status (Ruff 2005).

Diagnosing a history of combat-related mTBI presents even greater challenges. First, a brief period of altered mental status may go unreported in the midst of life-threatening events like close proximity to a detonated IED, an event that has been exceedingly common during the Iraq and Afghanistan conflicts (Gondusky and Reiter 2005; Terrio et al. 2009). Second, symptoms related to mTBI may be overlooked in the presence of other combat-related injuries that require immediate medical attention (e.g., traumatic amputations, lacerations, and burns). These first two diagnostic issues would result in an underidentification of a history of mTBI. Third, common diagnostic criteria with reasonable specificity in the civilian population, such as feeling dazed or confused, may result in insufficient levels of specificity when applied to injuries incurred during combat deployments. Conversely, a brief period of confusion or disorientation may represent a psychological reaction to an unexpected, highly stressful event rather than a manifestation of underlying brain injury. The third diagnostic issue would, thus, result in an overidentification of a history of mTBI.

Although there is a rich literature evaluating the sequelae of TBI and a general sense of agreement in terms of outcomes following moderate to severe TBI, there is less consensus in terms of outcomes following mTBI. Many studies evaluating the impact of mTBI have had widely different findings (e.g., Binder et al. 1997; Rimel et al. 1981) and this, in turn, is likely related to the inherent methodological difficulties in studying this population. For example, many people do not seek treatment following mTBI as there is likely perception that mTBI will have few meaningful consequences. This sharply contrasts against the established and adverse consequences that are associated with moderate to severe TBIs. For those patients that do seek emergent care, a GCS may be obtained, but this instrument is not suited to assess the more subtle cognitive changes that are likely to occur following an mTBI (Lezak et al. 2004). Historically, the lack of agreement about the mTBI classification has made comparisons between studies difficult and has the potential to skew data in a variety of ways. In both clinical and research settings, comprehensive neuropsychological evaluations in the period following mTBI are typically not undertaken and even fewer evaluations are likely to occur at more distal time points. For this reason, comparatively less is known about the impact that mTBI has on neuropsychological functioning relative to moderate to severe head injuries. Even the most promising prospective studies are often hampered by significant selection biases (i.e., oversampling from emergent care settings and attrition in longitudinal designs), less effective use of appropriate controls, and not controlling for potential confounds (Carroll et al. 1994). Despite these limitations regarding mTBI, there are several tenets that can be drawn from the literature and we address these below.

Tenet 1: Injury Severity is Related to Outcome

In a series of widely recognized studies (Dikmen et al. 1995a, b), it was demonstrated that both cognitive and functional outcomes following head injury are related to severity of TBI, with mTBI having better outcomes and severe TBI having the worst outcomes. The strength of these studies is that a large number of patients ($N=436$), with various injury severities, completed assessments at 1 month and 12 months post-injury with minimal attrition. In addition to the within-subjects comparisons, their patients were also compared to a matched trauma control sample ($N=132$) also evaluated at 1 month and 1 year post-injury. Patients with a history of TBI increasing in severity from moderate to severe, as measured by increased time to follow commands (the motor score from the GCS), had an incrementally greater chance of having more widespread and persisting neuropsychological and functional impairments 1 year post-injury. Among patients with a history of mild head injury (TFC < 1 h), however, baseline performance on neuropsychological testing was similar to trauma controls at 1 month (Dikmen et al. 1995a) and the vast majority were noted to experience good psychosocial outcomes 1 year post-injury (Dikmen et al. 1995b).

mTBI can occur in the context of other factors such as positive CT findings (e.g., "complicated mTBI" [focal brain lesion, skull fracture, etc.]) and this may further cause difficulties in recovery. In keeping with the inverse relationship between injury severity and outcome, patients with a history of complicated mTBI appear to have poorer cognitive function within the first month following mTBI (Williams et al. 1990). Kwok et al. (2008) evaluated complicated mTBI patients ($N=31$) with GCS scores ranging from 13 to 15 with abnormal CT scans (skull fractures, hematomas, subarachnoid hemorrhage) and found persisting impairments in attention at 3 months. The performance of patients with a history of complicated mTBI has also been compared to the performance of patients with a history of moderate TBI. In this study, patients with a history of complicated mTBI ($N=102$) and moderate TBI ($N=127$) underwent neuropsychological testing at discharge from a rehabilitation facility and after 1 year. At both time points, there were noteworthy similarities between the mTBI and moderate TBI groups, with mTBI patients evidencing less severely impaired cognitive processing speed. Both groups were also noted to have incomplete recovery in functional status at the 1 year follow-up, with no differences found between the groups (Kashluba et al. 2008). There remains some debate as to whether complicated and uncomplicated mTBI patients should be pooled together in studies, or if those with complications should be viewed as a separate diagnostic group.

Tenet 2: Symptoms Immediately Following an mTBI Are Varied and May Occur Across Cognitive, Physical, and Affective Domains

Self-report symptom inventories (e.g., Rivermead Post-Concussion Symptoms Questionnaire [RPQ], Standardized Assessment of Concussion [SAC], etc.) have been utilized in the period following mTBI and in a variety of different settings (Potter et al. 2006; McCrea et al. 2000, see Alla et al. 2009 for review of various inventories). The most frequent subjective complaints following mTBI include headache, dizziness, irritability, poor concentration, fatigue, and memory loss, with the majority of symptoms resolving within 1 month (Ryan and Warden 2003; McCrea 2008). Across multiple factor analytical studies, these varied symptoms have been noted to load onto cognitive, physical, and affective clusters, although there is some debate as to whether a single factor that some label "concussion" better accounts for the symptoms (Potter et al. 2006; Smith-Seemiller et al. 2003; Piland et al. 2006).

A similar pattern of symptoms has also been described in the sports concussion literature, with headache, dizziness, sensitivity to light, and cognitive difficulties (e.g., slowed cognitive processing speed, memory difficulty) reported in the period following mTBI (McCrea 2008). In a large sample of college football players prospectively evaluated prior to mTBI and at several time points post-injury, more severe symptoms were noted immediately following the mTBI and patterns of symptom recovery emerged as early as 3 h post-injury (McCrea et al. 2003). Within 7 days post-injury, there were no differences relative to baseline scores or matched controls. It is important to note that there are noteworthy differences between the general population and athletes evaluated in the sports concussion literature, as "motivation to return to play" in the latter may result in underreporting of mTBI symptoms. This likely explains the interesting finding that athletes report faster resolution of symptoms relative to those in the general population, as 85% of athletes reported full symptom recovery within 1 week and fewer than 3% reported symptoms beyond 1 month (see NCAA Concussion Study; McCrea et al. 2003) in contrast to an appreciably higher proportion reported in the non-sports concussion literature (e.g., 8–33%; Lees-Haley et al. 2001; Ryan and Warden 2003; Rimel et al. 1981).

Tenet 3: The Vast Majority of mTBI Patients Will Experience Full Cognitive Recovery Within 3 Months

It is generally accepted that among patients sustaining an mTBI the majority of symptoms resolve during the first week following the injury, with nearly complete resolution of most symptoms for most patients occurring within the first 3 months following the injury (e.g., Dikmen et al. 1986; Levin et al. 1987; Schretlen and Shapiro 2003). Consistent with this, the World Health Organization (WHO) has concluded the best evidence suggesting: "there are no mTBI-attributable, objectively measured, cognitive deficits beyond 1–3 months' post-injury in the majority of cases" (Carroll et al. 1994). The WHO based their conclusions on a critical review of the literature and parallels the findings from meta-analytic studies evaluating patient performance on cognitive testing following mTBI. Binder et al. (1997) included studies evaluating the cognitive functioning in adults (11 studies, 314 patients, 308 controls) at least 30 days following mTBI. The overall effect size was significant, but small ($d=0.18$), although a more conservative g statistic was notably smaller and not significant ($g=0.07$). Patient performance on cognitive testing was further analyzed using neuropsychological domains of attention, memory acquisition, and performance skills (only three domains were examined across enough of the studies to allow for meaningful analyses). Among these three, only attention emerged as impaired following mTBI with a small effect size ($g=0.17$). The authors also found it worthwhile to determine the positive and negative predictive values (PPV and NPV) of neuropsychological testing in patients with mTBI in the reviewed studies, as the detection of more subtle cognitive difficulties is more difficult than obvious neurological impairments. Given the low prevalence of persisting attention impairments based on their data (5%), the likelihood of accurately classifying mTBI with abnormal performance on cognitive measures, even with unrealistic sensitivity and specificity for the cognitive instruments (e.g., 0.9), was small at 0.32, and with smaller sensitivity and specificity test values the PPVs continued to decrease. In contrast, the NPV of these cognitive measures was consistently high at all sensitivity and specificity levels (>0.98), suggesting much higher accuracy when diagnosing no persisting brain injury following mTBI based on neuropsychological measures.

More pronounced impairments in attention following mTBI have been reported in recent prospective studies (e.g., Kwok et al. 2008; Landre et al. 2006). Landre et al. (2006) found mTBI patients ($N=37$) to perform worse on measures of vigilance, attention, and memory relative to trauma patients ($N=32$) approximately 5 days post-injury. The effect sizes for these group differences were in the moderate to large range. Interestingly, both mTBI and the trauma controls reported few concussion symptoms following their injury and pain levels were controlled for and found not to be associated with cognitive performance in either group. That more pronounced cognitive impairments are found in some studies (e.g., Landre et al. 2006) but not others (e.g., Binder et al. 1997) may, in part, be related to the timing of neuropsychological evaluations relative to the onset of the head injury. For example, in the Binder et al. (1997) meta-analysis, only studies evaluating cognitive performance 3 months post-injury, or later, were included, whereas other studies may focus on patient cognitive performance within the first or second week following mTBI. Consistent with this, Schretlen and Shapiro (2003) examined the effect of mTBI on cognitive performance across different time points post-injury. In their meta-analysis, cognitive performance varied as a function of time, with a significant medium effect size reported among patients tested during the first 6 days post-injury ($d=0.41$, mTBI patients performing at the 33rd percentile of matched controls) and a smaller but significant effect size reported among patients tested 7–29 days post-injury ($d=0.29$). Patients tested 1–3 months post-injury, and after 3 months post-injury, demonstrated no differences from controls. Belanger et al. (2005) demonstrated a similar finding, with small performance declines across seven of eight cognitive domains for mTBI patients evaluated acutely (<90 days) relative to those mTBI patients evaluated post-acutely (≥90 days). Interestingly, in this meta-analysis, there was variability in performance across domains for those mTBI patients evaluated acutely, with the most pronounced effects of mTBI for delayed memory and verbal fluency.

Tenet 4: A Significant Minority of Patients Will Experience Persisting Post-concussive Syndrome Symptoms

It is important to note that individual patients may experience variability, both in terms of rate of recovery during this time period as well as between various symptom clusters (Dikmen et al. 1995b; McCrea 2008). For a "significant minority," there may be mTBI symptoms that extend beyond the expected 3-month recovery period (Belanger et al. 2005; Binder et al. 1997). The persistence of symptoms following mTBI is known as post-concussion syndrome (PCS) (e.g., PCS, typically greater than 3 months post-injury), although the nature and reasons for persistence of these symptoms is the source of much debate. The relationship between reported symptoms immediately following mTBI and persistence of post-concussion symptoms remains unclear, in part because there are few studies consistently and systematically evaluating these factors in the literature (Carroll et al. 1994).

There is limited evidence to suggest that headache and dizziness in the ER, and dizziness 2 weeks post-injury, may be predictive of persisting concussion symptoms (De Kruijk et al. 2002; Yang et al. 2009). However, it is also important to note that many symptoms associated with concussion are also endorsed at high rates in other populations. Headache, fatigue, forgetfulness, frustration, irritability, concentration difficulty, and sleep disturbance are among many overlapping symptoms reported at high rates and varying severity in college (Wang et al. 2006), claimant (Lees-Haley et al. 2001), adult control (Paniak et al. 2002a), and chronic pain populations (Iverson and McCracken 1997; Smith-Seemiller et al. 2003), although typically at lesser severity levels than those with mTBI within the first month post-injury (Carroll et al. 1994). In a landmark study that supports a cognitive-behavioral conceptualization for PCS etiology and informs current mTBI treatments, Mittenberg et al. (1992) suggest that patients have pre-injury *expectations* about mTBI symptoms and these, in turn, have the potential to become self-fulfilling. This was based on their finding that healthy adults endorsed symptoms they would expect to have 6 months following an mTBI at similar levels to patients with PCS (i.e., both reported similar levels of anxiety, depression, irritability, fatigue, memory difficulty). Additionally, when PCS patients were asked to estimate the same symptoms prior to their own injuries, compared to a healthy adult sample rating current symptoms, the PCS patients consistently reported fewer pre-injury problems. Thus, it is hypothesized that PCS patients have expectations regarding TBI which have the potential to form internal representations about outcomes. These representations have the potential to become self-fulfilling and may augment perceived intensity and frequency of PCS symptoms (Miller and Mittenberg 1998).

While post-concussion symptoms have been weakly linked to prognosis, multiple studies have demonstrated that compensation-seeking behavior is associated with persistence and severity of impairments as well as a delayed return to work and slowed recovery following mTBI (Binder and Rohling 1996; Carroll et al. 1994; Paniak et al. 2002b). Belanger et al. (2005) found that across studies, clinic-based samples including patients engaged in litigation were likely to have greater cognitive sequelae ($d = 0.74$ after 3 months) and that litigation was negatively associated with improvement of cognitive functioning over time. Conclusions related to the nature of this relationship are not addressed by correlative studies; the association could plausibly reflect more severe impairment independently leading to compensation seeking. Other moderating factors that have been less reliably related to PCS include being female, off work due to injury, and history of psychiatric illness. Prior psychiatric illness has also been identified as a risk factor for acute stress disorder following a motor vehicle collision and this is, in turn, a predictor of the later development of PTSD (Carroll et al. 1994).

Complicated Comorbidity: Mild TBI and PTSD

Exposure to trauma, such as the potentially life-threatening events often associated with an mTBI (e.g., motor vehicle accidents and combat), places individuals at risk for various psychiatric disorders, most notably PTSD. As defined by the American Psychiatric Association, PTSD is a constellation of symptoms including reexperiencing the event, avoidance of reminders of the event, and chronic hyperarousal that persist 3 months or more after exposure to a life-threatening trauma (APA 2000). Physical injury to the body and brain associated with a life-threatening trauma has been shown to further increase the likelihood of developing PTSD. Given the increased risk of both trauma and TBI in combat, the recent wars in Iraq and Afghanistan have highlighted the complications associated with identifying TBI in the context of PTSD and vice versa. In a sample of 100 soldiers with similar combat experience, 16.7% of those who incurred a bodily injury during combat met the criteria for PTSD after deployment, while only 2.5% of those without injury were diagnosed with PTSD (Koren et al. 2005). The association between injury and later development of PTSD appears to be even greater in the case of mTBI relative to other bodily injuries. Hoge et al. (2008) noted a strong association between combat-related mTBI and screening positive for PTSD. In a stratified sample of soldiers who reported a history of no injury, non-brain injury, mTBI with altered mental status, and mTBI with loss of consciousness, the rate of positive post-deployment PTSD screens rose steadily from 9.1% in the non-brain injury group to 43.9% in the mTBI with loss of consciousness group. What remains unclear is if this relation between PTSD and history of mTBI would be changed if more stringent diagnostic standards for PTSD and mTBI (i.e., clinician-confirmed diagnosis) were employed. This frequent occurrence of PTSD symptomatology after mTBI is not unique to military populations. Estimated rates of PTSD following mTBI have ranged from 17 to 33% in civilians with TBI (Bryant and Harvey 1995, 1998; Middelboe et al. 1991; Ohry et al. 1996), a rate of PTSD considerably higher than 7.8% lifetime prevalence rate noted in the civilian population (Kessler et al. 1995).

The topic of PTSD following mTBI has caused considerable controversy for two reasons. First, the development of PTSD is assumed to stem from intense psychological trauma wherein the perceived potential for loss of life is present. From this perceived threat at the time of the traumatic event, the individual subsequently "cannot forget" the trauma as evidenced through reexperiencing the trauma, avoiding situations that serve as reminders of the trauma, and hypervigilance towards perceived threats. It has been questioned whether this psychological response to a traumatic event can occur in the context of a TBI associated with loss of memory for the event.

An early study on this topic appeared to validate the logical conclusion that mTBI should serve as a protective factor against later PTSD (Sbordone and Liter 1995). Of the 70 patients with either PTSD or a history of mTBI included in this study, none of the patients with a history of TBI reported any reexperiencing symptoms, consistent with the expectation that an amnestic state associated with an mTBI would preclude later recall of the event. Of note, the majority of patients in this study either reported loss of consciousness or amnesia for the event (i.e., 85.7% reported a positive loss of consciousness and 96.4% reported amnesia for the event), suggesting that this sample may have included a disproportionate number of patients with somewhat more significant mTBIs. Contemporary diagnostic standards now require only a period of disorientation or confusion to denote the presence of an mTBI (ACRM 1993), indicating that many individuals in the general population who are diagnosed with mTBI do not suffer loss of consciousness or amnesia for the event. A more recent study exploring the association between memory for the traumatic event and later development of PTSD suggested that those patients with mTBI without amnesia for the event were at increased risk of developing PTSD relative to those patients without memory for the event (Gil et al. 2005). The representativeness of the 120 patients in this study has also been called into question, however, since all the patients required hospitalization for observation.

Other studies, however, have failed to support the hypothesis that amnesia for the traumatic event surrounding the mTBI reduces the likelihood of developing PTSD. A large-scale study of consecutively evaluated civilians indicated that a history of mTBI with loss of consciousness does appear to be a risk factor for development of PTSD (Mayou et al. 2000). In this study, individuals with a definite loss of consciousness secondary to mTBI were more likely to be diagnosed with PTSD 3 months post-injury than those patients without a clear loss of consciousness. In a smaller but well-designed study of consecutively admitted patients with an average of 9 h of post-traumatic amnesia, Bryant and Harvey (1998) also found an elevated rate of PTSD at 6 months post-injury. King (2008) offered three explanations for the paradoxical appearance of PTSD (especially reexperiencing symptoms) following an mTBI with apparent loss of consciousness or post-traumatic amnesia proximal to the traumatic event. First, it is possible that islands of memory persist during the period of apparent amnesia. Second, an implicit fear response may still be evoked when a person is exposed to stimuli reminiscent of the traumatic event even if there was a clear loss of consciousness. Lastly, individuals without memory for the traumatic event may develop imagined or reconstructed memories based on information provided by others.

Although some consensus regarding the occurrence of PTSD following mTBI has been reached, a second problem concerns the considerable overlap in PTSD and PCS. Symptoms common to both disorders include sleep disturbance, irritability, memory and concentration difficulties, reduced speed of processing, depression, fatigue, headaches, and nausea (King 2008). As might be expected, the presence of PTSD following mTBI is associated with increased post-concussion symptoms' report, and PTSD symptoms are correlated with post-concussion symptoms. In a sample of 105 motor vehicle collision survivors with and without mTBI, the frequency of reported post-concussion symptoms was greatest in individuals who sustained an mTBI and had been diagnosed with PTSD and overall report of PTSD symptoms was significantly correlated with the report of post-concussion symptoms (Bryant and Harvey 1999).

In the context of combat-related mTBI, the controversy of mTBI as a risk factor for PTSD is different. Unlike the civilian population where a single event is theorized to precipitate both the mTBI and subsequent PTSD, the traumatic event that is associated with a combat-related mTBI often represents perhaps one in a series of psychologically traumatic events taking place over several months. A study of soldiers returning from the wars in Afghanistan and Iraq showed that a history of mTBI is associated with multiple injuries and exposure to heighted combat intensity (Hoge et al. 2008). In this context, a diagnosis of mTBI simply serves as a proxy indicating a likely history of exposure to repeated, traumatic events, any of which could have contributed to the later development of PTSD. In a theater of combat, the relationship between mTBI and PTSD is extremely complex. Although further research is needed to better delineate the interplay between these two disorders, it could be hypothesized that an mTBI occurring in the context of acute stress disorder or PTSD has the potential to worsen the anxiety disorder through a temporary reduction in cognitive resources used to process the ongoing trauma. Conversely, chronic stress associated with the presence of acute stress disorder or PTSD could impede or otherwise alter the trajectory of the course of spontaneous recovery of cognitive functioning following mTBI. Further research is needed to determine what other physical and psychological comorbidities (i.e., chronic pain, depression, etc.) may share in this complex interplay. Needless to say, the considerable symptom overlap and the high rates of PTSD and mTBI comorbidity in returning combatants from Afghanistan and Iraq present diagnostic challenges even to highly trained specialists (Kennedy et al. 2007).

Treatment of Behavioral Disorders Following TBI

Treatment of behavioral problems following TBI, including impulsive aggression (IA), a hair-trigger response to a threat with a behavioral loss of control (Barratt et al. 1991), has been recently reviewed by Warden et al. (2006). This and earlier reviews of therapy (e.g., Silver and Yudofsky 1995) demonstrate a paucity of large randomized trials that address behavioral outcomes. While there is little in the way of large randomized, long-term trials specifically in TBI patients to recommend most therapies, promising research implicates certain pharmacological approaches, such as beta-adrenergic receptor blocking agents. Other potential agents, in which most work has involved aggression in other conditions but with some support following TBI, include anticonvulsant agents such as carbamazepine and valproic acid (Silver and Yudofsky 1995). Our own work with phenytoin shows a very specific benefit in reducing the severity and frequency of IA acts (Barratt et al. 1991, 1997), although this work was in patients with no evidence of past symptomatic TBI and with normal EEG. It remains to be studied whether this work will translate to patients post-TBI. As with all of these agents, a thorough understanding of their side effects is necessary to individual assessments of risk and benefits.

Treatment recommendations of behavioral disorders in TBI patients generally involve targeting symptoms, such as attention, mood, and psychotic symptoms. Evidence on effectiveness in the treatment of other psychiatric disorders occurring in the TBI patients is similarly limited, but general treatment recommendations include agents shown to be beneficial in these conditions in non-TBI patients including selective serotonin reuptake inhibitors and anticonvulsants as well as non-pharmacological, behavioral therapies (Deb and Crownshaw 2004; Warden et al. 2006). There is currently great interest in the possibility of treatment of PTSD in combat veterans using the adrenergic agent, prazosin (Raskin 2003). Benefit for nightmares was particularly noted, while improvement in other symptoms is also being investigated in an ongoing clinical trial.

There are several reviews addressing the efficacy of treatment for persistent PCS symptoms of mTBI (e.g., Borg et al. 2004; Comper et al. 2005; Snell et al. 2009), although there are few well-designed studies. Treatments following mTBI vary depending on factors, such as time since injury and the symptoms experienced following the event. In general, mTBI treatments can be viewed as falling into one or more of the following four categories: cognitive behavioral therapy, cognitive remediation, pharmacotherapy for symptom-based management, and education and support, depending upon the symptoms present. We present a basic treatment algorithm (see Fig. 13.1) that describes mTBI interventions, both for symptom reduction and prevention of PCS, for military personnel and veterans at various time points post-injury. This model assumes the presence of unit and military medical personnel who are familiar enough with injury severity

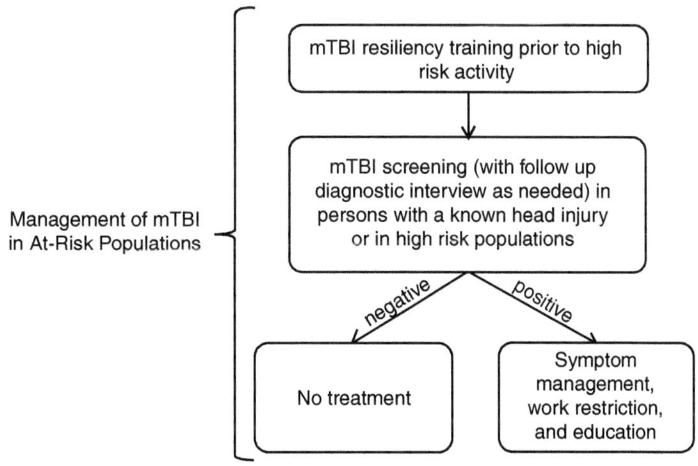

Fig. 13.1 Management of mTBI during acute recovery. The treatment algorithm for the management of mTBI during acute recovery is based on earlier work by Mittenberg et al. (1996), Paniak et al (1998), and others who have demonstrated the effectiveness of brief interventions for reducing the severity of symptoms following mTBI

characteristics to assist in classifying a suspected mTBI (see Fig. 13.1 level b).

Individual- and population-based mTBI screening instruments, such as the Standardized Assessment of Concussion (McCrea et al. 1998) upon which the more recent Military Acute Concussion Evaluation is based (Knuth et al. 2005) and the Brief Traumatic Brain Injury Screen (Schwab et al. 2007), have shown promise, although verification of the diagnosis through follow-up clinical interview is still necessary due to false-positive errors. As described earlier in this chapter, consensus criteria for concussion/mTBI are available to improve diagnostic accuracy (American Academy of Neurology 1997; ACRM 1993). Once the diagnosis has been verified and the specific symptoms have been detailed through clinical interview, symptom management and work restrictions should be considered, with the goals being to maximize functional recovery (Jaffee et al. 2009). While these first two aspects of treatment are meant to reduce the immediate impact of mTBI, the third component of treatment is aimed at reducing the subsequent development of PCS. It is during this period of time shortly following mTBI that psycho-education has been determined to be the most effective for the purpose of reducing subsequent PCS (Borg et al. 2004). However, it is important to note that in the WHO review of mTBI interventions, no treatments were found to provide clinically important effects on symptoms or disability, although there was some evidence to suggest that early education and limited support (e.g., information about common complaints and the likelihood for a good outcome) as to the effects of mTBI may reduce future symptom complaints (Borg et al. 2004). This approach of intervening after exposure to a trauma in order to reduce the likelihood of future maladjustment has also met with success in the management of PTS symptoms in military personnel following combat deployment (Adler et al. 2009).

Based upon their research regarding misappraisal of symptoms in mTBI patients (see above), Mittenberg et al. (1996) developed an effective, brief 1-h educational intervention. The effectiveness of this intervention in decreasing later post-concussive symptoms was demonstrated in 58 consecutive mTBI hospital admissions (GCS ≥ 13, Galveston Orientation and Amnesia Test score >75, no significant extracranial injuries). Half of the patients were randomized into a treatment arm during which time they met with a therapist to discuss symptoms for approximately 1 h and were provided with educational materials. The other patients received routine care and were provided with written discharge instructions that were verbally reviewed by a nurse. Six months after admission, mTBI patients in the treatment arm reported reduced symptom duration (33 days vs. 51 days) and a lower number of post-concussive symptoms (1.6 symptoms vs. 3.1) relative to the patients who received the standard of care (Mittenberg et al. 1996; Miller and Mittenberg 1998). More recently, psycho-education and support provided via telephone calls (four calls at 2, 4, 8, and 12 weeks post-injury) were also shown to be effective at reducing post-concussive symptoms 6 months post-mTBI relative to standard emergency room care (e.g., instruction handout) (Bell et al. 2008). The relative benefit of the follow-up telephone calls is difficult to determine due to the design of the study, although the results of other mTBI intervention studies indicate that more than one treatment session may not have an added benefit (Paniak et al. 1998, 2000).

Diagnostic criteria have also been developed to identify those individuals who experience an abnormal persistence of post-concussion symptoms following mTBI, otherwise known as PCS. The International Classification of Diseases, Tenth Revision, criteria include a history of TBI and the presence of three or more of the following eight symptoms: headache, dizziness, fatigue, irritability, insomnia, concentration difficulty, memory difficulty, and intolerance of stress, emotion, or alcohol (World Health Organization 1993). Proposed criteria for the diagnosis of post-concussional disorder have also been put forth for further research in the Diagnostic and Statistical Manual of Mental Disorder, Fourth Edition—Text Revision (American Psychiatric Association 2000). These criteria are as follows: (A) history of TBI causing "significant cerebral concussion;" (B) cognitive deficit in attention and/or memory; (C) presence of at least three of the following symptoms, e.g., fatigue, sleep disturbance, headache, dizziness, irritability, affective disturbance, personality change, and apathy, that appear after injury and persist for ≥3 months; (D) symptoms begin or worsen after injury; (E) symptoms interfere with social role functioning; and (F) exclusion of dementia due to head trauma and other disorders that better account for the symptoms. Boake et al. (2005) noted that the prevalence of diagnosed PCS was higher 3 months post-injury using the ICD-10 criteria (64%) relative to the DSM-IV-TR criteria (11%) in a sample of 178 adults with mild-to-moderate TBI, although both criteria showed poor specificity when tested with a control sample of 104 adults with extracranial injuries. The authors note that the relatively limited ICD-10 PCS criteria likely contributed to the higher diagnostic rates using that classification scheme, while the lack of specificity demonstrated by both classification schemes was due to the frequent endorsement of symptoms by patients without cranial injuries.

For military personnel who subsequently develop PCS, the Department of Veterans Affairs and Department of Defense recommend a combination of both psycho-education and symptom management (see Fig. 13.2) (Department of Veterans Affairs and Department of Defense 2009). The effectiveness of this treatment paradigm, especially the provision of psycho-education to veterans who may be several years post-injury, has yet to be determined. From a theoretical standpoint, it may be possible that allowing PCS to develop without early education allows patients to develop resistance to subsequent attempts at reducing PCS through education. That is, once erroneous expectations about consequences of mTBI are left unchecked for many months or years post-injury, patients may be reticent to consider other causes of their symptoms. Lastly, we also believe that there may be some benefit to early psycho-educational intervention for military personnel prior to deployment in that education at this level may provide resiliency in terms of subsequent development of PCS following mTBI. At present, there are no studies addressing the effectiveness of pre-deployment resiliency training. We believe, however, that this is a natural extension of the literature and is meant to augment, rather than replace, psycho-educational interventions that should occur immediately after a soldier sustains an mTBI.

Conclusion: Behavioral and Psychiatric Comorbidities of TBI

Extensive evidence associates TBI with psychiatric and behavioral sequelae. While the design of these studies makes it often difficult to differentiate symptoms based on severity of injury,

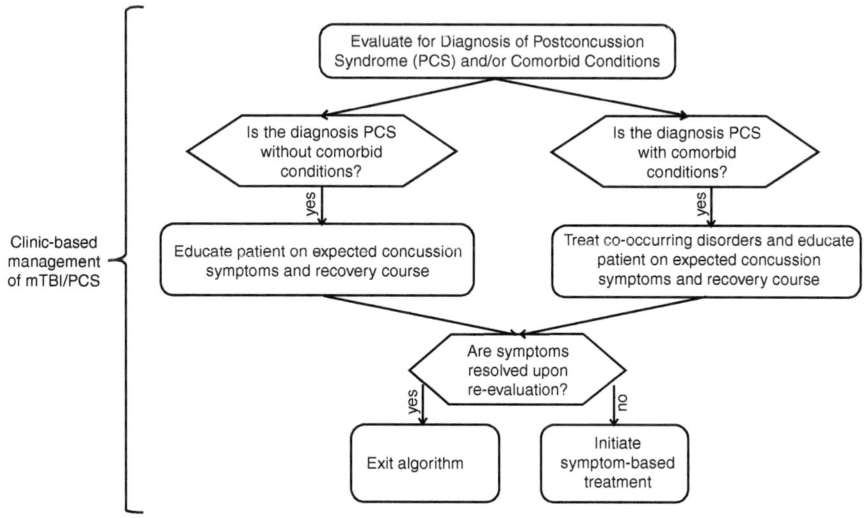

Fig. 13.2 Management of PCS. The treatment algorithm for the management of PCS is designed in part after the treatment recommendations offered by the Department of Veterans Affairs and Department of Defense (2009)

premorbid deficits, and functioning from the contribution of the TBI, it seems very likely that at the minimum, TBI is a risk for accentuating premorbid behaviors (Greve et al. 2001), and individual cases indicate the potential for profound behavioral change (Damasio et al. 1994). The mechanism of these effects has not been examined, although changes in self-regulation and social information processing may result from neurological insult, psychiatric symptoms, or substance use. On the other hand, it is also conceivable that psychiatric disorder and TBI become difficult to distinguish from an epidemiological perspective given that circumstances may put an individual at risk for both (Hoge et al. 2008). In this case, prospective studies and treatment interventions will be needed to identify the salient underlying disorders. Several research groups are pursuing a variety of imaging, neuropsychological, and treatment studies to identify characteristics that would contribute to this distinction. In the interim, it is important from a patient care perspective to identify treatable behaviors that are causing distress to the patients or those around them. While definitive evidence for efficacy is in many cases lacking, a number of reasonable suggestions or extrapolations from other conditions have been reported that provide a starting point to develop a treatment plan. However, lack of definitive evidence for efficacy or the possibility of a unique sensitivity to adverse events affecting TBI patients suggests that treatment should be approached with an appreciation for potential difficulties.

References

Adler AB, Bliese PD, McGurk D, Hoge CW, Castro CA. Battlemind debriefing and battlemind training as early interventions with soldiers returning from Iraq: randomization by platoon. J Consult Clin Psychol. 2009;77:928–40.

Alderman N, Knight C, Morgan C. Use of a modified version of the Overt Aggression Scale in the measurement and assessment of aggressive behaviours following brain injury. Brain Inj. 1997;11(7):503–23.

Alderman N. Prevalence, characteristics and causes of aggressive behaviour observed within a neurobehavioural rehabilitation service: Predictors and implications for management. Brain Injury. 2007;21(9):891–911.

Alexander MP. Mild traumatic brain injury: pathophysiology, natural history and clinical management. Neurology. 1995;45:1253–60.

Alla S, Sullivan S, Hale L, McCrory P. Self report scales/checklists for the measurement of concussion symptoms: a systematic review. Br J Sports Med. 2009;43:i3–12.

American Academy of Neurology. Practice parameter: the management of concussion in sports. Neurology. 1997;48:581–5.

American Congress of Rehabilitation Medicine. Definition of mild traumatic brain injury. J Head Trauma Rehabil. 1993;8:86–7.

American Psychiatric Association. Diagnostic and statistical manual of mental disorders, fourth edition, text revision. Washington, DC: American Psychiatric Association; 2000.

Arango-Lasprilla JC, Ketchum JM, Dezfulian T, Kreutzer JS, O'neil-Pirozzi TM, Hammond F, Jha A. Predictors of marital stability 2 years following traumatic brain injury. Brain Injury. 2008;22(7):565–74.

Baguley IJ, Cooper J, Felmingham KL. Aggressive behavior following traumatic brain injury: How common is common? Journal of Head Trauma Rehabilitation. 2006;21:45–57.

Barratt ES, Kent TA, Bryant SG, Felthous AR: A controlled trial of phenytoin in impulsive aggression. J Clin Psychopharmacol 1991;11:388–9.

Barratt ES, Stanford MS, Kent TA, et al: Neuropsychological and cognitive psychophysiological substrates of impulsive aggression. Biol Psychiatry 1997; 41:1045–1047.

Barratt ES, Stanford MS, Kent TA, et al. Neuropsychological and cognitive psychophysiological substrates of impulsive aggression. Biol Psychiatry. 1997a;41:1045–7.

Barratt ES, Stanford MS, Felthous AR, Kent TA. The effects of phenytoin on impulsive and premeditated aggression: a controlled study (1997a). J Clin Psychopharmacol. 1997b;17(5):341–9.

Bay E, Donders J. Risk factors for depressive symptoms after mild-to-moderate traumatic brain injury Brain Injury. 2008;22(3):233–41.

Beck AT, Steer RA, Garbin MG. Psychometric properties of the Beck Depression Inventory: twenty-five years of evaluation. Clin Psychol Rev. 1988;8:77–100.

Belanger HG, Curtiss G, Demery JA, Lebowitz BK, Vanderploeg RD. Factors moderating neuropsychological outcomes following mild traumatic brain injury: A meta-analysis. Journal of the International Neuropsychological Society. 2005;11:215–27.

Bell KR, Hoffman JM, Temkin NR, Powell JM, Fraser RT, Esselman PC, Barber JK, Dikmen S. The effect of telephone counseling on reducing post-injury traumatic symptoms after mild traumatic brain injury: a randomized trial. J Neurol Neurosurg Psychiatry. 2008;79:1275–81.

Binder LM, Rohling ML. Money matters: a meta-analytic review of the effects of financial incentives on recovery after closed head injury. Am J Psychiatry. 1996;153:7–10.

Binder LM, Rohling ML, Larrabee GL. A review of mild head trauma. Part I: meta-analytic review of neuropsychological studies. J Clin Exp Neuropsychol. 1997;19:421–31.

Boake C, McCauley SR, Levin HS, Pedroza C, Contant CF, et al. Diagnostic criteria for post-concussional syndrome after mild to moderate traumatic brain injury. J Neuropsychiatry Clin Neurosci. 2005;17:350–6.

Borg J, Holm L, Peloso PM, Cassidy JD, von Holst H, Cassidy JD, et al. Non-surgical intervention and cost for mild traumatic brain injury: results of the WHO collaborating centre task force in mild traumatic brain injury. J Rehabil Med. 2004;43:76–83.

Brain Injury Association of America. TBI Incidence Factsheet. Retrieved 11 April 2009 from: http://www.biausa.org/elements/aboutbi/factsheets/TBIincidence.pdf.

Brewer-Smyth, K., Burgess, AW, Shults, J. Physical and sexual abuse, salivary cortisol, and neurologic correlates of violent criminal behaviors in female prison inmates. Biological Psychiatry. 2004;55:21–31.

Bryant RA. Posttraumatic stress disorder and traumatic brain injury: Can they co-exist? Clinical Psychology Review. 2001;21:931–48.

Bryant RA, Harvey AG. Acute stress response: a comparison of head injured and non-head injured patients. Psychol Med. 1995;25:869–74.

Bryant RA, Harvey AG. Relationship between acute stress disorder and posttraumatic stress disorder following mild traumatic brain injury. Am J Psychiatry. 1998;155: 625–9.

Bryant RA, Harvey AG. Postconcussive symptoms and posttraumatic stress disorder after mild traumatic brain injury. J Nerv Ment Dis. 1999;187:302–5.

Buss AH, Perry M. The Aggression Questionnaire. J Pers Soc Psychol. 1992;63:452–9.

Carroll LJ, Cassidy D, Peloso PM, Borg J, Holst H, Holm L, Paniak C, Pepin M. Prognosis for mild traumatic brain injury: results of the WHO collaborating centre task force and mild traumatic brain injury. J Rehabil Med. 1994;43:84–105.

Cassidy JD, Carroll LJ, Peloso PM, Borg J, von Holst H, et al. Incidence, risk factors and prevention of mild traumatic brain injury: results of the WHO Collaborating Centre Task Force on Mild Traumatic Brain Injury. J Rehabil Med. 2004;43:28–60.

Centers for Disease Control and Prevention, National Center for Injury Prevention and Control. Report to Congress on mild traumatic brain injury in the United States: steps to prevent a serious public health problem. Atlanta, GA: Centers for Disease Control and Prevention; 2003.

Chamelian L, Feinstein A. The effects of major depression on subjective and objective cognitive deficits in mild to moderate traumatic brain injury; 2006.

Champion HR, Holcomb JB, Young LA. Injuries from explosions. Journal of Trauma. 2009;66(5):1468–76.

Comper P, Bisschop S, Carnide N, Triccio A. A systematic review of treatments for mild traumatic brain injury. Brain Inj. 2005;19:863–80.

Damasio H, Grabowski T, Frank R, Galaburda AM, Damasio AR. The return of Phineas Gage: clues about the brain from the skull of a famous patient. Science. 1994;264:1102–5.

Deb S, Crownshaw T. The role of pharmacotherapy in the management of behaviour disorders in traumatic brain injury patients. Brain Inj. 2004;18:1–31.

De Kruijk JR, Leffers P, Menheere P, Meerhoff S, Rutten J, Twijnstra A. Prediction of post-traumatic complaints after mild traumatic brain injury: early symptoms and biochemical markers. J Neurol Neurosurg Psychiatry. 2002;73:727–32.

DelBello MP, Soutullo CA, Zimmerman ME, Sax KW, Williams JR, McElroy SL, Strakowski SM. Traumatic brain injury in individuals convicted of sexual offenses with and without bipolar disorder. Psychiatry Research. 1999;89:281–86.

Department of Veterans Affairs & Department of Defense. VA/DOD clinical practice guideline for management of concussion/mild traumatic brain injury (v1.0); 2009.

Dikmen S, McLean A, Temkin N. Neuropsychological and psychosocial consequences of minor head injury. J Neurol Neurosurg Psychiatry. 1986;49:1227–32.

Dikmen S, Machamer J, Winn H, Temkin N. Neuropsychological outcome at 1-year post head injury. Neuropsychology. 1995a;9:80–90.

Dikmen S, Ross B, Machamer J, Tempkin N. One year psychosocial outcome in head injury. J Int Neuropsychol Soc. 1995b;1:67–77.

Draper K, Ponsford J, Schonberger M. Psychosocial and emotional outcomes 10 years following traumatic brain injury. Journal of Head Trauma Rehabilitation. 2007;22:278–87.

Dyer KFW, Bell R, McCann J, Rauch R. Aggression after traumatic brain injury: Analysing socially desirable responses and the nature of aggressive traits', Brain Injury. 2006;20(11):1163–73.

Fann JR, Katon WJ, Uomoto JM, Esselman PC. Psychiatric disorders and functional disability in outpatients with traumatic brain injuries. Am J Psychiatry. 1995;152(10): 1493–99.

Faul M, Xu L, Wald MM, Coronado VG. Traumatic brain injury in the United States: emergency department visits, hospitalizations, and deaths. Atlanta (GA): Centers for Disease Control and Prevention, National Center for Injury Prevention and Control; 2010.

Gil S, Caspi Y, Ben-Ari IZ, Koren D, Klein E. Does memory of a traumatic event increase the risk for posttraumatic stress disorder in patients with traumatic brain injury? A prospective study. Am J Psychiatry. 2005;162: 963–9.

Glenn MB, O'Neil-Pirozzi T, Goldstein R, Burke D, Jacob L. Depression amongst outpatients with traumatic brain injury. Brain Inj. 2001;15(9):811–18.

Gondusky JS, Reiter MP. Protecting military convoys in Iraq: an examination of battle injuries sustained by a mechanized battalion during Operation Iraqi Freedom II. Mil Med. 2005;170:546–9.

Grafman J, Schwab K, Warden D, Pridgen A, Brown HR, Salazar AM. Frontal lobe injuries, violence, and aggression: a report of the Vietnam Head Injury Study. Neurology. 1996;46:1231–38.

Greve KW, Sherwin E, Stanford MS, et al. Personality and neurocognitive correlates of impulsive aggression in long-term survivors of severe traumatic brain injury. Brain Inj. 2001;15:255–62.

Greve KW, Love J, Sherwin E, et al. Cognitive strategy usage in long term survivors of severe traumatic brain injury with persisting impulsive aggression. Pers Indiv Differ. 2002;32:639–47.

Hoge CW, Goldberg HM, Castro CA. Care of war veterans with mild traumatic brain injury-flawed perspective. N Engl J Med. 2009;360:1588–91.

Hoge CW, McGurk D, Thomas JL, Cox AL, Engel CC, et al. Mild traumatic brain injury in U.S. soldiers returning from Iraq. N Engl J Med. 2008;358:453–63.

Haller J, Kruk MR. Normal and abnormal aggression: human disorders and novel laboratory models. Neurosci Biobehav Rev. 2006;30(3):292–303.

Hibbard MR, Uysal S, Kepler K, Bogdany J, Silver J. Axis I psychopathology in individuals with traumatic brain injury. J Head Trauma Rehabil. 1998;13(4):24–39.

Hibbard MR, Ashman TA, Spielman LA, Chun D, Charatz HJ, Melvin S. Relationship between depression and psychosocial functioning after traumatic brain injury. Arch Phys Med Rehabil. 2004;85(4 suppl 2)43–53.

Hoaken PNS, Steward SH. Drugs of abuse and the elicitation of human aggressive behavior. Addict Behav. 2003;28:1533–54.

Horner, MD, Selassie, AW, Lineberry, L, Ferguson, PL, Labbate, LA. Predictors of psychological symptoms 1 year after traumatic brain injury: A population-based epidemiological study. Journal of Head Trauma Rehabilitation. 2008;23:74–83.

Iverson GL, McCracken LM. "Postconcussive" symptoms in persons with chronic pain. Brain Inj. 1997;11:783–90.

Jaffee MS, Helmick KM, Girard PD, Meyer KS, Dinegar K, et al. Acute clinical care and care coordination for traumatic brain injury within Department of Defense. J Rehabil Res Dev. 2009;46:655–66.

Johnson R, Balleny H. Behaviour problems after brain injury: incidence and need for treatment. Clin Rehabil. 1996;10:173–81.

Jorge R, Robinson RG. Mood disorders following traumatic brain injury. Neurorehabilitation. 2002;17(4):311–24.

Kashluba S, Hanks RA, Casey JE, Millis SR. Neuropsychologic and functional outcome after complicated mild traumatic brain injury. Arch Phys Med Rehabil. 2008;89:904–11.

Keiski MA, Shore DL, Hamilton, JM. The Role of Depression in Verbal Memory Following Traumatic Brain Injury. The Clinical Neuropsychologist. 2006; 21(5).744–61.

Kelly G, Brown S, Todd J, Kremer P. Challenging behaviour profiles of people with acquired brain injury living in community settings. Brain Injury. 2008; 22(6):457–70.

Kennedy JE, Jaffee MS, Leskin GA, Stokes JW, Leal FO, et al. Posttraumatic stress disorder and posttraumatic stress disorder-like symptoms and mild traumatic brain injury. J Rehabil Res Dev. 2007;44:895–920.

Kessler RC, Chiu WT, Demler O, Walters EE. Prevalence, severity, and comorbidity of twelve-month DSM-IV-TR disorders in the National Comorbidity Survey Replication (NCS-R). Arch Gen Psychiatry. 2005; 62(6):617–27.

Kessler RC, Sonnega A, Bromet E, Hughes M, Nelson CB. Posttraumatic stress disorder in the National Comorbidity Survey. Arch Gen Psychiatry. 1995;52: 1048–60.

Kim E. Agitation, aggression, and disinhibition syndromes after traumatic brain injury. Neurorehabilitation. 2002;17: 297–310.

King NS. PTSD and traumatic brain injury: folklore and fact? Brain Inj. 2008;22:1–5.

Knuth T, Letarte PB, Ling G, Moores LE, Rhee P, et al. Guidelines for the field management of combat related head trauma. New York, NY: Brain Trauma Foundation; 2005. p. 2005.

Koren D, Norman D, Cohen A, Berman J, Klein EM. Increased PTSD risk with combat-related injury: a matched comparison study of injured and uninjured soldiers experiencing the same combat events. Am J Psychiatry. 2005;162:276–82.

Kraus JF, Nourjah P. The epidemiology of mild, uncomplicated brain injury. J Trauma. 1988;28:1637–43.

Kwok FA, Lee TM, Leung CH, Poon WS. Changes of cognitive functioning following mild traumatic brain injury over a 3-month period. Brain Injury. 2008;22: 740–51.

Landre N, Poppe CJ, Davis N, Schmaus B, Hobbs SE. Cognitive functioning and postconcussive symptoms in trauma patients with and without mild TBI. Archives of Clinical Neuropsychology. 2006;21:255–73.

Lees-Haley PR, Fox DD, Courtney JC. A comparison of complaints by mild brain injury claimants and other claimants describing subjective experiences immediately following their injury. Arch Clin Neuropsychol. 2001;16:689–95.

Levin HS, Amparo E, Eisenberg HM, Williams DH, High Jr WM, et al. Magnetic resonance imaging and computerized tomography in relation to the neurobehavioral sequelae of mild and moderate head injuries. J Neurosurg. 1987;66:706–13.

Levin HS, et al. Depression and posttraumatic stress disorder at three months after mild to moderate traumatic brain injury. J Clin Exp Neuropsychol. 2001;23: 754–69.

Levin HS, McCauley SR, Pedroza Josic C, Boake C, Brown SA, Goodman HS, Merrit SG, Brundage SI. Predicting depression following mild traumatic brain injury. Arch Gen Psychiatry. 2005;62:523–8.

Lezak M, Howieson D, Loring D. Neuropsychological assessment. 4th ed. New York, NY: Oxford University Press; 2004.

Machamer JE, Temkin NR, Dikmen SS. Neurobehavioral outcome in persons with violent or normal traumatic brain injury. Journal of Head Trauma Rehabilitation. 2003;18;387–97.

Maiuro RD, Vitaliano PP, Chan TS. A brief measure of for the assessment of anger and aggression. J Interpers Violence. 1987;2:166–78.

Marsh NV, Martinovich WM. Executive dysfunction and domestic violence. Brain Inj. 2006;20(1):61–6.

Mayou RA, Black J, Bryant B. Unconsciousness, amnesia, and psychiatric symptoms following road traffic accident injury. Br J Psychiatry. 2000;177:540–5.

McCloskey MS, Noblett KL, Deffenbacher JL, Gollan JK, Coccaro EF. Cognitive-behavioral therapy for intermittent explosive disorder: A pilot randomized clinical trial. Journal of Consulting and Clinical Psychology. 2008;76:876–86.

McCrea M, Guskiewicz KM, Marshall SW. Acute effects and recovery time following concussion in collegiate football players: the NCAA concussion study. JAMA. 2003;290:2556–63.

McCrea M, Kelly JP, Randolph C, Kluge J, Bartolic E, et al. Standardized assessment of concussion (SAC): on-site mental status evaluation of the athlete. J Head Trauma Rehabil. 1998;13:27–35.

McCrea M. Mild traumatic brain injury and postconcussion syndrome: the new evidence base for diagnosis and treatment. New York, NY: Oxford University Press; 2008.

McCrea M, Randolph C, Kelly JP. Standardized Assessment for Concussion (SAC): manual for administration, scoring, and interpretation. 2nd ed. Waukesha, WI: CNS Inc.; 2000.

Mental Health Advisory Team V (2008). Full Report. Retrieved from: http://www.armymedicine.army.mil/reports/mhat/mhat_v/mhat-v.cfm.

Middelboe T, Anderson HS, Birket-Smith M, Friis ML. Minor head injury: impact on general health after 1 year. A prospective follow-up study. Acta Neurol Scand. 1991;85:5–9.

Miller L, Mittenberg W. Brief cognitive behavioral interventions in mild traumatic brain injury. Appl Neuropsychol. 1998;5:172–83.

Miller LA, Collins RL, Kent TA. Language and the modulation of impulsive aggression. The Journal of Neuropsychiatry and Clinical Neurosciences. 2008; 20:261–73.

Mittenberg W, DiGiulio DV, Perrin S, Bass AE. Symptoms following mild head injury: expectation as aetiology. J Neurol Neurosurg Psychiatry. 1992;55:200–4.

Mittenberg W, Tremont G, Zielinski RE, Fichera S, Rayls KR. Cognitive-behavioral prevention of postconcussion syndrome. Arch Clin Neuropsychol. 1996;11: 139–45.

Moeller FG, Barratt ES, Dougherty DM, Schmitz JM, Swann AC. Psychiatric aspect of impulsivity. Am J Psychiatry. 2001;158:1783–93.

Moldover JE, Goldberg KB, ProutMF. Depression after traumatic brain injury: a review of evidence for clinical heterogeneity. Neuropsychol Rev. 2004;14(3):143–54.

Mooney G, Speed J, Sheppard S. Factors related to recovery after mild traumatic brain injury. Brain Injury. 2005;19:12975–87.

Moore EL, Terryberry-Spohr L, Hope DA. Mild traumatic brain injury and anxiety sequelae: a review of the literature. Brain Inj. 2006;20:117–32.

National Institute of Neurological Disorders and Stroke. Traumatic Brain Injury: Hope through Research. Bethesda, MD: National Institute of Health; 2002.

Niemeier JP, Marwitz JH, Lesher K, Walker WC, Bushnik T. Gender differences in executive functions following traumatic brain injury. 2007;17:293–313.

Nott MT, Chapparo C, Baguley IJ. Agitation following traumatic brain injury: An Australian sample. Brain Injury. 2006;20(11):1175–82.

Ohry A, Rattok J, Solomon Z. Post-traumatic stress disorder in brain injury patients. Brain Inj. 1996;10:687–95.

Orth U, Wieland E. Anger, hostility, and posttraumatic stress disorder in trauma-exposed adults: a meta-analysis. J Consult Clin Psychol. 2006;74:698–706.

Oquendo MA, Friedman JH, Grunebaum MF, Burke A, Silver JM, Mann JJ. Suicidal behavior and mild traumatic brain injury in major depression. Journal of Nervous and Mental Disease. 2004;192:430–34.

Paniak C, Reynolds S, Phillips K, Toller-Lobe G, Melnyk A, Nagy J. Patient complaints within 1 month of mild traumatic brain injury: a controlled study. Arch Clin Neuropsychol. 2002a;17:319–34.

Paniak C, Reynolds S, Toller-Lobe G, Melnyk A, Nagy J. A longitudinal study of the relationship between financial compensation and symptoms after treated mild traumatic brain injury. J Clin Exp Neuropsychol. 2002b;24:187–93.

Paniak C, Toller-Lobe G, Durand J, Nagy J. A randomized trial of two treatments for mild traumatic brain injury. Brain Inj. 1998;12:1011–23.

Paniak C, Toller-Lobe G, Reynolds S, Melnyk A, Nagy J. A randomized trial of two treatments for mild traumatic brain injury: 1 year follow up. Brain Inj. 2000;14:219–26.

Pietrzak RH, Johnson DC, Goldstein MB, Malley JC, Southwick SM. Posttraumatic stress disorder mediates the relationship between mild traumatic brain injury and health and psychosocial functioning in veterans of Operations Enduring Freedom and Iraqi Freedom. J NervMent Dis. 2009;197:748–53.

Piland SG, Motl RW, Guskiewicz KM, McCrea M, Ferrara MS. Structural validity of a self-report concussion-related symptom scale. Med Sci Sports Exer. 2006;38:27–32.

Potter S, Leigh E, Wade D, Fleminger S. The Rivermead Post Concussion Symptoms Questionnaire: a confirmatory factor analysis. J Neurol. 2006;253:1603–14.

Rapoport MJ, McCullagh S, Streiner D, Feinstein A. Age and major depression after mild traumatic brain injury. Am J Geriatr Psychiatry. 2003;11:365–9.

Raskin MA. Reduction of nightmares and other PTSD symptoms in combat veterans by prazosin: a placebo-controlled study. Am J Psychiary. 2003;160:371–3.

Rimel RW, Giordani B, Barth JT, Boll TJ, Jane JA. Disability caused by minor head injury. Neurosurgery. 1981;9:221–8.

Rosenthal M, Christensen BK, Ross TP. Depression following traumatic brain injury. Arch Phys Med Rehabil. 1998;79(1):90–103.

Ruff R. Two decades of advances in understanding of mild traumatic brain injury. J Head Trauma Rehabil. 2005;20:5–18.

Ryan LM, Warden DL. Post concussion syndrome. Int Rev Psychiatry. 2003;15:310–6.

Sbordone RJ, Liter JC. Mild traumatic brain injury does not produce post-traumatic stress disorder. Brain Inj. 1995;9:405–12.

Schretlen DJ, Shapiro AM. A quantitative review of the effects of traumatic brain injury on cognitive functioning. Int Rev Psychiatry. 2003;15:341–9.

Schopp LH, Shigaki CL, Bounds TA, Johnstone B, Stucky RC, Conway, BA. Outcomes in TBI with violent versus nonviolent etiology in a predominantly rural setting. Journal of Head Trauma Rehabilitation. 2006;21:213–25.

Schwab KA, Warden D, Lux WE, Shupenko LA, Zitnay G. Defense and Veteran Brain Injury Center: Peacetime and wartime missions. Journal of Rehabilitation Research and Development. 2007; xiii–xxi.

Seel RT, Kreutzer JS, Rosenthal M, Hammond FM, Corrigan JD, Black K. Depression after traumatic brain injury: a National Institute on Disability and Rehabilitation Research Model Systems multicenter investigation. Arch PhysMed Rehabil. 2003;84(2):177–84.

Silver JM, Yudofsky SC. Organic mental disorders and impulsive aggression in impulsivity and aggression. In: Hollander E, Stein DJ, editors. John Wiley & Sons, Ltd; 1995.

Simpson G, Tate R. Suicidality in people surviving a traumatic brain injury: prevalence, risk factors and implications for clinical management. Brain Inj. 2007;21:1335–51.

Slaughter B, Fann JR, Ehde D. Traumatic brain injury in a county jail population: prevalence, neuropsychological functioning and psychiatric disorders. Brain Injury. 2003;17(9):731–41.

Smith-Seemiller L, Fow NR, Kant R, Franzen MD. Presence of post-concussion syndrome symptoms in patients with chronic pain vs mild traumatic brain injury. Brain Inj. 2003;17:199–206.

Snell DL, Surgenor LJ, Hay-Smith JC, Siegert RJ. A systematic review of psychological treatments for mild traumatic brain injury: an update on the evidence. J Clin Exp Neuropsychol. 2009;31:20–38.

Sosin DM, Sniezek JE, Thurman DJ. Incidence of mild and moderate brain injury in the United States, 1991. Brain Inj. 1996;10:47–54.

Stanford MS, Houston RJ, Mathias CW, Villemarette-Pittman NR, Helfritz LE, Conklin SM. Characterizing aggressive behavior. Assessment. 2003;10:183–90.

Stanford MS, Helfritz LE, Conklin SM, Villemarette-Pittman NR, Greve KW, Adams D, Houston RJ. A comparison of anticonvulsants in the treatment of impulsive aggression. Experimental and Clinical Psychopharmacology. 2005;13:72–77.

Stein DJ, Moeller FG. The man who turned bad. CNS Spectrums. 2005;10:88–90.

Tanielian T, Jaycox LH, editors. Invisible wounds of war: psychological and cognitive injuries, their consequences, and services to assist recovery. Santa Monica, CA: RAND; 2008.

Tateno A, Jorge RE, Robinson RG. Clinical correlates of aggressive behaviour after traumatic brain injury. The Journal of Neuropsychiatry and Clinical Neurosciences 2003;15:155–60.

Teasdale TW, Engberg AW. Suicide after traumatic brain injury: a population study. J Neurol Neurosurg Psychiatry. 2001;71:436–40.

Terrio H, Brenner LA, Ivins BJ, Cho JM, Helmick K, Schwab K, Scally K, Bretthauer R, Warden D. Traumatic brain injury screening: Preliminary findings

in a US Army brigade combat team. J Head Trauma Rehabil. 2009;24:14–23.
Teten AL, Miller LA, Stanford MS, Peterson N, Collins R, Bailey SD, Dunn NJ, Kent TA. Characterizing aggression and its association to anger and hostility among male veterans with posttraumatic stress disorder. Mil Med. 2010;175(6):405–10.
Teten AL, Miller LA, Bailey SD, Dunn NJ, Kent TA. Empathic deficits and alexithymia in trauma-related impulsive aggression. Behav Sci Law. 2008;26: 823–32.
Villemarette-Pittman NR, Stanford MS, Greve KW. Language and executive function in self-reported impulsive aggression. Pers Individ Dif. 2003;34:1533–44.
Wang Y, Chan RCK, Deng Y. Examination of postconcussion-like symptoms in healthy university students: Relationships to subjective and objective neuropsychological function performance. Arch Clin Neuropsychol. 2006;21:339–47.
Warden DL, Gordon B, McAllister TW, Silver JM, Barth JT, Bruns J, Drake A, Gentry T, Jagoda A, Katz DI, Kraus J, Labbate LA, Ryan LM, Sparling MB, Walters B, Whyte J, Zapata A, Zitnay G. Guidelines for the pharmacologic treatment of neurobehavioral sequelae of traumatic brain injury. J Neurotrauma. 2006;23(10):1468–501.
Wasserman L, Shaw T, Vu M, Ko C, Bollegala D, et al. An overview of traumatic brain injury and suicide. Brain Inj. 2008;22:811–9.
Williams DH, Levin HS, Eisenberg HM. Mild head injury classification. Neurosurgery. 1990;27:422–8.
Wood RL, Liossi C. Neuropsychological and neurobehavioral correlates of aggression following traumatic brain injury. Journal of Neuropsychiatry and Clinical Neurosciences. 2006;18:333–41.
World Health Organization. The ICD-10 classification of mental and behavioural disorders: diagnostic criteria for research. Geneva: World Health Organization; 1993.
Yang CC, Hua MS, Tu YK, Huang SJ. Early clinical characteristics of patients with persistent post-concussion symptoms: A prospective study. Brain Inj. 2009;23: 299–306.
Yudofsky SC, et al. The Overt Aggression Scale for the objective rating of verbal and physical aggression. Am J Psychiatry. 1986;143(1):35–9.

Rehabilitation Following TBI

14

Mel B. Glenn

Abstract

Rehabilitation following traumatic brain injury (TBI) is a complex endeavor requiring a coordinated team approach to the spectrum of medical, motor, cognitive, and behavioral issues that can develop. Used in the appropriate circumstances for the appropriate motor disorders, therapeutic exercise, physical modalities, medications, chemical denervation with botulinum toxin or phenol, intrathecal baclofen, and surgical techniques can all be helpful. Certain rehabilitation approaches have been found to improve cognitive deficits. While some medications can worsen cognition, there are drugs that can improve some aspects of cognition as well as diminished initiation and alertness. Depending on the individual, aggressive behavior can often be ameliorated by planned behavioral approaches, counseling, and/or psychopharmacological approaches. Depression and anxiety can be treated with psychotherapy and medications.

Keywords

Motor • Cognitive • Initiation • Alertness • Aggression • Medication • Mild traumatic brain injury • Post-concussion symptoms • Depression

Introduction

Traumatic brain injury (TBI) can cause a wide variety of motor, cognitive, behavioral, emotional, and medical problems. Rehabilitation following TBI is therefore a complex endeavor, requiring a team approach involving physicians, nurses, neuropsychologists, psychotherapists (e.g., psychologists, social workers, or mental health counselors), speech and language pathologists (SLPs), occupational therapists, physical therapists, vocational counselors, recreational

M.B. Glenn, M.D. (✉)
Department of Physical Medicine and Rehabilitation, Harvard Medical School, Boston, MA, USA

Outpatient and Community Brain Injury Rehabilitation, Spaulding Rehabilitation Hospital, Boston, MA, USA

NeuroRestorative-Massachusetts, Braintree, MA, USA

Community Rehab Care, Newton, MA, USA
e-mail: mglenn@partners.org

J.W. Tsao (ed.), *Traumatic Brain Injury: A Clinician's Guide to Diagnosis, Management, and Rehabilitation*,
DOI 10.1007/978-0-387-87887-4_14, © Springer Science+Business Media, LLC 2012

therapists, and case managers. This entails the need for strong communication among team members and considerable flexibility on the part of the team. Therapists often have to take roles that may not be required in other settings. For instance, physical therapists will treat the physical mobility issues, including community navigation skills and safety. However, they have to be tuned into how cognitive dysfunction will affect mobility and how best to address it. They will also be confronted with the behavioral disorders that are prominent among people with TBI: disinhibited behavior, including aggression, but also apathy. Occupational therapists (OTs) will work on activities of daily living (ADLs) and upper limb mobility, but will do so in the context of cognitive disability as well. Home and community skills, such as balancing a checkbook, meal preparation, and shopping, will take on greater importance in the rehabilitation of people with TBI because of the cognitive dimension. OTs, too, will have to treat behavioral disorders. SLPs will treat not only swallowing and language and speech deficits among people with TBI but cognitively based communication deficits as well. They will also treat problems with memory, attention, and executive skills, and may overlap with OTs in the areas of home and community skills such as scheduling and money management. Of course, SLPs will have to know how to manage behavioral issues as well. Nurses and the nurses' aides will have to deal with every dimension—medical, mobility, cognitive, and behavioral. Most TBI programs have neuropsychologists and/or behavioral psychologists who do neuropsychological assessments, guide the team with respect to cognitive, emotional, and behavioral treatments, and sometimes do counseling. The neuropsychologist has to apply his or her understanding of the cognitive and behavioral issues to pharmacology, mobility, ADLs, and home and community rehabilitation. Although important in all areas of rehabilitation, in rehabilitation following TBI, it is crucial that the physician listen to all team members. The physician is not going to learn all the details of what a patient is doing and saying with respect to emotional, behavioral, and cognitive status directly from the patient. The therapy and nursing staff will be the ones who observe the intricacies of the patient's inattention, disinhibition, and apathy, and hear about the patient's despairing thoughts, and so forth. At the same time, if the physician starts the patient on a medication for a cognitive, emotional, or behavioral issue, he or she will get a more complete perspective on the patient's response by hearing from other team members.

When it comes to treating physical issues, it is important that team members communicate their findings and concerns to one another. Disorders of muscle tone can change from moment to moment and differs with position. The therapists may see these changes manifested in different ways than will the physician. If the physician is going to intervene with medications or procedures, it is important that he or she understand the functional context in which the problem occurs. Again, the other team members' input will give the physician the information needed to make decisions about whether to try medications or whether or not they have been beneficial.

Medical problems, too, will affect the patient in every setting. It is important for the therapy staff to be aware of the medical status of the patient, which may change the person's physical, cognitive, and behavioral status. Therapy staff may be the first to see a change in a patient's status that will alert the physician to the possibility of medical issues or side effects of medications. Medical issues are covered in other chapters in this book.

Rehabilitation following TBI results in improved outcomes. Inpatient multidisciplinary rehabilitation beginning 4 weeks or less from the time of injury improved independence in mobility and ADLs in patients with severe TBI compared to a control group of inpatients in nonspecialty hospitals. Caregiver distress decreased more in the intervention group as well (Semlyen et al. 1998; Turner-Stokes et al. 2005). Salazar et al. (2000) did a randomized controlled trial (RCT) of inpatient cognitive rehabilitation versus education, advice, and weekly telephone follow-up in a population of independently ambulating military personnel with TBI who had a Glasgow Coma Scale (GCS) score of 13 or less at the time of injury and a current Rancho Los Amigos level of cognitive function of 7. They found no difference in gainful employment or fitness to return to military duty, nor in cognitive and behavioral/emotional performance between groups. However, a post hoc analysis found that among the more severely affected (loss of consciousness greater than 1 h), the inpatient rehabilitation group had a better rate of return to duty (Salazar et al. 2000). The appropriateness of this high-functioning group for inpatient rehabilitation has been questioned (Glenn et al. 2001). A single-blind RCT of community-based team rehabilitation for patients with severe TBI 3 months to 20 years after injury (mean 27 weeks) demonstrated improved mobility, ADLs, and participation level skills (Brain Injury Community Rehabilitation Outcome [BICRO]-39 scales) in 40% of patients compared to 27% of the controls given only written information (Turner-Stokes et al. 2005; Powell et al. 2002). In a single-blind RCT of a home-based multidisciplinary rehabilitation program for patients with severe TBI, improved mobility and ADLs were seen, as well as participation level outcomes on the BICRO-39 in the intervention group (Turner-Stokes et al. 2005; Slade et al. 2002). RCTs have found that additional therapies (Zhu et al. 2007) or the presence of an experienced brain injury professional on the rehabilitation team (Turner-Stokes et al. 2005; Shiel et al. 2001) results in more rapid gains, but does not seem to change the ultimate outcome (Turner-Stokes et al. 2005).

Motor Disorders

Definitions

There are a number of motor disorders commonly affecting people with TBI. Weakness is probably the most common disorder and can be addressed with strengthening exercises. There is mixed evidence for improved motor return in stroke with the administration of dextroamphetamine (Liepert 2008). This has not been studied in people with TBI. Weakness is often seen with other motor disorders. These disorders are often seen together in various combinations, so it is best to start with definitions and descriptions.

Signs of ataxia include intention tremor and postural tremor. These are perhaps the most difficult of all motor disorders to treat. Although buspirone may have some modest effects on ataxia (Trouillas et al. 1997), there are no medications that have been shown to have clear clinically significant benefit. Weighted extremities can help at times, but the effect is small. Velcro® wrist or ankle weights or ankle–foot orthoses with double metal uprights can be used. The only approach that is always worth trying is repetitive therapeutic exercise (e.g., reaching for a target or picking up a cup of water and bringing it to the mouth, or for the lower limbs, walking with as narrow a base as possible). Some patients will make slow gains with thousands of repetitions of the same activity. Others will be left frustrated by the lack of progress. Goals should be set that are achievable in order to minimize frustration.

Spasticity and rigidity are both disorders of muscle tone. Muscle tone is reflexive resistance to passive stretching of muscle. Spasticity is a manifestation of hyperactive stretch reflexes, one aspect of the upper motor neuron syndrome. It is characterized by a velocity-dependent increase in muscle tone (hypertonia) with a catch and release (the "clasp-knife" phenomenon), hyperactive deep tendon reflexes, and at times, clonus. It is often seen with other aspects of the upper motor neuron syndrome: weakness, impaired timing, and poor coordination (Gans et al. 1990; Barnes 2001; Lance 1980). Although treating spasticity may be helpful in some instances, it will not necessarily improve these other disorders. Spasticity can be useful as well as detrimental. Increased muscle tone in the hip and knee extensors may allow a person to bear weight on an otherwise weak extremity. Spasticity of the elbow flexors can make it possible for someone to carry a purse or shopping bag on the forearm. Increased tone in the finger flexors can allow a person to hold objects in the hand.

Rigidity is another form of hypertonia. In this case, the increase in muscle tone is not velocity dependent, and it is consistent throughout the available range of motion (Gans et al. 1990;

Sanger et al. 2003). Parkinsonian rigidity with cogwheeling can occur after TBI. In addition, gegenhalten or paratonia, in which there is a feeling of voluntary resistance (Glenn 1990a), can be seen as well.

Dystonia is also quite common. Dystonia occurs when involuntary muscle contractions result in intermittent or persistent posturing (Gans et al. 1990; Sanger et al. 2003; Abdo et al. 2010; Krauss et al. 2007). Dystonia is not necessarily a hypertonia, that is, it may or may not be elicited by a muscle stretch. It can be seen spontaneously or can be elicited by a sensory stimulus such as touch, perturbation, or even a loud noise. Technically, decerebrate and decorticate rigidity are dystonias. Spasticity can result in dystonic posturing. There is probably more than one neurophysiologic etiology.

Although more commonly seen in spinal cord disorders, involuntary flexor or extensor spasms of the limbs can be seen after TBI at times. These are sudden jerking movements that are manifestations of hyperactive cutaneous or soft tissue reflexes. Synergies and, less commonly, postural reflexes can be seen after TBI as well. These are obligate patterns of movement initiated by active (synergies and postural reflexes) or passive (postural reflexes) motion of a limb, or in the case of postural reflexes, at times the head and neck or trunk. The individual is unable to move joints in isolation (Gans et al. 1990; Soechting and Lacquaniti 1989).

Treatment

The mainstay of treatment of the upper motor neuron syndrome for all of these entities is therapeutic exercise and functional training done by physical and occupational therapists, including sustained stretching of muscles and soft tissues. EMG biofeedback can be helpful to facilitate isolation of the muscles that are most problematic, though the literature on its efficacy is limited (Jonsdottir et al. 2010; van Dijk et al. 2005). Although thus far the best evidence for its efficacy has been in subjects with stroke, constraint-induced movement therapy (CIMT) (Wolf et al. 2006) or a modification of the full therapy (Wu et al. 2007a, b) can be done for the hemiplegic individual with TBI who is capable of complying with the rigorous schedule (Shaw et al. 2005). It is most frequently used to facilitate movement of a partially impaired upper limb. In full CIMT, the patient receives therapy for the more impaired limb for 6 h a day, combining repetitive task practice with adaptive task practice. The latter involves practice of components of the task and eventually the entire sequence, with a gradual increase in task difficulty. The stronger limb is restrained with a mitt or other device for 90% of waking hours, forcing the patient to use the partially impaired extremity. The patient keeps a log of his/her activities as a check on compliance and to reinforce the behaviors. It has been successful in the subacute and chronic settings, where it has been shown to improve upper limb use following stroke (Wolf et al. 2006, 2007). However, limb restraint in the acute rehabilitation setting has been unsuccessful and even detrimental with a more intensive therapy group (Dromerick et al. 2009). CIMT is based on the hypothesis that people with hemiplegia make limited gains in the use of the impaired upper limb because of "learned disuse." This theory suggests that in the early days of rehabilitation people with hemiparesis who do not make rapid gains will limit the use of the impaired extremity and instead emphasize compensation using the stronger extremity because of the frustration and lack of positive reinforcement received from limited success. Thus, the full potential for recovery is not reached (Bonaiuti et al. 2007).

The initial approach to problems with spasticity includes treating provocative nociceptive influences, in particular, skin, bladder, and bowel problems. This decreases the noxious input into the central nervous system (CNS) that facilitates excitation of motor neurons (Gans et al. 1990; Glenn 1990a). Sustained stretch through range of motion exercises is also a key and generally needs to be done at least daily if there is a significant amount of spasticity. Positioning is also crucial for limiting spasticity. For instance, if when sitting in a wheelchair, a person is tending to slide out due to hip and knee extensor tone, a tilt-in-space wheelchair will take advantage of gravity to hold the hips in flexion. A seatbelt across the pelvis will help to keep the hips at 90°. If the toes are held down with toe loops, the knees will remain flexed. Maintaining this position will stretch the hip and knee extensors as well as the ankle plantar flexors, and the spasticity will decrease (Hallenborg 1990).

There are also a number of physical modalities that physical and occupational therapists use to treat spasticity that tend to work in the short term, so can be used before stretching or other therapeutic exercise. Warmth can decrease muscle tone. Cold generally increases spasticity in the short run, but after 15 or 20 min it will decrease the tone (Zafonte et al. 2004). Ultrasound is a deep heating method. If the elastic portions of the tendon and muscle are warmed, they become more flexible, and then more stretch can take place before the muscle spindle gets stretched. Electrical stimulation can be used, both in the antagonist and the agonist muscles. In the antagonist, reciprocal inhibition is leveraged to inhibit the muscle tone in the agonist muscle. In the targeted agonist muscle group, electrical stimulation over a period of time can deplete acetylcholine from the neuromuscular junction, thus fatiguing the spastic muscle (Zafonte et al. 2004). Low frequency generalized vibration can be used to decrease spasticity (Giebler 1990).

Casting and orthotics can decrease muscle tone, though casting tends to be more effective (Zafonte et al. 2004; Hylton 1990; Feldman 1990). If well applied, the soft tissues are held in a position for a sustained period of time, thus reducing muscle tone. However, a cast or orthotic that does not hold a joint well and allows for some movement will often provoke an increase in tone by acting as a noxious stimulus to the skin.

Medications can be helpful, though are used less frequently in people with brain injury than with spinal cord injury because many of them have deleterious cognitive side effects. Diazepam and other benzodiazepenes cause sedation, as well as attention and memory problems that may persist following withdrawal (Barker et al. 2005; Larson and Zollman 2010). They are generally to be avoided except in situations in which the hypertonia, dystonia, or muscle spasms are so severe as to be painful or otherwise disruptive, thus becoming a major distraction to the patient, and in which other approaches have either failed or are relatively contraindicated. They are not FDA approved for this use ("off-label"). Baclofen can be useful for treating spasticity and muscle spasms, but has been found to impair memory in animal experiments (Ogasawara et al. 1999; Dario et al. 2007). There is little evidence for its efficacy in people with spasticity caused by cerebral lesions (Zafonte et al. 2004), although anecdotally, individual clinicians have found it helpful at times. Cyproheptadine has been used to treat spasticity, but studies in people with spasticity resulting from cerebral lesions are extremely limited. Its sedating effect can be a major drawback (Zafonte et al. 2004). Clonodine was used more frequently in the past ("off-label") but has largely been replaced by tizanidine, which is also a central alpha-2 agonist that decreases spasticity, but with less effect on blood pressure. However, side effects, sedation in particular, often limit its use. Because of data suggesting that clonidine can inhibit recovery from CNS lesions, tizanidine is suspect as well (Zafonte et al. 2004). It also can cause elevated liver function tests (Zafonte et al. 2004). As an "off-label" use, gabapentin has been shown to be effective for treating spasticity in people with multiple sclerosis at doses of about 2,700 mg a day (Cutter et al. 2000), though individual dosing varies. Gabapentin can be sedating, but if titrated slowly, many patients accommodate to this effect. It is otherwise generally free of adverse cognitive effects (Cutter et al. 2000; Hoch and Daly 2003; Park and Kwon 2008). Dantrolene sodium is generally thought to be without deleterious cognitive effects, though studies in animals have shown an adverse effect on memory (Ohnuki and Nomura 1996; Edwards and Rickard 2006). Whereas the drugs previously mentioned work in the CNS at the reflex level, dantrolene works at the muscle itself by inhibiting the release of calcium from the sarcoplasmic reticulum. Hepatotoxicity is a serious potential problem, so liver function tests must be followed. However, efficacy appears to be optimal at doses of 200 mg daily or less, and at that dose the risk of hepatotoxicity is small. Dantrolene does tend to cause weakness in the non-spastic muscles (Zafonte et al. 2004). Because it acts peripherally, any muscle can be affected by it. This is generally not a problem if the muscle is unused or is strong, but in areas where the person is weak, dantrolene may tip them over the edge into weakness that affects function. This includes muscles involved in swallowing and speech.

When cogwheel rigidity is present, the same dopaminergic agents that are used in Parkinson's disease may be helpful ("off-label"), although this needs further study. Dystonia is very difficult to treat, and in patients with TBI, the pharmacologic approaches are "off-label." Anticholinergic agents can be used, though they are generally of limited benefit (Krauss et al. 2007). They can adversely affect memory and attention (Arciniegas 2003). Benzodiazapenes can be very effective, but as noted above, they can cause sedation and cognitive impairment (Barker et al. 2005; Larson and Zollman 2010).

Chemical denervation using botulinum toxin, phenol, or even alcohol will often provide a better risk:benefit ratio because of the lack of cognitive side effects. This is particularly the case when the hypertonia or dystonia is focal rather than generalized, or in situations in which the need for intervention is limited to a small number of areas. Chemical neurolysis with phenol destroys axons but weakness is not a common complication if used discretely. There is a very variable duration of action, from weeks to years. It often lasts longer than 6 months, which is in some ways an advantage and in other ways a disadvantage over botulinum toxin. It is most useful when the patient cannot or does not want to return frequently for injections, when the limit for the quantity of botulinum toxin has been reached and there are still areas in need of treatment, or when botulinum toxin is not effective. It can also be used as an adjunct to botulinum toxin. When only motor branches are blocked, then the common side effects are transient pain and occasionally swelling at the injection site, depending on how much is used and which muscles are injected. If mixed sensorimotor blocks are done, some patients (10–32%) will get dysesthesias in the sensory distribution of the nerve. This is usually a mild "pins and needles" sensation that lasts for 2 or 3 weeks and then resolves. Occasionally, these painful sensations need treatment with transcutaneous electrical nerve stimulation, a tricyclic antidepressant ("off-label"), or other medications until it has run its course. Rarely dysesthesias continue for longer periods of time. In such cases, reinjection with phenol at the same site will usually resolve the pain. The best approach to this issue is to prevent the problem entirely by doing motor branch blocks or injecting peripheral nerves that are largely motor such as the thoracodorsal or obturator nerves. Usually a motor branch block is sufficient to reduce spasticity, but mixed sensorimotor blocks are at times necessary to get a better result. Goals of treatment should be clear before injections are done (Glenn 1990b, 1994; Glenn and Elovic 1997). The use of phenol to treat hypertonia or dystonia is not FDA approved.

Botulinum toxin inhibits release of acetylcholine at the neuromuscular junction. There are several serotypes, but the only ones that are commercially available are botulinum toxin A and B. Within each serotype, there are preparations that differ according to the company that produced the toxin. The duration of effect (generally 2–6 months) is usually shorter than with a phenol block. This makes it a better choice when there is a concern that the procedure might adversely affect a person's function. There is a limit to how much botulinum toxin can be used in any given therapeutic period (approximately 3 months). If there are several muscle groups to cover, especially when bilateral procedures are necessary, it may not be possible to treat them all with botulinum toxin. There is a limit to how much phenol can be injected in a given day, but over a period of a few weeks, more can be used (Glenn and Elovic 1997). Botulinum toxin is relatively free of side effects and complications, although dysphagia and respiratory insufficiency have been reported even with therapeutic doses (Shaw et al. 2010; Coban et al. 2010). Dysphagia is more common when cervical muscles are injected. Rates of dysphagia and dry mouth may vary among different preparations/brands (Chapman et al. 2007). There can be diffusion of toxin to local muscles that are not targeted. As with phenol, it is important to clarify the specific goals of treatment prior to the procedure (Glenn and Elovic 1997). In a RCT, botulinum toxin A was been shown to improve muscle tone and performance on specific simple functional tasks, such as putting an arm through a sleeve, cleaning the palm of the hand, or cutting the fingernails in people with stroke (Shaw et al. 2010). The botulinum toxin preparations available in the USA are FDA approved for certain dystonias in adults. Onabotulinum toxin A is approved for spasticity of finger, wrist, and elbow flexors in adults, but not lower limb spasticity. Other uses are "off-label."

In an open study, selective tibial motor neurotomy was shown to decrease spasticity and improve dorsiflexion strength and gait on a long-term basis (at least 2 years) in patients with hemiplegia. Plantar flexion strength eventually returned to baseline due to collateral sprouting while decreased spasticity is maintained due to the inability of IA afferents to reconnect at the spinal cord level (Deltombe and Gustin 2010).

Local anesthetic nerve blocks can be used as a "test run" before using botulinum toxin, phenol, or neurotomy in order to ascertain whether or not reducing tone in a muscle or group of muscles will provide any benefit or adversely affect function. Local anesthetic blocks can be helpful when there is a question of whether the inability to move a joint beyond a certain range or motion is due to severe hypertonia or contracture. The local anesthetic trial is, of course, no guarantee, as it is not likely to be exactly comparable to the other procedures (Glenn 1990b; Glenn and Elovic 1997).

Baclofen pumps can also reduce spastic hypertonia in people with TBI (Meythaler et al. 1996, 1999) by delivering small quantities of baclofen directly to the intrathecal space, thus avoiding the systemic effects of baclofen. A potentially life-threatening withdrawal syndrome with high fever, altered mental status, and muscular rigidity can occur if the baclofen is suddenly cut off, either because the reservoir is depleted or there is a malfunction in the pump or catheter (Coffey et al. 2002). Regular visits for refills must be scheduled. Today's pumps have alarms that alert the patient that the pump is in danger of becoming empty.

There are also orthopedic procedures such as muscle and tendon lengthenings and transfers that help to decrease muscle tone. Lengthenings are done in the context of treating contractures, but transfers are usually done for the purpose of improving function. The split lateral anterior tibialis tendon transfer for the treatment of ankle–foot inversion is an example. The tibialis anterior tendon is split at its insertion, and half of it is taken from the medial side of the foot and implanted on the lateral foot such that it is now balancing the inversion with an eversion pull, thereby dorsiflexing the ankle in a neutral position (Keenan et al. 1999; Piazza et al. 2001). When ankle plantarflexion contracture accompanies inversion, the Achilles tendon is lengthened as well. In order to preserve the ankle plantar flexion strength, the flexor digitorum longus and flexor hallucis longus can be transferred to the calcaneus (Keenan et al. 1999). Surgeons and referring clinicians must beware of the possibility of overcorrection resulting in the dominance of antagonist muscles, both with lengthening and transfers (Piazza et al. 2001).

Persistent hypertonia and/or immobility can result in contractures. The main approaches to the prevention of contractures are range of motion exercises and proper positioning. Other approaches to spasticity and dystonia referred to above may be necessary as well. If contractures have developed, serial casting is an excellent way of reducing them. A cast is placed in close to the full range of motion achievable, and it is left on for 3–7 days. Muscle tone will be reduced. When the cast is removed, there will often be more passive range of motion available. Another cast is placed that takes advantage of these additional gains. This process continues until no additional range of motion is achieved (Giebler 1990; Marshall et al. 2007). However, the reduction of contractures in response to serial casting in patients with TBI may be transient (Singer et al. 2003; Moseley et al. 2008). Botulinum toxin injections to reduce spasticity prior to casting have been found to help to sustain the results in children with cerebral palsy (Ackman et al. 2005; Newman et al. 2007). Long-term studies of botulinum toxin injections combined with serial casting in adults or children with TBI need to be done.

When serial casting is not feasible, adjustable spring-loaded dynamic orthotics can be used to place maximum tolerable tension on the contracted soft tissues, with gradual changes in joint angle and tension being made over time (Charlton et al. 1999; Keeping and Major 1999). These orthotics have the advantage that the skin can more easily be observed for pressure ulcers, but they are not as effective as casting, partly because the patient can remove them. When these approaches fail, surgical lengthenings may be indicated.

Heterotopic ossification (HO) in the large joints is not uncommon among people with severe TBI, especially those who have been in a coma or minimally responsive for a significant period of time early in their course. HO can be extremely painful during range of motion exercises. Patients may be very resistant to range of motion exercises while HO is forming. HO often progresses to complete ankylosis of joints. It can entrap peripheral nerves with resultant neuropathy. Disodium etidronate and nonsteroidal anti-inflammatory drugs (NSAIDs) have both been used for prevention, although the evidence for their beneficial effect is largely from studies in other patient populations such as spinal cord injury and hip surgery (Cullen and Perera 2009; Cipriano et al. 2009). There is, in particular, an unanswered question as to whether the preventive effect of etidronate is only short-term (Haran et al. 2004). Although disodium etidronate is generally well-tolerated with serious side effects being rare, NSAIDs can cause gastric and duodenal ulcers and less commonly, adverse cardiac events (Cullen and Perera 2009). Some physicians use etidronate or NSAIDs prophylactically in people who have been in coma, vegetative state, or minimally conscious state for significant periods of time (the populations at increased risk of HO) (Spielman et al. 1983). Other clinicians will wait until there are symptoms. Usually HO begins with an inflammatory response resulting in a painful, warm, swollen, and erythematous area. It can be mistaken for a deep vein thrombosis (DVT), cellulitis, or deeper infection. Alkaline phosphatase and creatine phosphokinase will generally be elevated. At that point it will not show up on an X-ray, but a triple phase bone scan will be positive. It can take 3–4 weeks before it becomes calcified enough to see on an X-ray. Some physicians get bone scans when the inflammatory response is seen and DVT is ruled out, and if there is uptake on the bone scan in that area, then they will start disodium etidronate, an NSAID, or administer radiation, another treatment that has been effective in patients with SCI or following hip surgery. Once formed, the HO often restricts range of motion or fuses a joint. There is no evidence that waiting more than a year after injury to do a surgical excision is associated with a decreased chance of recurrence. Disodium etidronate, NSAIDs, and/or radiation can be effective for the prevention of recurrence after surgery (Cullen and Perera 2009; Cipriano et al. 2009; Chalidis et al. 2007).

Dysphagia

Dysphagia is a common disorder following TBI. Dysphagia is dependent on the status of the oral-motor musculature as evaluated by modified barium swallow (MBS) (Terre and Mearin 2007, 2009), but also on the patient's cognitive status (Mackay et al. 1999). Basic orientation and the ability to follow commands are predictive of aspiration (Leder and Suiter 2009). Even among patients with higher levels of cognitive function, poor self-monitoring and impulse control can affect swallowing ability due to difficulty in monitoring bolus size and speed of swallowing. Other predictors of dysphagia following TBI include Rancho Los Amigos level of cognitive function scale (RLAS) score, GCS score on admission, presence of a tracheostomy, and longer ventilation time (Terre and Mearin 2007; Mackay et al. 1999; Hansen et al. 2008). It is not necessary to be feeding orally to develop pneumonia in the early stages of recovery, and in fact one study found that 81% of people with TBI who developed pneumonia were not receiving anything by mouth (Hansen et al. 2008). One can aspirate secretions and refluxed or regurgitated stomach contents, and respiratory insufficiency, inadequate or absent cough, and lack of mobility can cause or contribute to pneumonia as well. Terre and Mearin (2007) found that 41% of patients with TBI who aspirated were found to do so silently, i.e., without coughing. Disability rating scale score, RLAS score, and oral-motor disorders on MBS are predictors of aspiration at 1 year after TBI (Terre and Mearin 2007, 2009). The MBS is considered the standard for evaluating swallowing. Even individuals with tracheostomy can undergo MBS and start treatment for swallowing (O'Neil-Pirozzi et al. 2003). Fiberoptic endoscopic evaluation of swallowing (FEES) can also be used for a better view of the pharynx (Logemann 2007).

The management of dysphagia involves trials of food and liquid consistencies as determined by MBS. Head and neck postural techniques and exercises, both tailored to the individual aspect of swallowing that is disordered, can improve performance (Logemann 2007).

Cognitive Disorders

Cognitive Rehabilitation

There are several aspects of cognition for which there is evidence for the benefit of therapeutic interventions. Hierarchical exercises in sustained, selective, alternating, and divided attention (attention process training) have been found to be helpful in the post-acute setting in people with TBI (Sohlberg et al. 2000) as well as in acute stroke (Barker-Collo et al. 2009) if the modalities and complexity are varied. The patient must be monitored and given feedback. Divided attention can be improved in people with TBI with dual-task training (Couillet et al. 2010).

For the treatment of memory disorders, there is some evidence for the benefit of teaching semantic strategies to people with TBI (Willis et al. 2006; O'Neil-Pirozzi et al. 2010). This includes semantic association, semantic clustering, and semantic elaboration. Training in visualization can be beneficial for people with mild memory problems (Kaschel et al. 2002). External aids such as notebooks and appointment books can be quite helpful and are recommended (Ownsworth and McFarland 1999; Cicerone et al. 2000, 2005). For those who can learn their use, even in a limited fashion, palmtop computers (personal digital assistants) are often more useful than notebooks (Depompei et al. 2008; Dowds et al. 2011). These can be programmed with reminder alarms and, therefore, do not rely on prospective memory as do appointment books. Palmtop computers may have to be programmed by somebody else if the person with TBI does not have the requisite skills. "Smart" mobile phones have also shown some promise as memory aids (Stapleton et al. 2007). Pagers are another external compensatory aid that have been found to be successful (Wilson et al. 2001, 2005). Although there is preliminary evidence that therapy to improve problem-solving skills may be beneficial (Levine et al. 2000), more study is needed in this area and other aspects of executive skills training.

The effectiveness of therapies to improve hemi-inattention and aphasia has been largely demonstrated in subjects with stroke. It is not unreasonable to tentatively extrapolate to people with TBI until the evidence is available with this population. Spatial neglect, usually of the left side, can be decreased with consistent cuing to scan to the neglected side (Cicerone et al. 2000; Niemeier 1998). Aphasia has been treated with functional language stimulation, cuing, and semantic analysis in people with strokes. The evidence suggests that such training is effective, but studies are not yet definitive (Cicerone et al. 2005; Cherney et al. 2008; Kelly et al. 2010). There is limited evidence for the effectiveness of constraint-induced language therapy (CILT) in the chronic phase after stroke (Cherney et al. 2008; Pulvermuller et al. 2001; Meinzer et al. 2007; Berthier et al. 2009). In CILT, the person being trained is not allowed to use gestures or to write and is forced to communicate during a simple card game, for instance. A screen can be put up so that gestures cannot be seen. The person being trained has to initially have some language function, such as the ability to say the number on a card. One study demonstrated a positive effect of CILT and the NMDA receptor antagonist memantine used separately for the treatment of aphasia, and a greater effect when used in combination (Berthier et al. 2009). There is limited evidence for the benefit of dextroamphetamine for the treatment of aphasia in the context of speech therapy (Liepert 2008).

There is also evidence for the efficacy of holistic cognitive rehabilitation programs in which the cognitive, emotional, motivational, and social function are addressed in a single program. Gains have been seen in employment and in community integration skills (Cicerone et al. 2004).

When a patient has problems with alertness, initiation, and/or attention, medical factors may need to be treated. Infection, electrolyte imbalance, and hydrocephalus can result in decreased arousal, attention, and initiation. Endocrine dysfunction is common and is addressed in Chap. 10. Insomnia and other sleep disorders are also frequently seen after TBI. This subject is addressed in Chap. 10. Seizures can result in postictal lethargy and is also addressed (Chap. 10).

Pharmacological Treatment of Cognitive Disorders

Pharmacological approaches can be useful, particularly for treating arousal, attention, initiation, and other aspects of executive skills. The first pharmacologic intervention to consider is withdrawing offending agents such as phenobarbital (Hoch and Daly 2003; Park and Kwon 2008; Zaccara 2008), phenytoin (Park and Kwon 2008; Zaccara 2008; Smith et al. 1994), carbamazepine (Park and Kwon 2008; Smith et al. 1994; Meador et al. 2007), topiramate (Hoch and Daly 2003; Park and Kwon 2008; Blum et al. 2006; Tang et al. 2007; Mills et al. 2008; Smith et al. 2006; Lee et al. 2006; Gomer et al. 2007; Meador 2008), zonisamide (Park and Kwon 2008), pregabalin (Park and Kwon 2008; Salinsky et al. 2010), baclofen (Ogasawara et al. 1999; Dario et al. 2007), tizanidine (Zafonte et al. 2004), benzodiazapines (Tsunoda et al. 2010), tricyclic antidepressants (Writer and Schillerstrom 2009), opiates (Gruber et al. 2007), and antipsychotics (especially the typical antipsychotics, such as haloperidol, chlorpromazine, and thiothixene) (Writer and Schillerstrom 2009). Among the anticonvulsants, levetiracetam (Meador 2008; Meador et al. 2007), gabapentin (Park and Kwon 2008), tiagabine (Park and Kwon 2008), vigabatrin (Park and Kwon 2008), and lamotrigine (Park and Kwon 2008) are relatively free of adverse cognitive effects, although sedation can be an issue with levetiracetam (Zaccara 2008) and gabapentin. Studies on valproic acid (Park and Kwon 2008; Dikmen et al. 2000) and oxcarbazepine (Park and Kwon 2008) are mixed with respect to their effect on cognition.

The benefit that a medication is providing must be weighed against the probability that it is causing cognitive impairment. Individual responses to medications vary considerably, so that any change seen or not seen when the patient started the medication is important in determining whether it is causing adverse effects.

Insomnia is often a contributor to daytime sleepiness and cognitive impairment. When simple sleep hygiene approaches are not working, medications may be helpful. However, for the long-term, if the patient is capable of participating effectively, cognitive behavioral therapy is usually more beneficial than medications (Jacobs et al. 2004). See Chap. 10 for further discussion of sleep disorders.

When other causes of attention, arousal, or initiation problems have been addressed to whatever extent possible, stimulants or stimulant-like drugs can be useful. The use of all of the medications discussed here are "off-label." This includes methyphenidate, amphetamines, modafinil, atomoxetine, dopaminergic drugs, the NMDA inhibitors such as amantadine and memantine, and cholinesterase inhibitors. Methylphenidate has the best evidence for effectiveness in treating attention following TBI, especially on-task behavior and speed of processing (Whyte et al. 1997; Wilmont et al. 2009; Chew and Zafonte 2009). Methylphenidate comes in both immediate release and long-acting formulations (see Table 14.1) (Glenn and Wroblewski 2005; Focalin XR for

Table 14.1 Some long-acting formulations of methylphenidate (Glenn and Wroblewski 2005; Focalin XR for ADHD 2009; The PDR® Electronic Library from Thomson Micromedex 2009)

Drug taken once daily	Mechanism	Peaks (h)[a]	Duration of action (h)[a]
Metadate CD (UCB)	Beaded MP, double pulse release, second release at 3 h, IR/ER	1.5, 4.5	8–12
Ritalin LA (Novartis)	Beaded MP, double pulse release, IR/DR	1–3, 6–7	8–12
Concerta (McNeil)	ER via osmotic pump coated with IR	1–2, 6–8	10–12
Daytrana transdermal patch (Noven-Shire)	Multipolymeric adhesive transdermal absorption	7.5–10.5	11.5[b]
Focalin XR (Novartis) (dexmethylphenidate)	Beaded MP, double pulse release, second release at 4 h, IR/DR	1.5, 6.5	8–12

MP methylphenidate, *IR* immediate release, *ER* extended release, *DR* delayed release
[a]Most studies have been done in children
[b]Assuming 9-h wearing time; includes 3-h delay until MP appears in plasma

ADHD 2009; The PDR® Electronic Library from Thomson Micromedex 2009). Amphetamines have a similar mechanism of action, but have not been as well-studied for the treatment of attention, initiation, or arousal deficits in people with brain injury (Whyte et al. 2002).

Amantadine can be effective for hastening, and perhaps improving, the responsiveness of individuals in a minimally conscious state during the first few months after injury (Katz et al. 2011; Giacino et al. 2012). There is more limited for an effect of amantadine on the outcome of inpatient rehabilitation (Chew and Zafonte 2009; Meythaler et al. 2002). Although modafinil did not bring about improvement in fatigue and alertness following TBI in one small RCT (Jha et al. 2008), in another RCT sleepiness but not fatigue improved (Kaiser et al. 2010).

There is some evidence that acetylcholinesterase inhibitors can have a positive effect on sustained attention and anterograde memory in people with TBI (Liepert 2008; Chew and Zafonte 2009; Ballesteros et al. 2008; Zhang et al. 2004). A study of rivastigmine in subjects with TBI showed no benefit for the group as a whole, but positive results for visual processing speed latency and memory among those with moderate-to-severe injury in a secondary analysis (Silver et al. 2006). Bromocriptine was shown to help dual-task attention in an early study (McDowell et al. 1998), but this result was not replicated by Whyte et al. (2008). In the later study, and other aspects of attention also did not improve with bromocriptine. Protriptyline is a stimulating antidepressant that can be activating (Glenn 1993), but has not been well-studied.

Behavioral and Emotional Disorders

Treating behavioral and emotional disorders requires an evaluation of the underlying contributing factors. Medical conditions such as electrolyte disturbance, endocrine disorders, infection, hydrocephalus, epilepsy, and others can cause behavioral changes. The loss of control that comes with being physically or cognitively disabled often results in depression and anxiety. Pre-injury psychiatric issues often continue to play a role after a TBI. Staff, family, or friends may inadvertently reinforce aggressive and disruptive behaviors by paying undue attention to them. Antecedents to aggression must be evaluated to determine the triggers to such behavior.

Mood Disorders

Depression is extremely common following TBI (Ashman et al. 2009; Bombardier et al. 2010), and is associated with anxiety (Bombardier et al. 2010). Some people with TBI can benefit from individual counseling despite some cognitive impairment (Alderfer et al. 2005). Cognitive behavioral therapy has been found to be helpful in treating distress following acquired brain injury (Bradbury et al. 2008). However, problems with executive function, attention, and memory can be limiting factors. Group treatments can sometimes be helpful as well. A periodic telephone call inquiring about problems, providing needed information, and facilitating problem-solving has been found to be preventive of future depression and also to treat preexisting depression (Bombardier et al. 2009). Medications can be used when depressive symptoms and/or anxiety interfere with quality of life and/or rehabilitation over a sustained period of time. Depression is best treated with the low or nonsedating antidepressants—the SSRIs and SNRIs (Chew and Zafonte 2009)—although there is a dearth of studies in people with TBI. A recent RCT of sertraline failed to conclusively demonstrate benefit in people with TBI, possibly related to an inadequate number of subjects (Ashman et al. 2009). Antidepressants should be used cautiously, especially in the elderly, as SSRIs (and tricyclic antidepressants) have been associated with increased mortality and hemorrhagic stroke in postmenopausal women. This fact, however, must be weighed against quality of life issues and the known risk of cardiovascular disease in untreated depression (Smoller et al. 2009). Anxiety can also be treated with these medications. Benzodiazepines are best avoided when possible due to their adverse effect on alertness, attention, and memory, though occasionally the trade-off can be in favor of their use since anxiety itself can affect cognition. Buspirone is unlikely to cause cognitive side effects (Chamberlain et al. 2008).

Differential Diagnosis of Behavioral Disorders

There are a number of behavioral disorders that are often seen after TBI. Disinhibition, aggression, and emotional dyscontrol are extremely common, usually as a result of frontal lobe lesions. Lack of initiation and expression, depression, and anxiety—often as a reaction to the disability once the person becomes aware enough—are also seen frequently. Psychotic behaviors are unusual but do occur. New onset of mania is seen rarely. Clinicians must be careful not to mistake the influences of cognitive and perceptual deficits for psychiatric syndromes. For instance, reduplicative phenomena caused by frontal dysfunction often includes the belief that certain people are imposters. However, this can easily be mistaken for delusional thinking as seen in more classical psychiatric settings. Memory disorders can cause what appear to be hallucinations or delusions. A person with a severe memory disorder may, for instance, believe that someone important to them who has died is actually alive because he or she has no memory of the person's death, particularly if it occurred shortly before the injury. Visual-perceptual impairment, especially in the context of executive dysfunction, can result in hallucinatory-like experiences. There can be a fine line between these sorts of behaviors and manifestations of actual psychosis. This is an important consideration because it may involve a decision about whether or not to use antipsychotic medication. There are no studies that address this issue, so the clinician has to use his or her best judgment. One consideration is whether or not there is significant emotion, in particular, fear, surrounding a belief. For example, if the person with TBI fears that they will be hurt by someone or something that they see or believe to exist, one would be more apt to treat it as a psychotic behavior than if the person is unconcerned. Other combinations of cognitive, behavioral, and perceptual problems can mimic psychiatric syndromes. Neurologically based apathy can mimic depression, except that the withdrawn, apathetic patient will not feel sad or be tearful (Glenn 2002).

Nursing and therapy staff or other caregivers will often be in the best position to provide information to physicians, psychologists, and social workers that may provide clues to the etiology of behaviors. They will often be the ones to hear the despairing words of a depressed patient, to observe that a patient does not initiate and shows little affect, to see the circumstances under which a person becomes aggressive, or to see whether fearfulness is associated with hallucinatory or delusional-like behaviors. They can see the degree to which a behavior is interfering with rehabilitation or causing disruption to the patient or to others' lives. Of course this does not mean that the clinician should rely entirely upon others to evaluate behavior. Interviewing even very impaired patients can turn up clues that aid in diagnosis and observing them in therapies or on the nursing unit can also be revealing.

Behavioral Approaches to Treatment

Treating behavioral issues following TBI requires understanding and addressing both antecedents to and consequences of an individual's behavior (Ylvisaker 2003). Treating other aspects of disability, facilitating communication, and providing opportunities for enjoyable and productive activities can resolve some of the causes of disruptive behaviors, improve mood, and allow the person with TBI to feel more in control, with resultant decreases in aggressive and disruptive behavior. Along these lines, a review of approaches to social and behavioral dysfunction after acquired brain injury concluded that comprehensive holistic rehabilitation programs are more effective than both cognitive behavioral therapy and applied behavioral analysis (Cattelani et al. 2010). A patient's environment should be considered as well, including reduction of physical barriers to function and addressing the influences of those around him or her who may be provoking antisocial behavior. Behavioral interventions to address aggressive behavior should provide natural consequences (e.g., cleaning up and paying for broken items) whenever possible, and should avoid reinforcing disruptive behavior. The individual must be taught alternative approaches to expressing him/herself and getting his/her needs met (Ylvisaker 2003). Positive consequences for pro-social behavior can be put in place by exploring what would be rewarding to the person in question. Some programs use point systems or tokens that can be exchanged for rewards. There is a natural tendency for health care professionals and family members to pay attention to patients who are, for instance, shouting and shaking the bed rails or demanding something that cannot be provided. If, after addressing antecedents and consequences, a disruptive behavior continues, caregivers may have to give the patient "time outs" from reinforcement of those disruptive behaviors (Wood 1987). To treat the executive dysfunction that is behind aggressive behavior, therapists must increase the awareness of the patient's own internal reactions by teaching self-monitoring techniques, providing feedback, and having them do self-evaluations. This type of training has been shown to result in decreased expression of anger and improved socialization in one study (Medd and Tate 2000). Paradoxically, the person's awareness of his or her reactions did not have to increase for the therapy to be effective. This finding requires verification.

Pharmacologic Treatment

At times pharmacologic intervention is helpful. Treating underlying problems with arousal, initiation, and attentional disorders can have a secondary effect on irritability and disruptive behavior. Studies of methylphenidate to treat aggression ("off-label") have been of limited quality and mixed in their outcomes (Levy et al. 2005). Treating depression and anxiety can also have an ameliorating effect on irritability and aggressive and disruptive behavior. The treatment of depression and anxiety are discussed above. The effect of antidepressants on aggressive behavior (not necessarily in the context of depression, therefore "off-label") has been studied, but the evidence for their efficacy is limited (Levy et al. 2005). The pharmacologic treatment of aggression caused by disinhibition has been poorly studied (Chew and Zafonte 2009) and all pharmacological uses are "off-label." Therefore, among the medications that may be useful for this condition, it is best to start with medications that have the fewest cognitive side effects. Some anticonvulsants (valproic acid, carbamazepine, and gabapentin) have been used for treating aggression, and as noted above (see section on "Cognitive Rehabilitation" above), some of them are relatively free of such effects. Levetiracetam can cause impulsive, irritable, and aggressive behavior (Hoch and Daly 2003). However, there are no well-controlled studies demonstrating the efficacy of anticonvulsants (Levy et al. 2005; Fleminger et al. 2006). There are studies suggesting that beta-blockers can be helpful (Meador et al. 2007), but high doses were used in most of the studies. It can take considerable time to reach high doses while the patient accommodates to the changes in blood pressure and heart rate (Levy et al. 2005; Fleminger et al. 2006). Furthermore, beta-blockers have been found to cause cognitive decline in the elderly (Paran et al. 2010), and they can also cause fatigue and sedation (Dimsdale et al. 1989). Buspirone (Levy et al. 2005; Fleminger et al. 2006) and lithium (Chew and Zafonte 2009; Glenn and Josephs 1987; Glenn et al. 1989) have been used as well, although controlled studies in people with brain injury are lacking (Levy et al. 2005; Fleminger et al. 2006). The antipsychotics (Chew and Zafonte 2009) can be used for more severe aggressive behaviors when other medications have not been effective or when relatively rapid control of behavior is needed because of the danger that someone will be harmed. There is some limited evidence for their efficacy in treating aggressive behavior (Elovic et al. 2008). However, they can cause Parkinsonian symptoms, dystonias, and tardive dyskinesia (Levy et al. 2005). The atypical antipsychotics, which may have fewer motor side effects, can result in weight gain, dyslipidemia, and insulin resistance (Stahl et al. 2009). Both typical and atypical antipsychotics have been found to be associated with sudden death in elderly populations (Glenn 2010; Ray et al. 2009; Douglas and Smeeth 2008). If they are to be used for an extended period of time, it is best to get a fasting blood sugar, lipid profile, and EKG before or shortly after starting them. Benzodiazepenes are sometimes also used for situations in which relatively rapid control of aggressive behavior is needed. However, some authors believe that benzodiazepines can themselves cause disinhibition and agitated behavior (Fava 1997). As noted above, they can result in memory and attentional dysfunction and increase confusion. Even when they are helpful in the short term, this is often due to their sedating effect (Levy et al. 2005). Their use can result in a pattern in which the patient is either sleepy or agitated. This results in other medications needing to be used to replace the benzodiazepine, and/or behavior plans must be put in place to reduce the aggressive behavior.

Social Support and Motivation

Social support is also an important element to success in rehabilitation, as it provides incentive and motivation to continue with what is usually a difficult ordeal. Motivation and engagement are key to the success in rehabilitation, yet can be elusive, particularly following TBI when initiation, insight, or self-awareness are impaired (Lequerica and Kortte 2010). Motivational interviewing, which is a non-confrontational approach that allows the patient to take the lead and, thereby, fosters self-efficacy, can be effective with some individuals (Medley and Powell 2010). Bell et al. (2005) found that a periodic telephone call that included motivational interviewing, counseling, education, and follow-up of various aspects of care resulted in improved functional outcomes and quality of life.

Families of people with TBI are often under considerable emotional stress, especially when in caregiver roles. It is important to educate them about TBI and to provide them with lists of resources (e.g., brain injury associations, governmental programs, health care providers) that they may find useful so that they are equipped to cope with whatever issues arise. They should be encouraged to seek support via support groups, counseling, religious institutions, and friends (Kreutzer et al. 2009, 2010).

Mild Traumatic Brain Injury

Definition and Diagnosis

The definition of mild traumatic brain injury (mTBI) found in the literature has varied somewhat, but the most widely used definition is that formulated by the Mild TBI Task Force of the American Congress of Rehabilitation Medicine:

> A traumatically induced physiological disruption of brain function, as manifested by *at least* one of the following:
> 1. Any period of loss of consciousness;
> 2. Any loss of memory for events immediately before or after the accident;
> 3. Any alteration in mental state at the time of the accident (e.g., feeling dazed, disoriented, or confused);
> 4. Focal neurologic deficit(s) which may or may not be transient;
>
> but where the severity of injury does not exceed the following: loss of consciousness of approximately 30 min or less; after 30 min, an initial GCS of 13–15; and post-traumatic amnesia not greater than 24 h (Mild Traumatic Brain Injury Committee of the Head Injury Interdisciplinary Special Interest Group of the American Congress of Rehabilitation Medicine 1993).

Making the diagnosis of mTBI can be a difficult undertaking with a number of potential pitfalls. The patient's memory of or deductions about what occurred may be inaccurate. Medical records may not reflect a period of LOC or post-traumatic amnesia (PTA) that occurred before medical personnel arrived at the scene. The GCS may not have been assessed or reassessed until more than 30 min has passed. There is a potential problem with the overlap of the acute signs and symptoms of mTBI with acute stress reactions that commonly cause people to be "dazed, disoriented, or confused" after a major physical and/or psychological trauma that may include a brush with death. The clinician must obtain the most objective information available (e.g., emergency medical records, accounts of observers), ask probing questions, and listen carefully to the patient's account, and then use his or her judgment to sort out the etiology(ies) (Ruff et al. 2009). There are times when it is impossible to make the distinction.

Post-concussion Symptoms

mTBI can be associated with a variety of symptoms, and the term "post-concussion syndrome" has frequently been used to describe the complex of cognitive, physical, and emotional complaints that can occur. Some have argued that these symptoms do not manifest in a specific set, but rather can occur in various combinations of one or two symptoms to many symptoms, and should, therefore, not be referred to as a "syndrome" (Cicerone and Kalmar 1995). They are probably best referred to as "post-concussion symptoms" (PCS) or "post-concussion disorders." The most frequent complaints are fatigue, forgetfulness, difficulty in concentrating, headaches, dizziness, irritability, insomnia, depression, and anxiety. They have generally been found to persist in 10–15% of people with mTBI (Stein and McAllister 2009), but higher and lower estimates exist as well (Iverson et al. 2007). Symptom frequency diminishes over time, and it is controversial whether the symptoms can continue indefinitely or are the result of litigation or other factors when persistent. They can, of course, be seen in people with moderate or severe TBI, and are in fact common complaints of people who have never had a TBI (Fear et al. 2009). A study of people with mTBI occurring 22–35 months earlier and sex and age-matched controls who had presented to the emergency room with minor non-head injuries (also matched by time from injury) was done in Lithuania, where compensation is not much of an issue. It was found that there was no significant difference between the frequency of complaints that could be attributed to a TBI in the group that had mTBI compared with the control group, except for depression, alcohol intolerance, and worry about having a brain injury. However, there were trends toward more complaints of "sporadic memory problems" in the mTBI group ($p=0.052$) and toward more frequent endorsement of "no concentration problems" in the control group ($p=0.079$) (Mickeviciene et al. 2002). In a study by Wilk et al. (2010), blast injuries in a military context that resulted in mTBI without loss of consciousness were not associated with PCS 3–6 months after the injury, whereas TBIs with LOC were associated with headaches and tinnitus, but not other PCS. Studies have shown that healthy control subjects or controls with minor non-head injuries report the frequency of PCS at a rate higher than the frequency retrospectively reported by people with mTBI to have been present before their injuries. This has been interpreted to indicate that people with mTBI tend to attribute to the injury symptoms that were in fact present beforehand (Mickeviciene et al. 2002; Mittenberg et al. 1992; Iverson et al. 2010).

It is important to recognize that many of the physical and emotional symptoms associated with mTBI can, themselves, result in cognitive impairment even outside the context of mTBI. Some of the cognitive complaints following concussion may therefore have their origin at least in part from pain, insomnia, depression, and anxiety (Glenn 2008).

Many studies have found persistent PCS (often said to be those symptoms that continue for at least 3 months) to be associated with both pre- and post-injury psychological issues (Iverson et al. 2007; Fear et al. 2009; Rosenfeld and Ford 2010; Fenton et al. 1993; Alexander 1995; Hoge et al. 2008). Depression is a frequent associated condition. PCS overlap considerably with the symptoms of post-traumatic stress disorder (PTSD) (Stein and McAllister 2009; Iverson et al. 2007; Fear et al. 2009; Rosenfeld and Ford 2010; Hoge et al. 2008). This is a major issue in the treatment of military populations, many of whom have blast injuries. As noted above, this is complicated by the fact that acute stress reactions are probably the norm at the time of a blast injury, when the service member may have had a brush with death, may have had severe bodily injury such as loss of a limb, and may have seen other service members killed and/or injured around him or her. Military combatants are likely to feel "dazed" and perhaps confused from emotional trauma at such times. When screened at a later date (Government Accountability Office 2010), they may endorse these symptoms and be screened positive on that basis (without clinician confirmation) for mTBI, setting in motion a process that may result in an incorrect diagnosis and treatment if they are actually experiencing PTSD or depression or a combination of mTBI with one or more mental health disorders (Stein and McAllister 2009; Rosenfeld and Ford 2010; Hoge et al. 2008, 2009). The case can be made that some such people would never have sought help for their emotional struggles due to an inability to face their emotional problems and/or the stigma attached to mental health disorders. PTSD is to some extent preventable in people with mTBI with the use of cognitive behavioral therapy during the period of acute stress reaction (Bryant et al. 2003).

Symptoms, such as headaches and dizziness, should be treated symptomatically (see below), particularly in the early weeks and months following a mTBI. However, if such symptoms, in particular the cognitive, persist beyond a few months in the absence of other contributing factors (e.g., older age, previous concussions, history of attention deficit disorder or learning disability—see below), the treating clinician should *consider* a psychological etiology or component and/or exaggeration related to litigation. However, as is the case with conversion disorder, such diagnoses are often met with considerable resistance and may result in the patient looking elsewhere for care until finding someone who believes them. In the case of psychological etiology, it can be helpful to have a program addressing persistent PCS in place that includes a psychological treatment component (Iverson et al. 2007) so that the patient with persistent PCS can enter this program.

Rehabilitation following mTBI or concussion is associated with considerable controversy revolving around the expectation for cognitive recovery. The controversy stems from the fact that prospective, controlled studies of unselected populations that use neuropsychological testing as an outcome measure have indicated that recovery is completed by 3 months after a first concussion (Dikmen et al. 1995; Schretlen and Shapiro 2003; Belanger et al. 2005). Samples taken from outpatient clinics or those including participants in litigation are associated with cognitive impairment beyond 3 months (Belanger et al. 2005). However, clinicians do see patients with residual cognitive complaints that continue indefinitely, even among non-litigators, leading some to believe that long-term cognitive deficits are possible in a group of outliers. Rehabilitation after mTBI is difficult to discuss without reference to this controversy.

There is an argument to be made that indeed a small number of people may have long standing residual cognitive impairment as a result of mTBI apart from any other influences. If such mild impairment existed in one in several hundred people who have concussions, it might take thousands of subjects before a statistically significant effect could be seen in a controlled study or meta-analysis. However, the number of people who have concussions has been estimated by the CDC to be approximately 1,275,000 annually in the USA (75% of the 1.7 million TBIs) (CDC 2003; Faul et al. 2010), so that the few clinicians who treat large numbers of people with mTBI still might see such patients more than occasionally.

There are a few lines of evidence suggesting the possibility that concussion could cause such residual cognitive impairment: (1) It has been established that multiple concussions can cause permanent findings on neuropsychological testing (Collins et al. 1999; Guskiewicz et al. 2005; Belanger et al. 2010; De Beaumont et al. 2009). In order for this to be the case there has to be a certain amount of neuronal loss in a single concussion that is additive with each new concussion. Similarly, people with preexisting learning disabilities are more likely to have lasting cognitive effects from multiple concussions (Collins et al. 1999). Concussion has been found to result in worse functional outcomes (Mosenthal et al. 2004; Jacobs et al. 2010) and to be more likely to cause permanent cognitive deficits in older adults (Mazzucchi et al. 1992), though there is a study suggesting the contrary (Goldstein et al. 2001). This subject is in need of further investigation. (2) Some studies of diffusion tensor imaging done in people with mTBI have demonstrated diminished axonal integrity months or years after the injury (Kraus et al. 2007; Lipton et al. 2008; Lo et al. 2009). Kraus et al. (2007) found that there was an overlap between the degree of white matter disruption found in people with mTBI and that of people with moderate TBI. They found that performance on neuropsychological testing was inversely correlated with white matter integrity. (3) There have been studies that have looked at more subtle aspects of cognition after mTBI than are generally evaluated in the studies that showed no change (Bleiberg et al. 1998). Subjects with mTBI (more than 3 months and even greater than 1 year post-injury) have been found to have longer reaction times than controls (Bleiberg et al. 1998). Pare et al. (2009) found that reaction time in a dual-task paradigm was still prolonged at 3 months post-injury compared with healthy controls. Another study found subtle learning differences in a sample of non-litigating, working people following mTBI compared with controls (Malojcic et al. 2008). (4) There is evidence that there may be real differences in cognitive complaints of people who have had mTBI in the distant past compared with controls. One study of consecutive patients with mTBI 6 months after injury found fatigue, which could reflect additional attentional resources being mobilized to accomplish the same tasks, to be a more common complaint (32%) among those with mTBI than among controls with minor injuries (Stulemeijer et al. 2006). The Lithuanian study cited above found trends toward complaints of memory and attention problems in people long after mTBI compared to controls (Mickeviciene et al. 2002). With a higher number of subjects, these trends may have been significant.

It is possible that a very mild decline in cognitive capacity that would not be clinically significant for most people can play a larger role in the context of diminished cognitive reserve. The cognitive reserve hypothesis suggests individuals with traits that are associated with lower cognitive function would have a worse cognitive outcome than others with the same injury (Stein and McAllister 2009; Ropacki and Elias 2003; Green et al. 2008). Advancing age has been associated with worse outcomes following TBI (Ropacki and Elias 2003; Livingston et al. 2005). As noted above, among those with mTBI, previous concussions, preexisting learning disability, and perhaps older age are risk factors for persistent neuropsychological decline. As also discussed above, other factors that affect cognition, such as sleep disorders (e.g., insomnia, sleep apnea), persistent pain, or psychological factors (e.g., depression, PTSD) can diminish cognitive reserve such that a mTBI would result in persistent neuropsychological deficits that may not otherwise have been manifested (Ropacki and Elias 2003).

Rehabilitation of PCS

When a clinician first sees a patient with mTBI, it is important to begin an educational process. The patient will be considerably more open to such intervention if seen shortly after the injury. At that time, the individual can be told that it is extremely likely that the outcome will be complete cognitive recovery over a period of days or weeks. Such an educational process has been shown to improve the outcome in patients with mTBI (Mittenberg et al. 1996; Ponsford 2005; Ponsford et al. 2002). In a single-blind RCT of patients with injuries mostly on the milder side (all patients who presented at the hospital with TBI), a telephone follow-up for advice and referral as needed 7–10 days following injury improved social disability and reduced PCS compared with a control group with no specific intervention, though subgroup analysis demonstrated benefit only in those with length of PTA less than 7 days (Turner-Stokes et al. 2005; Wade et al. 1998). It seems likely that the more severely injured needed a more intensive intervention. However another single-blind RCT of all patients with mTBI presenting to the hospital found that there was no difference in the change in symptoms, community skills or self-perception of general health among those who received rehabilitation interventions as needed versus education (including that a good outcome could be expected) and advice (Turner-Stokes et al. 2005; Paniak et al. 1998).

The patient can be told that dizziness, headaches, insomnia, and other PCS are also likely to resolve over time, and that pain, emotional factors, and insomnia can exacerbate or cause cognitive impairment. Although educational interventions seem to be beneficial for the mTBI group as a whole, it is not clear how best to approach those at risk for persistent PCS. If the symptoms, including cognitive problems, have been continuing for more than a 10–14 days, it can be worthwhile to caution the patient that it can be quite stressful to experience these symptoms, especially cognitive dysfunction, and that this stress can itself further exacerbate the symptoms. Such education is as much an art as a science at this point in time, and what the clinician says, and how and to whom it is said depend to a certain extent on the feeling that he or she picks up from the patient. In another study of patients with mTBI, there was no difference in PCS at 1 year between those who received a telephone call or letter with advice and referral for rehabilitation as needed 2–8 weeks after injury versus no intervention. In the intervention group, those with few PCS declined rehabilitation and returned to work. Those with several PCS accepted rehabilitation, but had not recovered after 1 year (Elgmark Andersson et al. 2007).

When one suspects that an extended recovery is possible due to psychological issues, it may help to take it a step further and tell the patient that some people with PCS experience an extended course of recovery as a result of the stress involved, and that if his or her recovery takes more than a few months, psychological issues are a possible cause and should be explored in greater depth at that time. Having anticipated this process makes it easier to broach the subject of psychological issues at a later date, whereas usually patients are otherwise quite resistant to accepting a psychological etiology for their symptoms. Having normalized the possible emergence of psychological problems will make it easier for patients to confront their anxious or depressive feelings and to accept treatment if they do occur. For patients who may be susceptible to the cognitive equivalent of a conversion disorder, it also creates a conscious or unconscious bind in which the patient, by allowing psychological issues to influence the recovery process, will precipitate a psychological evaluation and possibly a psychiatric diagnosis, something that is often repugnant to such individuals. This is an approach that has been successfully used to treat people with conversion disorder (Teasell and Shapiro 1994). As noted above (see section on "Behavioral and Emotional Disorders" above), cognitive behavioral therapy can be successful in treating anxiety and depression following TBI, including mTBI (Soo and Tate 2007). Symptoms such as dizziness may be influenced by cognitive behavioral therapy (Andersson et al. 2006). A study of individual cognitive behavioral psychotherapy combined with cognitive remediation in participants with persistent PCS found that those in the experimental group showed better emotional functioning and also did better on a measure of divided attention than a waitlist control group (Tiersky et al. 2005). Although not yet studied in mTBI, contextual behavior therapy and acceptance and commitment therapy is preferred by one group (Iverson et al. 2007). As noted (see section on "Behavioral and Emotional Disorders" above), if pharmacological intervention becomes necessary, depression is best treated with the SSRIs and the non-sedating SNRIs. Anxiety can be treated with these medications as well.

If cognitive symptoms do persist, patients may benefit from cognitive rehabilitation to learn strategies for managing problems with arousal, attention, memory, and executive function (see section on "Cognitive Rehabilitation" above). There is no published data to assist the clinician in determining when it is best to begin these interventions in people with mTBI, and there are no specific guidelines available. Clinicians must be careful not to contribute to some patient's exaggerated belief that all of their problems are caused by brain injury (Iverson et al. 2007). Therapies should address the functional tasks that the individual is involved in everyday life and may need to include community outings. Pharmacological interventions can be helpful (see section on "Cognitive Rehabilitation" above), and again there is no information available on the timing of such treatment. Foam earplugs or sunglasses can be tried for those sensitive to noise and light, respectively (Zasler 1992). When sleep apnea is contributing to attention or arousal problems, positive airway pressure therapy or a custom oral device designed to open the airway are indicated. Insomnia is also a common contributor to cognitive symptoms following mTBI. See Chap. 10 for a discussion of insomnia and other sleep disorders following TBI. Endocrine dysfunction should also be addressed if present. See Chap. 10 for a discussion of endocrine disorders after TBI.

As noted above, if PCS persist beyond a few months, psychological intervention may be indicated, whether for assistance with reactive depression and anxiety or for pre-existing issues. Instruction on sleep hygiene should be given for those with insomnia. Relaxation techniques can be helpful as well. Clinicians should continue to educate the patient and significant others with respect to the interaction between the cognitive, psychological, and physical sequelae. Support groups are often useful. Family counseling is indicated when there is evidence of stress on family members or dysfunctional family dynamics.

There are several common types of post-traumatic headaches, and in any given individual more than one can be at play (Fenton et al. 1993; Martelli et al. 1999; Hines 1999; Lew et al. 2006; Zafonte and Horn 1999). They should, therefore, be addressed on multiple levels, with the emphasis depending on the headache type. When patients have tension headaches, treating problems with attention, sleep disorders, and psychological stresses may reduce symptoms. Patients with myofascial pain originating in the neck, upper back, or temporomandibular (TMJ) joints generally benefit from physical therapy, including stretching and strengthening exercises; postural retraining; trigger point massage; modalities such as heat or cold (some respond better to one or the other) or electrical stimulation; electromyographic biofeedback; or massage. A workplace or other environmental evaluation can identify remediable factors that may be contributing. Trigger point injections can be helpful, as can pharmacological approaches (e.g., some antidepressants, gabapentin, milnacipran—all "off-label"). Patients with TMJ problems can be treated with myofascial techniques, mouth guards, and exercises. Those headaches with an apparent vascular component (e.g., migraine headaches) may respond to acetaminophen, NSAIDs, or vasoconstrictive agents commonly used to abort migraine headaches (e.g., sumatriptan), but over-reliance on these agents can cause medication overuse headaches (MOH) ("rebound headaches"). Patients must be educated about MOH and told to restrict the use of such drugs for the worst headaches if they are frequent. For prophylaxis, some beta-blockers (e.g., propranolol), calcium-channel blockers (e.g., verapamil), antidepressants (e.g., amitriptyline, nortriptyline, venlafaxine), and anticonvulsants (e.g., valproic acid, gabapentin, topirimate) can be helpful (all "off-label"). Tension headaches may respond to some of these agents as well, though not to calcium-channel blockers. Injection of local anesthetics and/or corticosteroids can be considered for greater or lesser occipital neuralgia that does not respond to more conservative approaches. Injection should be done at the site along the nerve that replicates the headache when palpated (Hines 1999; Lew et al. 2006; Bell et al. 1999). Botulinum toxin A injections into pericranial musculature have been approved by the FDA for migraine prophylaxis, though may have only marginal benefit (Cady and Schreiber 2008). There may also be a role for botulinum toxin injections as prophylaxis against rebound headaches ("off-label") (Sandrini et al. 2011). See Chap. 10 for further discussion for the treatment of headaches following TBI.

Dizziness following mTBI is often of the vertiginous type, with sensations of spinning or, more commonly, movement. When vertiginous dizziness persists beyond 3 months, vestibular rehabilitation can bring about CNS accommodation under controlled circumstances, thus reducing symptoms. The therapist can also instruct the patient in learning compensatory strategies when accommodation is not successful (Wrisley and Pavlou 2005). Repositioning maneuvers can provide relief from benign paroxysmal positional vertigo by displacing and dispersing calcium stones (White et al. 2005). Cervicogenic dizziness is addressed by treating the underlying cervical musculoskeletal dysfunction. Suppressive medications (e.g., clonazepam, scopolamine, meclizine, gabapentin), if used at all, should only be tried when other approaches have failed (Tusa and Brown 1996). The evidence for their efficacy is extremely limited, and some of them can cause an exacerbation of problems with attention and memory. Occasionally perilymph fistula is the cause of persistent vertigo, but the diagnosis is difficult to make. Pressure-induced vertigo or disequilibrium and sensorineural hearing loss are often present. A promising diagnostic test for the presence of perilymph has been developed (Ikezono et al. 2010). The outcomes with respect to vertigo are reported to be good in 82–95% of cases, but only case series have been published. Recurrence rates are reported at 8–27%, but others believe the recurrence rate is considerably higher, as much as 67% (Seltzer and McCabe 1986; Black et al. 1992; Gyo et al. 1994; Hain 2010; Goto et al. 2001). See Chap. 10 for further discussion of balance disorders.

Vocational Rehabilitation

The extent to which an employer is supportive following a TBI can be crucial to successful return to work for all severities. Vocational counselors can facilitate communication between the patient and the workplace. Therapies should attempt to simulate workplace tasks, although if the employer is cooperative it may be better to return the person to work and have them coached and trained on the job. A gradual return to work can ease the transition (Kay 1993). Assistance with coordinating the return to work will often be needed, including on-the-job training and contact with the employer (Fadyl and McPherson 2009; Wehman et al. 1994).

References

Abdo WF, van de Warrenburg BP, Burn DJ, Quinn NP, Bloem BR. The clinical approach to movement disorders. Nat Rev Neurol. 2010;6(1):29–37.

Ackman JD, Russman BS, Thomas SS, et al. Comparing botulinum toxin A with casting for treatment of dynamic equinus in children with cerebral palsy. Dev Med Child Neurol. 2005;47(9):620–7.

Alderfer BS, Arciniegas DB, Silver JM. Treatment of depression following traumatic brain injury. J Head Trauma Rehabil. 2005;20(6):544–62.

Alexander MP. Mild traumatic brain injury: pathophysiology, natural history, and clinical management. Neurology. 1995;45(7):1253–60.

Andersson G, Asmundson GJ, Denev J, Nilsson J, Larsen HC. A controlled trial of cognitive-behavior therapy combined with vestibular rehabilitation in the treatment of dizziness. Behav Res Ther. 2006;44(9):1265–73.

Arciniegas DB. The cholinergic hypothesis of cognitive impairment caused by traumatic brain injury. Curr Psychiatry Rep. 2003;5(5):391–9.

Ashman TA, Cantor JB, Gordon WA, et al. A randomized controlled trial of sertraline for the treatment of depression in persons with traumatic brain injury. Arch Phys Med Rehabil. 2009;90(5):733–40.

Ballesteros J, Guemes I, Ibarra N, Quemada JI. The effectiveness of donepezil for cognitive rehabilitation after traumatic brain injury: a systematic review. J Head Trauma Rehabil. 2008;23(3):171–80.

Barker MJ, Greenwood KM, Jackson M, Crowe SF. An evaluation of persisting cognitive effects after withdrawal from long-term benzodiazepine use. J Int Neuropsychol Soc. 2005;11(3):281–9.

Barker-Collo SL, Feigin VL, Lawes CM, Parag V, Senior H, Rodgers A. Reducing attention deficits after stroke using attention process training: a randomized controlled trial. Stroke. 2009;40(10):3293–8.

Barnes MP. An overview of the clinical management of spasticity. In: Barnes MP, Johnson GR, editors. Upper motor neuron syndrome and spasticity: clinical management and neurophysiology. New York: Cambridge University Press; 2001. p. 1–11.

Belanger HG, Curtiss G, Demery JA, Lebowitz BK, Vanderploeg RD. Factors moderating neuropsychological outcomes following mild traumatic brain injury: a meta-analysis. J Int Neuropsychol Soc. 2005;11(3):215–27.

Belanger HG, Spiegel E, Vanderploeg RD. Neuropsychological performance following a history of multiple self-reported concussions: a meta-analysis. J Int Neuropsychol Soc. 2010;16(2):262–7.

Bell KR, Kraus EE, Zasler ND. Medical management of posttraumatic headaches: pharmacological and physical treatment. J Head Trauma Rehabil. 1999;14(1):34–48.

Bell KR, Temkin NR, Esselman PC, et al. The effect of a scheduled telephone intervention on outcome after moderate to severe traumatic brain injury: a randomized trial. Arch Phys Med Rehabil. 2005;86(5):851–6.

Berthier ML, Green C, Lara JP, et al. Memantine and constraint-induced aphasia therapy in chronic poststroke aphasia. Ann Neurol. 2009;65(5):577–85.

Black FO, Pesznecker S, Norton T, et al. Surgical management of perilymphatic fistulas: a Portland experience. Am J Otol. 1992;13(3):254–62.

Bleiberg J, Halpern EL, Reeves D, Daniel JC. Future directions for the neuropsychological assessment of sports concussion. J Head Trauma Rehabil. 1998;13(2):36–44.

Blum D, Meador K, Biton V, et al. Cognitive effects of lamotrigine compared with topiramate in patients with epilepsy. Neurology. 2006;67(3):400–6.

Bombardier CH, Bell KR, Temkin NR, Fann JR, Hoffman J, Dikmen S. The efficacy of a scheduled telephone intervention for ameliorating depressive symptoms during the first year after traumatic brain injury. J Head Trauma Rehabil. 2009;24(4):230–8.

Bombardier CH, Fann JR, Temkin NR, Esselman PC, Barber J, Dikmen SS. Rates of major depressive disorder and clinical outcomes following traumatic brain injury. JAMA. 2010;303(19):1938–45.

Bonaiuti D, Rebasti L, Sioli P. The constraint induced movement therapy: a systematic review of randomised controlled trials on the adult stroke patients. Eura Medicophys. 2007;43(2):139–46.

Bradbury CL, Christensen BK, Lau MA, Ruttan LA, Arundine AL, Green RE. The efficacy of cognitive behavior therapy in the treatment of emotional distress after acquired brain injury. Arch Phys Med Rehabil. 2008;89(12 Suppl):S61–8.

Bryant RA, Moulds M, Guthrie R, Nixon RD. Treating acute stress disorder following mild traumatic brain injury. Am J Psychiatry. 2003;160(3):585–7.

Cady R, Schreiber C. Botulinum toxin type A as migraine preventive treatment in patients previously failing oral prophylactic treatment due to compliance issues. Headache. 2008;48(6):900–13.

Cattelani R, Zettin M, Zoccolotti P. Rehabilitation treatments for adults with behavioral and psychosocial disorders following acquired brain injury: a systematic review. Neuropsychol Rev. 2010;20(1):52–85.

Centers for Disease Control and Prevention (CDC). Report to Congress on mild traumatic brain injury in the United States: steps to prevent a serious public health problem. Atlanta: Centers for Disease Control and Prevention (CDC); 2003.

Chalidis B, Stengel D, Giannoudis PV. Early excision and late excision of heterotopic ossification after traumatic brain injury are equivalent: a systematic review of the literature. J Neurotrauma. 2007;24(11):1675–86.

Chamberlain SR, Müller U, Deakin JB, et al. Lack of deleterious effects of buspirone on cognition in healthy male volunteers. J Psychopharmacol. 2008;22(6):699.

Chapman MA, Barron R, Tanis DC, Gill CE, Charles PD. Comparison of botulinum neurotoxin preparations for the treatment of cervical dystonia. Clin Ther. 2007;29(7):1325–37.

Charlton P, Ferguson D, Peacock C, Stallard J. Preliminary clinical experience of a contracture correction device. Prosthet Orthot Int. 1999;23(2):163–8.

Cherney LR, Patterson JP, Raymer A, Frymark T, Schooling T. Evidence-based systematic review: effects of intensity of treatment and constraint-induced language therapy for individuals with stroke-induced aphasia. J Speech Lang Hear Res. 2008;51(5):1282–99.

Chew E, Zafonte RD. Pharmacological management of neurobehavioral disorders following traumatic brain injury–a state-of-the-art review. J Rehabil Res Dev. 2009;46(6):851–79.

Cicerone KD, Kalmar K. Persistent postconcussion syndrome: the structure of subjective complaints after mild traumatic brain injury. J Head Trauma Rehabil. 1995;10(3):1–17.

Cicerone KD, Dahlberg C, Kalmar K, et al. Evidence-based cognitive rehabilitation: recommendations for clinical practice. Arch Phys Med Rehabil. 2000;81(12):1596–615.

Cicerone KD, Mott T, Azulay J, Friel JC. Community integration and satisfaction with functioning after intensive cognitive rehabilitation for traumatic brain injury. Arch Phys Med Rehabil. 2004;85(6):943–50.

Cicerone KD, Dahlberg C, Malec JF, et al. Evidence-based cognitive rehabilitation: updated review of the

literature from 1998 through 2002. Arch Phys Med Rehabil. 2005;86(8):1681–92.
Cipriano CA, Pill SG, Keenan MA. Heterotopic ossification following traumatic brain injury and spinal cord injury. J Am Acad Orthop Surg. 2009;17(11):689–97.
Coban A, Matur Z, Hanagasi HA, Parman Y. Iatrogenic botulism after botulinum toxin type a injections. Clin Neuropharmacol. 2010;33(3):158–60.
Coffey RJ, Edgar TS, Francisco GE, et al. Abrupt withdrawal from intrathecal baclofen: recognition and management of a potentially life-threatening syndrome. Arch Phys Med Rehabil. 2002;83(6):735–41.
Collins MW, Grindel SH, Lovell MR, et al. Relationship between concussion and neuropsychological performance in college football players. JAMA. 1999; 282(10):964–70.
Couillet J, Soury S, Lebornec G. Rehabilitation of divided attention after severe traumatic brain injury: a randomised trial. Neuropsychol Rehabil. 2010;3:1–19.
Cullen N, Perera J. Heterotopic ossification: pharmacologic options. J Head Trauma Rehabil. 2009;24(1):69–71.
Cutter NC, Scott DD, Johnson JC, Whiteneck G. Gabapentin effect on spasticity in multiple sclerosis: a placebo-controlled, randomized trial. Arch Phys Med Rehabil. 2000;81(2):164–9.
Dario A, Pisani R, Sangiorgi S, Pessina F, Tomei G. Relationship between intrathecal baclofen and the central nervous system. Acta Neurochir Suppl. 2007;97(Pt 1):461–4.
De Beaumont L, Theoret H, Mongeon D, et al. Brain function decline in healthy retired athletes who sustained their last sports concussion in early adulthood. Brain. 2009;132(Pt 3):695–708.
Deltombe T, Gustin T. Selective tibial neurotomy in the treatment of spastic equinovarus foot in hemiplegic patients: a 2-year longitudinal follow-up of 30 cases. Arch Phys Med Rehabil. 2010;91(7):1025–30.
Depompei R, Gillette Y, Goetz E, Xenopoulos-Oddsson A, Bryen D, Dowds M. Practical applications for use of PDAs and smartphones with children and adolescents who have traumatic brain injury. NeuroRehabilitation. 2008;23(6):487–99.
Dikmen S, Machamer JE, Winn HR, Temkin NR. Neuropsychological outcome at 1-year post head injury. Neuropsychology. 1995;9(1):80–90.
Dikmen SS, Machamer JE, Winn HR, Anderson GD, Temkin NR. Neuropsychological effects of valproate in traumatic brain injury: a randomized trial. Neurology. 2000;54(4):895–902.
Dimsdale JE, Newton RP, Joist T. Neuropsychological side effects of beta-blockers. Arch Intern Med. 1989; 149(3):514–25.
Douglas IJ, Smeeth L. Exposure to antipsychotics and risk of stroke: self controlled case series study. BMJ. 2008;337:a1227.
Dowds MM, Lee P, Sheer JB, et al. Electronic reminding technology following traumatic brain injury: effects on timely task completion. J Head Trauma Rehabil. 2011;26:339–47.
Dromerick AW, Lang CE, Birkenmeier RL, et al. Very Early Constraint-Induced Movement during Stroke Rehabilitation (VECTORS): a single-center RCT. Neurology. 2009;73(3):195–201.
Edwards TM, Rickard NS. Pharmaco-behavioural evidence indicating a complex role for ryanodine receptor calcium release channels in memory processing for a passive avoidance task. Neurobiol Learn Mem. 2006;86(1):1–8.
Elgmark Andersson E, Emanuelson I, Bjorklund R, Stalhammar DA. Mild traumatic brain injuries: the impact of early intervention on late sequelae. A randomized controlled trial. Acta Neurochir (Wien). 2007;149(2):151–9. discussion 160.
Elovic EP, Jasey Jr NN, Eisenberg ME. The use of atypical antipsychotics after traumatic brain injury. J Head Trauma Rehabil. 2008;23(2):132–5.
Fadyl JK, McPherson KM. Approaches to vocational rehabilitation after traumatic brain injury: a review of the evidence. J Head Trauma Rehabil. 2009;24(3):195–212.
Faul M, Xu L, Wald MM, Coronado V. Traumatic brain injury in the United States: emergency department visits, hospitalizations and deaths 2002–2006. Atlanta: Centers for Disease Control and Prevention, National Center for Injury Prevention and Control; 2010.
Fava M. Psychopharmacologic treatment of pathologic aggression. Psychiatr Clin North Am. 1997;20(2): 427–51.
Fear NT, Jones E, Groom M, et al. Symptoms of post-concussional syndrome are non-specifically related to mild traumatic brain injury in UK Armed Forces personnel on return from deployment in Iraq: an analysis of self-reported data. Psychol Med. 2009;39(8): 1379–87.
Feldman PA. Upper extremity casting and splinting. In: Glenn MB, Whyte J, editors. The practical management of spasticity in children and adults. Philadelphia: Lea and Febiger; 1990. p. 149–66.
Fenton G, McClelland R, Montgomery A, MacFlynn G, Rutherford W. The postconcussional syndrome: social antecedents and psychological sequelae. Br J Psychiatry. 1993;162:493–7.
Fleminger S, Greenwood RJ, Oliver DL. Pharmacological management for agitation and aggression in people with acquired brain injury. Cochrane Database Syst Rev. 2006(4):CD003299.
Focalin XR for ADHD. Med Lett Drugs Ther. 2009;51(1308):22–24.
Gans BM, Glenn MB. Introduction. In: Glenn MB, Whyte J, editors. The practical management of spasticity in children and adults. Philadelphia: Lea and Febieger; 1990. p. 1.
Giacino JT, Whyte J, Bagiella E, et al. Placeto-controlled trial of amantadine for severe traumatic brain injury. N Engl J Med. 2012;366(9):819–26.
Giebler KB. Physical modalities. In: Glenn MB, Whyte J, editors. The practical management of spasticity in children and adults. Philadelphia: Lea and Febiger; 1990. p. 118–48.

Glenn MB. The management of spasticity after traumatic brain injury. In: Glenn MB, Whyte J, editors. The practical management of spasticity in children and adults. Philadelphia: Lea and Febieger; 1990a. p. 296.
Glenn MB. Nerve blocks. In: Glenn MB, Whyte J, editors. The practical management of spasticity in children and adults. Philadelphia: Lea and Febieger; 1990b. p. 227.
Glenn MB. Update on pharmacology: Etidronate disodium: effects on heterotopic ossification and osteoporosis. J Head Trauma Rehabil. 1993;8(3):99–103.
Glenn MB. A differential diagnostic approach to the pharmacologic treatment of cognitive, behavioral, and affective disorders after traumatic brain injury. J Head Trauma Rehabil. 2002;17(4):273–83.
Glenn MB. Post-concussion disorders. In: Frontera WR, Silver J, editors. Essentials of rehabilitation medicine. 2nd ed. Philadelphia: Hanley & Blefus; 2008. p. 801–6.
Glenn MB. Update on pharmacology: sudden cardiac death and stroke with the use of antipsychotic medications: implications for clinicians treating individuals with traumatic brain injury. J Head Trauma Rehabil. 2010;25(1):68–70.
Glenn MB. Nerve blocks for the treatment of spasticity. In: Katz R, editor. Spasticity. Phys Med Rehabil State Art Rev. vol 3. Philadelphia: Hanley & Belfus; 1994. p. 481.
Glenn MB, Elovic E. Chemical denervation in the treatment of hypertonia and other motor disorders: Phenol and botulinum toxin. J Head Trauma Rehabil. 1997;12(6):40–62.
Glenn MB, Josephs AB. The use of lithium for behavioral and affective disorders after traumatic brain injury. J Head Trauma Rehabil. 1987;2(4):68–76.
Glenn MB, Wroblewski B. Twenty years of pharmacology. J Head Trauma Rehabil. 2005;20(1):51–61.
Glenn MB, Wroblewski B, Parziale J, Levine L, Whyte J, Rosenthal M. Lithium carbonate for aggressive behavior or affective instability in ten brain-injured patients. Am J Phys Med Rehabil. 1989;68(5):221–6.
Glenn MB, Yablon SA, Whyte J, Zafonte R. Letter to the editor. Re: a home program of rehabilitation for moderately severe traumatic brain injury patients. J Head Trauma Rehabil. 2001;16(1):vii–ix.
Goldstein FC, Levin HS, Goldman WP, Clark AN, Altonen TK. Cognitive and neurobehavioral functioning after mild versus moderate traumatic brain injury in older adults. J Int Neuropsychol Soc. 2001;7(3):373–83.
Gomer B, Wagner K, Frings L, et al. The influence of antiepileptic drugs on cognition: a comparison of levetiracetam with topiramate. Epilepsy Behav. 2007;10(3): 486–94.
Goto F, Ogawa K, Kunihiro T, Kurashima K, Kobayashi H, Kanzaki J. Perilymph fistula–45 case analysis. Auris Nasus Larynx. 2001;28(1):29–33.
Government Accountability Office. DOD health care: mental health and traumatic brain injury screening efforts implemented, but consistent pre-deployment medical record review policies needed. http://www.gao.gov/new.items/d08615.pdf. Accessed 4 April 2010.
Green RE, Colella B, Christensen B, et al. Examining moderators of cognitive recovery trajectories after moderate to severe traumatic brain injury. Arch Phys Med Rehabil. 2008;89(12 Suppl):S16–24.
Gruber SA, Silveri MM, Yurgelun-Todd DA. Neuropsychological consequences of opiate use. Neuropsychol Rev. 2007;17(3):299–315.
Guskiewicz KM, Marshall SW, Bailes J, et al. Association between recurrent concussion and late-life cognitive impairment in retired professional football players. Neurosurgery. 2005;57(4):719–26. discussion 719–726.
Gyo K, Kobayashi T, Yumoto E, Yanagihara N. Postoperative recurrence of perilymphatic fistulas. Acta Otolaryngol Suppl. 1994;514:59–62.
Hain TC. Perilymph fistula. http://www.dizziness-and-balance.com/disorders/unilat/fistula.html. Accessed 23 July 2010.
Hallenborg SC. Positioning. In: Glenn MB, Whyte J, editors. The practical management of spasticity in children and adults. Philadelphia: Lea and Febiger; 1990. p. 97–117.
Hansen TS, Larsen K, Engberg AW. The association of functional oral intake and pneumonia in patients with severe traumatic brain injury. Arch Phys Med Rehabil. 2008;89(11):2114–20.
Haran M, Bhuta T, Lee B. Pharmacological interventions for treating acute heterotopic ossification. Cochrane Database Syst Rev. 2004(4):CD003321.
Hines ME. Posttraumatic headaches. In: Varney NR, Roberts RJ, editors. The evaluation and treatment of mild traumatic brain injury. Mahwah: Lawrence Erlbaum Associates; 1999. p. 375–410.
Hoch DB, Daly L. Anticonvulsants. J Head Trauma Rehabil. 2003;18(4):383–6.
Hoge CW, McGurk D, Thomas JL, Cox AL, Engel CC, Castro CA. Mild traumatic brain injury in U.S. Soldiers returning from Iraq. N Engl J Med. 2008;358(5): 453–63.
Hoge CW, Goldberg HM, Castro CA. Care of war veterans with mild traumatic brain injury–flawed perspectives. N Engl J Med. 2009;360(16):1588–91.
Hylton N. Dynamic casting and orthotics. In: Glenn MB, Whyte J, editors. The practical management of spasticity in children and adults. Philadelphia: Lea and Febiger; 1990. p. 167–200.
Ikezono T, Shindo S, Sekiguchi S, et al. The performance of Cochlin-tomoprotein detection test in the diagnosis of perilymphatic fistula. Audiol Neurootol. 2010;15(3):168–74.
Iverson GL, Zasler ND, Lang RT. Post-concussive disorder. In: Zasler ND, Katz DI, Zafonte R, editors. Brain injury medicine: principles and practice. New York: Demos Medical Publishing, LLC; 2007. p. 373–405.
Iverson GL, Lange RT, Brooks BL, Rennison VL. "Good old days" bias following mild traumatic brain injury. Clin Neuropsychol. 2010;24(1):17–37.
Jacobs GD, Pace-Schott EF, Stickgold R, Otto MW. Cognitive behavior therapy and pharmacotherapy for insomnia: a randomized controlled trial and direct comparison. Arch Intern Med. 2004;164(17):1888–96.
Jacobs B, Beems T, Stulemeijer M, et al. Outcome prediction in mild traumatic brain injury: age and clinical

variables are stronger predictors than CT abnormalities. J Neurotrauma. 2010;27(4):655–68.
Jha A, Weintraub A, Allshouse A, et al. A randomized trial of modafinil for the treatment of fatigue and excessive daytime sleepiness in individuals with chronic traumatic brain injury. J Head Trauma Rehabil. 2008;23(1):52–63.
Jonsdottir J, Cattaneo D, Recalcati M, et al. Task-oriented biofeedback to improve gait in individuals with chronic stroke: motor learning approach. Neurorehabil Neural Repair. 2010;24:478–85.
Kaiser PR, Valko PO, Werth E, et al. Modafinil ameliorates excessive daytime sleepiness after traumatic brain injury. Neurology. 2010;75(20):1780–5.
Kaschel R, Sala SD, Cantagallo A, Fahlbock A, Laaksonen R, Kazen M. Imagery mneumonics for the rehabilitation of memory: a randomised group controlled trial. Neuropsychol Rehabil. 2002;12(2):127–53.
Katz DI, Giacino JT, Whyte J. The effectiveness of amantadine hydrochloride in improving level of consciousness and functional recovery of patients in the vegetative or minimally conscious state after traumatic brain injury. Neurology. 2011;76 Suppl 4:A345.
Kay T. Neuropsychological treatment of mild traumatic brain injury. J Head Trauma Rehabil. 1993;8(3):74–85.
Keenan MA, Lee GA, Tuckman AS, Esquenazi A. Improving calf muscle strength in patients with spastic equinovarus deformity by transfer of the long toe flexors to the Os calcis. J Head Trauma Rehabil. 1999;14(2):163–75.
Keeping P, Major R. Use of a gas spring contracture correction orthosis for the management of a fixed flexion contracture of the elbow. Prosthet Orthot Int. 1999; 23(1):82–4.
Kelly H, Brady MC, Enderby P. Speech and language therapy for aphasia following stroke. Cochrane Database Syst Rev. 2010;5:CD000425.
Kraus MF, Susmaras T, Caughlin BP, Walker CJ, Sweeney JA, Little DM. White matter integrity and cognition in chronic traumatic brain injury: a diffusion tensor imaging study. Brain. 2007;130(Pt 10):2508–19.
Krauss JK, Jankovic J. Movement disorders after TBI. In: Zasler ND, Katz DI, Zafonte R, editors. Brain injury medicine: principles and practice. New York: Demos Medical Publishing, LLC; 2007. p. 469–89.
Kreutzer JS, Rapport LJ, Marwitz JH, et al. Caregivers' well-being after traumatic brain injury: a multicenter prospective investigation. Arch Phys Med Rehabil. 2009;90(6):939–46.
Kreutzer JS, Marwitz JH, Godwin EE, Arango-Lasprilla JC. Practical approaches to effective family intervention after brain injury. J Head Trauma Rehabil. 2010;25(2):113–20.
Lance JW. The control of muscle tone, reflexes, and movement: Robert Wartenberg Lecture. Neurology. 1980;30(12):1303–13.
Larson EB, Zollman FS. The effect of sleep medications on cognitive recovery from traumatic brain injury. J Head Trauma Rehabil. 2010;25(1):61–7.
Leder SB, Suiter DM, Lisitano Warner H. Answering orientation questions and following single-step verbal commands: effect on aspiration status. Dysphagia. 2009;24(3):290–5.
Lee HW, Jung DK, Suh CK, Kwon SH, Park SP. Cognitive effects of low-dose topiramate monotherapy in epilepsy patients: a 1-year follow-up. Epilepsy Behav. 2006;8(4):736–41.
Lequerica AH, Kortte K. Therapeutic engagement: a proposed model of engagement in medical rehabilitation. Am J Phys Med Rehabil. 2010;89(5):415–22.
Levine B, Robertson IH, Clare L, et al. Rehabilitation of executive functioning: an experimental-clinical validation of goal management training. J Int Neuropsychol Soc. 2000;6(3):299–312.
Levy M, Berson A, Cook T, et al. Treatment of agitation following traumatic brain injury: a review of the literature. NeuroRehabilitation. 2005;20(4):279–306.
Lew HL, Lin PH, Fuh JL, Wang SJ, Clark DJ, Walker WC. Characteristics and treatment of headache after traumatic brain injury: a focused review. Am J Phys Med Rehabil. 2006;85(7):619–27.
Liepert J. Pharmacotherapy in restorative neurology. Curr Opin Neurol. 2008;21(6):639–43.
Lipton ML, Gellella E, Lo C, et al. Multifocal white matter ultrastructural abnormalities in mild traumatic brain injury with cognitive disability: a voxel-wise analysis of diffusion tensor imaging. J Neurotrauma. 2008;25(11):1335–42.
Livingston DH, Lavery RF, Mosenthal AC, et al. Recovery at one year following isolated traumatic brain injury: a Western Trauma Association prospective multicenter trial. J Trauma. 2005;59(6):1298–304. discussion 1304.
Lo C, Shifteh K, Gold T, Bello JA, Lipton ML. Diffusion tensor imaging abnormalities in patients with mild traumatic brain injury and neurocognitive impairment. J Comput Assist Tomogr. 2009;33(2):293–7.
Logemann JA. Evaluation and treatment of swallowing problems after TBI. In: Zasler ND, Katz DI, Zafonte R, editors. Brain injury medicine: principles and practice. New York: Demos Medical Publishing, LLC; 2007. p. 887–94.
Mackay LE, Morgan AS, Bernstein BA. Swallowing disorders in severe brain injury: risk factors affecting return to oral intake. Arch Phys Med Rehabil. 1999;80(4):365–71.
Malojcic B, Mubrin Z, Coric B, Susnic M, Spilich GJ. Consequences of mild traumatic brain injury on information processing assessed with attention and short-term memory tasks. J Neurotrauma. 2008;25(1): 30–7.
Marshall S, Teasell R, Bayona N, et al. Motor impairment rehabilitation post acquired brain injury. Brain Inj. 2007;21(2):133–60.
Martelli MF, Grayson RL, Zasler ND. Posttraumatic headache: neuropsychological and psychological effects and treatment implications. J Head Trauma Rehabil. 1999;14(1):49–69.
Mazzucchi A, Cattelani R, Missale G, Gugliotta M, Brianti R, Parma M. Head-injured subjects aged over

50 years: correlations between variables of trauma and neuropsychological follow-up. J Neurol. 1992;239(5):256–60.

McDowell S, Whyte J, D'Esposito M. Differential effect of a dopaminergic agonist on prefrontal function in traumatic brain injury patients. Brain. 1998;121(Pt 6):1155–64.

Meador KJ. Cognitive effects of levetiracetam versus topiramate. Epilepsy Curr. 2008;8(3):64–5.

Meador KJ, Gevins A, Loring DW, et al. Neuropsychological and neurophysiologic effects of carbamazepine and levetiracetam. Neurology. 2007;69(22):2076–84.

Medd J, Tate RL. Evaluation of an anger management therapy programme following ABI: a preliminary study. Neuropsychol Rehabil. 2000;10:185–201.

Medley AR, Powell T. Motivational Interviewing to promote self-awareness and engagement in rehabilitation following acquired brain injury: a conceptual review. Neuropsychol Rehabil. 2010;18:1–28.

Meinzer M, Elbert T, Djundja D, Taub E, Rockstroh B. Extending the Constraint-Induced Movement Therapy (CIMT) approach to cognitive functions: Constraint-Induced Aphasia Therapy (CIAT) of chronic aphasia. NeuroRehabilitation. 2007;22(4):311–8.

Meythaler JM, DeVivo MJ, Hadley M. Prospective study on the use of bolus intrathecal baclofen for spastic hypertonia due to acquired brain injury. Arch Phys Med Rehabil. 1996;77(5):461–6.

Meythaler JM, Guin-Renfroe S, Grabb P, Hadley MN. Long-term continuously infused intrathecal baclofen for spastic-dystonic hypertonia in traumatic brain injury: 1-year experience. Arch Phys Med Rehabil. 1999;80(1):13–9.

Meythaler JM, Brunner RC, Johnson A, Novack TA. Amantadine to improve neurorecovery in traumatic brain injury-associated diffuse axonal injury: a pilot double-blind randomized trial. J Head Trauma Rehabil. 2002;17(4):300–13.

Mickeviciene D, Schrader H, Nestvold K, et al. A controlled historical cohort study on the post-concussion syndrome. Eur J Neurol. 2002;9(6):581–7.

Mild Traumatic Brain Injury Committee of the Head Injury Interdisciplinary Special Interest Group of the American Congress of Rehabilitation Medicine. Definition of mild traumatic brain injury. J Head Trauma Rehabil. 1993;8(3):86–7.

Mills KC, Drazkowski JF, Hammer AE, Caldwell PT, Kustra RP, Blum DE. Relative influences of adjunctive topiramate and adjunctive lamotrigine on scanning and the effective field of view. Epilepsy Res. 2008;78(2–3):140–6.

Mittenberg W, DiGiulio DV, Perrin S, Bass AE. Symptoms following mild head injury: expectation as aetiology. J Neurol Neurosurg Psychiatry. 1992;55(3):200–4.

Mittenberg W, Tremont G, Zielinski RE, Fichera S, Rayls KR. Cognitive-behavioral prevention of postconcussion syndrome. Arch Clin Neuropsychol. 1996;11(2):139–45.

Moseley AM, Hassett LM, Leung J, Clare JS, Herbert RD, Harvey LA. Serial casting versus positioning for the treatment of elbow contractures in adults with traumatic brain injury: a randomized controlled trial. Clin Rehabil. 2008;22(5):406–17.

Mosenthal AC, Livingston DH, Lavery RF, et al. The effect of age on functional outcome in mild traumatic brain injury: 6-month report of a prospective multicenter trial. J Trauma. 2004;56(5):1042–8.

Newman CJ, Kennedy A, Walsh M, O'Brien T, Lynch B, Hensey O. A pilot study of delayed versus immediate serial casting after botulinum toxin injection for partially reducible spastic equinus. J Pediatr Orthop. 2007;27(8):882–5.

Niemeier JP. The Lighthouse Strategy: use of a visual imagery technique to treat visual inattention in stroke patients. Brain Inj. 1998;12(5):399–406.

O'Neil-Pirozzi TM, Momose KJ, Mello J, et al. Feasibility of swallowing interventions for tracheostomized individuals with severely disordered consciousness following traumatic brain injury. Brain Inj. 2003;17(5):389–99.

O'Neil-Pirozzi TM, Strangman GE, Goldstein R, et al. A controlled treatment study of internal memory strategies (I-MEMS) following traumatic brain injury. J Head Trauma Rehabil. 2010;25(1):43–51.

Ogasawara T, Itoh Y, Tamura M, et al. Involvement of cholinergic and GABAergic systems in the reversal of memory disruption by NS-105, a cognition enhancer. Pharmacol Biochem Behav. 1999;64(1):41–52.

Ohnuki T, Nomura Y. 1-[[[5-(4-Nitrophenyl)-2-furanyl] methylene]imino]-2,4-imidazolidinedione (dantrolene), an inhibitor of intracellular Ca2+ mobilization, impairs avoidance performance and spatial memory in mice. Biol Pharm Bull. 1996;19(8):1038–40.

Ownsworth TL, McFarland K. Memory remediation in long-term acquired brain injury: two approaches in diary training. Brain Inj. 1999;13(8):605–26.

Paniak C, Toller-Lobe G, Durand A, Nagy J. A randomized trial of two treatments for mild traumatic brain injury. Brain Inj. 1998;12(12):1011–23.

Paran E, Anson O, Lowenthal DT. Cognitive function and antihypertensive treatment in the elderly: a 6-year follow-up study. Am J Ther. 2010;17:358–64.

Pare N, Rabin LA, Fogel J, Pepin M. Mild traumatic brain injury and its sequelae: characterisation of divided attention deficits. Neuropsychol Rehabil. 2009;19(1).110–37.

Park SP, Kwon SH. Cognitive effects of antiepileptic drugs. J Clin Neurol. 2008;4(3):99–106.

Piazza SJ, Adamson RL, Sanders JO, Sharkey NA. Changes in muscle moment arms following split tendon transfer of tibialis anterior and tibialis posterior. Gait Posture. 2001;14(3):271–8.

Ponsford J. Rehabilitation interventions after mild head injury. Curr Opin Neurol. 2005;18(6):692–7.

Ponsford J, Willmott C, Rothwell A, et al. Impact of early intervention on outcome following mild head injury in adults. J Neurol Neurosurg Psychiatry. 2002;73(3):330–2.

Powell J, Heslin J, Greenwood R. Community based rehabilitation after severe traumatic brain injury: a randomised controlled trial. J Neurol Neurosurg Psychiatry. 2002;72(2):193–202.

Pulvermuller F, Neininger B, Elbert T, et al. Constraint-induced therapy of chronic aphasia after stroke. Stroke. 2001;32(7):1621–6.

Ray WA, Chung CP, Murray KT, Hall K, Stein CM. Atypical antipsychotic drugs and the risk of sudden cardiac death. N Engl J Med. 2009;360(3):225–35.

Ropacki MT, Elias JW. Preliminary examination of cognitive reserve theory in closed head injury. Arch Clin Neuropsychol. 2003;18(6):643–54.

Rosenfeld JV, Ford NL. Bomb blast, mild traumatic brain injury and psychiatric morbidity: a review. Injury. 2010;41(5):437–43.

Ruff RM, Iverson GL, Barth JT, Bush SS, Broshek DK. Recommendations for diagnosing a mild traumatic brain injury: a National Academy of Neuropsychology education paper. Arch Clin Neuropsychol. 2009;24(1) :3–10.

Salazar AM, Warden DL, Schwab K, et al. Cognitive rehabilitation for traumatic brain injury. A randomized trial: Defense and Veterans Head Injury Program (DVHIP) Study Group. JAMA. 2000;283(23): 3075–81.

Salinsky M, Storzbach D, Munoz S. Cognitive effects of pregabalin in healthy volunteers: a double-blind, placebo-controlled trial. Neurology. 2010;74(9):755–61.

Sandrini G, Perrotta A, Tassorelli C. Botulinum toxin type-A in the prophylactic treatment of medication-overuse headache: a multicenter, double-blind, randomized, placebo-controlled, parallel group study. J Headache Pain. 2011;12(4):427–33.

Sanger TD, Delgado MR, Gaebler-Spira D, Hallett M, Mink JW. Classification and definition of disorders causing hypertonia in childhood. Pediatrics. 2003; 111(1):e89–97.

Schretlen DJ, Shapiro AM. A quantitative review of the effects of traumatic brain injury on cognitive functioning. Int Rev Psychiatry. 2003;15(4):341–9.

Seltzer S, McCabe BF. Perilymph fistula: the Iowa experience. Laryngoscope. 1986;94:37–49.

Semlyen JK, Summers SJ, Barnes MP. Traumatic brain injury: efficacy of multidisciplinary rehabilitation. Arch Phys Med Rehabil. 1998;79(6):678–83.

Shaw SE, Morris DM, Uswatte G, McKay S, Meythaler JM, Taub E. Constraint-induced movement therapy for recovery of upper-limb function following traumatic brain injury. J Rehabil Res Dev. 2005;42(6):769–78.

Shaw L, Rodgers H, Price C, et al. BoTULS: a multicentre randomised controlled trial to evaluate the clinical effectiveness and cost-effectiveness of treating upper limb spasticity due to stroke with botulinum toxin type A. Health Technol Assess. 2010;14(26):1–113. iii–iv.

Shiel A, Burn JP, Henry D, et al. The effects of increased rehabilitation therapy after brain injury: results of a prospective controlled trial. Clin Rehabil. 2001;15(5): 501–14.

Silver JM, Koumaras B, Chen M, et al. Effects of rivastigmine on cognitive function in patients with traumatic brain injury. Neurology. 2006;67(5):748–55.

Singer BJ, Jegasothy GM, Singer KP, Allison GT. Evaluation of serial casting to correct equinovarus deformity of the ankle after acquired brain injury in adults. Arch Phys Med Rehabil. 2003;84(4):483–91.

Slade A, Tennant A, Chamberlain MA. A randomised controlled trial to determine the effect of intensity of therapy upon length of stay in a neurological rehabilitation setting. J Rehabil Med. 2002;34(6):260–6.

Smith Jr KR, Goulding PM, Wilderman D, Goldfader PR, Holterman-Hommes P, Wei F. Neurobehavioral effects of phenytoin and carbamazepine in patients recovering from brain trauma: a comparative study. Arch Neurol. 1994;51(7):653–60.

Smith ME, Gevins A, McEvoy LK, Meador KJ, Ray PG, Gilliam F. Distinct cognitive neurophysiologic profiles for lamotrigine and topiramate. Epilepsia. 2006;47(4): 695–703.

Smoller JW, Allison M, Cochrane BB, et al. Antidepressant use and risk of incident cardiovascular morbidity and mortality among postmenopausal women in the Women's Health Initiative study. Arch Intern Med. 2009;169(22):2128–39.

Soechting JF, Lacquaniti F. An assessment of the existence of muscle synergies during load perturbations and intentional movements of the human arm. Exp Brain Res. 1989;74(3):535–48.

Sohlberg MM, McLaughlin KA, Pavese A, Heidrich A, Posner MI. Evaluation of attention process training and brain injury education in persons with acquired brain injury. J Clin Exp Neuropsychol. 2000;22(5): 656–76.

Soo C, Tate R. Psychological treatment for anxiety in people with traumatic brain injury. Cochrane Database Syst Rev. 2007(3):CD005239.

Spielman G, Gennarelli TA, Rogers CR. Disodium etidronate: its role in preventing heterotopic ossification in severe head injury. Arch Phys Med Rehabil. 1983;64(11):539–42.

Stahl SM, Mignon L, Meyer JM. Which comes first: atypical antipsychotic treatment or cardiometabolic risk? Acta Psychiatr Scand. 2009;119(3):171–9.

Stapleton S, Adams M, Atterton L. A mobile phone as a memory aid for individuals with traumatic brain injury: a preliminary investigation. Brain Inj. 2007;21(4):401–11.

Stein MB, McAllister TW. Exploring the convergence of posttraumatic stress disorder and mild traumatic brain injury. Am J Psychiatry. 2009;166(7):768–76.

Stulemeijer M, van der Werf S, Bleijenberg G, Biert J, Brauer J, Vos PE. Recovery from mild traumatic brain injury: a focus on fatigue. J Neurol. 2006;253(8): 1041–7.

Tang V, Warden J, Cullen N, Rutledge E. Topiramate in traumatic brain injury: adverse effects on cognitive function. J Head Trauma Rehabil. 2007;22(6): 409–10.

Teasell RW, Shapiro AP. Strategic-behavioral intervention in the treatment of chronic nonorganic motor disorders. Am J Phys Med Rehabil. 1994;73(1):44–50.

Terre R, Mearin F. Prospective evaluation of oro-pharyngeal dysphagia after severe traumatic brain injury. Brain Inj. 2007;21(13–14):1411–7.

Terre R, Mearin F. Evolution of tracheal aspiration in severe traumatic brain injury-related oropharyngeal dysphagia: 1-year longitudinal follow-up study. Neurogastroenterol Motil. 2009;21(4):361–9.

The PDR® Electronic Library from Thomson Micromedex. 2009. Revised 01/2008. http://www.micromedex.com/products/pdrlibrary/. Accessed 24 July 2010.

Tiersky LA, Anselmi V, Johnston MV, et al. A trial of neuropsychologic rehabilitation in mild-spectrum traumatic brain injury. Arch Phys Med Rehabil. 2005;86(8):1565–74.

Trouillas P, Xie J, Adeleine P, et al. Buspirone, a 5-hydroxytryptamine1A agonist, is active in cerebellar ataxia. Results of a double-blind drug placebo study in patients with cerebellar cortical atrophy. Arch Neurol. 1997;54(6):749–52.

Tsunoda K, Uchida H, Suzuki T, Watanabe K, Yamashima T, Kashima H. Effects of discontinuing benzodiazepine-derivative hypnotics on postural sway and cognitive functions in the elderly. Int J Geriatr Psychiatry. 2010;25:1259–65.

Turner-Stokes L, Disler PB, Nair A, Wade DT. Multidisciplinary rehabilitation for acquired brain injury in adults of working age. Cochrane Database Syst Rev. 2005(3):CD004170.

Tusa RJ, Brown SB. Neuro-otologic trauma and dizziness. In: Rizzo M, Tranel D, editors. Head injury and postconcussive syndrome. New York: Churchill Livingstone; 1996. p. 177–200.

van Dijk H, Jannink MJ, Hermens HJ. Effect of augmented feedback on motor function of the affected upper extremity in rehabilitation patients: a systematic review of randomized controlled trials. J Rehabil Med. 2005;37(4):202–11.

Wade DT, King NS, Wenden FJ, Crawford S, Caldwell FE. Routine follow up after head injury: a second randomised controlled trial. J Neurol Neurosurg Psychiatry. 1998;65(2):177–83.

Wehman P, Booth M, Stallard D, et al. Return to work for persons with traumatic brain injury and spinal cord injury: three case studies. Int J Rehabil Res. 1994;17(3):268–77.

White J, Savvides P, Cherian N, Oas J. Canalith repositioning for benign paroxysmal positional vertigo. Otol Neurotol. 2005;26(4):704–10.

Whyte J, Hart T, Schuster K, Fleming M, Polansky M, Coslett HB. Effects of methylphenidate on attentional function after traumatic brain injury. A randomized, placebo-controlled trial. Am J Phys Med Rehabil. 1997;76(6):440–50.

Whyte J, Vaccaro M, Grieb-Neff P, Hart T. Psychostimulant use in the rehabilitation of individuals with traumatic brain injury. J Head Trauma Rehabil. 2002;17(4):284–99.

Whyte J, Vaccaro M, Grieb-Neff P, Hart T, Polansky M, Coslett HB. The effects of bromocriptine on attention deficits after traumatic brain injury: a placebo-controlled pilot study. Am J Phys Med Rehabil. 2008;87(2):85–99.

Wilk JE, Thomas JL, McGurk DM, Riviere LA, Castro CA, Hoge CW. Mild traumatic brain injury (concussion) during combat: lack of association of blast mechanism with persistent postconcussive symptoms. J Head Trauma Rehabil. 2010;25(1):9–14.

Willis SL, Tennstedt SL, Marsiske M, et al. Long-term effects of cognitive training on everyday functional outcomes in older adults. JAMA. 2006;296(23): 2805–14.

Wilmont J, Ponsford J. Efficacy of methylphenidate in the rehabilitation of attention following traumatic brain injury: a randomised, crossover, double-blind, placebo controlled inpatient trial. J Neurol Neurosurg Psychiatry. 2009;80:552–7.

Wilson BA, Emslie HC, Quirk K, Evans JJ. Reducing everyday memory and planning problems by means of a paging system: a randomised control crossover study. J Neurol Neurosurg Psychiatry. 2001;70(4):477–82.

Wilson BA, Emslie H, Quirk K, Evans J, Watson P. A randomized control trial to evaluate a paging system for people with traumatic brain injury. Brain Inj. 2005;19(11):891–4.

Wolf SL, Winstein CJ, Miller JP, et al. Effect of constraint-induced movement therapy on upper extremity function 3 to 9 months after stroke: the EXCITE randomized clinical trial. JAMA. 2006;296(17):2095–104.

Wolf SL, Newton H, Maddy D, et al. The Excite Trial: relationship of intensity of constraint induced movement therapy to improvement in the wolf motor function test. Restor Neurol Neurosci. 2007;25(5–6): 549–62.

Wood RL. Brain injury rehabilitation: a neurobehavioural approach. Rockville: An Aspen Publication; 1987.

Wrisley DM, Pavlou M. Physical therapy for balance disorders. Neurol Clin. 2005;23(3):855–74. vii–viii.

Writer BW, Schillerstrom JE. Psychopharmacological treatment for cognitive impairment in survivors of traumatic brain injury: a critical review. J Neuropsychiatry Clin Neurosci. 2009;21(4):362–70.

Wu CY, Chen CL, Tsai WC, Lin KC, Chou SH. A randomized controlled trial of modified constraint-induced movement therapy for elderly stroke survivors: changes in motor impairment, daily functioning, and quality of life. Arch Phys Med Rehabil. 2007a;88(3): 273–8.

Wu CY, Lin KC, Chen HC, Chen IH, Hong WH. Effects of modified constraint-induced movement therapy on movement kinematics and daily function in patients with stroke: a kinematic study of motor control mechanisms. Neurorehabil Neural Repair. 2007b;21(5): 460–6.

Ylvisaker M, Jacobs HE, Feeney T. Positive supports for people who experience behavioral and cognitive disability after brain injury: a review. J Head Trauma Rehabil. 2003;18(1):7–32.

Zaccara G, Gangemi PF, Cincotta M. Central nervous system adverse effects of new antiepileptic drugs. A meta-analysis of placebo-controlled studies. Seizure. 2008;17(5):405–21.

Zafonte RD, Horn LJ. Clinical assessment of posttraumatic headaches. J Head Trauma Rehabil. 1999;14(1): 22–33.

Zafonte R, Lombard L, Elovic E. Antispasticity medications: uses and limitations of enteral therapy. Am J Phys Med Rehabil. 2004;83(10 Suppl):S50–8.

Zasler ND. Neuromedical diagnosis and management of post-concussive disorders. Rehabilitation of post-concussive disorders. Phys Med Rehabil State Art Rev. 1992; 6(1):33–67.

Zhang L, Plotkin RC, Wang G, Sandel ME, Lee S. Cholinergic augmentation with donepezil enhances recovery in short-term memory and sustained attention after traumatic brain injury. Arch Phys Med Rehabil. 2004;85(7):1050–5.

Zhu XL, Poon WS, Chan CC, Chan SS. Does intensive rehabilitation improve the functional outcome of patients with traumatic brain injury (TBI)? A randomized controlled trial. Brain Inj. 2007;21(7):681–90.

Interventions to Improve Cognitive Functioning After TBI

15

Anthony J.-W. Chen and Tatjana Novakovic-Agopian

Abstract

Traumatic injury to the brain can affect the core of what makes us human—our cognition and emotion. The injuries are acute but may result in chronic burdens for individuals and families as well as society. Effective approaches to improving functioning are needed, and the benefits may be far-reaching. We discuss some basic principles to guide current practice, as well as major directions for continuing advancement of ways to improve functioning after injury. Interventions are more likely to be effective when we take into account multiple levels of brain functioning, from neurons to pharmacological systems to social networks. Training of cognitive functions is of special importance, and benefits may synergize with pharmacologic and other approaches that modify biology. The combination of physical and experiential trauma deserves special consideration, with effects on cognition, emotion, and other substrates of behavior. Directing further research toward key frontiers that bridge neuroscience and rehabilitation will advance the development of clinically effective interventions.

Keywords

Traumatic brain injury • Rehabilitation • Cognitive training • Cognitive neuroscience • Frontal lobes • Attention • Memory • Executive control

A.J.-W. Chen, M.D. (✉)
Department of Neurology, VA Northern California Health Care System and University of California at San Francisco, San Francisco, CA, USA
e-mail: anthony.chen@ucsf.edu

T. Novakovic-Agopian, Ph.D.
Department of Neurology, University of California at San Francisco and Martinez VAMC, San Francisco, CA, USA

J.W. Tsao (ed.), *Traumatic Brain Injury: A Clinician's Guide to Diagnosis, Management, and Rehabilitation*,
DOI 10.1007/978-0-387-87887-4_15, © Springer Science+Business Media, LLC 2012

Outline

I. Introduction and Overview
   - Brain injuries and cognition
   - Acute injuries, chronic consequences
   - A combined combat neurotrauma syndrome (TBI–PTSD)?

II. Approaches to Intervention
   - Overview of potential targets of therapy: overlapping layers of brain functioning
   - Targeting the outer layers: modulators of cognition
   - Targeting core cognitive processes
   - Integrating behavioral and pharmacologic therapies
   - Special considerations for TBI–PTSD and frontiers for the interactions between cognition and emotion

III. Directions and Imperatives for Future Work
   - A long-term view
   - Challenges for implementation
   - Bridges between neuroscience and rehabilitation

A service member returning from active duty deployment to the Middle East states on a screening questionnaire that he was exposed to multiple blasts in combat. In one incident, while he was riding in a convoy, his truck was struck by a blast from a roadside improvised explosive device. A wheel was caught in the crater and the vehicle dove into a ditch. "I think my head struck the side of the truck, and I may have blacked out—I'm not sure how long." He admits to feeling dazed and somewhat confused. This seemed to resolve within a day, and the soldier returned to full duty. However, he was exposed to several more blasts during his deployment. While he cannot recall the details of each incident clearly, he endorses feeling dazed with each episode. He complains that he has had many difficulties since returning home. He has had trouble getting organized for job applications and other tasks—"I would get started, but then I always ended up doing something else." He complains of feeling highly distractible and easily overwhelmed, and states that his memory is like "swiss cheese." Others describe him as irritable and easily angered. He has difficulty in sleeping, feels depressed, and avoids leaving his home.

Introduction and Overview

Cognitive Dysfunction from Traumatic Brain Injury

This individual's experience is quite common among veterans who have served in active duty. Approximately 7,000 military personnel with traumatic brain injury (TBI) were admitted annually to military and Veterans Hospitals based on a 2003 report by the Defense and Veterans Brain Injury Center. Recent combat-related activities in the Middle East have resulted in an increased incidence of TBI, and TBI has been called a "hallmark injury" of current combat activities. It has been estimated that 59% of soldiers exposed to blasts will have some form of closed head injury (Okie 2005). Head injury is commonly caused by other combat and non-combat-related causes, such as motor vehicle collisions, falling objects, altercations, or projectile strikes to helmets. According to Walter Reed's Brain Injury Center, 31% of battle-injured soldiers admitted between January 2003 and April 2005 had TBIs.

The impact of these injuries may be at once basic and far-reaching, yet difficult to recognize.

From Acute to Chronic Cognitive Dysfunction

In the moment of an instant, an injury to the brain can cause changes that affect a person for a lifetime. Although the injuries are acute, functional deficits that result from TBI may produce tremendous *chronic* burden on individuals, families, and health care systems. This discussion will focus on problems that persist to become debilitating on a chronic basis. This is an important area to address for several reasons. The intrinsic importance of problems that are persistent (not resolving spontaneously or not responsive to therapies) is obvious. Acquired brain injuries have been a leading cause of long-term disability in the USA, even before the current conflicts (Thurman et al. 1999) and a leading contributor to increasing health care costs in the VA (Yu et al. 2003). Individuals with TBI are at risk for being unable to live independently. Surveillance for TBI across 14 states showed that approximately one-third of patients continue to require assistance with daily activities 1 year after injury (Langlois et al. 2003). For patients hospitalized for TBI, cognitive status is a major factor in determining whether individuals are discharged to institutions (van Baalen et al. 2008). A more dire but difficult to quantify consequence is the cascade that may lead to homelessness.

For less severe dysfunction, patients may have symptoms that are not recognized by health care providers without specific screening, but which are significant and need to be addressed (Hux et al. 2009). One specific challenge for combat-related injury is that some of the "milder" effects of brain injury may not be immediately detected. Detection may be particularly complicated as some individuals experience problems that only become apparent with a change in setting, new cognitive demands, loss of supportive social structure, and demands to learn new skills or knowledge. For example, cognitive dysfunction may become particularly debilitating during transitions from the familiar structure of military life to civilian life, including adjustments to school or new occupations.

TBI, if recognized at all, is predominantly addressed during acute stages. Ironically, *chronic* cognitive problems tend to receive relatively little medical attention. The issue of insurance coverage in the private sector has been raised as one barrier to care that has even been recognized by public press (Burton 2007). However, another fundamental factor is the need for improved guidance for treating chronic cognitive dysfunction. Treatment needs tend to be complex and individual, and few general guidelines have been available to guide treatment. However, an evidence base for cognitive rehabilitation interventions is being progressively strengthened.

A long-term view is needed and major long-term issues need to be taken into account in clinical programs (Chen and D'Esposito 2010). The far-reaching impact of these seemingly "invisible" deficits is often not recognized. For example, individuals who cannot pay attention, hold information in mind, and actively participate in learning activities will have reduced benefit from other rehabilitation efforts, such as those directed toward motor or speech functions (Prigatano and Wong 1999). Individuals who have suffered a TBI may also be at increased risk for developing cognitive changes later in life (Mauri et al. 2006; Van Den Heuvel et al. 2007; Schwartz 2009).

Injuries and Cognitive Symptoms

Although it is commonly understood that TBI can result in almost any neurologic deficit, the most common and persistent deficits tend to be in cognitive functions. Among cortical regions, prefrontal and mesial temporal structures are vulnerable to contusions and hemorrhages. These correspond to deficits in frontal executive functions and declarative memory, as well as other aspects of behavioral and emotional self-regulation. Diffuse or multifocal axonal injury may affect commissural, callosal, association as well as particularly vulnerable long fibers, including those carrying neuromodulators in projections from the brainstem to cerebral end targets and those that connect the prefrontal cortex (PFC) with other brain regions. Some of the most common deficits with distributed axonal injury, even in the absence of cortical lesions, are in speed of processing, frontal executive functions, and memory (Scheid et al. 2006). The nature of cognitive dysfunction with TBI and intervention approaches for these symptoms are discussed in greater detail in this chapter.

Are cognitive deficits important in mild TBI? The occurrence of cognitive deficits in moderate and severe TBI is well-recognized, but cognitive deficits may also be a significant problem after so-called "mild" TBI (Binder et al. 1997; Mathias and Coats 1999; Cicerone and Azulay 2002; Mathias et al. 2004; Belanger et al. 2005; Frencham et al. 2005; Vanderploeg et al. 2005). Delineation of cognitive dysfunction has been more problematic, however. The controversies and debates have been extensive. We argue that it is particularly important to define the severity of dysfunction, rather than the severity of initial injury. It is clear that traditional labels of "mild, moderate, or severe" are poor characterizations of individuals with TBI (Saatman et al. 2008). Furthermore, injury history is often not clear for many veterans who suffered injury(ies) in the field, making these labels even more imprecise. Current functional status is measurable. For the current discussion, an emphasis is placed on considering "mild" cognitive dysfunction as a persistent problem, not "mild TBI." In other words, we emphasize the targeting of interventions to current functioning, not the diagnostic label for the historical acute injury.

Although self-reported symptoms and outcomes from cognitive testing vary greatly, deficits in control processes, including attention and working memory, and also reflected in speed of processing are commonly reported and may be the most affected domains in mild TBI (Binder et al. 1997; Mathias and Coats 1999; Cicerone and Azulay 2002; Mathias et al. 2004; Belanger et al. 2005; Frencham et al. 2005; Vanderploeg et al. 2005). Aspects of executive control may be important factors in determining successful return to work after mild TBI (Drake et al. 2000). Deficits from blast injury are still being defined, though preliminary evidence suggests that similar issues occur with blasts as other forms of TBI (Belanger et al. 2009). As will be discussed in this chapter, there may be a number of contributors to poor cognitive functioning, asides from the physical brain injury per se.

Spontaneous recovery? Despite their importance, chronic deficits in cognitive functions are often poorly addressed. Patients with mild TBI, but also patients with more severe initial injuries, are commonly advised that recovery will simply occur with time. This can be reassuring, and, fortunately, the recovery trajectory for most patients who survive TBI is positive over time. Most individuals with mild TBI improve to baseline. However, there is significant variability in the rate and end point of recovery. A significant minority (10–20% in nonmilitary settings) report persistent deficits that can last months and years post-injury, leaving chronic, residual disabilities that have a wide-ranging impact on an individual's life (Binder et al. 1997; Ruff 2005). Additional data from tracking of military veterans will be needed in order to understand the long-term effects of combat-related TBI, which commonly results in forms of "mild TBI."

Approaching treatment of post-TBI cognitive dysfunction is complicated by the frequent occurrence of multiple and varied symptoms. For example, the existence of a "post-concussive syndrome" (PCS) is now widely accepted, though this remains a somewhat difficult to define entity or entities even in the better studied nonmilitary settings, with variable presentations, sources, and possible courses. The syndrome is characterized by headaches, dizziness, general malaise, excessive fatigue, or noise intolerance; irritability, emotional lability, depression, or anxiety; subjective complaints of concentration or memory difficulty; insomnia; reduced tolerance to alcohol; preoccupation with these symptoms and fear of permanent brain damage. Documentation of cognitive dysfunction on "objective" testing is not required for diagnosis, though altered cognitive functioning may accompany these symptoms. Although these symptoms are, by definition, occurring after a concussion, this does not necessarily mean that brain injury directly causes these symptoms. The pathogenetic factors that lead a persistence of symptoms are not fully understood and remain controversial. It is not clear that imaging findings are predictive of persistence of symptoms. However, it is likely that psychological factors play an important role—this is a particularly important consideration given the contexts in which physical trauma and recovery periods occur, including the associated traumatic experiences in combat or even in medical settings. These factors may be important in formulating interventions to improve functioning.

Beyond Post-concussive Symptoms: A Combined Combat Neurotrauma Syndrome

It is increasingly recognized that a large portion of individuals returning from combat activities suffer from both TBI and post-traumatic stress disorder (PTSD) or at least symptoms. A 2005 survey of Iraq/Afghanistan veterans found that for the 12% of 2,235 respondents with a history of mild TBI, the strongest factor associated with persistent post-concussive symptoms was PTSD, even after removing overlapping symptoms from the PTSD score (Schneiderman et al. 2008). A cross-sectional survey of Army veterans, 3–4 months after return from Iraq in 2006, revealed the highest prevalence of PTSD among those with a history of loss of consciousness (LOC) (Hoge et al. 2008). LOC was also associated with major depression. Mild TBI (defined by a history of traumatically induced disruption of brain function accompanied by LOC or alteration of mental status) was associated with post-concussive symptoms—but not after controlling for PTSD and depression. In examining the incidence of PTSD, rates increase in relationship to the occurrence of TBI, with increased incidence of PTSD along the gradient of no TBI to altered mental status to LOC (Taber and Hurley 2009). A study by examining TBI and PTSD service utilization of OIF veterans found that 1-year post-deployment, 65% of those with "mild TBI"–PTSD reported seeking treatment for concerns related to re-integration (Polusny et al. 2011). All of these epidemiological findings raise questions about the interactions between TBI and PTSD.

The interactions between TBI and PTSD are undoubtedly complex and multilayered. Trauma may alter an individual's brain functioning via many routes. Direct physical injury may certainly be caused by traumatic forces, leading not only to contusions, hemorrhages, and even strokes but also injuries to the white matter fibers that connect brain regions. However, severe distress from the traumatic experience may also have immediate as well as long-term effects on brain functioning. Post-traumatic stress effects are increasingly recognized as being mediated by altered brain functions and possibly structure. Both physical and experiential trauma may contribute to acute disruption of function as well as ongoing cascades of sequelae that layer upon the initial injury. Understanding that these mechanisms of injury interact at multiple levels is of great importance for understanding, diagnosing, and managing the effects of these injuries. This may have particularly important ramifications for the formulation of interventions, and this is discussed in detail in this chapter.

The story told by the veteran above is likely to raise a number of important questions in a clinician's mind, including questions of etiology, diagnosis, and diagnostics, but perhaps the most important question is this: What can be done to improve this person's functioning?

Approaches to Intervention

Synopsis of Intervening to Improve Cognitive Functioning

The following are key points to consider in determining interventions for improving cognitive functioning after brain injury.

- The most common difficulties after TBI involve complex attention, learning, memory, organization, and other processes important for goal-directed behavior.
- Sources of dysfunction may be multifactorial. Sources include not only deficits in specific neural processes but also functional difficulties

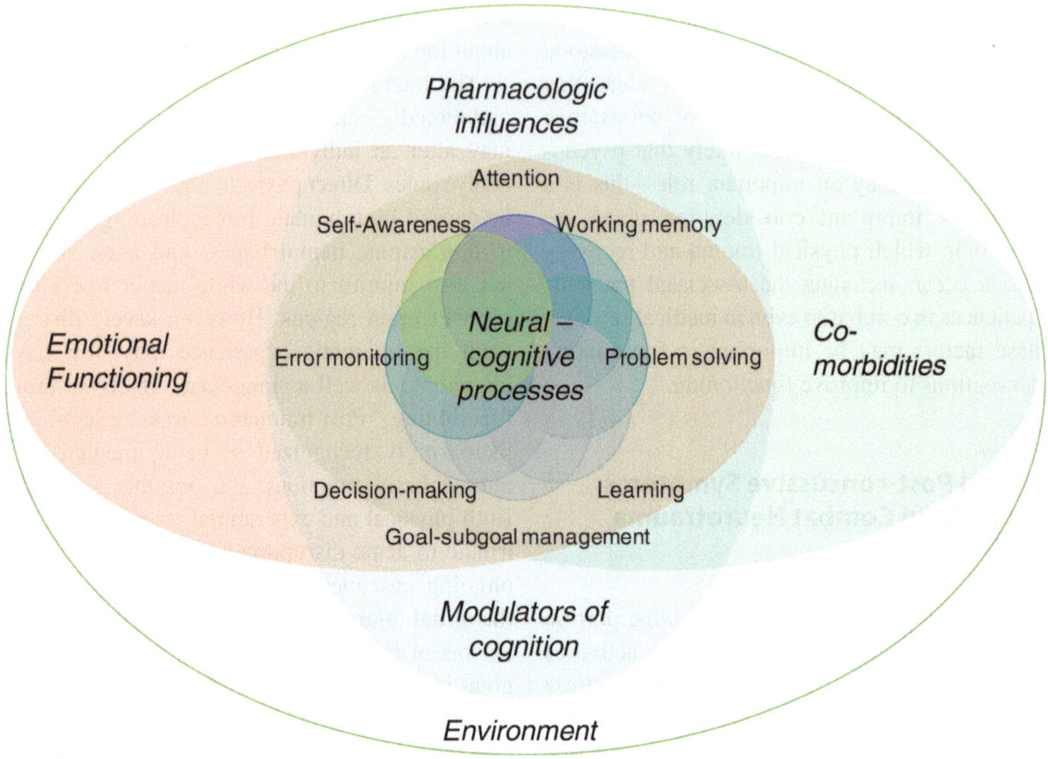

Fig. 15.1 Multiple sources of dysfunction lead to multiple tiers of intervention. Core targets of intervention include specific neural-cognitive processes important for healthy, goal-directed functioning after brain injuries. However, these processes may also be affected by modulators that alter cognitive state or cognitive performance (e.g., sleep, fatigue), pharmacologic influences (e.g., medications, other drugs), emotional functioning (e.g., irritability, anger, depression), and other comorbidities (e.g., chronic pain). All of these are potential targets for interventions to improve cognitive functioning

in engaging cognitive processes for goal-relevant activities, factors that modulate physiologic brain states, emotional factors that interact with cognitive functioning, pharmacologic and other biological modifiers, and interactions of cognition with specific environments. The interactive nature of these factors is illustrated in the overlapping layers in Fig. 15.1. Any or all of the above may have to be taken into account for a therapeutic intervention to be effective. Each of these layers is discussed in this chapter.

- Interventions may be targeted to specific cognitive processes, specific sources of dysfunction, supportive processes, specific modulating or exacerbating factors, and/or an integrated approach that addresses multiple targets concurrently based on a particular therapeutic goal.
- Some processes may be worth targeting even if "deficits" are not detectable, including processes that are "gateways" to learning and change. Although a wide range of cognitive processes may be affected by injury, a core set of cognitive processes may be considered central to enhancing the rehabilitation process itself. These include "meta-cognitive" processes such as self-awareness (awareness of one's abilities, strengths, weaknesses, and goals, with the ability to monitor and review one's actions in these contexts), and functions for regulating attention, learning, and memory in an organized, goal-directed manner. These processes will also be crucial for continued learning and adaption outside of clinician-guided settings.
- Behavioral approaches for modifying behavior include training, i.e., the guidance of learning

through activities with specific learning goals. Training forms the most fundamental core of post-injury rehabilitation, but may be combined with biological approaches (e.g., pharmacotherapy).

- A number of factors may need to be accounted for in synergizing therapies to optimize improvements in functioning. These include not only understanding the immediate effects and side effects of pharmacologic agents but also the potential influences on processes of learning and change and relationships between the underlying neural systems modified by these agents vs. training. Different drugs, as well as different doses of the same drug, may have differential effects for specific neural subsystems and the behaviors they subserve.
- Engagement of active participation for each individual in treatment is a major factor in treatment outcome. Elements of enhancing engagement include raising awareness of one's abilities and difficulties, opportunities for self-direction during treatment, and active attempts at applying and transferring learned skills to personally relevant situations and goals. These are basic, almost mundane considerations that become all the more important when patient have deficits affecting awareness, motivation, attention, and other aspects of self-regulation. Issues of active avoidance or negative reactions to intervention may be further heightened when TBI is combined with PTSD or other psychological health conditions.
- Transfer of the gains achieved during treatment to new contexts, and generalization to each individual's personal life must be taken into account when considering intervention approach as well as measurement of outcomes.

Overarching Considerations in Intervening to Improve Cognitive Functioning After Brain Injury

Interventions may be considered along a number of major axes. Various axes may be used to characterize these approaches. Each of these axes briefly highlights particular considerations in determining optimal interventions, discussed briefly in this overview and in more detail in subsequent sections. Considering the spectrum along each axis may be helpful in determining the best approach for each patient.

Targeting the environment vs. the patient: Managing an individual's environment (organization of the physical environment, work, and time demands, etc.) is a common approach to post-injury care. This may be particularly valuable during acute phases of injury or with more severe deficits in self-management. This approach may sometimes be taken alone for at least two reasons. There may be an interest in maximizing function in a specific environment, given the least amount of time and effort. Second, there may be an assumption that the patient's functioning is "static" (at least within the time allotted.) However, increasing evidence supports significant functional plasticity over long periods of time, although the time course may not be conducive to standard practice parameters. Significant expertise is available in various fields of rehabilitation therapy; this chapter focuses more on patient-targeted approaches, where one of the ultimate goals is to alter the abilities of an individual to adapt to or manage their own environment.

Targeting of ancillary health factors vs. directly targeting central neural-cognitive processes: As will be discussed, a number of ancillary factors may be addressed that may have dramatic effects on cognitive functioning, with or without detailed consideration of deficits in central neural-cognitive processes or systems. It may sometimes be advantageous to address these contributing factors first, revealing a clearer picture of the underlying status of an individual's cognitive functioning. However, this approach alone will not resolve underlying deficits.

Application of external tools vs. internalized skills and strategies: Within an individual's "personal environment," one may consider external tools vs. internal tools available for a patient's use. The use of external tools is clearly a valuable aspect of human functioning and has an important role in improving functioning post-injury.

Tools may provide immediate benefits as external "signals" or orthotics (e.g., paging systems for alerts or reminders, Fish et al. 2008a, b), but they may also include training to leverage external tools to compensate for one's deficits or augment one's abilities (e.g., using a planner to improve organizational skills). Strong evidence supports the use of external tools for improving an individual's ability to accomplish intended actions. An important question for continued investigation is the extent to which use of any of these tools may improve an individual's intrinsic abilities. This chapter emphasizes approaches that may alter an individual's neurologic functioning.

Behavioral modification vs. biological modification: Methods for modifying biological underpinnings of behavior may be applied separately or in combination with behavioral modification. Biological modification approaches, considered broadly, may include not only pharmacotherapy but also identification and targeting of factors that influence the neural systems that support cognition. These may include factors such as sleep, pain, physical activity, circadian systems, nutrition, and more. It is valuable to keep in mind that biological approaches will more likely aid in accomplishing therapeutic goals when applied in the context of a behavioral modification plan (e.g., goal-driven rehabilitation training), rather than in isolation.

Integrating pharmacotherapy with rehabilitation: Careful application of pharmacotherapy can play an important role in improving cognitive functioning after brain injury. Clinical evidence to support particular medications is slowly accumulating (reviewed in Warden et al. 2006), and the approach is generally empiric, with little information to guide a clinician's prescription of one drug or another for any given individual. Determining the benefit of any given medication remains dependent on trial-and-error. Systematic trials involving step-wise dose adjustments of medications may be helpful.

There are a number of reasons to consider neuromodulator systems of the brain as therapeutic targets. These include findings that TBI tends to affect cognitive functions dependent on these neuromodulators, such as dopamine, norepinephrine, acetylcholine, and serotonin, and the predilection for TBI to affect the cortical termination zones as well as the long projection fibers that carry these neuromodulators. Almost all of the major neuromodulators of the brain are produced in small nuclei at the base of the brain or in the brain stem and project to distributed cerebral structures. Acetylcholine from the basal forebrain is projected to cortex throughout the brain. Dopamine from the ventral tegmental area is projected primarily to PFC. Norepinephrine from the locus coeruleus is projected to cortex throughout the brain, as well as thalamus, cerebellum, and spinal cord. Serotonin (5-HT) is also predominantly produced in brainstem and rostral nuclei (in the pons and midbrain) projections throughout the brain, with prominent targets including frontal lobes and hippocampus. On the other hand, GABA neurons are distributed throughout the brain, in particular as inhibitory inter-neurons. Disruption in one or more of these systems presumably contributes to neurologic symptoms seen in TBI.

A number of drugs that affect neuromodulator systems have been used in clinical practice for years. Each pharmacotherapeutic agent is, in theory, targeted to particular neural systems, whether defined by particular receptor types, synthesis of or metabolism of particular neurotransmitters, or other drug-specific mechanisms. The delineation of the targets of a particular drug, and the relation to cognitive functioning, is an area in need of further investigation. Helpful and hurtful effects of drugs must be considered, and these may occur simultaneously. For example, more detailed examination may reveal domain-specific effects (as described in McDowell et al. 1998) or simultaneous helpful vs. detrimental effects on separable brain systems (i.e., "double-edged sword" effects) (Cools et al. 2001). An important frontier will be to determine the pharmacology of each patient, potentially providing guidance for therapy.

It is also valuable to consider separately immediate effects of pharmacologic modulation, e.g., altering current behavior, vs. longer-term effects. Attending to longer-term effects raises considerations of effects on learning and response to other therapies. Drug effects may be supportive for current issues, but may also be detrimental for longer-term goals. For example, medications have long been used to address problematic behavior post-injury. The immediate effects may seem helpful (e.g., reducing behavioral instability), but the same medication may adversely affect functioning in a cumulative manner (e.g., by altering attention and learning during training).

New approaches to biological modification may actually have no beneficial immediate effects, but may help to accomplish long-term therapeutic goals but altering the plasticity of neural systems. Such approaches may include using stem cells, growth factors, small molecules, or other novel approaches (Zhang and Chopp 2009). However, the effectiveness of these methods for helping to accomplish therapeutic goals will depend on effectively augmenting the specific changes guided by training.

Factors That Modulate Cognitive Functioning and "Brain State" on a Dynamic Basis: Important Targets of Therapy

Medications

Medications may have both beneficial and detrimental effects on cognition. Patients may have prescriptions for issues that arise during the many phases from acute injury to chronic recovery. Polypharmacy is a common problem, likely due to factors such as multiple comorbidities with TBI (e.g., anxiety, PTSD, insomnia, pain) and attempts to treat some post-TBI sequelae (e.g., behavioral dysregulation, seizures, headaches). A valuable first-step in clinical decision-making is a review of medications that may contribute to poor cognitive functioning. Unfortunately, numerous medications commonly used for patients with TBI have adverse effects on cognition.

Post-traumatic epilepsy, especially with complex partial seizures, is a treatable potential contributor to cognitive dysfunction. However, medications may need to be managed with attention to cognitive side effects. Phenytoin has been shown to impair cognitive function in patients with severe TBI (Dikmen et al. 1991, 2000). Carbemazepine may also have cognitive side effects (Smith et al. 1994). Among older antiepileptic agents, valproate may be preferable. Among newer agents, topiramate may be particularly concerning for cognitive side effects.

Benzodiazepines and baclofen are GABA agonists, and these may reduce the rate of recovery from TBI (Zafonte et al. 2004). The use of these medications should be minimized in the context of cognitive dysfunction after TBI. In certain circumstances, spasticity may be treated by more localized means (e.g., intrathecal baclofen or targeted botulinum toxin).

Dopamine antagonists, such as haloperidol, have been shown to impede learning and recovery (Stanislav 1997; Wilson et al. 2003; Meintzschel and Ziemann 2006; Hoffman et al. 2008; Kline et al. 2008). These agents are commonly used for managing behavioral dysregulation, but should be used sparingly, and continual use should be avoided as much as possible.

In sum, it is important to repeatedly review the rationale, necessity, and dosage of each medication at each clinical juncture, with a concern for potential adverse effects on cognition and recovery. In general, when medications are deemed necessary, cognitive functioning should be monitored while dosing is adjusted. It is often necessary to discontinue medications before reliable determination of sources of dysfunction can be made. Indeed, cessation of medication is often as valuable as starting any medications in the rehabilitation course.

Alertness and Arousal State

Optimal alertness may be considered a prerequisite for effectively activating and engaging other cognitive functions. The concept of alertness is integrally tied to the sustainment of attention. The translation of alertness or arousal to task-related attention may lead to greater neural-cognitive processing (Spitzer et al. 1988). Tonic alertness refers to the ongoing state of intrinsic arousal that is intimately involved in sustaining engagement during higher-order functions such as selective attention, working memory, and executive control (Sturm et al. 1999; Posner

2008). Although the term "attention" is commonly used in this context, it should be distinguished from the many other meanings of attention, as separable neural systems appear to subserve alertness vs. other "attention" functions (Sturm et al. 1999; Posner 2008). Alertness may influence performance in almost all cognitive domains, including during rehabilitation (Sohlberg et al. 2000). Improving regulation of this "gateway" function may improve the "readiness" state of individuals for participation in rehabilitation.

Alertness and arousal need to be considered in terms of optimizing balance. Patients with more severe TBI may exhibit marked deficits in alertness (Whyte et al. 1995; Manly et al. 1999). Noradrenergic systems involving inter-connected regions of brainstem and frontal cortex, in particular, have been proposed to be particularly important mediators of alertness state (Aston-Jones and Cohen 2005). The importance of long distance connections, both for delivering noradrenergic signals from brainstem to cortex as well as regulation of brainstem nuclei, may help to explain why alertness is so often dysregulated after TBI. High levels of arousal may also be maladaptive. This is a significant problem with TBI–PTSD, for example. Thus, therapies may need to focus on the concept of optimizing the *regulation* of alertness, rather than simply increasing or decreasing arousal per se.

Approaches to regulating arousal state may involve behavioral regulation, training, and pharmacologic treatments. Recent training approaches may provide methods for improving regulation of arousal and are discussed in more detail with other training approaches. A number of pharmacologic agents that affect alertness and arousal are already in common use. However, the effects of each agent can be quite individual, especially given underlying issues with variability in alertness state, i.e., lability, rather than a simple uni-directional deficit. Thus, each agent needs to be considered carefully based on patient goals and treatment contexts. Multifactorial considerations become particularly challenging when TBI is combined with post-traumatic stress symptoms, behavioral lability, anxiety, or depression.

Commonly used pharmacologic agents that affect neuromodulator function include methylphenidate and amphetamines as well as newer stimulants. For example, methylphenidate has been shown to alter sustained attention in patients with TBI (Whyte et al. 1997). Modafinil is a newer agent that promotes alertness. Atomoxetine works selectively on noradrenergic systems. "Antidepressants" with noradrenergic targets and possible "activating" effects, such as venlafaxine or duloxetine, may be helpful for some individuals. These agents could be considered for use as agents satisfying multiple therapeutic goals, minimizing the total number of different medications. Reuptake inhibitors for serotonin as well as norepinephrine are perhaps among the few agents that may improve stability of arousal state.

As always, the effects of medications, prescribed for other reasons, must be evaluated. A number of medications commonly used after TBI, as well as for post-traumatic stress and anxiety symptoms, affect alertness. Other factors that modulate cognitive state that are related to alertness are fatigue and sleep. These are discussed separately, given some distinct considerations.

Fatigue

Fatigue is likely the most commonly reported symptom after TBI, reported in 21–73% of patients with TBI (Olver et al. 1996; Hillier et al. 1997), and is also common after other types of brain injury (Staub and Bogousslavsky 2001; De Groot et al. 2003). Fatigue is a subjective complaint. There is no standard definition of fatigue, but the key elements include a requirement for increased effort to maintain mental activities and difficulty sustaining goal-directed efforts (Fellus and Elovic 2007). Central fatigue is the concern in TBI, and should be distinguished from peripheral fatigue, which refers to muscular or other sources outside the brain. Central fatigue is itself a major cause of poor functioning, adding to other physical or cognitive deficits. Failure to sustain cognitive effort is a major limitation for effective cognitive functioning even when brief assessments reveal intact abilities. Just as distractibility might cut short an effort before a goal is completed, so might fatigue. Fatigue affects functional recovery, emotional well-being, cognitive functioning, quality of life, and ability to perform daily activities (Bushnik et al. 2008a, b).

Assessment of fatigue is complicated by its dynamic nature. Characterization of fatigue needs to take into account fluctuations and the contexts in which an individual functions. A key goal of the assessment is to determine potential sources or factors that exacerbate fatigue, as these may be targets for management. Clinical assessments of fatigue are often brief and subjective. Questionnaires querying subjective report may be helpful in characterizing an individual's fatigue (reviewed elsewhere) (Borgaro et al. 2004; Fellus and Elovic 2007; Bushnik et al. 2008a, b). Assessment of associated factors, such as sleep, depression, and pain, may be particularly valuable. The development of objective measurements, as an adjunct to subjective report, may be helpful for identifying underlying sources of fatigue or tracking fatigue more closely when self-awareness is limited.

Interventions for improving post-injury fatigue remain very basic and general at the current time. Regular physical exercise is one of the first recommendations. Adherence to an exercise regimen is a major obstacle, with factors including motivation, pain, and other physical limitations. Overcoming these problems may require creative problem-solving, with expert guidance in individualizing exercise activities. Compensatory strategies to manage energy use may be helpful for a person to achieve desired functional goals given limited capacity for activity. The patient may require assistance identifying situations or behaviors that exacerbate fatigue that could be modified. Addressing sleep disturbances is an obvious and crucial step to improving energy levels. Sleep history, and in some cases, polysomnography may help diagnose sleep disturbances. Reduction of distractions, thereby reducing the amount of cognitive effort required to accomplish tasks, may be beneficial. Improved self-regulation of attention and other aspects of cognitive processing may help improve the efficiency (reducing the work load) for accomplishing tasks. Similarly, improving regulation of emotions, such as anger, may also reduce fatigue.

Medications such as beta-blockers, anti-dopaminergics, and anti-epileptics may all contribute to feelings of tiredness. Pharmacotherapy with agents that improve alertness, attention, and concentration, such as methylphenidate, amantadine, dextroamphetamine, atomoxetine, or modafinil, may improve fatigue. Activating antidepressants may be helpful. Systematic evidence to support the effectiveness of any given therapy for fatigue remains limited, and studies may be complicated by the heterogeneity of fatigue sources and symptoms. This is a major frontier for development with potentially wide-reaching benefits for individuals with brain injury.

Sleep

Sleep disturbances are a major issue after TBI (Mahmood et al. 2004; Castriotta et al. 2007; Watson et al. 2007; Zeitzer et al. 2009) and insomnia is particularly common for combat veterans, whether related to TBI, PTSD, or other causes (Lewis et al. 2009). Poor sleep adversely affects cognitive function, particularly for frontal systems and memory functions (Muzur et al. 2002; Yoo et al. 2007), including sustained attention after TBI (Bloomfield et al. 2009). Chronic lack of sleep may also be associated with anxiety and depression (Neckelmann et al. 2007), another pathway by which poor sleep may worsen functioning after TBI. Dopamine may play a role in compensating for cognitive changes after sleep deprivation (Volkow et al. 2008). This again highlights the importance of considering multiple levels of factors in determining treatment prescription.

Sleep regulation and adequate sleep may be of fundamental importance for learning and recovery after brain injury. As mentioned, sleep deprivation may have adverse effects on functions that are crucial for learning, such as alertness, attention, and memory (Mahmood et al. 2004). In addition, sleep, including naps, has been shown to benefit learning of information or skills learned prior to sleeping (Mednick et al. 2003; Tucker et al. 2006). Thus, thinking of sleep in both a retrospective direction (sleep deprivation) and a prospective direction (planned sleep after learning activities) may significantly alter one's approach to sleep in rehabilitation.

Management of sleep as a direct, explicit target of therapy is an important frontier for further development. There remains a major need for defining optimal approaches for improving sleep duration and quality after TBI, as well as determining how best to integrate sleep into rehabilitation treatment regimens. Asides from basic considerations of sleep hygiene and the effects of substances (e.g., caffeine, alcohol, or other drugs), more complex issues may need to be addressed. Dysregulation in sleep cycles may occur from physical injury to the brain (Ayalon et al. 2007), medications or even intensive military training and experiences. Insomnia is a major symptom of PTSD, and barriers to sleep may include not only hyper-arousal but also active resistance to sleep due to feelings of fear and nightmares. Intensive schedule regularization may be necessary, but not sufficient, and individualized trials combining scheduling with efforts to augment sleep or wake signaling (e.g., melatonin supplementation at night; sunlight, exercise, possibly stimulants in the morning) may be valuable.

Pharmacologic agents for inducing or prolonging sleep all have potential side effects, and balancing becomes more complex when cognitive dysfunction, pain (and associated medications), substance abuse, psychopathology, and other factors inter-mix. Furthermore, medication-induced sleep does not replace normal physiologic sleep, and use of such drugs would ideally be limited in time. For example, such drugs may be used during initial phases of therapy, to temporarily address extreme sleep deprivation and associated complications of cognitive and emotional dysfunction that may impede initiation of other therapies with longer-term benefits. In the long term, addressing underlying psychological issues (e.g., anxiety, PTSD) will be particularly important for achieving restful sleep without medication assistance.

Identifying and treating sleep apnea is another major priority. Sleep apnea may contribute to cognitive dysfunction not only from disruption of the regular sleep cycle but also potentially from hypoxia itself (Canessa and Ferini-Strambi 2011; Yaffe et al. 2011). Prescription of sleep-inducing medications such as benzodiazepines may actually exacerbate these issues.

Pain

Pain is a common accompaniment of TBI. Chronic pain, in particular, may have wide-ranging effects on well-being, emotional, and social functioning as well as cognitive functioning. Some of the effects of pain on cognition may be mediated by influences on sleep, mood, and energy levels. For example, chronic pain may lead to irritability and poor frustration tolerance, reducing cognitive effort for cognitive tasks that are challenging. Pain may also modulate cognitive functioning via increased fatigue or poor sleep. On the other hand, treatments for chronic pain, such as with opioid analgesics, may contribute to poor cognitive functioning. Although opioid medications may play an important role in pain management, especially in settings of acute injury, other approaches may be particularly valuable in the long term.

Multidisciplinary collaboration in an intensive program may be necessary, especially given the multifactorial nature of chronic pain. Approaches to pain management that include strengthening of self-regulation and coping (e.g., with mindfulness-based training or biofeedback), as well as localized interventions (e.g., transcutaneous electrical stimulation, injections), with a goal of minimizing systemic opiates, may be particularly valuable.

Training to Improve Cognitive Functioning

Training of Neurologic Functions

Training forms the most fundamental core of post-injury rehabilitation. Training involves specific activities that guide changes in brain functioning based on specific learning goals. Within the training approaches, different learning goals may be defined.

Training may emphasize the learning and application of cognitive skills and/or strategies. Strategies help to organize behavior may be helpful in improving the efficiency or effectiveness of accomplishing particular tasks. Strategies, once internalized, may be thought of as providing intrinsic "tools" available to an individual to help accomplish particular tasks. Examples of cognitive strategies are discussed in this chapter. Effective application of a strategy typically results in an immediate beneficial effect; however, the long-term benefits depend on a number of factors. Factors to consider include to what extent the strategies are context-specific or transferable to other contexts, to what extent the individual can learn and remember the strategy, and to what extent the individual will be able to prospectively initiate use of the strategy in the appropriate situations. For example, it is not uncommon for an individual to be able to learn a strategy during therapy (e.g., a method for breaking problems into manageable steps), but then fail to apply this strategy when faced with a real-world problem. Such failures of transfer may be directly related to an individual's cognitive deficits.

Available literature on treatment of combat-related "mild TBI" is sparse. A recent pilot study examined strategy training in combat veterans with mild cognitive dysfunction and a history of TBI (Huckans et al. 2010). Training involved a variety of compensatory internal and external cognitive strategies, including day planner usage in a structured group-based format. Following training, participants reported increased use of compensatory cognitive strategies and day planners, increased perception that these strategies were useful to them, increased life satisfaction, and decreased depressive, memory, and cognitive symptom severity.

A skills-based approach may also be taken. Though the distinctions between strategies and skills may blur, skills may generally be considered as the integrated use of particular neurologic functions or processes for the accomplishment of functional tasks. Skill training is generally considered a more gradual process, with improvements accumulating over repetitive practice. Skills may be further divided into the concepts of "neurologic skills" (based on definable neurocognitive processes, such as working memory, which are applicable to multiple specific tasks or situations) or "functional skills" (procedures for accomplishing a task, such as making a sandwich). The latter may blur the borders between potentially separable cognitive processes, but this is ecologically relevant as real-life tasks typically require the integration of multiple neurologic processes.

These differing approaches may help to achieve different goals in rehabilitation. For example, it is theorized that if fundamental neural-cognitive processes are improved, then the benefits will more likely carry over to tasks and contexts outside the training. On the other hand, training on specific actions (functional tasks) may be thought of as consolidating a particular task-specific skill or procedure. As such, the behavioral improvements may be more immediately apparent as patients improve in task performance, but the improvements may be task- or context-specific. The choice of approach may depend on the nature and severity of cognitive deficits. It has been argued that functional approaches may be more effective for patients with severe deficits (Giles 2010).

The utility of training that targets specific neurologic processes remains controversial, and this is an active area of research and development. Process-targeted methods have typically involved practice on tasks "isolated" from complex real-world situations. The development of training programs that target neurologic processes and result in effective and ecologically relevant gains remains an important frontier for further advancement in intervention development. Optimization of methods for higher level cognitive functions continues to be a challenge. Advances in neuroscience, informed by clinical concerns, provide a foundation for defining, targeting, and training cognitive functions. In the next section, we outline the foundations for process-targeted, neuroscience-driven interventions.

Cognitive Neuroscience Foundations for Rehabilitation Training

Although a wide range and variety of deficits can result from TBI, symptoms in two general areas stand out as some of the most common and disruptive to patients—"executive control" and memory. The abilities of paying attention, holding information in mind, organizing, and developing efficient strategies for completing activities seem to be particularly vulnerable to TBI. These processes come together in the regulation and control of other, more basic neurologic processes based on goals, and are often referred to as "executive control" functions (Hecaen and Albert 1978; Lezak 1995). Although problems with memory are some of the most commonly reported complaints after TBI, the actual deficits may be quite varied. Processes important for goal-directed behavior, learning, and memory will receive special focus in this section.

Functional Impacts of Cognitive Dysfunction and the Impetus to Address Them

Processes important for goal-directed behavior, learning, and memory are fundamental for successful independent living, and deficits may directly contribute to poor outcomes. At the broadest level, poor executive control leads to disorganized behavior that affects numerous aspects of personal functioning. Executive control functions are crucial for the pursuit of educational and occupational goals (Drake et al. 2000; Ownsworth and McKenna 2004; Doctor et al. 2005; Machamer et al. 2005) with TBI resulting in an increased rate of job turnover and reduced job status (Machamer et al. 2005). However, the effects may be even more fundamental in the process of recovery from brain injury.

As empirically observed by rehabilitation clinicians, if certain cognitive functions are not intact, other attempts at rehabilitation are made much more difficult. Who, after all, are the most difficult individuals to teach? Which patients are most likely to be labeled as "not ready" for intensive rehabilitation efforts? Individuals who cannot pay attention, hold information in mind, and actively participate in learning activities may have reduced benefit from rehabilitation training efforts for other neurologic domains (Tatemichi et al. 1994; Prigatano and Wong 1999; Ozdemir et al. 2001; Hyndman and Ashburn 2003; Fischer et al. 2004). As a frontier reaching beyond simply triaging patients, the remediation of these functions may be valuable for influencing learning and recovery in other neurologic domains. For example, improved goal-directed functioning may enhance an individual's ability to actively participate in attempts to rehabilitate motor functions, allowing an individual to hold learning goals in mind, selectively focusing attention to learning activities, and solve problems in the numerous intervening steps between a current state and achieving a learning goal. Finally, individuals with brain injury spend a much larger amount of time on their own than with a therapist; thus, the importance of executive control and memory functions translates to an individual's ability to self-teach skills, remember strategies and self-adjust to residual deficits in any domain.

Foundations for Training: Neural Bases of Cognitive Functions Important After TBI

It is conceptually simple to understand how one might train motor strength by training particular muscles, but how would one prescribe training for "executive control" functions? Reviews of interventions have noted a gap between theories about subsystems of executive functions and intervention design and practice (Kennedy et al. 2008; Levine et al. 2008). A better understanding of the nature of the specific underlying neural processes, as well as mechanisms of learning and recovery specific to these functions may help advance treatment development (Chen et al. 2006; D'Esposito and Chen 2006; D'Esposito and Gazzaley 2006).

Neurologic deficits caused by TBI are not unique to trauma per se, but certain patterns of dysfunction are more common with TBI than other causes of injury. While these patterns are partially explained by traditional neurologic localization with focal cerebral lesions, the localization approach has left many TBI sequelae poorly explained. Basic abilities, such as ambulation and speech, may be spared, and the impact of deficits may only become clear when individuals are challenged by the complexities of real-life. Deficits in executive control functions are generally attributable to damage to prefrontal systems, which include not only PFC per se but also extensive interconnections with subcortical and posterior cortical structures (D'Esposito and

Chen 2006). The importance of axonal injuries in TBI highlights the need to understand brain functioning in terms of distributed but coordinated network processes (Chen et al. 2006). "Diffuse axonal injury" without focal cortical lesions has been shown to lead to changes in executive working memory processing activity (Levine et al. 2008).

PFC is involved in multiple major networks (Goldman-Rakic and Friedman 1991). One major network involves connections with posterior parietal cortex as well as anterior and posterior cingulate and medial temporal lobe regions (Selemon and Goldman-Rakic 1988). Another major network involves cortical–subcortical connections between the PFC and the striatum, globus pallidus, substantia nigra, and mediodorsal nucleus of the thalamus (Ilinisky et al. 1985). Additional interactions with other more posterior brain regions such as sensory or motor cortex are likely important for the domain-specificity of control processes (Postle 2006; Ranganath 2006). Deficits may also be related to damage to neuromodulatory pathways from the base of the brain to the cortex. These interactions are crucial for the modulatory control of distributed neuronal activity in order to facilitate processes that are relevant to internal goals while suppressing nonrelevant processes (Fuster 2000; Miller and Cohen 2001; Curtis and D'Esposito 2003).

How is goal-directed control implemented in neural systems? At the simplest level, neural aspects of control involve modulation of neural activity from the "top-down" based on goals, as well as coordination and monitoring of distributed neural networks in the brain. Without such control, activity would be either driven by low-level processes, such as by "stimulus-response" principles, or generally disorganized, with poorly coordinated activity that lacks guidance by a higher level goal structure. The modulation of neurologic processes from the "top-down" is accomplished by at least two important general mechanisms: *selection* (enhancement and suppression) of neural activity based on goal-direction and active *maintenance* of goal-relevant neural activity for the accomplishment of tasks. The functional integration of neurons within local networks is also important. The neural representations of information appear to be coded not in single neurons, but rather in networks of neurons. For example, representations of the myriad possible visual objects, including household objects, faces etc., have been shown to be encoded in a distributed architecture (Haxby et al. 2001). This organizational architecture allows for a much wider range of information to be encoded with a limited number of neurons. Otherwise, if a separate neuron were needed for every item or variation of information stored, the number of neurons needed would far exceed what exists in the human brain. Distributed injury, atrophy, or degeneration could disrupt neural processing even in the absence of obvious cortical lesions. Examples of this may occur in age-related degeneration (Park et al. 2004) and is likely to occur in TBI as well.

Thus, understanding the importance of network interactions is an important foundation for understanding the functional consequences of TBI, which might otherwise be labeled "nonfocal." This also has implications for the measurement methodologies to be used to understand neural mechanisms of injury, learning, and recovery in rehabilitation studies. Examples of this frontier are discussed at the end of this chapter.

Cognitive Functions as Potential Targets of Therapy

Functions for Goal-Directed Control: Attention and Other Components Processes of "Executive Control"

Control over neurologic functions to accomplish goals may involve control over perception and information processing, motor actions, emotional functioning, as well as other aspects of behavior. One way to organize our conceptualization of control functions is to consider the components required for successful goal attainment. (For additional discussion, anatomically based schema for subdividing frontal functions (Stuss and Alexander 2007; Levine et al. 2008) and goal management steps have been reviewed by others (Levine et al. 2000; Rath et al. 2003).) Deficits in any component may disrupt efficient and effective goal attainment.

- At the outset, a *goal* needs to be generated and/or selected. Whether the goal is simple or complex (e.g., make a cup of coffee vs. apply for college), inability to generate clear goals, or deficiencies in evaluating and selecting a manageable goal, will obviously result in poor goal attainment.
- This goal will then be important for guiding all subsequent processes. An *attentional set* based on the selected goal needs to be established, framing all upcoming information or actions (Banich et al. 2000a, b; Luks et al. 2002). Poor establishment of the appropriate set will make it more likely that the individual will be distracted or take the wrong path.
- Goal attainment activities need to be *initiated*, and this depends on motivation and an appropriate level of alertness or arousal. Apathy, depression, low arousal (such as from fatigue) may lead to poor initiation.
- Goal attainment activities including determining the optimal *plans* to accomplish the main goal. Planning includes more in-depth analysis of the goal, and breakdown of the goal into an appropriately sequenced series of subgoals (steps), including re-organization of potential actions in relation to the main goal. These processes may require interactions across a hierarchy of prefrontal networks (Badre and D'Esposito 2009).
- *Strategy* determination and related processes of planning are crucial for efficient goal attainment, especially with more complex tasks. This higher level function is relevant for learning, memory, and problem-solving. Patients with frontal injuries show impairments in strategic planning and organization of information (Baldo et al. 2004; Yochim et al. 2009).
- Some goals may require more complex levels of planning, and *maintenance of the goal* during this process can be important. The planning process can be thrown off track with forgetting of the main goal or disconnection of planning from the goal (one form of "goal neglect") (Duncan et al. 1996).
- Translation of the imagined cognitive sequences (plans) into action requires a step of *initiation of action* that is separable from the initiation of planning and decision-making, and is another point at which an individual may stall.
- Once actions are initiated, goals and plans need to be maintained to accomplish each subgoal and the sequence of subgoals that build toward the main goal. *Goal maintenance* becomes increasingly important with goals that require multiple steps over extended periods of time, as the risk of going "off track" increases (Shallice and Burgess 1991; Gouveia et al. 2007). This may be another form of "goal neglect" (Duncan et al. 1996).
- Throughout the goal attainment process, the individual will likely be exposed to vast amounts of information (from perception or memory)—some of this will be relevant and some non-relevant to the goal. Positive selection of goal-relevant information for deeper processing (with the complementary negative selection of non-relevant information) at the outset and at every stage of the goal attainment process will be necessary to reach the goal, else the individual may be distracted or even overwhelmed. Selected information needs to be maintained, at the exclusion of other competing information, to accomplish each step toward the goal. The *selection and maintenance of goal-relevant information* involves processes often referred to as selective attention and working memory, functions that are integrally related (D'Esposito et al. 1995; D'Esposito and Postle 1999; D'Esposito et al. 1999; Bunge et al. 2001; Thompson-Schill et al. 2002; Gazzaley et al. 2005; Gilbert et al. 2006; Chen et al. 2007).
- Similarly, a plethora of actions is possible at any moment in time, but only a selected few will be goal-relevant. *Response selection and inhibition* refers to the ability to select between competing alternatives and to inhibit inappropriate response tendencies (Bunge et al. 2002a, b).
- The selection of actions also needs to be framed by *rules* (e.g., do not drive across the double-yellow lines while trying to get across the street). Making use of rules includes processes for the retrieval, maintenance, selection,

and implementation of relevant rules that guide behavior on a task (Bunge et al. 2003; Donohue et al. 2005; Crone et al. 2006).

- In determining appropriate actions, multiple considerations may need to be integrated. Relational integration requires the ability to integrate multiple relationships, and is crucial in problem-solving and reasoning (Bunge et al. 2005; Bunge and Zelazo 2006).
- There may be a need to transition between tasks, such as to move to the next subgoal or to deal with an interruption and yet return back to the goal-relevant path. *Direction and re-direction* of attention, information processing, and actions is necessary for successfully making these transitions. Patients with frontal lesions are relatively impaired on tests that require switching between tasks or attentional sets (Yochim et al. 2007).
- Once actions are taken, the results that follow may or may not be relevant to goal attainment. Comparison of results with the original goals and detection of disparities or errors is necessary for correction of the above series of processes to ultimately achieve the goal. However, neglect of the goal, deficits in awareness of errors, as well as failure to take corrective actions are major impediments to successful goal attainment.
- Independence in the above processes, and cognitive functioning in general, requires some ability to *generate* ideas and information with minimal cuing, especially for processes that require creativity and/or problem-solving. Aspects of generative ability may be impaired with brain injuries (Baldo and Shimamura 1998; Baldo et al. 2001, 2006). Overall, frontal systems appear to be broadly important for core abilities that allow a person to flexibly and adaptively solve problems across multiple contexts (Duncan et al. 1995; Kane and Engle 2002).

Pharmacotherapy: Bromocriptine has been recommended for use in enhancing aspects of executive functioning (e.g., divided attention/central executive functions) in patients with severe TBI (McDowell et al. 1998; Warden et al. 2006). Other agents that modulate catecholamine function, such as dextroamphetamine, methylphenidate, amantadine, are also commonly used. However, there is less direct evidence to support positive clinical effects on executive control functions. As a general rule, agents that modulate dopaminergic function should be considered to be dosed based on individual response, as dopamine modulation of function tends to follow a "U-shaped" curve that varies in dose-relationship for each individual (Kimberg et al. 1997; Cools et al. 2003, 2008).

Although difficult to isolate to a specific process, the efficiency and speed with which an individual can process information and accomplish cognitive tasks is commonly affected by TBI. Although the neural substrates of speed of processing are not well understood, one underlying pathophysiologic factor may be damage to interconnecting systems in the brain, as would occur with axonal injury, reducing the efficiency of computations that require interregional interactions. As a general theme, first, medications should be reviewed for potential contribution to slow processing. Medications, such as dopamine antagonists, benzodiazepines, and opiates, may also contribute to slow processing. Other contributors may be of concern as well, e.g., sleep deprivation. Practice guidelines support the use of the stimulant methylphenidate in the treatment of deficits in attention and speed of information processing following TBI (Warden et al. 2006). The evidence for methylphenidate is strongest for an effect on speed of cognitive processing and sustained attention/vigilance (Whyte et al. 1997, 2004). The cholinesterase inhibitor donepezil has also been recommended for enhancing attention in patients with moderate-to-severe TBI in subacute and chronic periods of recovery. Dextroamphetamine and amantadine may also be considered. To what extent these medications are indicated for "mild TBI," such as from blasts, needs to be further tested.

The specific effects of each medication on each of the specific component functions is not yet clear, and further work will be valuable for providing specific guidance on how best to combine pharmacotherapies with any particular rehabilitation training regimen.

Learning and Memory

Functions of *learning and memory* are integrally intertwined with all of the above process of goal-direction. Thus, this discussion treats these processes as part of the ensemble of functions needed for goal attainment. For example, information, strategies, and skills need to be learned and remembered so that they may be applied to problem-solving and goal attainment. Conversely, learning and memory are also dependent on many of the control processes discussed. Indeed, one of the most common subjective complaints after TBI is of problems with "memory."

The underlying sources of these complaints may vary. Deficits related to declarative or episodic memory may be related to damage to medial temporal structures. The basal forebrain and long tracts that connect the forebrain to other structures are also important for memory processing. The basal forebrain, a major source of cholinergic projections throughout the brain, is particularly vulnerable to injury, and, furthermore, long projections may be vulnerable to shearing injury (Salmond et al. 2005). However, complaints of problems with "memory" do not necessarily equate to problems with these structures systems.

Problems with memory encoding and retrieval may also be related to attention and "frontal executive" functions that influence the selectivity and depth of information processing, as well as the ability to organize information to be encoded and strategically retrieve information to be recalled (Blumenfeld and Ranganath 2007). Encoding and retrieval of information from memory may be impaired in individuals with frontal systems dysfunction. Important aspects of encoding and retrieval of information from memory appear to be mediated by the role of PFC in activating, maintaining, and organizing information in working memory, as well as in re-activating and retrieving stored information (Ranganath et al. 2003, 2007). A common deficit seen is that a patient has difficulty on free delayed recall, but when provided with a retrieval strategy (cue) his performance improves. An additional set of functions is important for the "prospective" memory of upcoming events or actions (Burgess et al. 2011).

Behavioral approaches to compensating for or training memory have been reviewed elsewhere (e.g., Raskin 2000). For patients with severe deficits in declarative memory related to mesial temporal injury, external aids are particularly valuable. Evidence to date argues against significant potential for remediation of such memory deficits, though this has mainly been examined in the context of hypoxic injury. However, memory problems related to deficits in controlled aspects of encoding and retrieval, related to executive control functions, may respond well to training, such as with strategies for selecting or organizing information for memory. Thus, distinguishing the underlying etiologies of memory complaints may be highly valuable in therapeutic decision-making.

Pharmacotherapy: The cholinesterase inhibitor donepezil (5–10 mg/day) has been recommended as a practice guideline to enhance aspects of memory function for patients with moderate-to-severe TBI in subacute and chronic periods of recovery (Zhang et al. 2004; Warden et al. 2006). There is support for rivastigmine improving memory deficits as well, in a subgroup of patients with moderate-to-severe memory impairment at baseline (Silver et al. 2006). In general, these cholinesterase inhibitors appear to be safe and well-tolerated in patients with TBI (Gualtieri and Evans 1988). Although the rationale for these agents was previously focused on bolstering "memory systems," effects on attention and registration of information may be particularly important contributors to the amelioration of symptoms. Methylphenidate, amphetamines, and other agents that enhance attention or executive control may also improve learning and memory functioning after TBI. To what extent these medications are indicated for mild TBI, such as from blasts, needs to be further tested, and additional considerations of the interaction with anxiety and PTSD need to be considered.

Targeting Cognitive Functions: Integration of Component Processes

In sum, each component process provides a potential target for intervention. This is summarized in a schematic in Fig. 15.2.

Discussed as separate processes, the above may seem like a confusing and complex array of

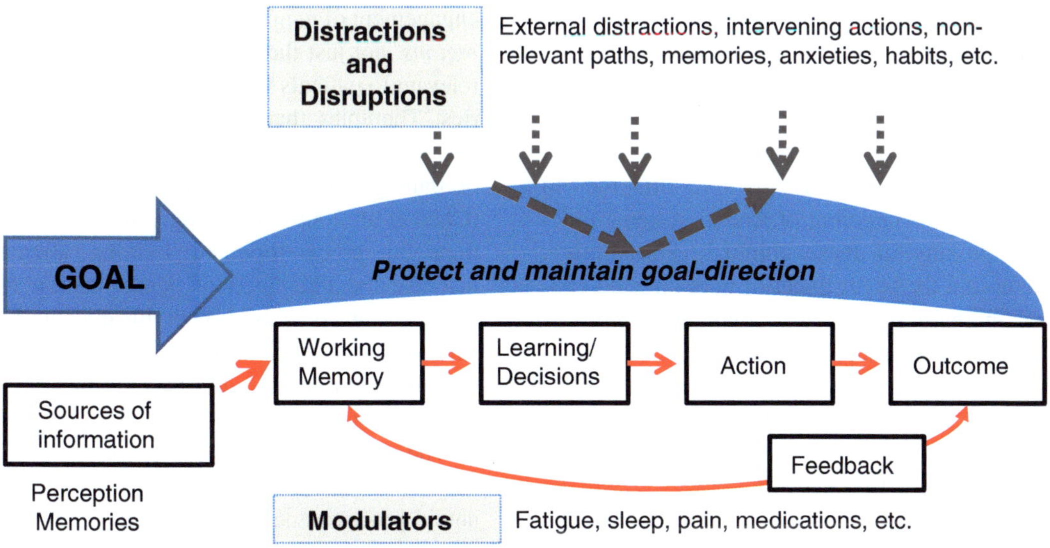

Fig. 15.2 Component processes in pathways to goal attainment: targets for intervention. All the main processes, *connected in red*, work together for goal attainment and are potential targets for interventions. An overarching target for strengthening involves abilities to protect and maintain goal-directed processes from distractions and disruptions, which may otherwise affect any component in the pathway. As discussed separately, other potential modulators may influence the central processes and are also potential targets for other forms of intervention

functions that are difficult to understand or target. However, an important principle is that the component processes need to be *coordinated* or *functionally integrated* in the accomplishment of any particular goal. Goals may be conceptualized as serving to functionally organize the multiple neural processes necessary for accomplishing the goal, including selecting the relevant pathways or processes (while excluding others), coordinating them at any given moment in time, and dynamically adjusting this coordination while maintaining the central goal across time to eventually accomplish the goal. Thus, not only the components but also their functional coordination may be important targets for intervention. Process-based approaches may be analogous to isolating and working out the biceps muscle, while functional approaches may be analogous to training the coordination of multiple muscles to accomplish basketball shots. A more advanced question is whether training that involves functionally integrated approaches may actually serve as an effective, more motivating way to improve underlying component processes.

Principles for Training and Improving Functions of Goal-Directed Control

Functions that subserve goal-directed behavior are a particularly important training target for individuals with TBI. This encompasses functions that have far-reaching influence on neural processes in almost any neurologic domain, crucial to navigating the challenges of learning and adaptation after injury. Given the difficulty in understanding and designing interventions to improve goal-directed cognitive functioning, we have proposed some basic principles of training could be incorporated into interventions to target and maximize improvements in these functions (D'Esposito and Chen 2006).

Many of the methods applied in clinical rehabilitation are designed for the learning of strategies that compensate for deficits. We focus here on possible approaches for remediation of goal-directed control deficits, a challenging but worthwhile goal that remains at the frontiers of clinical rehabilitation. As introduced above, the extensive research on the neural mechanisms underlying goal-directed control functions may provide a useful theoretical foundation for the development of interventions for remediation. These principles may not only bolster therapies where goal-directed cognition is the primary target of therapy but may also be incorporated into cognitive, motor, speech, or other therapies in order to maximize the targeting of frontal systems functions in any of these contexts. Furthermore, increasing the engagement of goal-directed control in these settings may maximize improvements across domains.

1. Training of process, not content: cognitive training tasks should challenge patients to engage "top-down" modulatory processes mediated by PFC networks.

   As delineated above, there are a number of cognitive processes that could be targeted by training. Functional imaging studies aimed at investigating normal brain-behavior relationships may provide a relatively new source of guidance for the type of tasks that can engage PFC networks. For example, tasks that require selective processing of competing information based on task-relevance (selective attention), working memory (e.g., the maintenance of information over a short period of time and especially manipulation of that information), performance of dual tasks, as well as goal–subgoal management have all been shown to engage the PFC networks (D'Esposito et al. 1995; Banich et al. 2000a, b; Curtis et al. 2004; D'Esposito and Chen 2006). During the performance of these tasks, it is the processing demands, and not the specific contents of stimuli per se, that engage PFC networks. For example, PFC networks are engaged during working memory tasks regardless of the type of information (e.g., words or objects) that must be remembered (D'Esposito et al. 1998; Collette et al. 2005). Thus, training needs to target specific top-down control *processes,* and not *specific task content.* This contrasts with training that emphasizes repetition of task content, which promotes a shift toward automatic processing and disengagement of PFC-mediated control (Petersen et al. 1998). Importantly, examination of the neural substrates of these functions emphasizes the engagement of *networks across multiple brain regions*, not just the PFC. This is particularly relevant to patients with "disconnection" injuries. Therapies that target control processes may be a way of promoting the "re-integration" of damaged brain into functional networks (Chen et al. 2006). Targeting core PFC functions in process-oriented training should increase the likelihood of generalization of gains to new contexts, though this may not be sufficient without additional considerations.

2. Cognitive training should explicitly include a goal-based approach.

   The role of goal-based executive processes may be to functionally organize the multiple neural processes necessary for accomplishing the goal, including selecting the relevant pathways or processes (while excluding others), coordinating them at any given moment in time, and dynamically adjusting this coordination while maintaining the central goal across time to eventually accomplish the goal. In the development of a training protocol, it is important to consider the processes required for accomplishment of any specific goals during training. These processes will differ depending on the nature of the goals. For example, if the goal is to make a quick decision regarding a left vs. right button press based on an image on a computer screen in an isolated setting, then the engaged processes and the level of integration necessary will be very different than what is engaged by a more complex task, such as paying attention to one's supervisor in a noisy office in order to accomplish an extended project. Thus, the opportunity for the greatest engagement of goal-direction processes will be provided with complex goals.

   A goal-based approach will allow training of multiple goal-direction processes. Who sets the goals? *Goal-generation* involves the highest levels of goal-directed control, requiring generation de novo, or retrieval and appraisal of potential goals that will guide behavior. Training that involves an active role for the trainee in defining the goals and subgoals of the tasks being learned may differ in effect from when goals are "assigned." Coordination of the many steps required for goal attainment may critically rely on the protection and maintenance of the goal. Thus, goals which require greater lengths of time and multiple tasks to accomplish will provide greater challenge to *maintenance* of goal information. What is the *personal relevance* of the goals to the individual? It is important for several reasons that the goals of training are of significance to the patient: this will increase motivation, encourage application of skills to ("real-life") goals that are often more complex than "artificial" goals, and allow for increased practice of goal processing in daily life. There is also the potential for increased positive feedback from accomplishment of goals that are important to the trainee. Incorporation of some or all of these features would significantly affect the nature of the intervention and likely benefits.

3. Cognitive training tasks should progressively challenge the patient.

   The importance of progressive increases in challenge is underscored by the ability of the brain to adapt to tasks. Even tasks that engage goal-directed control processes may become less challenging with practice, and thus less effective at encouraging learning in the targeted domain. As a patient's level of function improves for a specific process, tasks may need to be adjusted such that demands for that process are increased. This is more specific than simply increasing the general "difficulty" of the task, as parameters that are adjusted should quantitatively vary the level of engagement of specific processes, such as working memory, multitasking (Erickson et al. 2007), updating (Dahlin et al. 2008), or interference control (Persson and Reuter-Lorenz 2008). However, again, practicing on isolated tasks that are designed to engage control mechanisms may improve performance, but in a way limited to the specific tasks practiced. Extensive studies on the effects of practice of well-known cognitive control tasks have documented context-specific improvements (MacLeod and Dunbar 1988; MacLeod 1991). Thus, simply practicing isolated, purportedly process-targeted tasks may not be sufficient to improve functioning in a significant way, even if the trainee is challenged progressively.

4. Training should enhance the transfer and generalization of training effects to new and real-world contexts.

   A major gauge of the success of any training-based therapy is the extent to which benefits actually extend beyond the training tasks and context. As mentioned above, if functions of the core PFC networks for goal-directed control are effectively improved, then generalization of benefits should be more likely. How would this be accomplished? To effectively target core PFC functions, and not simply context-specific abilities, it is arguably important to train the target processes in multiple modalities and multiple settings. PFC is multimodal association cortex, and PFC networks serve to integrate information from multiple modalities (Schumacher et al. 1996; Collette et al. 2005; Postle 2006; Zelano et al. 2005). Training across *multiple modalities* may maximize engagement of core PFC networks leading to improved functioning across contexts. The above simplified process-oriented view of PFC involvement in goal-directed control raises a question regarding the importance of the *context(s)* in which these functions are engaged. Any training context carries with it important cues and inherent structure, which may provide scaffolding for an injured individual. Most deficits in goal-directed control are only apparent in contexts that lack strong external cues for action, requiring hierarchical organization that allows top-down goal-directed signals to out-compete bottom-up signals encouraging engagement with the environment (Duncan et al. 1995, 1996). Thus, the opportunity for the greatest engagement of goal-direction processes will be provided in *unstructured* settings. Furthermore, learning a skill within a specific context does not guarantee that that the skill will be applied to other contexts, where scaffolding is no longer present. Indeed, certain rehabilitation approaches emphasize the training of context-specific "functional" skills (such as getting dressed). This is highly valuable as a clinical approach for patients who have severe limitations in cognition, but this is also the antithesis of training underlying abilities to accomplish adaptive behavior. To potentially remediate goal-directed control functions, training would ideally occur in as many contexts as possible.

5. Meta-cognitive strategy training may provide a form of goal-directed control function remediation.

   Meta-cognitive strategies are proposed to play an important role in achieving generalizable improvements in goal-directed functioning. One hallmark of prefrontal networks dysfunction is difficulty in structuring cognition and behavior by employing strategies to efficiently and effectively accomplish goals. Increasing clinical evidence supports the proposition that training-based therapies targeting problem-solving, involving the use of meta-cognitive strategies, may improve functioning in individuals with brain injury (Cicerone et al. 2005; Kennedy et al. 2008). Several interventions have been developed and implemented with such an approach (D'Zurilla and Goldfried 1971; Kabat-Zinn 1990; VonCramon et al. 1991; Cicerone 2002; Rath et al. 2003; Robertson et al. 2005; Nezu et al. 2007). For example, in goal management training (Levine et al. 2000), patients are trained to clearly define a goal, learn the steps required to achieve it, and then regularly check their progress. Engagement of PFC appears to play an important role in the successful application of strategies (Newman et al. 2003; Miotto et al. 2006). Thus, meta-cognitive strategy training may enhance PFC-mediated control processes, rather than simply being compensatory. The neural mechanisms underlying successful improvement with meta-cognitive strategy training will be worth further investigation.

6. Training of goal-directed control of brain states.

   Goal-directed control may also be improved via improved regulation of brain states. At a neural level, modulation of brain states alters signal and noise properties of information processing systems in the brain that support abilities such as goal-directed control functions (Arnsten and Goldman-Rakic 1998; Gold and Shadlen 2001; Jazayeri 2008). Thus, training that improves regulation of brain states may also improve cognitive function following brain injury. A full understanding of the regulation of brain states that is translatable to treatment considerations still needs to be developed; however, certain aspects of state regulation are understood to be important for cognitive functioning.

   It is clear that brain states established by alertness and arousal, attentional sets, emotional states, and motivation can affect cognitive functioning. For example, a state of hyper-arousal may lead to rapid shifts of attention (distractibility) while low arousal may lead to poor activation and maintenance of attention. Patients with TBI–PTSD may show severe hyper-arousal, while patients with more severe TBI may exhibit marked deficits in alertness (Manly et al. 1999; Sturm et al. 1999; Posner 2008). Interventions that improve the regulation of arousal state may improve goal-directed functioning. External cues may help (Manly et al. 2002; Fish et al. 2008a, b), but training to improve self-regulation, from mindfulness exercises to more recent developments with computer-assisted techniques, may also be helpful (Degutis and Van Vleet 2010; Van Vleet et al. 2011). Mindfulness-based training approaches may train regulation of arousal state, reduce the load of non-relevant cognitive or emotional processing on limited neuro-cognitive resources, and improve an individual's ability to re-direct attention to goal-relevant processes (Posner et al. 2006; Jha et al. 2007; Slagter et al. 2007; Novakovic-Agopian et al. 2011). It is often presumed that individuals with goal-directed control function deficits due to brain injuries would not be good candidates for such training, given difficulty with attention regulation. We have found that cognitive training that incorporates principles of mindfulness can improve attention, working memory, and goal-directed functioning for individuals with brain injury (Novakovic-Agopian et al. 2011).

It is worth noting that improvements in state regulation may improve implicitly during any training intervention. For example, it is likely that trainees develop self-regulatory skills during intensive training when tasks are challenging (cognitively or physically), requiring the ability to regulate one's cognitive and emotional states (Paulus et al. 2009). Thus, even tasks that are described as task-based (e.g., computer games) may result in improvements in functioning that are due to improvements in state regulation.

7. Interactions of emotion and cognition.

   Special consideration needs to be made for the importance of emotion regulation for optimal cognitive functioning. Poor emotional control can significantly affect cognition and goal attainment. Emotional and cognitive control are directly tied together in that the underlying neural systems interact significantly in achieving self-regulatory control necessary for goal-directed behavior.

   Dysregulation of emotion can occur at multiple levels. An individual experiencing feelings of anxiety, irritability, and/or distress will be less able to effectively complete tasks that require overcoming challenges and solving problems, especially unexpected ones. Even further, she may negatively "over-react" to challenging situations, and the emotional reaction may impede the clear cognition needed for effective goal attainment. It is also likely that reduced cognitive control would contribute to poorer emotional control. Individuals with TBI, with reduced self-regulatory control, may have more difficulty in managing and altering negative and/or traumatic associations and the "triggered" emotions. For example, an inability to filter out information and demands that are not directly related to a current goal (additional "cognitive noise") may lead to increased feelings of being overwhelmed. Indeed, given the known limitations of neural processing resources, it seems logical that an increase in "load," whether from cognitive or emotional sources, would lead to less efficient overall functioning. Interventions that improve attentional self-regulation may also improve emotional self-regulation, and vice versa.

   Thus, in order to improve an individual's ability to learn, change, and adapt in the process of goal attainment, it will often be necessary to address both cognitive and emotional self-regulation. These issues are discussed in more detail in the next section, with a focus on the combination of TBI and PTSD, perhaps the "hallmark" syndrome of recent combat activities.

Cognition, Emotion, and Combined TBI–PTSD: Frontiers for Treatment

Interactions of TBI–PTSD

Either TBI or PTSD alone may alter cognitive, emotional, and behavioral functioning. The co-occurrence of TBI and PTSD raises the question of how the two entities interact, and whether the combination of physical and experiential trauma results in consequences not simply explained by additive effects of TBI or PTSD alone.

PTSD and mild TBI may have independent and additive roles (Vanderploeg et al. 2009), but may also interact at multiple levels, including at the genesis of injury, the maintenance of symptoms, various aspects of cognitive-emotional functioning, and at the level of neural mechanisms. Features of each may interact to worsen functioning and/or make treatment more difficult. Approaching TBI–PTSD will require a multifactorial approach that addresses multiple, interacting layers of functioning. Furthermore, potential special features of the combination may need to be addressed. Defining certain core targets of intervention, such as processes of self-regulatory control important for both TBI and PTSD, may provide a gateway to enhance the success of other aspects of therapy. Special considerations are discussed in more depth in each section below.

Interactions Between Cognitive and Emotional Functioning with TBI–PTSD

Although TBI can result in dysfunction in almost any neurologic domain, the most common and persistent deficits tend to be in the *control* of cognitive-emotional functions. Indeed, injured individuals may be able to engage basic functions, but the disrupted regulation of these functions leads to variability, lability, inconsistency. As a classic example, some individuals with TBI display emotional lability, in one instant cooperative and friendly, in the next instant irritable and angry. This may be due to cognitive factors, such as misinterpreting or overreacting to environmental stimuli, as well as issues in the control of emotions or behavioral expression. This characterization overlaps greatly with PTSD. Effective regulation of emotion is crucial for optimal cognitive functioning. Dysfunction in emotional control, leading to frustration, irritability, anger, or even apathy, may significantly alter cognitive performance.

In another example, individuals may commonly complain of reduced ability to pay attention and hold information in mind, affecting many aspects of life functioning. However, attentional processes may be disrupted by "noise" from both "external" and "internal" sources. For example, it may be difficult to concentrate on a single conversation when other conversations are being heard in a crowded room, or it may be difficult to focus on a lecture during class when emotion-laden thoughts are also distracting from processing that goal-relevant stream of information. Should these symptoms be attributed to TBI or PTSD? Or is that the wrong question?

The Occurrence of PTSD May Add to the Cognitive Dysfunction Associated with TBI

The addition of PTSD to TBI may contribute to cognitive difficulties. The most common cognitive deficits associated with PTSD involve attention, executive functions, and memory (Vasterling and Brewin 2005). Attention and executive functions deficits commonly found in PTSD include working memory difficulties (Brandes et al. 2002; Gilbertson et al. 2001), problems in sustaining attention over time (Vasterling et al. 2002), response inhibition (Leskin and White 2007; Vasterling et al. 1998), and impaired ability to gate, monitor, and regulate the flow of incoming information and environmental stimuli (Vasterling et al. 1998).

A number of studies have documented impairment in learning and remembering new information in PTSD patients. With respect to learning new information, impairments in PTSD have been noted on both verbal and visual memory tasks but are more pronounced on verbal memory tasks (Brewin et al. 2007). PTSD-related deficits have been observed at different stages of memory processing, including the initial registration of new information and, somewhat less commonly, in retaining the newly learned information over time (Vasterling and Brewin 2005; Verfaellie and Vasterling 2009).

Could TBI Contribute to the Development and Sustainment of PTSD Symptoms?

There are clearly commonalities in terms of the external events that generate physical and experiential trauma. Could TBI contribute to the development and sustainment of PTSD symptoms? The occurrence of TBI could actually increase the risk of development of PTSD. Repeated exposure to experiences involving fear, horror, or helplessness in situations of threat to life or well-being is common in combat. In the post-deployment health assessment and re-assessment of 88,000 soldiers, 53% witnessed someone wounded or killed, 49% felt in danger of being killed, up to 42% required mental health treatment, PTSD reported in up to 25% (Milliken et al. 2007). There is an increased risk of PTSD with personal physical injury. In particular, there is an increased rate of PTSD for those with TBI (RR 1.8) (van Reekum et al. 2000). In examining the incidence of PTSD, rates increase in relationship to the occurrence of TBI, with increased incidence of PTSD along the gradient of no TBI to altered mental status to LOC (Taber and Hurley 2009). All of these numbers argue that some aspect of TBI contributes to the development or sustainment of PTSD symptoms. From the initial instant of injury mechanism, physical and experiential injuries are intertwined. However, there are likely additional interactions that contribute to symptom maintenance across time.

Cognitive Dysfunction May Impede Treatment for Emotional Problems, and Emotional Dysregulation May Impede Treatment of Cognitive Dysfunction

Severe emotional control dysfunction, including anxiety, hyper-vigilance, and avoidance, may become significant barriers to treatment of cognitive issues. On the other hand, cognitive deficits, especially those affecting aspects of attention, learning, and memory, may become barriers to effective treatment of emotional issues. Existing interventions designed for TBI rehabilitation or PTSD alone may need to be modified in order to maximize effectiveness. The modifications may require crossing the boundaries between traditional disciplines, creating a significant challenge in care systems designed to address single diagnoses.

Modifications to Existing Treatments

In current practice, most interventions are directed toward a diagnosis of PTSD or TBI, but not both. Treating PTSD, in the context of TBI, may differ from treating PTSD alone. For individuals in the chronic phase of the disorder, the PTSD treatments with the strongest evidence are cognitive-behavioral psychotherapies (Cahill et al. 2009) such as cognitive processing therapy, as well as prolonged exposure (Monson et al. 2006; Schnurr et al. 2007). Preliminary data also suggest that these therapies will be helpful for OEF/OIF veterans. A small, ongoing trial of prolonged exposure among OEF/OIF veterans has shown a 50% reduction in PTSD symptoms following treatment (Rauch et al. 2009). There is some evidence supporting the effectiveness of CBT for treatment of acute stress disorder following mild TBI and CBT combined with neurorehabilitation for targeting general anxiety symptomatology in people with mild-to-moderate TBI (Soo and Tate 2007).

Modification of these approaches for individuals with cognitive dysfunction remains an important frontier for intervention development. Current experience suggests that PTSD in individuals who also sustain a TBI may be a more complicated, and the chronicity of symptoms may be extended. Patients with TBI–PTSD may respond differently to standard treatments compared to those with only TBI or PTSD. Cognitive limitations may make it necessary to modify cognitive-behavioral therapies, and emotion regulation and impulse control problems may complicate the use of exposure techniques. Physical pain, which frequently occurs after TBI, may limit the extent to which patients can engage in PTSD treatments that involve in-person exposure to anxiety producing situations (Bryant and Hopwood 2006; Nampiaparampil 2008). Conversely, the emotional dysregulation, avoidance, and potential for triggering may impede engagement in cognitive rehabilitation therapies. Reduction of PTSD and management of severe TBI may be facilitated by teaching patients more adaptive coping strategies (Bryant et al. 2000).

Interventions for TBI–PTSD

Recognizing complexities with regards to TBI diagnosis and attribution of symptoms, a recent VA directive stated the following: "The assessment of an individual with persistent concussion/mild TBI-related symptoms should be directed to the *specific nature of the symptoms regardless of their etiology*. The *management* of an individual who has sustained a documented concussion/mild TBI and has *persistent* cognitive and behavioral symptoms after 1 month should not differ *based on the specific underlying etiology of their symptoms* (i.e., concussion vs. pain, concussion vs. stress disorder)."

To date, there are no empirically validated therapies to treat comorbid PTSD and TBI. Therapeutic formulations may also need to address associated issues with substance use disorders, pain, and the other issues discussed in this chapter. Combined approaches for co-treating the variety of emotional/behavioral and cognitive sequelae may need to involve mental health/PTSD specialists and TBI rehabilitation specialists (Vanderploeg et al. 2009).

Vanderploeg et al. discuss the need to intervene early after military post-deployment with social and emotional adjustment interventions, including the development of mindfulness-based relaxation and stress management skills, improved sleep hygiene, and education regarding substance use/abuse and alternative coping supports (Vanderploeg et al. 2009). They further suggest that early symptom-based adjustment and stress management interventions may minimize the development or prolongation of PTSD and additionally may serve to reduce residual symptoms associated with TBI. Current findings also suggest that PTSD treatment likely should be prioritized after combat or other types of injury, regardless of TBI status, to decrease symptom complaints and enhance outcomes.

Targeting Core Self-Regulatory Control Functions Involved in TBI–PTSD

These considerations argue strongly that treatments that effectively improve cognitive and emotional self-regulatory functions may be particularly valuable in treating the combined neurotrauma syndrome. The issues from TBI–PTSD include disruption of core cognitive and emotional regulation mechanisms that are essential for goal-directed functioning in life. Interventions that strengthen the goal-directed control functions, such as the selection of relevant information along with inhibition of distracting information, may be particularly helpful. Dorsolateral PFC and ventromedical PFC interact in the regulation of emotions, with modulation of amygdala (Phelps et al. 2004). These interacting circuits are likely to be important for cognitive and emotional self-regulation training such as mindfulness-based attention regulation. This forms an important foundation for further development of interventions for TBI–PTSD.

Neural Bases of TBI–PTSD and Frontiers in Intervention Development

Treating individuals with TBI–PTSD symptomatically, regardless of diagnosis, is important initial approach. However, it is possible that intervention approaches may be refined as more is learned about the underlying biology of the disorders. Consideration of potential interrelationships between traumatic and experiential injury at neural levels generates important hypotheses for guiding research and intervention development. Direct interactions may be understood based on structural neuroanatomy, functional neural network circuitry, and neuropharmacology. Neurologic abnormalities associated with TBI may complicate abnormalities associated with PTSD. Limbic structures, including the amygdala, are thought to be integral to emotions (e.g., anxiety) involved in the fear response. As a "modulator" on the limbic system, the medial PFC is thought to play a significant inhibitory role, allowing higher-order cognitive functions to moderate less volitional limbic-based fear responses. Because TBI may involve damage to prefrontal circuits, the additional loss of inhibitory control of the limbic system related to the TBI may play a role in exacerbating and maintaining PTSD symptoms.

Investigations that focus on neural mechanisms of learning and plasticity in particular will be valuable for better understanding the pathogenesis of symptoms and dysfunction as well as providing foundations for treatment approaches. Neural level considerations suggest that certain treatment approaches used for TBI or PTSD may need to be modified in order to maximize beneficial effects and reduce potential for unexpected harm in individuals with the combined syndrome. This applies to pharmacologic and other biological approaches, as well as behavioral approaches.

On a broader level, all of the above interactions argue for a re-consideration of a combined combat neurotrauma syndrome as an entity distinct from TBI or PTSD, with features that are not simply the addition of the two. Definition of this syndrome has implications for guiding future research, defining new research questions as well as requiring new approaches and methodologies. Regardless of whether we can define a definitive syndrome and its etiology, it is clear that the combinations of symptoms that veterans experience after combat do need to be addressed with available tools immediately. Addressing these symptoms will require a multifactorial approach that takes into account contributory environmental, personal, social, emotional, and cognitive factors as well as changes in underlying neural systems. In particular, a much greater emphasis on cognitive, emotional, and behavioral self-regulation may be needed, even in individuals with so-called "mild" TBI.

Tested Theory-Driven Cognitive Interventions for Attention, Working Memory, and Other Control Processes

A variety of innovations have been developed for targeting aspects of cognitive functioning. Individualization is a key tenet for optimizing rehabilitation. Thus, each therapist may provide a different intervention for each patient, and systematically studying such interventions is challenging. A small number of structured intervention protocols have been directly studied. Increasing evidence supports the proposition that training-based therapies have utility for rehabilitation in the chronic phase of TBI, including training for attention, working memory, problem-solving, and other strategic aspects of goal management.

Even within the domain of attention, there may be many varieties of approaches to training. Selected handful of theory-driven interventions are highlighted here. A new paradigmatic example is attention process training, originally formulated by Sohlberg and Mateer (Sohlberg and Mateer 1987; Sohlberg et al. 2000). Versions of APT train a hierarchy of attention processes using guided exercises. This method, along with other clinically based approaches, has been reviewed in multiple reviews and meta-analyses (Cicerone et al. 2000, 2005; Kennedy et al. 2008; Levine et al. 2008; Rohling et al. 2009), and there is significant evidence to support their use for patients with brain injury. This and other approaches that target specific processes, including a number using computer-based tasks, have been demonstrated to improve functioning on targeted measures. However, the transfer and generalization of gains from task practice have turned out to be an important barrier (D'Esposito and Gazzaley 2006). This raises important questions regarding the nature of transfer beyond practiced tasks, and the development of approaches to enhance generalization remains an important goal.

Some recent approaches have shown promise in not only improving the targeted processes but also showing transfer of benefits to other tasks that were not included in training. In a series of studies utilizing computer-based practice of tasks that progressively engage spatial working memory, Klingberg and colleagues have shown improvements in working memory functioning as well as transfer to higher level cognitive functions that presumably rely on working memory (Klingberg 2010; Westerberg et al. 2007). In healthy subjects, improvements correlated with increases in activation in PFC and parietal regions, as well as changes in dopamine receptor binding (Olesen et al. 2004; McNab et al. 2009). Other recent studies, testing computer-based tasks with health individuals, have generated excitement by demonstrating improvements in aspects of goal-directed control and even general fluid intelligence (Erickson et al. 2007; Dahlin et al. 2008; Jaeggi et al. 2008; Persson and Reuter-Lorenz 2008). To what extent process-targeted, computer-based approaches may be helpful for individuals with brain injury, with improvements that generalize to real-world functioning will be worth further investigation.

Approaches that train the use of meta-cognitive strategies have demonstrated utility for individuals with brain injury. Noting that many individuals with brain injury have difficulties with specific aspects of goal management, including making absent-minded slips, going off track, and having difficulty completing multi-step tasks, goal management training emphasizes the cessation of ongoing activity, and a meta-cognitive strategy for breaking down goals into manageable substeps. This approach attempts to ameliorate deficits related to goal neglect, and studies testing training protocols have shown that learning of these strategies may improve goal management for individuals with brain injury, as well as healthy older adults (Levine et al. 2000, 2007).

Another intervention that combines attention and problem-solving as targets of therapy in a group-based training protocol was recently described by Evans (2001, 2005). Initial group sessions address attentional difficulties, and later sessions introduce and practice the use of problem-solving strategies. Participants are encouraged to adopt a systematic approach to solving problems and to manage and monitor goal achievement through periodic mental checking. In a study by Miotto et al. (2009), participants with chronic frontal lesions showed improvement on a measure of functional performance with multiple tasks, and on caregiver ratings of executive functioning, though not on neuropsychological tests, after the implementation of training relative to control conditions.

We are all constantly faced with sources of information that either contain too much information or are ambiguous with respect to one's goals. The ability to synthesize core meaning from incoming information (i.e., "get the gist") is important for goal-directed behavior in everyday life, and relies on the integration of a number of cognitive processes. Chapman and colleagues have developed protocols to train gist-based strategic reasoning, guiding individuals through steps that engage attention (repeating and filtering the information), working memory (integration of information), and higher level elaborative reasoning (expanding, extracting). Training has been shown to improve the ability to extract gist, as well as other aspects of learning and reasoning for children, as well as adults with brain injury (Vas et al. 2011). Performance on tests of attention and working memory also improved. This raises the interesting possibility that training in higher level integrative abilities may improve more basic functions.

Bridges to Improved Interventions

Defining neurologic processes as specific therapeutic targets facilitates the "vertical integration" of developments in neuroscience and rehabilitative therapies. Of particular interest in this discussion are studies that "close the loop," testing not only the behavioral and clinical effects of these interventions but also hypothesized neural mechanisms. The nature of plasticity within prefrontal networks remains one of the frontiers of neuroscience (Miller and Cohen 2001) as well as rehabilitation. On the one hand, defining mechanisms of neural plasticity may provide potential targets for treatment. On the other hand, rehabilitation interventions may provide powerful tools to probe mechanisms of plasticity, especially when matched with appropriate neurophysiologic measurements. It would be ideal for interventions and measurements to be drawn from a unified neuroscience framework, opening the potential for well-integrated studies to test the mechanisms that support improvements in cognition. This is the essence of a rehabilitation neuroscience approach.

Two general and complementary directions for development are worth pointing out. First, any approach should be designed to enhance neural mechanisms of control. The foundations in cognitive neuroscience discussed earlier may help. Second, cognitive training must lead to improvement in function in activities of everyday living. Patients are most in need of functional improvements for navigating the complexities and ambiguities of daily life in low-structure settings of the real-world. Computer-based "brain training games" have staged a resurgence in interest recently, and provide a timely example for considering whether the offered cognitive training approaches maximize generalization of improvements. In general, there has been little evidence to support transfer and generalization of benefits from practice on basic tasks, such as computer games, to improved functioning in real-life situations (D'Esposito and Gazzaley 2006). However, computer, Internet, and other technologies may provide valuable tools to augment training, if applied appropriately in interventions that are well-informed by neuroscience and best clinical practice. We provide one example of a rehabilitation neuroscience study that utilizes a theory-driven intervention to test hypotheses regarding functional, behavioral, and neural changes.

Targeting the Selection Gateway

The regulation of information processing in the brain deserves special emphasis. Selective processing of goal-relevant information, a central component of executive control, is a crucial gateway that filters what information gains access to more in-depth processing (Baddeley 2001; Vogel et al. 2005; Cowan and Morey 2006; Repovs and Baddeley 2006; Awh and Vogel 2008). The integrity of information processing, whether from perception or through other steps to action, requires mechanisms of selection, maintenance, and protection from disruption during working memory, learning, decision-making, and/or problem-solving. The protection of information processing from distractions anywhere along this pathway is crucial to efficient and effective goal attainment, especially when extended time or multiple steps are required.

The general principles proposed earlier in this chapter for optimally training control functions would ideally be applied with this specific "selection" gateway as a target. In one example of a rehabilitation neuroscience study, our particular interest was in examining neural-behavioral changes with an intervention that targets goal-oriented attention regulation (Novakovic-Agopian et al. 2011). Participants with chronic brain injury and executive dysfunction completed a training intervention for goal-oriented attentional self-regulation that takes into account the links connecting attention, working memory, and goal-based direction of behavior in daily life. In contrast to training via practice on isolated tasks, this training protocol involved application of attention regulation skills and strategies to participant-defined goals in real-life, ecologically valid settings.

Two conceptual lines converged to delineate target processes for intervention. First, pathways from perception to action require mechanisms for the selection of information for in-depth processing, as well as the maintenance and protection of this information from disruption during working memory and subsequent learning, decision-making, and/or problem-solving. Second, many patients with brain injuries show an overall "life disorganization," with poor ability to manage and attain goals, even when they may be able to describe their intentions at the outset. Duncan and others have described this phenomenon as "goal neglect" (Duncan et al. 1995, 1996). We reasoned that selective maintenance of goal-related information is important for guiding sequences of steps (subgoals) required to accomplish the goal. Therefore, intervening on these processes may help to ameliorate symptoms of goal neglect. The experimental training protocol was based on training interventions that have been applied to patients with brain injury as well as other populations (D'Zurilla and Goldfried 1971; VonCramon et al. 1991; Levine et al. 2000, 2007; Rath et al. 2003; Nezu et al. 2007) with special emphasis on mindfulness-based attention regulation strategies applied to daily life situations and complex, project-based functional tasks. An overarching hypothesis was that training that improves goal-directed control over neural processing would benefit all subsequent stages of goal-based processing, helping by making damaged, poorly integrated collections of neurons into more efficient, better integrated functional networks for the performance of relevant tasks, and ultimately, goal attainment in real-life contexts.

It may be argued that the ecologically valid measurement of executive control functioning requires observation and quantification of performance with real-life, functional tasks in a low-structure environment. We therefore assessed training-related changes in participant functioning on measures of performance in "real-life" low-structure settings. Following training, participants showed improvements in accomplishing tasks, confirming generalization of training effects to complex, real-life settings. In testing whether functional improvements might be related to improvements in the targeted cognitive functions, we also assessed domain-specific changes utilizing neuropsychological testing. Participants who completed a course of goal-oriented attentional self-regulation training improved on neuropsychological measures of complex attention and executive functions, including working memory, mental flexibility, inhibition, and sustained attention. Long-term follow-up is particularly helpful in determining what aspects of an intervention have enduring benefits. In a follow-up conducted 6 months-to-2 years post-training, 87% of participants indicated continuing to use at least one trained strategy in their daily life.

Understanding the neural bases of cognition, including the mechanisms by which improvements occur, may provide guidance for the development of treatments to enhance functioning (Chen et al. 2006; D'Esposito and Chen 2006;

Kennedy et al. 2008; Levine et al. 2008). Intervening via rehabilitation provides an opportunity to probe such mechanisms. Functional neuroimaging studies examining changes associated with various forms of training in neurologically intact individuals have shown different patterns of results, primarily in terms of increases or decreases in regional brain activation, and the significance of these results remains unclear (Kelly and Garavan 2005; Kelly et al. 2006; Hillary 2008). It is also unclear from functional neuroimaging studies of patients with acquired brain injuries as to what neural changes support improved recovery of cognitive function (Rosen et al. 2000; Corbetta et al. 2005; Chen et al. 2008; Sanchez-Carrion et al. 2008). Information regarding neural mechanisms of improvement in executive control functions is particularly sparse. Even the extent to which the neural systems that underlie executive control are plastic, if at all, has remained an open question. Only a handful of fMRI studies to date have examined cognitive rehabilitation following brain injury (Laatsch et al. 2004; Strangman et al. 2009) and even fewer have examined the effects of rehabilitation interventions on executive control functions (Kim et al. 2009). We attempted to identify neural mechanisms that underlie improvements in attention and executive control with the above described rehabilitation training.

We hypothesized that training in attention regulation improves cognitive performance by enhancing goal-based modulatory control of neural processing. Functional MRI methods adapted for testing the effects of intervention for patients with varied injury pathology were used to index modulatory control of neural processing (Chen et al. 2011). Another important paradigm shift is supported by measurements that "read the *information*" coded in brain networks, rather than simply quantifying activity levels. Information is represented in the brain through the coordinated activity of distributed networks. Methods for decoding neural information representations may provide valuable tools for gauging the functional integration of these networks, particularly important in individuals who have suffered brain injury and potentially a "disintegration" of brain networks. We hypothesized that attention regulation training would lead to changes in tuning of neural representations such that the balance of representation would favor goal-relevant information. Our findings with training were consistent with this prediction. Modulation of neural processing in extrastriate cortex was significantly enhanced by attention regulation training.

As discussed above, the lateral PFC has been strongly implicated as a source of attentional control signals that could bias neural processing in extrastriate cortex (Desimone 1998; Miller and Cohen 2001; Miller and D'Esposito 2005). The pattern of findings within lateral PFC showed that changes in function depended on the baseline state of any given individual. One particularly important but challenging question for further investigation is to understand the individual variability in mechanisms by which different individuals may achieve improvement in functioning after brain injury.

A training study with veterans with chronic TBI, some of whom have co-morbid PTSD and depression, is currently ongoing. This study, as well as future studies with veterans with PTSD, will help test not only whether goal-directed cognitive functioning may be improved, but also to what extent emotional functioning may be improved with training in attentional self-regulation. We are also working on methods that leverage the advantages of computer game-based formats to augment training. The intervention protocols are designed based on the principles discussed in this chapter, bridging the neuroscience and clinical rehabilitation of goal-directed control functions.

Directions and Imperatives for Future Work

A Long-Term View on Brain Injury Sequelae

Functional deficits from TBI may produce tremendous *chronic* burden on individuals, families, and health care systems. The far-reaching impact of these seemingly "invisible" deficits is often not recognized. Beyond the immediate effects of injury on cognition, or even the effects on engagement in rehabilitation, school, or work, there may be ramifications across the lifespan (Chen and D'Esposito 2010). Individuals who have suffered a TBI may be at increased risk for developing cognitive changes later in life. For example, individuals who have suffered moderate or severe TBI may be at 2.3 and 4.5 times increased risk of developing Alzheimer's disease (Plassman et al. 2000). Risk may be increased for those with certain apolipoprotein E genotypes (Van Den Heuvel et al. 2007).

What are the mechanisms by which TBI may contribute to worsened cognitive functioning with aging? Does TBI simply change an individual's cognitive baseline, thereby reducing the threshold at which detectable dementia later in life would occur? This effect could be mediated by a relatively simple mechanism that is related to the concept of "cognitive reserve" (Kesler et al. 2003; Nithianantharajah and Hannan 2009). If an individual's baseline functioning is "knocked down" a notch after a TBI, leaving a reduced reserve, then that person is more likely to fall below some "threshold" during the aging process.

Could TBI actually alter the course and rate of age-related cognitive decline? It is possible that there could be a more dynamic "cumulative" effect of TBI across time. One must consider the dynamic nature of brain functioning, where development and learning vs. degradation and forgetting are constantly countering each other to determine an individual's current level of functioning. After a brain injury, an individual may not learn as quickly or as effectively as without the injury. Even small, possibly undetectable "deficits" in cognitive functioning may have a magnified effect over the course of aging, as the effects of poor learning accumulate over time. This has significant implications for the development of interventions that address long-term brain health after brain injury.

Translation to Intervention Implementation and Delivery in Systems of Care

The considerations discussed in this chapter suggest important changes in the organization of existing systems of care. How integrated is the overall approach to the patient? The organization of care needs to be considered given the complex nature of cognitive dysfunction after brain injury, and the approaches that are needed to improve functioning. The effective integration of any or all of the neural-cognitive processes and modulators illustrated in Fig. 15.1 is a particularly important determinant of overall cognitive functioning. Intervention approaches may need to target not only separate processes but also the effective integration of these processes. Thus, at a systems level, expert care may require the integration of expertise that is typically divided across many disciplines.

Care may need to be re-organized to more efficiently and effectively address the multiple issues faced by individuals with brain injuries. This may involve team members addressing and reinforcing common themes and issues that cross psychological and emotional functioning, psychiatric health, social work, case management, pharmacotherapy, vocational or educational assistance, family interactions, and more. Taking into account interactions between emotions and cognition is particularly relevant given the frequent co-occurrence of TBI and post-traumatic stress symptoms. Specific themes or approaches may be implemented by multiple team members, increasing the chances of accomplishing a therapeutic goal. Individual practitioners may need to expand their range of expertise, for example, incorporating strategies that bridge cognitive rehabilitation with mental health, pain management, and substance abuse. Given the combined issues of potentially reduced awareness, vulnerability to confusion, and potential difficulty mentally integrating multiple approaches, it would be ideal to take an integrated, patient-centered approach.

Certain issues in the implementation and delivery for military veterans deserve special consideration. Treatment implementation and delivery methods need to be adapted to take into account issues related to geographic distribution of veterans, the "culture" of military as well as community settings for post-military life, a high level of comorbidity with PTSD and other mental health conditions, individual goals after military service (e.g., educational or occupational), and more.

The wide geographic distribution of veterans creates challenges for treatment delivery and implementation. For example, one of the largest catchment areas for veterans returning from the combat in the Middle East spans thousands of square miles of Northern California, Nevada, and Hawaii, from oceans to mountains and desert as well as cities. The majority of veterans are not within easy travel distance to specialty medical centers. This limits the applicability of intensive on-site therapies, and raises challenges to achieving integrated, interdisciplinary care. Furthermore, many of the cognitive, emotional, or behavioral problems that occur with TBI, even without deficits in other physical functions, have not been standard indications for inpatient or residential treatment. Expansion of inpatient or in-residence programs may be necessary.

Telemedicine approaches may extend therapeutic range, and new tools for augmenting therapeutic interventions at a distance will be valuable. The development of telemedicine implementation for treatments for complex issues such as cognitive dysfunction is still in its infancy. Computer-assisted therapy tools may help bridge the distances, though issues of engagement, compliance, and monitoring need to be taken into account to maximize treatment effectiveness. For example, the development of computer-assisted cognitive training regimens that are remotely administered, yet supervised by expert therapists via telecommunication technologies, may help.

Another important barrier is the divide between "medical care" and community. An important goal of many younger veterans is successful re-integration into civilian communities, with goals involving family, education, and/or new occupations. Care traditionally centered within medical facilities will need to better connect with each individual's community setting. Telecommunication technologies (e.g., video interactions from therapist to a patient's house) and formulation of therapy programs that cross the borders between medical center and home, school, or work may be valuable.

Conclusions

The effects of TBI on cognition are complex and have challenged clinicians throughout history, as well as deterred neuroscientists from pursuing studies in this "messy" area of inquiry. The complexity is compounded by combinations of physical and experiential injury, as well as other comorbidities. Much work will need to be done to better define effective therapies for cognitive dysfunction caused by brain injuries. Research and development along several key directions will be crucial.

Building a strong theoretical and scientific foundation will be valuable for guiding the development of new therapies. Understanding the brain systems that underlie the cognitive changes associated with brain injury should help in the delineation of targets in the rehabilitation of an individual with TBI. In particular, this knowledge will open the way for therapies that target biological systems and synergistically augment the beneficial specific effects of training.

Pharmacotherapy and other biological modification therapies may be integrated into rehabilitation to help augment learning by changing specific brain systems or altering the plasticity of the brain in a more general way. Much work needs to be done to define the specific effects of drugs at multiple levels of nervous system function, in order to best define combined behavioral-pharmacotherapeutic prescriptions. Mechanisms of plasticity to be harnessed may range from changes in intracellular signaling, cellular proliferation, alterations of dendritic or axonal structures, and more, but these changes, occurring in isolation, will not necessarily be beneficial. Ultimately, for any neuronal changes to beneficially affect neurological functioning, they must lead to functional changes in neuronal networks. Training provides a crucial set of methods to guide or sculpt plasticity to achieve functionally integrated networks and improvements in behavioral functioning.

Approaches that bridge the basic neuroscience of neural-cognitive functioning with the practical realities of clinical rehabilitation will be valuable in intervention development. It will be particularly important to consider the relationships between multiple levels of individual functioning, from neurons to neural networks all the way up to social networks, each providing complementary targets for therapy.

Improved measures of the effects and mechanisms of interventions are sorely needed. The lack of adequate measurements has limited intervention development. Measurement development needs to progress in at least two directions. First, biomarkers of the neural processes that mediate cognitive functions affected by brain injuries would be valuable for determining mechanisms. Cognitive neuroscience can serve as a foundation for development of these biomarkers. Measurements informative of cognitive processes, especially higher-order cognitive functioning, are also needed. These measurements of neural-cognitive processes will be crucial for elucidating mechanisms of the benefits (or lack thereof) for any intervention. Just as importantly, measurements that reflect cognitive functioning in ecologically relevant, real-life contexts are needed. Most tests of cognitive functioning, including neuropsychological tests and most cognitive neuroscience measures, are designed to isolate the processes of interest. This is analogous to judging how accurate a basketball player will be at shooting foul shots by measuring isolated biceps strength. On the other hand, the few functional assessment measures available are not linked in any clear way to the underlying neural-cognitive component processes affected by TBI. The development of ecologically relevant, neuroscience-driven interventions will benefit greatly from measurements that bridge neural-cognitive processes to real-world behavior.

Taking a long term view on TBI in the context of the lifespan may lead to a major paradigm shift for the field. We will need to consider the enhancement of ongoing learning, recovery, and/or maintenance as a long-term goal of post-injury "brain health." Keeping in mind the benefits of bridging across levels of human functioning, across disciplines, and across the lifespan will significantly alter the emphasis of research and intervention development, expanding the horizons for improving cognitive functioning for individuals who have suffered brain injury.

Acknowledgment Special thanks to Katelyn Begany for assistance with editing.

References

Arnsten AF, Goldman-Rakic PS. Noise stress impairs prefrontal cortical cognitive function in monkeys: evidence for a hyperdopaminergic mechanism. Arch Gen Psychiatry. 1998;55(4):362–8.

Aston-Jones G, Cohen JD. An integrative theory of locus coeruleus-norepinephrine function: adaptive gain and optimal performance. Annu Rev Neurosci. 2005;28:403–50.

Awh E, Vogel EK. The bouncer in the brain. Nat Neurosci. 2008;11(1):5–6.

Ayalon L, Borodkin K, et al. Circadian rhythm sleep disorders following mild traumatic brain injury. Neurology. 2007;68(14):1136–40.

Baddeley AD. Is working memory still working? Am Psychol. 2001;56(11):851–64.

Badre D, D'Esposito M. Is the rostro-caudal axis of the frontal lobe hierarchical? Nat Rev Neurosci. 2009;10(9):659–69.

Baldo JV, Shimamura AP. Letter and category fluency in patients with frontal lobe lesions. Neuropsychology. 1998;12(2):259–67.

Baldo JV, Shimamura AP, et al. Verbal and design fluency in patients with frontal lobe lesions. J Int Neuropsychol Soc. 2001;7(5):586–96.

Baldo JV, Delis DC, et al. Is it bigger than a breadbox? Performance of patients with prefrontal lesions on a new executive function test. Arch Clin Neuropsychol. 2004;19(3):407–19.

Baldo JV, Schwartz S, et al. Role of frontal versus temporal cortex in verbal fluency as revealed by voxel-based lesion symptom mapping. J Int Neuropsychol Soc. 2006;12(6):896–900.

Banich MT, Milham MP, et al. fMri studies of Stroop tasks reveal unique roles of anterior and posterior brain systems in attentional selection. J Cogn Neurosci. 2000a;12(6):988–1000.

Banich MT, Milham MP, et al. Prefrontal regions play a predominant role in imposing an attentional 'set': evidence from fMRI. Brain Res Cogn Brain Res. 2000b;10(1–2):1–9.

Belanger HG, Curtiss G, et al. Factors moderating neuropsychological outcomes following mild traumatic brain injury: a meta-analysis. J Int Neuropsychol Soc. 2005;11(3):215–27.

Belanger HG, Kretzmer T, et al. Cognitive sequelae of blast-related versus other mechanisms of brain trauma. J Int Neuropsychol Soc. 2009;15(1):1–8.

Binder LM, Rohling ML, et al. A review of mild head trauma. Part I: meta-analytic review of neuropsychological studies. J Clin Exp Neuropsychol. 1997;19(3):421–31.

Bloomfield IL, Espie CA, et al. Do sleep difficulties exacerbate deficits in sustained attention following traumatic brain injury? J Int Neuropsychol Soc. 2009;16(1):17–25.

Blumenfeld RS, Ranganath C. Prefrontal cortex and long-term memory encoding: an integrative review of findings from neuropsychology and neuroimaging. Neuroscientist. 2007;13(3):280–91.

Borgaro SR, Gierok S, et al. Fatigue after brain injury: initial reliability study of the BNI Fatigue Scale. Brain Inj. 2004;18(7):685–90.

Brandes D, Ben-Schachar G, et al. PTSD symptoms and cognitive performance in recent trauma survivors. Psychiatry Res. 2002;110(3):231–8.

Brewin CR, Kleiner JS, et al. Memory for emotionally neutral information in posttraumatic stress disorder: a meta-analytic investigation. J Abnorm Psychol. 2007;116(3):448–63.

Bryant R, Hopwood S. Commentary on "Trauma to the Psyche and Soma". Cogn Behav Pract. 2006;13(1):17–23.

Bryant RA, Marosszeky JE, et al. Coping style and post-traumatic stress disorder following severe traumatic brain injury. Brain Inj. 2000;14(2):175–80.

Bunge SA, Zelazo PD. A brain-based account of the development of rule use in childhood. Curr Dir Psychol Sci. 2006;15(3):118–21.

Bunge SA, Ochsner KN, et al. Prefrontal regions involved in keeping information in and out of mind. Brain. 2001;124(Pt 10):2074–86.

Bunge SA, Dudukovic NM, et al. Immature frontal lobe contributions to cognitive control in children: evidence from fMRI. Neuron. 2002a;33(2):301–11.

Bunge SA, Hazeltine E, et al. Dissociable contributions of prefrontal and parietal cortices to response selection. Neuroimage. 2002b;17(3):1562–71.

Bunge SA, Kahn I, et al. Neural circuits subserving the retrieval and maintenance of abstract rules. J Neurophysiol. 2003;90(5):3419–28.

Bunge SA, Wendelken C, et al. Analogical reasoning and prefrontal cortex: evidence for separable retrieval and integration mechanisms. Cereb Cortex. 2005;15(3):239–49.

Burgess PW, Gonen-Yaacovi G, et al. Functional neuroimaging studies of prospective memory: what have we learnt so far? Neuropsychologia. 2011;49(8):2246–57.

Burton, T. Why some patients get no help after brain injury. Wall St j. January 8, 2007. http://online.wsj.com/article/SB116822903868669978.html.

Bushnik T, Englander J, et al. The experience of fatigue in the first 2 years after moderate-to-severe traumatic brain injury: a preliminary report. J Head Trauma Rehabil. 2008a;23(1):17–24.

Bushnik T, Englander J, et al. Patterns of fatigue and its correlates over the first 2 years after traumatic brain injury. J Head Trauma Rehabil. 2008b;23(1):25–32.

Cahill S, Rothbaum B, et al. Cognitive-behavioral therapy for adults. In: Foa EB, Keane TM, Friedman MJ, Cohen JA, editors. Effective treatments for PTSD: practice guidelines for the international society for traumatic stress studies. New York: Guilford Press; 2009. p. 139–222.

Canessa N, Ferini-Strambi L. Sleep-disordered breathing and cognitive decline in older adults. JAMA. 2011;306(6):654–5.

Castriotta RJ, Wilde MC, et al. Prevalence and consequences of sleep disorders in traumatic brain injury. J Clin Sleep Med. 2007;3(4):349–56.

Chen AJ-W, D'Esposito M. Traumatic brain injury: from bench to beside to society. Neuron. 2010;66(1):11–4.

Chen AJ-W, Abrams GM, et al. Functional re-integration of prefrontal neural networks for enhancing recovery after brain injury. J Head Trauma Rehabil. 2006;21(2):107–18.

Chen AJ-W, Britton M, et al. Sharpening of neural representations: a mechanism of top-down control over information processing by selective attention. New York City: Cognitive Neuroscience Society; 2007.

Chen JK, Johnston KM, et al. Recovery from mild head injury in sports: evidence from serial functional magnetic resonance imaging studies in male athletes. Clin J Sport Med. 2008;18(3):241–7.

Chen AJW, Novakovic-Agopian T, et al. Training of goal-directed attention regulation enhances control over neural processing for individuals with brain injury. Brain. 2011.

Cicerone KD. Remediation of "working attention" in mild traumatic brain injury. Brain Inj. 2002;16(3):185–95.

Cicerone KD, Azulay J. Diagnostic utility of attention measures in postconcussion syndrome. Clin Neuropsychol. 2002;16(3):280–9.

Cicerone KD, Dahlberg C, et al. Evidence-based cognitive rehabilitation: recommendations for clinical practice. Arch Phys Med Rehabil. 2000;81(12):1596–615.

Cicerone KD, Dahlberg C, et al. Evidence-based cognitive rehabilitation: updated review of the literature from 1998 through 2002. Arch Phys Med Rehabil. 2005;86(8):1681–92.

Collette F, Van der Linden M, et al. Exploring the unity and diversity of the neural substrates of executive functioning. Hum Brain Mapp. 2005;25(4):409–23.

Cools R, Barker RA, et al. Enhanced or impaired cognitive function in Parkinson's disease as a function of dopaminergic medication and task demands. Cereb Cortex. 2001;11(12):1136–43.

Cools R, Barker RA, et al. L-Dopa medication remediates cognitive inflexibility, but increases impulsivity in patients with Parkinson's disease. Neuropsychologia. 2003;41(11):1431–41.

Cools R, Gibbs SE, et al. Working memory capacity predicts dopamine synthesis capacity in the human striatum. J Neurosci. 2008;28(5):1208–12.

Corbetta M, Kincade MJ, et al. Neural basis and recovery of spatial attention deficits in spatial neglect. Nat Neurosci. 2005;8(11):1603–10.

Cowan N, Morey CC. Visual working memory depends on attentional filtering. Trends Cogn Sci. 2006;10(4):139–41.

Crone EA, Donohue SE, et al. Brain regions mediating flexible rule use during development. J Neurosci. 2006;26(43):11239–47.

Curtis CE, D'Esposito M. Persistent activity in the prefrontal cortex during working memory. Trends Cogn Sci. 2003;7(9):415–23.

Curtis CE, Rao VY, et al. Maintenance of spatial and motor codes during oculomotor delayed response tasks. J Neurosci. 2004;24(16):3944–52.

D'Esposito M, Gazzaley A. Neurorehabilitation and executive function. In: Selzer ME, Cohen L, Gage FH, Clarke S, Duncan PW, editors. Neural rehabilitation and repair. Cambridge, UK: Cambridge University Press, 2006 p. 475–87.

D'Esposito M, Postle BR. The dependence of span and delayed-response performance on prefrontal cortex. Neuropsychologia. 1999;37(11):1303–15.

D'Esposito M, Detre JA, et al. The neural basis of the central executive system of working memory. Nature. 1995;378(6554):279–81.

D'Esposito M, Aguirre GK, et al. Functional MRI studies of spatial and non-spatial working memory. Cogn Brain Res. 1998;7:1–13.

D'Esposito M, Postle BR, et al. Maintenance versus manipulation of information held in working memory: an event-related fMRI study. Brain Cogn. 1999;41(1):66–86.

D'Esposito M, Chen AJW. Neural mechanisms of prefrontal cortical function: implications for cognitive rehabilitation. In: Moller A, Chapman SB, Lomber SG, editors. Reprogramming the human brain: progress in brain research. Elsevier; 2006. 157.

D'Zurilla TJ, Goldfried M. Problem solving and behavior modification. J Abnorm Psychol. 1971;78:107–26.

Dahlin E, Neely AS, et al. Transfer of learning after updating training mediated by the striatum. Science. 2008;320(5882):1510–2.

De Groot MH, Phillips SJ, et al. Fatigue associated with stroke and other neurologic conditions: implications for stroke rehabilitation. Arch Phys Med Rehabil. 2003;84(11).1714–20.

Degutis JM, Van Vleet TM. Tonic and phasic alertness training: a novel behavioral therapy to improve spatial and non-spatial attention in patients with hemispatial neglect. Front Hum Neurosci. 2010;4:60.

Desimone R. Visual attention mediated by biased competition in extrastriate visual cortex. Philos Trans R Soc Lond B Biol Sci. 1998;353(1373):1245–55.

Dikmen SS, Temkin NR, et al. Neurobehavioral effects of phenytoin prophylaxis of posttraumatic seizures. JAMA. 1991;265(10):1271–7.

Dikmen SS, Machamer JE, et al. Neuropsychological effects of valproate in traumatic brain injury: a randomized trial. Neurology. 2000;54(4):895–902.

Doctor JN, Castro J, et al. Workers' risk of unemployment after traumatic brain injury: a normed comparison. J Int Neuropsychol Soc. 2005;11(6):747–52.

Donohue SE, Wendelken C, et al. Retrieving rules for behavior from long-term memory. Neuroimage. 2005;26(4):1140–9.

Drake AI, Gray N, et al. Factors predicting return to work following mild traumatic brain injury: a discriminant analysis. J Head Trauma Rehabil. 2000;15(5):1103–12.

Duncan J, Burgess P, et al. Fluid intelligence after frontal lobe lesions. Neuropsychologia. 1995;33(3):261–8.

Duncan J, Emslie H, et al. Intelligence and the frontal lobe: the organization of goal-directed behavior. Cognit Psychol. 1996;30(3):257–303.

Erickson KI, Colcombe SJ, et al. Training-induced functional activation changes in dual-task processing: an FMRI study. Cereb Cortex. 2007;17(1):192–204.

Evans J. Rehabilitation of the dysexecutive syndrome. In: Wood R, McMillan T, editors. Neurobehavioural disability and social handicap. London: Psychology Press; 2001. p. 209–27.

Evans J. Can executive impairments be effectively treated? In: Effectiveness of rehabilitation for cognitive deficits. New York, Oxford University Press; 2005. p. 247–57.

Fellus JL, Elovic EP. Fatigue: assessment and treatment. In: Zasler ND, Katz DI, Zafonte R, editors. Brain injury medicine. New York: Demos Medical Publishing; 2007.

Fischer S, Gauggel S, et al. Awareness of activity limitations, goal setting and rehabilitation outcome in patients with brain injuries. Brain Inj. 2004;18(6):547–62.

Fish J, Manly T, et al. Compensatory strategies for acquired disorders of memory and planning: differential effects of a paging system for patients with brain injury of traumatic versus cerebrovascular aetiology. J Neurol Neurosurg Psychiatry. 2008a;79(8):930–5.

Fish J, Manly T, et al. Long-term compensatory treatment of organizational deficits in a patient with bilateral frontal lobe damage. J Int Neuropsychol Soc. 2008b;14(1):154–63.

Frencham KA, Fox AM, et al. Neuropsychological studies of mild traumatic brain injury: a meta-analytic review of research since 1995. J Clin Exp Neuropsychol. 2005;27(3):334–51.

Fuster JM. Executive frontal functions. Exp Brain Res. 2000;133(1):66–70.

Gazzaley A, Cooney JW, et al. Top-down enhancement and suppression of the magnitude and speed of neural activity. J Cogn Neurosci. 2005;17(3):507–17.

Gilbert SJ, Spengler S, et al. Functional specialization within rostral prefrontal cortex (area 10): a meta-analysis. J Cogn Neurosci. 2006;18(6):932–48.

Gilbertson MW, Gurvits TV, et al. Multivariate assessment of explicit memory function in combat veterans with posttraumatic stress disorder. J Trauma Stress. 2001;14(2):413–32.

Giles GM. Cognitive versus functional approaches to rehabilitation after traumatic brain injury: commentary on a randomized controlled trial. Am J Occup Ther. 2010;64(1):182–5.

Gold JI, Shadlen MN. Neural computations that underlie decisions about sensory stimuli. Trends Cogn Sci. 2001;5(1):10–6.

Goldman-Rakic PS, Friedman HR. The circuitry of working memory revealed by anatomy and metabolic imaging. In: Levin H, Eisenberg H, Benton A, editors. Frontal lobe function and dysfunction. New York: Oxford University Press; 1991. p. 72–91.

Gouveia PA, Brucki SM, et al. Disorders in planning and strategy application in frontal lobe lesion patients. Brain Cogn. 2007;63(3):240–6.

Gualtieri CT, Evans RW. Stimulant treatment for the neurobehavioural sequelae of traumatic brain injury. Brain Inj. 1988;2(4):273–90.

Haxby JV, Gobbini MI, et al. Distributed and overlapping representations of faces and objects in ventral temporal cortex. Science. 2001;293(5539):2425–30.

Hecaen H, Albert ML. Human neuropsychology. New York: Wiley; 1978.

Hillary FG. Neuroimaging of working memory dysfunction and the dilemma with brain reorganization hypotheses. J Int Neuropsychol Soc. 2008;14(4): 526–34.

Hillier SL, Sharpe MH, et al. Outcomes 5 years post-traumatic brain injury (with further reference to neurophysical impairment and disability). Brain Inj. 1997;11(9):661–75.

Hoffman AN, Cheng JP, et al. Administration of haloperidol and risperidone after neurobehavioral testing hinders the recovery of traumatic brain injury-induced deficits. Life Sci. 2008;83(17–18):602–7.

Hoge CW, McGurk D, et al. Mild traumatic brain injury in U.S. Soldiers returning from Iraq. N Engl J Med. 2008;358(5):453–63.

Huckans M, Pavawalla S, et al. A pilot study examining effects of group-based Cognitive Strategy Training treatment on self-reported cognitive problems, psychiatric symptoms, functioning, and compensatory strategy use in OIF/OEF combat veterans with persistent mild cognitive disorder and history of traumatic brain injury. J Rehabil Res Dev. 2010;47(1):43–60.

Hux K, Schneider T, et al. Screening for traumatic brain injury. Brain Inj. 2009;23(1):8–14.

Hyndman D, Ashburn A. People with stroke living in the community: attention deficits, balance, ADL ability and falls. Disabil Rehabil. 2003;25(15):817–22.

Ilinisky IA, Jouandet ML, et al. Organization of the nigrothalamocortical system in the rhesus monkey. J Comp Neurol. 1985;236:315–30.

Jaeggi SM, Buschkuehl M, et al. Improving fluid intelligence with training on working memory. Proc Natl Acad Sci USA. 2008;105(19):6829–33.

Jazayeri M. Probabilistic sensory recoding. Curr Opin Neurobiol. 2008;18(4):431–7.

Jha AP, Krompinger J, et al. Mindfulness training modifies subsystems of attention. Cogn Affect Behav Neurosci. 2007;7(2):109–19.

Kabat-Zinn J. Full catastrophe living. New York, NY: Delacorte Press; 1990.

Kane MJ, Engle RW. The role of prefrontal cortex in working-memory capacity, executive attention, and general fluid intelligence: an individual-differences perspective. Psychon Bull Rev. 2002;9(4):637–71.

Kelly AM, Garavan H. Human functional neuroimaging of brain changes associated with practice. Cereb Cortex. 2005;15(8):1089–102.

Kelly C, Foxe JJ, et al. Patterns of normal human brain plasticity after practice and their implications for neurorehabilitation. Arch Phys Med Rehabil. 2006;87(12 Suppl 2):S20–9.

Kennedy MR, Coelho C, et al. Intervention for executive functions after traumatic brain injury: a systematic review, meta-analysis and clinical recommendations. Neuropsychol Rehabil. 2008;18(3):257–99.

Kesler SR, Adams HF, et al. Premorbid intellectual functioning, education, and brain size in traumatic brain injury: an investigation of the cognitive reserve hypothesis. Appl Neuropsychol. 2003;10(3):153–62.

Kim YH, Yoo WK, et al. Plasticity of the attentional network after brain injury and cognitive rehabilitation. Neurorehabil Neural Repair. 2009;23(5):468–77.

Kimberg DY, D'Esposito M, et al. Effects of bromocriptine on human subjects depend on working memory capacity. Neuroreport. 1997;8(16):3581–5.

Kline AE, Hoffman AN, et al. Chronic administration of antipsychotics impede behavioral recovery after experimental traumatic brain injury. Neurosci Lett. 2008;448(3):263–7.

Klingberg T. Training and plasticity of working memory. Trends Cogn Sci. 2010;14(7):317–24.

Laatsch LK, Thulborn KR, et al. Investigating the neurobiological basis of cognitive rehabilitation therapy with fMRI. Brain Inj. 2004;18(10):957–74.

Langlois JA, Kegler SR, et al. Traumatic brain injury-related hospital discharges. Results from a 14-state surveillance system, 1997. MMWR Surveill Summ. 2003;52(4):1–20.

Leskin LP, White PM. Attentional networks reveal executive function deficits in posttraumatic stress disorder. Neuropsychology. 2007;21(3):275–84.

Levine B, Robertson IH, et al. Rehabilitation of executive functioning: an experimental-clinical validation of goal management training. J Int Neuropsychol Soc. 2000;6(3):299–312.

Levine B, Stuss DT, et al. Cognitive rehabilitation in the elderly: effects on strategic behavior in relation to goal management. J Int Neuropsychol Soc. 2007;13(1): 143–52.

Levine B, Turner G, et al. (2008). Cognitive rehabilitation of executive dysfunction In : Cognitive Neurorehabilitation: Evidence & Applications (2nd Edition). D. T. Stuss, G. Winocur and I. H. Robertson Editors. Cambridge Unuversity Press; pp 464–87.

Lewis V, Creamer M, et al. Is poor sleep in veterans a function of post-traumatic stress disorder? Mil Med. 2009;174(9):948–51.

Lezak MD. Neuropsychological assessment. New York: Oxford University Press; 1995.

Luks TL, Simpson GV, et al. Evidence for anterior cingulate cortex involvement in monitoring preparatory attentional set. Neuroimage. 2002;17(2):792–802.

Machamer J, Temkin N, et al. Stability of employment after traumatic brain injury. J Int Neuropsychol Soc. 2005;11(7):807–16.

MacLeod CM. Half a century of research on the Stroop effect: an integrative review. Psychol Bull. 1991;109(2):163–203.

MacLeod CM, Dunbar K. Training and Stroop-like interference: evidence for a continuum of automaticity. J Exp Psychol Learn Mem Cogn. 1988;14(1):126–35.

Mahmood O, Rapport LJ, et al. Neuropsychological performance and sleep disturbance following traumatic brain injury. J Head Trauma Rehabil. 2004;19(5):378–90.

Manly T, Robertson IH, et al. The absent mind: further investigations of sustained attention to response. Neuropsychologia. 1999;37(6):661–70.

Manly T, Hawkins K, et al. Rehabilitation of executive function: facilitation of effective goal management on complex tasks using periodic auditory alerts. Neuropsychologia. 2002;40:271–81.

Mathias JL, Coats JL. Emotional and cognitive sequelae to mild traumatic brain injury. J Clin Exp Neuropsychol. 1999;21(2):200–15.

Mathias JL, Beall JA, et al. Neuropsychological and information processing deficits following mild traumatic brain injury. J Int Neuropsychol Soc. 2004;10(2): 286–97.

Mauri M, Sinforiani E, et al. Interaction between Apolipoprotein epsilon 4 and traumatic brain injury in patients with Alzheimer's disease and Mild Cognitive Impairment. Funct Neurol. 2006;21(4):223–8.

McDowell S, Whyte J, et al. Differential effect of a dopaminergic agonist on prefrontal function in traumatic brain injury patients. Brain. 1998;121(Pt 6):1155–64.

McNab F, Varrone A, et al. Changes in cortical dopamine D1 receptor binding associated with cognitive training. Science. 2009;323(5915):800–2.

Mednick S, Nakayama K, et al. Sleep-dependent learning: a nap is as good as a night. Nat Neurosci. 2003;6(7): 697–8.

Meintzschel F, Ziemann U. Modification of practice-dependent plasticity in human motor cortex by neuromodulators. Cereb Cortex. 2006;16(8):1106–15.

Miller EK, Cohen JD. An integrative theory of prefrontal cortex function. Annu Rev Neurosci. 2001;24: 167–202.

Miller BT, D'Esposito M. Searching for "the top" in top-down control. Neuron. 2005;48(4):535–8.

Milliken CS, Auchterlonie JL, et al. Longitudinal assessment of mental health problems among active and reserve component soldiers returning from the Iraq war. JAMA. 2007;298(18):2141–8.

Miotto EC, Savage CR, et al. Bilateral activation of the prefrontal cortex after strategic semantic cognitive training. Hum Brain Mapp. 2006;27(4):288–95.

Miotto E, Evans J, et al. Rehabilitation of executive dysfunction: a controlled trial of an attention and problem solving treatment group. Neuropsychol Rehabil. 2009;19:517–40.

Monson C, Schnurr P, et al. Cognitive processing therapy for veterans with military-related posttraumatic stress disorder. J Consult Clin Psychol. 2006;74(5): 898–907.

Muzur A, Pace-Schott EF, et al. The prefrontal cortex in sleep. Trends Cogn Sci. 2002;6(11):475–81.

Nampiaparampil D. Prevalence of chronic pain after traumatic brain injury: a systematic review. JAMA. 2008;300(6):711–9.

Neckelmann D, Mykletun A, et al. Chronic insomnia as a risk factor for developing anxiety and depression. Sleep. 2007;30(7):873–80.

Newman SD, Carpenter PA, et al. Frontal and parietal participation in problem solving in the Tower of London: fMRI and computational modeling of planning and high-level perception. Neuropsychologia. 2003;41(12):1668–82.

Nezu AM, Nezu CM, et al. Solving life's problems. New York: Springer Publishing Company; 2007.

Nithianantharajah J, Hannan AJ. The neurobiology of brain and cognitive reserve: mental and physical activity as modulators of brain disorders. Prog Neurobiol. 2009;89(4):369–82.

Novakovic-Agopian T, Chen A, et al. Rehabilitation of executive functioning with training in attention regulation applied to individually defined goals: a pilot study bridging theory, assessment and treatment. J Head Trauma Rehabil. 2011;26(5):325–38.

Okie S. Traumatic brain injury in the war zone. N Engl J Med. 2005;352(20):2043–7.

Olesen PJ, Westerberg H, et al. Increased prefrontal and parietal activity after training of working memory. Nat Neurosci. 2004;7(1):75–9.

Olver JH, Ponsford JL, et al. Outcome following traumatic brain injury: a comparison between 2 and 5 years after injury. Brain Inj. 1996;10(11):841–8.

Ownsworth T, McKenna K. Investigation of factors related to employment outcome following traumatic brain injury: a critical review and conceptual model. Disabil Rehabil. 2004;26(13):765–83.

Ozdemir F, Birtane M, et al. Cognitive evaluation and functional outcome after stroke. Am J Phys Med Rehabil. 2001;80(6):410–5.

Park DC, Polk TA, et al. Aging reduces neural specialization in ventral visual cortex. Proc Natl Acad Sci USA. 2004;101(35):13091–5.

Paulus MP, Potterat EG, et al. A neuroscience approach to optimizing brain resources for human performance in extreme environments. Neurosci Biobehav Rev. 2009;33(7):1080–8.

Persson J, Reuter-Lorenz PA. Gaining control: training executive function and far transfer of the ability to resolve interference. Psychol Sci. 2008;19(9):881–8.

Petersen SE, van Mier H, et al. The effects of practice on the functional anatomy of task performance. Proc Natl Acad Sci USA. 1998;95(3):853–60.

Phelps EA, Delgado MR, et al. Extinction learning in humans: role of the amygdala and vmPFC. Neuron. 2004;43(6):897–905.

Plassman BL, Havlik RJ, et al. Documented head injury in early adulthood and risk of Alzheimer's disease and other dementias. Neurology. 2000;55(8):1158–66.

Polusny MA, Kehle SM, et al. Longitudinal effects of mild traumatic brain injury and posttraumatic stress disorder comorbidity on postdeployment outcomes in national guard soldiers deployed to Iraq. Arch Gen Psychiatry. 2011;68(1):79–89.

Posner MI. Measuring alertness. Ann N Y Acad Sci. 2008;1129:193–9.

Posner MI, Sheese BE, et al. Analyzing and shaping human attentional networks. Neural Netw. 2006;19(9): 1422–9.

Postle BR. Working memory as an emergent property of the mind and brain. Neurosci. 2006;139:23–38.

Prigatano GP, Wong JL. Cognitive and affective improvement in brain dysfunctional patients who achieve inpatient rehabilitation goals. Arch Phys Med Rehabil. 1999;80(1):77–84.

Ranganath C. Working memory for visual objects: complementary roles of inferior temporal, medial temporal, and prefrontal cortex. Neuroscience. 2006;139(1):277–89.

Ranganath C, Johnson MK, et al. Prefrontal activity associated with working memory and episodic long-term memory. Neuropsychologia. 2003;41(3):378–89.

Ranganath C, Heller AS, et al. Dissociable correlates of two classes of retrieval processing in prefrontal cortex. Neuroimage. 2007;35(4):1663–73.

Raskin SA. Memory. In: Raskin SA, Mateer C, editors. Neuropsychological management of mild traumatic brain injury. Oxford: Oxford University Press; 2000.

Rath J, Simon D, et al. Group treatment of problem-solving deficits in outpatients with traumatic brain injury: a randomised outcome study. Neuropsychol Rehabil. 2003;13(4):461–88.

Rauch S, Defever E, et al. Prolonged exposurefor PTSD in a Veterans Health Administration PTSD clinic. J Trauma Stress. 2009;22(1):60–4.

Repovs G, Baddeley A. The multi-component model of working memory: explorations in experimental cognitive psychology. Neuroscience. 2006;139(1):5–21.

Robertson IH. Goal management training: a clinical manual. Cambridge: PsyConsult. 1996.

Rohling ML, Faust ME, et al. Effectiveness of cognitive rehabilitation following acquired brain injury: a meta-analytic re-examination of Cicerone et al'.s (2000, 2005) systematic reviews. Neuropsychology. 2009;23(1):20–39.

Rosen HJ, Petersen SE, et al. Neural correlates of recovery from aphasia after damage to left inferior frontal cortex. Neurology. 2000;55(12):1883–94.

Ruff R. Two decades of advances in understanding of mild traumatic brain injury. J Head Trauma Rehabil. 2005;20(1):5–18.

Saatman KE, Duhaime AC, et al. Classification of traumatic brain injury for targeted therapies. J Neurotrauma. 2008;25(7):719–38.

Salmond CH, Chatfield DA, et al. Cognitive sequelae of head injury: involvement of basal forebrain and associated structures. Brain. 2005;128(Pt 1):189–200.

Sanchez-Carrion R, Fernandez-Espejo D, et al. A longitudinal fMRI study of working memory in severe TBI patients with diffuse axonal injury. Neuroimage. 2008;43(3):421–9.

Scheid R, Walther K, et al. Cognitive sequelae of diffuse axonal injury. Arch Neurol. 2006;63(3):418–24.

Schneiderman AI, Braver ER, et al. Understanding sequelae of injury mechanisms and mild traumatic brain injury incurred during the conflicts in Iraq and Afghanistan: persistent postconcussive symptoms and posttraumatic stress disorder. Am J Epidemiol. 2008;167(12):1446–52.

Schnurr P, Friedman M, et al. Cognitive behavioral therapy for posttraumatic stress disorder in women: a randomized controlled trial. JAMA. 2007;297(8): 820–30.

Schumacher EH, Lauber E, et al. PET evidence for an amodal verbal working memory system. Neuroimage. 1996;3:79–88.

Schwartz A. New sign of brain damage in N.F.L. New York: New York Times; 2009.

Selemon RD, Goldman-Rakic PS. Common cortical and subcortical targets of the dorsolateral prefrontal and posterior parietal cortices in the rhesus monkey: evidence for a distributed neural network serving spatially guided behavior. J Neurosci. 1988;8: 4049–68.

Shallice T, Burgess PW. Deficits in strategy application following frontal lobe damage in man. Brain. 1991;114:727–41.

Silver JM, Koumaras B, et al. Effects of rivastigmine on cognitive function in patients with traumatic brain injury. Neurology. 2006;67(5):748–55.

Slagter HA, Lutz A, et al. Mental training affects distribution of limited brain resources. PLoS Biol. 2007;5(6):e138.

Smith Jr KR, Goulding PM, et al. Neurobehavioral effects of phenytoin and carbamazepine in patients recovering from brain trauma: a comparative study. Arch Neurol. 1994;51(7):653–60.

Sohlberg MM, Mateer CA. Effectiveness of an attention-training program. J Clin Exp Neuropsychol. 1987;9(2): 117–30.

Sohlberg MM, McLaughlin KA, et al. Evaluation of attention process training and brain injury education in persons with acquired brain injury. J Clin Exp Neuropsychol. 2000;22(5):656–76.

Soo C, Tate R. Psychological treatment for anxiety in people with traumatic brain injury. Cochrane Database Syst Rev. 2007(3): CD005239.

Spitzer H, Desimone R, et al. Increased attention enhances both behavioral and neuronal performance. Science. 1988;240(4850):338–40.

Stanislav SW. Cognitive effects of antipsychotic agents in persons with traumatic brain injury. Brain Inj. 1997;11(5):335–41.

Staub F, Bogousslavsky J. Fatigue after stroke: a major but neglected issue. Cerebrovasc Dis. 2001;12(2):75–81.

Strangman GE, Goldstein R, et al. Neurophysiological alterations during strategy-based verbal learning in traumatic brain injury. Neurorehabil Neural Repair. 2009;226–236.

Sturm W, de Simone A, et al. Functional anatomy of intrinsic alertness: evidence for a fronto-parietal-thalamic-brainstem network in the right hemisphere. Neuropsychologia. 1999;37(7):797–805.

Stuss DT, Alexander MP. Is there a dysexecutive syndrome? Philos Trans R Soc Lond B Biol Sci. 2007;362(1481):901–15.

Taber KH, Hurley RA. PTSD and combat-related injuries: functional neuroanatomy. J Neuropsychiatry Clin Neurosci. 2009;21(1):1p. preceding 1, 1–4.

Tatemichi TK, Paik M, et al. Dementia after stroke is a predictor of long-term survival. Stroke. 1994;25(10): 1915–9.

Thompson-Schill SL, Jonides J, et al. Effects of frontal lobe damage on interference effects in working memory. Cogn Affect Behav Neurosci. 2002;2(2):109–20.

Thurman D, Alverson C, et al. Traumatic brain injury in the United States: a public health perspective. J Head Trauma Rehabil. 1999;14(6):602–15.

Tucker MA, Hirota Y, et al. A daytime nap containing solely non-REM sleep enhances declarative but not procedural memory. Neurobiol Learn Mem. 2006;86(2):241–7.

van Baalen B, Odding E, et al. Cognitive status at discharge from the hospital determines discharge destination in traumatic brain injury patients. Brain Inj. 2008;22(1):25–32.

Van Den Heuvel C, Thornton E, et al. Traumatic brain injury and Alzheimer's disease: a review. Prog Brain Res. 2007;161:303–16.

van Reekum R, Cohen T, et al. Can traumatic brain injury cause psychiatric disorders? J Neuropsychiatry Clin Neurosci. 2000;12(3):316–27.

Van Vleet TM, Hoang-Duc AK, et al. Modulation of non spatial attention and the global/local processing bias. Neuropsychologia. 2011;49(3):352–9.

Vanderploeg RD, Curtiss G, et al. Long-term neuropsychological outcomes following mild traumatic brain injury. J Int Neuropsychol Soc. 2005;11(3):228–36.

Vanderploeg RD, Belanger HG, et al. Mild traumatic brain injury and posttraumatic stress disorder and their associations with health symptoms. Arch Phys MedRehabil. 2009;90:1084–93.

Vas A, Chapman S, et al. Higher-order reasoning training years after traumatic brain injury in adults. J Head Trauma Rehabil. 2011;26(3):224–39.

Vasterling JJ, Brewin CR. Neuropsychology of PTSD. New York: The Guilford Press; 2005.

Vasterling JJ, Brailey K, et al. Attention and memory dysfunction in posttraumatic stress disorder. Neuropsychology. 1998;12(1):125–33.

Vasterling JJ, Duke LM, et al. Attention, learning, and memory performances and intellectual resources in Vietnam veterans: PTSD and no disorder comparisons. Neuropsychology. 2002;16(1):5–14.

Verfaellie M, Vasterling JJ. Memory in PTSD: a neurocognitive approach. In: Shiromani P, Keane TM, LeDoux J, editors. Neurobiology of PTSD. Totowa, NJ: Humana Press; 2009. p. 105–32.

Vogel EK, McCollough AW, et al. Neural measures reveal individual differences in controlling access to working memory. Nature. 2005;438(7067):500–3.

Volkow ND, Wang GJ, et al. Sleep deprivation decreases binding of [11C]raclopride to dopamine D2/D3 receptors in the human brain. J Neurosci. 2008;28(34): 8454–61.

VonCramon D, Matthes-Von Cramon G, et al. Problem-solving deficits in brain-injured patients: a therapeutic approach. Neuropsychol Rehabil. 1991;1:45–64.

Warden DL, Gordon B, et al. Guidelines for the pharmacologic treatment of neurobehavioral sequelae of traumatic brain injury. J Neurotrauma. 2006;23(10): 1468–501.

Watson NF, Dikmen S, et al. Hypersomnia following traumatic brain injury. J Clin Sleep Med. 2007;3(4): 363–8.

Westerberg H, Jacobaeus H, et al. Computerized working memory training after stroke – a pilot study. Brain Inj. 2007;21(1):21–9.

Whyte J, Polansky M, et al. Sustained arousal and attention after traumatic brain injury. Neuropsychologia. 1995;33(7):797–813.

Whyte J, Hart T, et al. Effects of methylphenidate on attentional function after traumatic brain injury. A randomized, placebo-controlled trial. Am J Phys Med Rehabil. 1997;76(6):440–50.

Whyte J, Hart T, et al. Effects of methylphenidate on attention deficits after traumatic brain injury: a multidimensional, randomized, controlled trial. Am J Phys Med Rehabil. 2004;83(6):401–20.

Wilson MS, Gibson CJ, et al. Haloperidol, but not olanzapine, impairs cognitive performance after traumatic brain injury in rats. Am J Phys Med Rehabil. 2003;82(11):871–9.

Yaffe K, Laffan AM, et al. Sleep-disordered breathing, hypoxia, and risk of mild cognitive impairment and dementia in older women. JAMA. 2011; 306(6):613–9.

Yochim B, Baldo J, et al. D-KEFS Trail Making Test performance in patients with lateral prefrontal cortex lesions. J Int Neuropsychol Soc. 2007;13(4):704–9.

Yochim BP, Baldo JV, et al. D-KEFS Tower Test performance in patients with lateral prefrontal cortex lesions: the importance of error monitoring. J Clin Exp Neuropsychol. 2009;31(6):658–63.

Yoo SS, Hu PT, et al. A deficit in the ability to form new human memories without sleep. Nat Neurosci. 2007;10(3):385–92.

Yu W, Ravelo A, et al. Prevalence and costs of chronic conditions in the VA health care system. Med Care Res Rev. 2003;60(3 Suppl):146S–67.

Zafonte R, Lombard L, et al. Antispasticity medications: uses and limitations of enteral therapy. Am J Phys Med Rehabil. 2004;83(10 Suppl):S50–8.

Zeitzer JM, Friedman L, et al. Insomnia in the context of traumatic brain injury. J Rehabil Res Dev. 2009;46(6): 827–36.

Zelano C, Bensafi M, et al. Attentional modulation in human primary olfactory cortex. Nat Neurosci. 2005; 8(1):114–20.

Zhang ZG, Chopp M. Neurorestorative therapies for stroke: underlying mechanisms and translation to the clinic. Lancet Neurol. 2009;8(5):491–500.

Zhang L, Plotkin RC, et al. Cholinergic augmentation with donepezil enhances recovery in short-term memory and sustained attention after traumatic brain injury. Arch Phys Med Rehabil. 2004;85(7): 1050–5.

Current Diagnostic and Therapeutic Challenges

16

Donald W. Marion

Abstract

Traumatic brain injury (TBI) is a common cause of death and disability in the USA. Progress has been made in improving outcomes for those with moderate and severe TBI, but for those with mild TBI (concussion) significant diagnostic and therapeutic challenges remain. Concussion typically causes physiologic injury that results in an alteration of the level of consciousness, often associated with headaches, balance problems, and difficulties concentrating. While these symptoms typically clear within hours or days, there is increasing evidence that sustaining a second concussion before fully recovering from the first can lead to prolonged or permanent neurologic injury. Because the diagnosis of concussion currently relies on patient self-report, and the culture in groups most at risk for concussion (e.g., high school and college athletes and the military) is to withhold symptoms in order to return to play or duty as quickly as possible, there is an urgent need for a point-of-care battery of tests that can provide an objective, highly reliable diagnosis of concussion. This chapter reviews innovative technologies currently being evaluated for the objective diagnosis of concussion, and innovative TBI therapies currently in clinical trial.

Keywords

TBI • Concussion • mTBI • Diagnosis • Clinical trials • Head injury • Physiologic abnormalities • Diffusion tensor imaging • qEEG • Tau protein • Progesterone

D.W. Marion, M.D. (✉)
The Defense and Veterans Brain Injury Center,
Henry M. Jackson Foundation for the Advancement
of Military Medicine, 11300 Rockville Pike, Suite 1100,
Rockville, MD 20852, USA
e-mail: Donald.Marion@us.army.mil

J.W. Tsao (ed.), *Traumatic Brain Injury: A Clinician's Guide to Diagnosis, Management, and Rehabilitation*,
DOI 10.1007/978-0-387-87887-4_16, © Springer Science+Business Media, LLC 2012

Introduction

Traumatic brain injury (TBI) is the leading cause of death and disability among people in their first 4 decades of life. The National Center for Injury Prevention and Control estimates that 53,000 people (18.4/100,000 population) die each year from TBI-related injuries (Coronado et al. 2011). At present, the diagnosis of TBI is typically based on a clinical evaluation by a healthcare provider. The patient either presents to the provider, as with concussion, or is brought to the provider in the case of severe or moderate TBI. The hallmark of concussion is physiologic injury not associated with physical disruption or damage to CNS tissues, at least as can be detected with conventional imaging studies, due to an external event that imparts a concussive energy to the brain. There is an associated alteration of consciousness with or without amnesia for the event. Concomitant symptoms may include headache, insomnia, dizziness, and/or diminished attention or reaction time.

There is an urgent need for new diagnostic technology that will allow for the objective acute diagnosis of TBI, and especially of concussion. Patients with moderate and severe TBI typically have obvious neurologic signs and symptoms, and the brain injury can be identified utilizing conventional imaging studies, such as CT scanning. But concussion, or mild TBI, presents a unique diagnostic challenge because the neurologic signs and symptoms are much more subtle and typically require the patients to volunteer information to their provider, and to answer subjective questions about their recovery. The culture in subgroups of individuals most at risk, such as high school and college athletes and active duty military, is to minimize or ignore symptoms of concussion and not be forthcoming about such symptoms so that they can quickly return to play or battle. But if a person still symptomatic from a concussion sustains a second concussion before full recovery from the first, he or she is at an increased risk for prolonged or permanent neurologic injury. In part, this is because there is a significant mismatch of cerebral blood flow and metabolism immediately following a TBI which can be observed for several days (Barkhoudarian et al. 2011). More recent investigations also find that compensatory sodium channel metabolism following a concussion imposes a significant metabolic burden on the axon, and this too may contribute to the vulnerability of the tissue to prolonged or permanent damage following a second impact.

Recent findings from the Glasgow Traumatic Brain Bank are especially alarming (Johnson et al. 2010). Among the vast majority of TBI patients who survive, there is ongoing white matter degeneration for up to 10 years after injury. This includes thinning of the corpus collosum with up to 25–30% loss of volume. Others have documented amyloid precursor protein and, to a lesser extent, neurofibrillary tangles, as frequent findings in subjects with a history of multiple concussions who die from other causes (McKee et al. 2009). The concussions appear to cause hyperphosphorlyation and misfolding of tau protein leading to the abnormal deposition of the amyloid and neurofibrillary tangles, as well as stress granules. This pathology has been linked to the early onset of an Alzheimer's-like dementia, and is most common with multiple concussions.

There appears to be a general association between the presence of this metabolic mismatch and symptoms of TBI so that after the individual is completely symptom free he or she may no longer be at risk for significant neurologic injury from a subsequent concussion. Thus, an objective test or group of tests that can reliably diagnose concussion would be useful not only for the acute diagnosis, but also for return-to-duty or return-to-play decision making. This chapter reviews contemporary methods for diagnosing TBI and discusses new or experimental technology with a focus on novel imaging techniques, physiologic and cognitive testing, and serum biomarkers. Novel TBI therapies that currently are being considered for or are already in clinical trials also are described.

Innovative Diagnostic Techniques

The optimal test for the acute diagnosis of concussion will likely include a combination of three or more tests of neurologic or physiologic dysfunction (Marion et al. 2011). Diagnostic technology that can provide an objective evaluation for TBI and eliminate the need for the affected individual to volunteer symptoms is being developed in several areas: subtle neurologic and physiologic abnormalities, cognitive abnormalities, electrophysiologic abnormalities, imaging, and molecular biomarkers.

Physical Abnormalities

Concussion can result in a number of oculomotor problems manifesting as abnormal saccades, difficulty with smooth pursuit, or an abnormal vestibulo-ocular reflex. Technology is currently in development that will automate and computerize testing of this reflex in a device that is portable, quantitative, and requires minimal subject cooperation. The test is not capable of differentiating concussion from damage to the vestibular nerve or the peripheral vestibular apparatus, however. Olfaction also is impaired in a large proportion of people affected by TBI and is very easy to test—a person smells a scented card and is asked to identify the smell. Association of olfactory injury with concussion is not clear, however, and this may be a more common problem for those with moderate or severe injury where the olfactory fibers are severed at the cribriform plate. Damage to olfaction also can be caused by chemical or blast exposure to the airway making it nonspecific to TBI.

Physiologic Abnormalities

Autonomic dysfunction is a common acute manifestation of concussion (Hendricks et al. 2010). An automated system to monitor and analyze heart rate variability has been developed, but because heart rate variability also is seen with non-CNS trauma, it is not a very specific finding. Such a device would likely be most helpful for informing return to duty/play rather than as a diagnostic test. Moreover, it would likely be most useful as a component of a test battery that assessed other variables. Measurement of pupil size, and especially reactivity to light, is an alternative test of autonomic instability that also would require an automation and analysis package. A portable "pupillometer" has been developed but would need to be validated in concussion particularly because pupil abnormalities can be due to injury or compression of the optic or oculomotor cranial nerves in the absence of a concussion. Abnormalities with sweating have been described as an autonomic dysfunction associated with TBI, but clinically significant hyperhydrosis has only been reported in those with severe injuries (Hendricks et al. 2010).

Dizziness and balance disturbances are common problems associated with concussion, and together with headaches were identified as among the top three most common acute manifestations of sports-related concussion by NCAA sports medicine specialists (McCrory et al. 2009). It was recommended by this group that balance testing should be a component of any acute assessment of concussion. The Balance Error Scoring System (BESS), which utilizes a foam plate on which you have to balance and includes an easy-to-use scoring system, was introduced as a practical test of balance that could be used on the sideline of an athletic competition, or in combat medical facilities (Iverson et al. 2008). Sensitivity of the BESS to symptomatic concussion has not yet been adequately studied, so it would have to be clinically validated.

Cognitive Deficits

In order to standardize concussion evaluation for active duty Service Members, the Military Acute Concussion Evaluation (MACE) was developed as a screening algorithm for use by all military medical personnel, including those with very basic medical training. The MACE is composed of three parts that include a Standardized Assessment of Concussion (SAC), which is essentially a cognitive test of working memory, an evaluation of neurologic signs, and an evaluation of symptoms typically associated with concussion. Although the three parts of the MACE used together have not been formally validated, the SAC portion of the MACE has been in a cohort of civilians (McCrea et al. 2003). Its use currently is mandated as a first assessment for all Service Members who have a potentially concussive event, but there is some controversy about the cognitive portion of the MACE regarding its sensitivity and specificity when administered more than 12 h after concussion (Coldren et al. 2010). The Sports Concussion Assessment Tool (SCAT) 2 is a quasi-neurological exam that is slightly more standardized than the MACE, contains a symptom rating section that is on a continuum, and, most importantly, contains a balance test (McCrory et al. 2009). However, SCAT2 requires considerably more time to administer than the MACE and may therefore not be practical.

More recently, the Military implemented an "incident-based" directive for the evaluation of Service Members at risk for concussion which mandates concussion evaluation for all those exposed to a blast. While this circumvents the problem of Service Members not volunteering concussion-related symptoms, it does not address the lack of an objective diagnostic for concussion. A similar problem exists for civilian athletic teams in making return-to-play decisions. In the most recent NCAA International Symposia on Concussion in Sport, experts concluded that management and return-to-play decisions remained as a clinical judgment on an individual basis (McCrory et al. 2009).

Computerized neurocognitive assessment tools (NCATs) have been developed as convenient sideline methods for assessing cognitive deficits associated with sports-related concussions. Ideally, baseline studies are obtained preseason, and the results of the baseline can then be compared to post-injury studies. Following a concussion, changes in scores from the subject's own pre-injury baseline are more helpful for defining true cognitive deficits than are comparisons of post-injury tests with population norms. In the military, and pursuant to a congressional mandate, baseline NCATs have been obtained for deploying Service Members for more than 3 years and are available for comparison with post-injury studies. A comprehensive set of clinical recommendations for the indications and conditions for in-theater post-injury NCATs have been published by the Defense Centers of Excellence for Psychological Health and Traumatic Brain Injury, and provide specific guidance to providers on how and when to use the tests. NCAT performance is independently influenced by environmental factors, especially sleep deprivation, fatigue, and medications, so such guidance should significantly improve the quality of the studies obtained in the Military.

Smooth pursuit eye tracking also has been promoted as a measure of attention and working memory. Ocular movements can be tracked and quantified according to speed, direction, and delay, with much of the variation attributed to attention deficits. This technology will need clinical validation in theater and in civilian mTBI. Sleep deprivation and stress may also confound the results.

Electrophysiology

Conventional EEG is most useful for evaluating brain death, seizures, and sleep disorders. Certain EEG changes could be unique to concussion, but they will need to be well defined. A simplified cap-based 12-lead dry electrode array with a highly automated detection analysis system has been developed. But there are concerns about obtaining good signal-to-noise ratio in the field. Sleep deprivation and diet also can affect EEG, along with external 60-cycle interference. There will be a need to validate a well-defined concussion signature.

Quantitative EEG (qEEG) has the potential for summarizing the large amount of electrophysiologic data obtained from multiple leads over hours of monitoring. However, experience to date has shown that the study is highly sensitive to a variety of brain electrical activity, not all of which is pathologic, and it therefore is not very specific. There also is a lack of standardization for obtaining and interpreting qEEG.

Event-related potentials (ERPs), both auditory and visual induced, have been shown to be abnormal with mTBI. One of the most common TBI-induced abnormalities is the appearance of the P50 wave, which normally is suppressed. An ERP device for medic use has been developed and needs to be refined for field-deployable testing. There also is a need to validate ERPs in concussion, and determine if concussion is associated with a well-defined signature. Maximizing the signal-to-noise ratio, and avoiding artifact, is a primary concern with acquisition of good-quality, interpretable data.

Structural and Functional Imaging

Imaging of TBI patients with CT, and more recently MRI, is standard practice for those with moderate or severe injuries, and for concussed patients with severe or persistent symptoms or signs. In the acute setting, the primary concern is to identify intracranial mass lesions such as hematomas that require immediate surgical evacuation. Structural imaging may also help explain neurologic signs and symptoms associated with TBI by revealing areas of the brain that have been damaged by the trauma.

Head-only MRI is under development and may have utility in forward theater military treatment facilities. Since the average time for medical evacuation of injured Service Members is estimated at less than an hour, such imaging in theater may now be practical. In the last decade, diffusion tensor imaging (DTI) has been refined as an MRI technique with potential to assess subtle axonal injury not detectable on conventional T1, T2, or flair MRI sequences. With DTI, some of the most useful data are focal measures of the fractional anisotropy (FA) and apparent diffusion coefficient (ADC). Investigators have demonstrated a strong correlation between ADC values and verbal memory and processing speed, two cognitive areas frequently affected by concussion. But recent studies have not found as clear an association of DTI abnormalities with post-concussive disorder. In their study of 63 Service Members who had a clinical diagnosis of mild, uncomplicated TBI, and who underwent DTI within 90 days of their injury, MacDonald et al. found that only 18, or 29%, had abnormalities on DTI that were consistent with multifocal traumatic axonal injury (Mac Donald et al. 2011). In a DTI study of 60 civilian patients with mTBI evaluated within 1–2 months of injury, Lange and colleagues found no association between white matter integrity in the corpus callosum and self-reported postconcussion symptoms (Lange et al. 2011).

Moreover, the utility and reliability of DTI are limited by technical issues that include a lack of equivalency among centers, or even within a center. Thus, a DTI evaluation of an individual will vary depending on the magnet strength, magnet manufacturer, software used for data analysis, acquisition parameters, gradient number and directions, and several other variables. Many of these issues would be resolved with development of an appropriate phantom for systematic calibration of the machines.

Diffusion kurtosis imaging (DKI) has recently been developed as an MR imaging technique that accounts for the non-Gaussian properties of water diffusion in the brain. With DTI, the diffusion of water molecules through brain structures assumes monoexponential diffusion-weighted signal attenuation (Gaussian movement). The estimated diffusion parameters depend on the diffusion weighting strength, the *b*-value, which hampers the interpretation and comparison of various diffusion tensor imaging studies (Veraart et al. 2011). In contrast, the DKI model provides a *b*-value-independent estimation of the diffusion tensor parameters by measuring water diffusion in 15 or more directions. Data analysis utilizes a four-dimensional matrix referred to as the diffusion kurtosis tensor. As a result, DKI allows for the evaluation of gray matter which was not possible with DTI. It also has been found to be better for imaging astrogliosis, and an association between DKI abnormalities and elevated serum GFAP has been demonstrated.

Functional MRI (fMRI) can be used to image the regional or local cerebral metabolic changes associated with motor or cognitive activity. Blood oxygen level-dependent (BOLD) measurements following a cognitive challenge typically reveal enlargement of the area of BOLD activation, though not necessarily increase in the intensity of the activation, following a concussion. However, calibration of challenge fMRI studies is difficult, and there is substantial instability of the studies. Specifically, test-retest reliability is poor, so multicenter trials are currently not possible (Maitra et al. 2002). Resting fMRI has recently been proposed as a more stable protocol than challenge fMRI, and has been found to be especially helpful for evaluating functional connectivity between various regions of the brain (Jack et al. 2010).

Near-infrared spectroscopy (NIRS) can be used to detect abnormal patterns of metabolic activity similar to fMRI, and superficial hemorrhage, following TBI (van Rossem et al. 1999). Easy-to-use portable devices are available and are being used in studies of hemorrhage and task-related brain activation. Validation for use in detection of metabolic changes characteristic of concussion is the challenge, and may not be feasible with such subtle injury.

Several other imaging studies that provide valuable metabolic information, such as magnetic resonance spectroscopy and PET, are primarily research tools and will not have a practical role in the routine evaluation of TBI patients for the foreseeable future.

Molecular Biomarkers

Serum or whole blood biomarkers have been identified that are uniquely associated with TBI. Targeted proteins from neural tissue are furthest along the development path, but endothelial proteins also are associated with TBI. Ubiquitin C-terminal hydrolase 1 (UCHL1) was first detected as a brain-specific protein over 25 years ago, and currently is being tested as a promising biomarker for mTBI (Hausmann et al. 1999). S100B and glial fibrillary acidic protein (GFAP) have the potential to predict inflammatory injury to glia, and are both undergoing validation in humans (Pelinka et al. 2004; Wiesmann et al. 2010; Stranjalis et al. 2004; Mussack et al. 2000). Neuron-specific enolase (NSE) is associated with neuronal damage following TBI and serum levels are elevated, but primarily with moderate or severe TBI (Begaz et al. 2006; Stalnacke et al. 2004). In addition, copper, ceruloplasmin, and cuprizone have been proposed as potential biomarkers because of a key role they play in transmembrane calcium transport (Dash et al. 2010). Serum concentrations of peripherally produced apolipoprotein A-I (ApoA-I) are elevated within 6 h of mTBI. The increase is specific to brain injury, and associated with favorable short-term outcome. Other promising candidates for serum protein biomarkers are Tau (total and phosphorylated), alpha II spectrin breakdown protein (SBDP145—generated by calpain; SBDP120—generated by caspace), and beta amyloid precursor protein.

Metabolomics, transcriptomics, and unbiased proteomics are expected to reveal other protein and nonprotein biomarker candidates, including several inflammatory molecules. In addition, there currently are studies evaluating biomarkers in urine and saliva as alternative fluids for testing. Those fluids have the advantage of avoiding finger stick or venipuncture. But micro levels of the proteins being investigated are often undetectable in fluids other than serum or cerebrospinal fluid, and the latter is not practical to obtain in most settings. Serum levels of some of the promising molecular biomarkers, and especially those associated with the inflammatory response, can vary significantly with exposure to a myriad of environmental variables such as sleep deprivation, diet, non-CNS injury, and medications, so the clinical context in which the post-traumatic testing occurs needs to be thoroughly defined.

Energy Sensors

Impact or blast dosimeters have now been developed for detection of the degree and direction of mechanical energy exposure. The sensor data can be transmitted to a laptop computer or PDA, and allows providers to define the actual severity of impact to the helmet. Prototype devices are being used in high school and college football. However, there is some concern that while these detectors may reliably sense the energy imparted to the helmet, this may not reflect the energy imparted to the head because of independent movement of the helmet (Guskiewicz et al. 2007). Several studies of high school and college football players found no significant relationship between impact biomechanics measures, including linear acceleration and rotational acceleration, and post-concussive symptoms or cognitive performance change scores on a computerized neurocognitive assessment test (Guskiewicz et al. 2007; Broglio et al. 2011).

Studies currently underway are examining devices embedded in ear plugs and mouthguards, or attached directly to the head at the mastoid prominences.

Future Therapies for TBI

Current care of patients with a TBI is focused on the early identification of metabolic and physiologic dysfunction, and effective treatment of that dysfunction so as to limit or prevent permanent neurologic and functional damage. The pathobiology of TBI involves multiple biochemical, metabolic, inflammatory, and even genetic mechanisms. Failure of most previous therapies to benefit patients with TBI is likely because they targeted only one of these mechanisms responsible for secondary brain injury and not others that played a significant role. Drugs or other therapies most likely to be successful in future clinical trials must target multiple key mechanisms responsible for secondary brain injury. Those that are considered most promising, and are either currently or soon to be studied in clinical trials, include erythropoietin, statins, progesterone, and cyclosporine A.

Erythropoietin

Erythropoietin (EPO) is a 165 amino acid glycoprotein manufactured using recombinant human DNA technology. It has undergone extensive clinical testing and is approved by the FDA for the treatment of anemia due to renal failure. Preclinical studies of several models of TBI have consistently found that it has neuroprotective properties, acting via EPO receptors on cerebrovascular endothelia and ischemic neurons. EPO was shown to reduce hippocampal cell loss, enhance angiogenesis and neurogenesis, and improve functional outcome following TBI in rats (Xiong et al. 2010). In a similar TBI model, others found that EPO led to inhibition of the composition and secretion of S100B protein and IL-6 levels, suggesting that it may decrease the inflammatory reaction in the brain which may, in part at least, mediate the neuroprotective effect of EPO after TBI (Bian et al. 2010). These effects appear to be independent of the well-known increase in hematocrit associated with EPO therapy (Zhang et al. 2009). A Phase II clinical trial of EPO in 80 patients with aneurysmal subarachnoid hemorrhage was completed and found that the drug reduced the incidence of delayed cerebral ischemia by decreasing the severity of vasospasm and shortening the duration of impaired autoregulation (Tseng et al. 2009).

A randomized controlled clinical trial of recombinant human EPO for the treatment of severe TBI is currently underway (Baylor), and aims to enroll 200 patients (ClinicalTrials.gov Identifier: NCT00313716). The primary outcome measure is a set of biomarkers of cerebrovascular function, and the study is estimated to be completed by February 2013. The Australia–New Zealand Intensive Care Research Center also has initiated a clinical trial of EPO and plans to enroll 606 patients with moderate to severe TBI (GCS 3–12) at 15 hospitals in Australia, 3 hospitals in New Zealand, and 1 in Saudi Arabia, with an estimated study completion date of August 2014 (ClinicalTrials.gov Identifier: NCT00987454).

Statins

The statins are 3-hydroxy-3-methylglutaryl coenzyme A reductase inhibitors, and are thought to have neuroprotective effects because of their antioxidant and anti-inflammatory properties. Several statin formulations have been investigated; in a rat controlled cortical injury model, pre-injury treatment with lovastatin significantly improved functional outcomes, reduced contusion volume, and led to a significant reduction of levels of TNF-alpha and IL-1beta (Chen et al. 2007). Atorvastatin was shown to be effective in a weight drop rodent TBI model for reducing brain edema, lipid peroxidation, and ultrastructural changes (Turkoglu et al. 2009). There is some evidence that simvastatin may be more effective than the others: in a rodent study comparing atorvastatin with simvastatin, post-injury treatment was associated with better recovery of spatial learning in the group that received simvastatin

(Lu et al. 2007). In addition, simvastatin has been shown to reduce TBI-induced increases in A beta, reduce hippocampal damage and microglial activation, and improve behavioral outcomes (Abrahamson et al. 2009; Mahmood et al. 2009). Reduction of the A beta load following TBI may result in a reduced incidence of chronic traumatic encephalopathy over time.

In a mouse TBI model, the synergistic effects of EPO and simvastatin were investigated, and EPO was more effective than simvastatin in promoting cell proliferation, while simvastatin was more effective than EPO in restoring axonal damage (Chauhan and Gatto 2010). Combined treatment with simvastatin and EPO maximally restored axonal integrity while simultaneously inducing greater proliferation of newly formed cells, resulting in better functional recovery after TBI than treatment with either alone.

The University of Texas, Houston, and Baylor currently are conducting a Phase II randomized clinical trial of 200 subjects with concussion to evaluate atorvastatin therapy for 7 days after injury (ClinicalTrials.gov Identifier: NCT01013870). The study is scheduled to be completed by July of 2013.

Progesterone

Preclinical studies have found that progesterone decreases inflammation, reduces oxidative stress, decreases edema, and improves functional outcome following experimental TBI (Shahrokhi et al. 2010). These studies have also found a significant reduction in lesion volume associated with progesterone treatment of either cerebral ischemia or TBI, in a dose-dependent manner (Gibson et al. 2008). Progesterone appears to exert its protective effects by protecting or rebuilding the blood–brain barrier, decreasing the development of cerebral edema, down-regulating the inflammatory cascade, and limiting cellular necrosis and apoptosis (Hu et al. 2009).

A Cochrane Database review in January of 2011 identified three randomized controlled clinical trials of progesterone that had enrolled a total of 315 TBI patients (Junpeng et al. 2011). That meta-analysis found that progesterone treatment was associated with a pooled relative risk for mortality of 0.61; the relative risk for severe disability or death was 0.77. At present, the largest active clinical trial of a therapy for TBI is the Progesterone for the Treatment of Traumatic Brain Injury (ProTECT) III trial (ClinicalTrials.gov identifier: NCT00822900). That study began enrollment in March of 2010 and intends to enroll 1,140 adults with moderate or severe TBI by June of 2015.

Cyclosporin A

Cyclosporin A (CsA) inhibits the opening of the mitochondrial permeability transition pore, thereby maintaining mitochondrial homeostasis by inhibiting calcium influx, and preserving the mitochondrial membrane potential and cellular respiration. Murine models of TBI have found that post-injury treatment with CsA significantly reduces alpha-spectrin degradation, preserves mitochondrial integrity (Mbye et al. 2009), and restores *N*-acetylaspartate and ATP, two sensitive markers of mitochondrial dysfunction (Signoretti et al. 2004). In a large animal model, post-injury CsA treatment resulted in a significant reduction in amyloid precursor protein (APP) mRNA, and neuronal perikaryal APP antigen expression (Van Den Heuvel et al. 2004).

A prospective, randomized, placebo-controlled Phase I/II trial was published in 2009 with the aim to evaluate the safety, tolerability, and pharmacokinetics of a single intravenous infusion of CsA in patients with severe TBI (Mazzeo et al. 2009). Fifty adult patients with severe TBI were enrolled over a 22-month period and received treatment within 12 h of the injury. Compared with placebo, CsA was not associated with significant adverse events. However, there also was no significant difference in neurological outcomes. A clinical study of 50 adults with severe TBI examined the effect of 24 h of CsA treatment on brain extracellular metabolites using in vivo microdialysis (Mazzeo et al. 2008). That study found that CsA was associated with significantly higher extracellular levels of glucose and pyruvate, and a lower lactate/

pyruvate ratio, as compared to placebo. These findings suggested a positive effect of CsA treatment on post-traumatic brain energy metabolism.

Other Therapies

Stem cells, singularly or in combination with biomaterials that act as a scaffold, are being investigated in preclinical studies to reduce brain injury via neuroprotection, and promote brain remodeling via angiogenesis, neurogenesis, and synaptogenesis (Stabenfeldt and Irons 2011). Tissue engineering, using a bioactive scaffold, can help to counter some of the hostile host inflammatory factors that have limited the successful structural and functional integration of these transplants in the past. The scaffold can chaperone donor cells into the brain and promote differentiation of the cells into neurons, astrocytes, or oligodendrocytes as might be appropriate for the specific needs of the brain location. The cell source (i.e., embryonic, umbilical cord, bone marrow), scaffold composition, and delivery methods are all areas of intense investigation. In addition, enriched environment and voluntary physical exercise show promise in promoting functional outcome after TBI, and should be evaluated alone or in combination with other treatments as therapeutic approaches for TBI (Xiong et al. 2009).

Disclaimer The views expressed in this document are those of the author, and do not reflect official policy of the US Department of Defense, Department of Veterans Affairs, or the US Government.

References

Abrahamson EE, Ikonomovic MD, Dixon CE, DeKosky ST. Simvastatin therapy prevents brain trauma-induced increases in beta-amyloid peptide levels. Ann Neurol. 2009;66(3):407–14.

Barkhoudarian G, Hovda DA, Giza CC. The molecular pathophysiology of concussive brain injury. Clin Sports Med. 2011;30(1):33–48. vii–iii.

Begaz T, Kyriacou DN, Segal J, Bazarian JJ. Serum biochemical markers for post-concussion syndrome in patients with mild traumatic brain injury. J Neurotrauma. 2006;23(8):1201–10.

Bian XX, Yuan XS, Qi CP. Effect of recombinant human erythropoietin on serum S100B protein and interleukin-6 levels after traumatic brain injury in the rat. Neurol Med Chir (Tokyo). 2010;50(5):361–6.

Broglio SP, Eckner JT, Surma T, Kutcher JS. Post-concussion cognitive declines and symptomatology are not related to concussion biomechanics in high school football players. J Neurotrauma. 2011;28(10): 2061–8.

Chauhan NB, Gatto R. Synergistic benefits of erythropoietin and simvastatin after traumatic brain injury. Brain Res. 2010;1360:177–92.

Chen SF, Hung TH, Chen CC, Lin KH, Huang YN, Tsai HC, et al. Lovastatin improves histological and functional outcomes and reduces inflammation after experimental traumatic brain injury. Life Sci. 2007; 81(4):288–98.

Coldren RL, Kelly MP, Parish RV, Dretsch M, Russell ML. Evaluation of the Military Acute Concussion Evaluation for use in combat operations more than 12 hours after injury. Mil Med. 2010;175(7):477–81.

Coronado VG, Xu L, Basavaraju SV, McGuire LC, Wald MM, Faul MD, et al. Surveillance for traumatic brain injury-related deaths – United States, 1997–2007. MMWR Surveill Summ. 2011;60(5):1–32.

Dash PK, Redell JB, Hergenroeder G, Zhao J, Clifton GL, Moore A. Serum ceruloplasmin and copper are early biomarkers for traumatic brain injury-associated elevated intracranial pressure. J Neurosci Res. 2010; 88(8):1719–26.

Gibson CL, Gray LJ, Bath PM, Murphy SP. Progesterone for the treatment of experimental brain injury; a systematic review. Brain. 2008;131(Pt 2):318–28.

Guskiewicz KM, Mihalik JP, Shankar V, Marshall SW, Crowell DH, Oliaro SM, et al. Measurement of head impacts in collegiate football players: relationship between head impact biomechanics and acute clinical outcome after concussion. Neurosurgery. 2007;61(6):1244–52. discussion 52–3.

Hausmann R, Kaiser A, Lang C, Bohnert M, Betz P. A quantitative immunohistochemical study on the time-dependent course of acute inflammatory cellular response to human brain injury. Int J Legal Med. 1999; 112(4):227–32.

Hendricks HT, Heeren AH, Vos PE. Dysautonomia after severe traumatic brain injury. Eur J Neurol. 2010; 17(9):1172–7.

Hu Z, Li Y, Fang M, Wai MS, Yew DT. Exogenous progesterone: a potential therapeutic candidate in CNS injury and neurodegeneration. Curr Med Chem. 2009;16(11):1418–25.

Iverson GL, Kaarto ML, Koehle MS. Normative data for the balance error scoring system: implications for brain injury evaluations. Brain Inj. 2008;22(2):147–52.

Jack Jr CR, Bernstein MA, Borowski BJ, Gunter JL, Fox NC, Thompson PM, et al. Update on the magnetic resonance imaging core of the Alzheimer's disease

neuroimaging initiative. Alzheimers Dement. 2010;6(3): 212–20.
Johnson VE, Stewart W, Smith DH. Traumatic brain injury and amyloid-beta pathology: a link to Alzheimer's disease? Nat Rev Neurosci. 2010;11:361–70.
Junpeng M, Huang S, Qin S. Progesterone for acute traumatic brain injury. Cochrane Database Syst Rev. 2011(1):CD008409.
Lange RT, Iverson GL, Brubacher JR, Madler B, Heran MK. Diffusion tensor imaging findings are not strongly associated with postconcussional disorder 2 months following mild traumatic brain injury. J Head Trauma Rehabil. 2011 [Epub ahead of print].
Lu D, Qu C, Goussev A, Jiang H, Lu C, Schallert T, et al. Statins increase neurogenesis in the dentate gyrus, reduce delayed neuronal death in the hippocampal CA3 region, and improve spatial learning in rat after traumatic brain injury. J Neurotrauma. 2007;24(7): 1132–46.
Mac Donald CL, Johnson AM, Cooper D, Nelson EC, Werner NJ, Shimony JS, et al. Detection of blast-related traumatic brain injury in US military personnel. N Engl J Med. 2011;364(22):2091–100.
Mahmood A, Goussev A, Kazmi H, Qu C, Lu D, Chopp M. Long-term benefits after treatment of traumatic brain injury with simvastatin in rats. Neurosurgery. 2009;65(1):187–91. discussion 91–2.
Maitra R, Roys SR, Gullapalli RP. Test-retest reliability estimation of functional MRI data. Magn Reson Med. 2002;48(1):62–70.
Marion DW, Curley KC, Schwab K, Hicks RR. Proceedings of the military mTBI diagnostics workshop, St. Pete Beach, August 2010. J Neurotrauma. 2011;28(4): 517–26.
Mazzeo AT, Alves OL, Gilman CB, Hayes RL, Tolias C, Niki Kunene K, et al. Brain metabolic and hemodynamic effects of cyclosporin A after human severe traumatic brain injury: a microdialysis study. Acta Neurochir (Wien). 2008;150(10):1019–31. discussion 31.
Mazzeo AT, Brophy GM, Gilman CB, Alves OL, Robles JR, Hayes RL, et al. Safety and tolerability of cyclosporin a in severe traumatic brain injury patients: results from a prospective randomized trial. J Neurotrauma. 2009;26(12):2195–206.
Mbye LH, Singh IN, Carrico KM, Saatman KE, Hall ED. Comparative neuroprotective effects of cyclosporin A and NIM811, a nonimmunosuppressive cyclosporin A analog, following traumatic brain injury. J Cereb Blood Flow Metab. 2009;29(1):87–97.
McCrea M, Guskiewicz KM, Marshall SW, Barr W, Randolph C, Cantu RC, et al. Acute effects and recovery time following concussion in collegiate football players: the NCAA Concussion Study. JAMA. 2003;290(19):2556–63.
McCrory P, Meeuwisse W, Johnston K, Dvorak J, Aubry M, Molloy M, et al. Consensus statement on concussion in sport – the Third International Conference on Concussion in Sport held in Zurich, November 2008. Phys Sportsmed. 2009;37(2):141–59.
McKee AC, Cantu RC, Nowinski CJ, Hedley-Whyte ET, Gavett BE, Budson AE, et al. Chronic traumatic encephalopathy in athletes: progressive tauopathy after repetitive head injury. J Neuropathol Exp Neurol. 2009;68(7):709–35.
Mussack T, Biberthaler P, Wiedemann E, Kanz KG, Englert A, Gippner-Steppert C, et al. S-100b as a screening marker of the severity of minor head trauma (MHT) – a pilot study. Acta Neurochir Suppl. 2000;76:393–6.
Pelinka LE, Kroepfl A, Leixnering M, Buchinger W, Raabe A, Redl H. GFAP versus S100B in serum after traumatic brain injury: relationship to brain damage and outcome. J Neurotrauma. 2004;21(11):1553–61.
Shahrokhi N, Khaksari M, Soltani Z, Mahmoodi M, Nakhaee N. Effect of sex steroid hormones on brain edema, intracranial pressure, and neurologic outcomes after traumatic brain injury. Can J Physiol Pharmacol. 2010;88(4):414–21.
Signoretti S, Marmarou A, Tavazzi B, Dunbar J, Amorini AM, Lazzarino G, et al. The protective effect of cyclosporin A upon N-acetylaspartate and mitochondrial dysfunction following experimental diffuse traumatic brain injury. J Neurotrauma. 2004; 21(9): 1154–67.
Stabenfeldt SE, Irons HR, Laplaca MC. Stem cells and bioactive scaffolds as a treatment for traumatic brain injury. Curr Stem Cell Res Ther. 2011;6(3):208–20.
Stalnacke BM, Tegner Y, Sojka P. Playing soccer increases serum concentrations of the biochemical markers of brain damage S-100B and neuron-specific enolase in elite players: a pilot study. Brain Inj. 2004;18(9):899–909.
Stranjalis G, Korfias S, Papapetrou C, Kouyialis A, Boviatsis E, Psachoulia C, et al. Elevated serum S-100B protein as a predictor of failure to short-term return to work or activities after mild head injury. J Neurotrauma. 2004;21(8):1070–5.
Tseng MY, Hutchinson PJ, Richards HK, Czosnyka M, Pickard JD, Erber WN, et al. Acute systemic erythropoietin therapy to reduce delayed ischemic deficits following aneurysmal subarachnoid hemorrhage: a Phase II randomized, double-blind, placebo-controlled trial. Clinical article. J Neurosurg. 2009;111(1):171–80.
Turkoglu OF, Eroglu H, Okutan O, Gurcan O, Bodur E, Sargon MF, et al. Atorvastatin efficiency after traumatic brain injury in rats. Surg Neurol. 2009;72(2):146–52. discussion 52.
Van Den Heuvel C, Donkin JJ, Finnie JW, Blumbergs PC, Kuchel T, Koszyca B, et al. Downregulation of amyloid precursor protein (APP) expression following post-traumatic cyclosporin-A administration. J Neurotrauma. 2004;21(11):1562–72.
van Rossem K, Garcia-Martinez S, De Mulder G, Van Deuren B, Engelborghs K, Van Reempts J, et al. Brain oxygenation after experimental closed head injury. A NIRS study. Adv Exp Med Biol. 1999;471:209–15.
Veraart J, Poot DH, Van Hecke W, Blockx I, Van der Linden A, Verhoye M, et al. More accurate estimation of diffusion tensor parameters using diffusion Kurtosis imaging. Magn Reson Med. 2011;65(1):138–45.

Wiesmann M, Steinmeier E, Magerkurth O, Linn J, Gottmann D, Missler U. Outcome prediction in traumatic brain injury: comparison of neurological status, CT findings, and blood levels of S100B and GFAP. Acta Neurol Scand. 2010;121(3):178–85.

Xiong Y, Mahmood A, Chopp M. Emerging treatments for traumatic brain injury. Expert Opin Emerg Drugs. 2009;14(1):67–84.

Xiong Y, Mahmood A, Meng Y, Zhang Y, Qu C, Schallert T, et al. Delayed administration of erythropoietin reducing hippocampal cell loss, enhancing angiogenesis and neurogenesis, and improving functional outcome following traumatic brain injury in rats: comparison of treatment with single and triple dose. J Neurosurg. 2010;113(3):598–608.

Zhang Y, Xiong Y, Mahmood A, Meng Y, Qu C, Schallert T, et al. Therapeutic effects of erythropoietin on histological and functional outcomes following traumatic brain injury in rats are independent of hematocrit. Brain Res. 2009;1294:153–64.

Coding for TBI

Theresa B. Lattimore

International Classification of Diseases, Ninth Revision, Clinical Modification (ICD-9-CM) Codes Used in Traumatic Brain Injury

Acute Injury Codes

Note that codes in categories 800, 801, 803, 804, 851, 852, 853, and 854 require a fifth digit as follows:

0. Unspecified state of consciousness
1. With no loss of consciousness
2. With brief [less than 1 h] loss of consciousness
3. With moderate [1–24 h] loss of consciousness
4. With prolonged [more than 24 h] loss of consciousness and return to preexisting conscious level
5. With prolonged [more than 24 h] loss of consciousness without return to preexisting conscious level

   Use fifth-digit 5 to designate when a patient is unconscious and dies before regaining consciousness, regardless of the duration of loss of consciousness
6. With loss of consciousness of unspecified duration
7. With concussion, unspecified

Note that these extenders do not apply to the 850xx series or 802xx series codes.

T.B. Lattimore, M.S.N., N.P.-C. (✉)
Traumatic Brain Injury Programs (M96), Wounded, Ill, & Injured (M96), & Injured Directorate, US Navy Bureau of Medicine and Surgery, Washington, DC, USA
e-mail: tracie.lattimore@gmail.com

Traumatic Brain Injury with Skull Fracture

800.00–800.09	Fracture of vault of skull, closed, without mention of intracranial injury
800.10–800.19	Fracture of vault of skull, closed, with cerebral laceration and contusion
800.20–800.29	Fracture of vault of skull, closed, with subarachnoid, subdural, and extradural hemorrhage
800.30–800.39	Fracture of vault of skull, closed, with other and unspecified intracranial hemorrhage
800.40–800.49	Fracture of vault of skull, closed, with intracranial injury of other and unspecified nature
800.50–800.59	Fracture of vault of skull, open, without mention of intracranial injury
800.60–800.69	Fracture of vault of skull, open, with cerebral laceration and contusion
800.70–800.79	Fracture of vault of skull, open, with subarachnoid, subdural, and extradural hemorrhage
800.80–800.89	Fracture of vault of skull, open, with other and unspecified intracranial hemorrhage
800.90–800.99	Fracture of vault of skull, open, with intracranial injury of other and unspecified nature
801.00–801.09	Fracture of base of skull, closed, without mention of intracranial injury
801.10–801.19	Fracture of base of skull, closed, with cerebral laceration and contusion
801.20–801.29	Fracture of base of skull, closed, with subarachnoid, subdural, and extradural hemorrhage
801.30–801.39	Fracture of base of skull, closed, with other and unspecified intracranial hemorrhage

J.W. Tsao (ed.), *Traumatic Brain Injury: A Clinician's Guide to Diagnosis, Management, and Rehabilitation*,
DOI 10.1007/978-0-387-87887-4, © Springer Science+Business Media, LLC 2012

801.40–801.49	Fracture of base of skull, closed, with intracranial injury of other and unspecified nature
801.50–801.59	Fracture of base of skull, open, without mention of intracranial injury
801.60–801.69	Fracture of base of skull, open, with cerebral laceration and contusion
801.70–801.79	Fracture of base of skull, open, with subarachnoid, subdural, and extradural hemorrhage
801.80–801.89	Fracture of base of skull, open, with other and unspecified intracranial hemorrhage
801.90–801.99	Fracture of base of skull, open, with intracranial injury of other and unspecified nature
802.0	Closed fracture of the nasal bones
802.1	Open fracture of the nasal bones
802.20–802.29	Closed fracture of the mandible
803.00–803.09	Other and unqualified skull fractures, closed, without mention of intracranial injury
803.10–803.19	Other and unqualified skull fractures, closed, with cerebral laceration and contusion
803.20–803.29	Other and unqualified skull fractures, closed, with subarachnoid, subdural, and extradural hemorrhage
803.30–803.39	Other and unqualified skull fractures, closed, with other and unspecified intracranial hemorrhage
803.40–803.49	Other and unqualified skull fractures, closed, with intracranial injury of other and unspecified nature
803.50–803.59	Other and unqualified skull fractures, open, without mention of intracranial injury
803.60–803.69	Other and unqualified skull fractures, open, with cerebral laceration and contusion
803.70–803.79	Other and unqualified skull fractures, open, with subarachnoid, subdural, and extradural hemorrhage
803.80–803.89	Other and unqualified skull fractures, open, with other and unspecified intracranial hemorrhage
803.90–803.99	Other and unqualified skull fractures, open, with intracranial injury of other and unspecified nature
804.00–804.09	Multiple fractures involving skull or face with other bones, closed, without mention of intracranial injury
804.10–804.19	Multiple fractures involving skull or face with other bones, closed, with cerebral laceration and contusion
804.20–804.29	Multiple fractures involving skull or face with other bones, closed, with subarachnoid, subdural, and extradural hemorrhage
804.30–804.39	Multiple fractures involving skull or face with other bones, closed, with other and unspecified intracranial hemorrhage
804.40–804.49	Multiple fractures involving skull or face with other bones, closed, with intracranial injury of other and unspecified nature
804.50–804.59	Multiple fractures involving skull or face with other bones, open, without mention of intracranial injury
804.60–804.69	Multiple fractures involving skull or face with other bones, open, with cerebral laceration and contusion
804.70–804.79	Multiple fractures involving skull or face with other bones, open, with subarachnoid, subdural, and extradural hemorrhage
804.80–804.89	Multiple fractures involving skull or face with other bones, open, with other and unspecified intracranial hemorrhage
804.90–804.99	Multiple fractures involving skull or face with other bones, open, with intracranial injury of other and unspecified nature

Traumatic Brain Injury Without Skull Fracture

850.0	Concussion with no loss of consciousness
850.11	Concussion with brief loss of consciousness of 30 min or less
850.12	Concussion with brief loss of consciousness of 31–59 min
850.2	Concussion with moderate loss of consciousness (1–24 h)
850.3	With prolonged loss of consciousness (more than 24 h) and return to preexisting conscious level (complete recovery)
850.4	Concussion with prolonged loss of consciousness without return to preexisting conscious level
850.5	With loss of consciousness of unspecified duration
850.9	Concussion, unspecified
851.00–851.09	Cortex (cerebral) contusion without mention of open intracranial wound

851.10–851.19	Cortex (cerebral) contusion with open intracranial wound
851.20–851.29	Cortex (cerebral) laceration without mention of open intracranial wound
851.30–851.39	Cortex (cerebral) laceration with open intracranial wound
851.40–851.49	Cerebellar or brain stem contusion without mention of open intracranial wound
851.50–851.59	Cerebellar or brain stem contusion with open intracranial wound
851.60–852.69	Cerebellar or brain stem laceration without mention of open intracranial wound
851.70–851.79	Cerebellar or brain stem laceration with open intracranial wound
851.80–851.89	Other and unspecified cerebral laceration and contusion, without mention of open intracranial wound
851.90–851.99	Other and unspecified cerebral laceration and contusion, with open intracranial wound
852.00–852.09	Subarachnoid hemorrhage following injury without mention of open intracranial wound
852.10–852.19	Subarachnoid hemorrhage following injury with open intracranial wound
852.20–852.29	Subdural hemorrhage following injury without mention of open intracranial wound
852.30–852.39	Subdural hemorrhage following injury with open intracranial wound
852.40–852.49	Extradural hemorrhage following injury without mention of open intracranial wound
852.50–852.59	Extradural hemorrhage following injury with open intracranial wound
853.00–853.09	Other and unspecified intracranial hemorrhage following injury, without mention of open intracranial wound (This is the default code for *Traumatic cerebral hemorrhage*)
853.10–853.19	Other and unspecified intracranial hemorrhage following injury, with open intracranial wound
854.00–854.09	Intracranial injury of other and unspecified nature without mention of open intracranial wound (This is the default code for *Traumatic brain injury but other codes more accurately reflect the degree of injury*)
854.10–854.19	Intracranial injury of other and unspecified nature with open intracranial wound
959.01	Head injury, unspecified

Manifestation Codes

Coding manifestation is encouraged since there is not one common presentation for traumatic brain injury (TBI). The "coma" codes from 780.0 to 780.93 may NOT be used with TBI. Likewise, memory loss, 780.93, may NOT be used with TBI. The manifestation codes should be listed after the primary TBI code from the preceding list during the acute hospitalization.

Following is a list of relatively new or little known TBI code manifestations:

310.0	Frontal lobe syndrome (due to brain damage)
310.2	Postconcussion syndrome
310.8	Other specified nonpsychotic mental disorders following organic brain damage Mild memory disturbance due to organic brain damage
339.20	Posttraumatic headache, unspecified
339.21	Acute posttraumatic headache
339.22	Chronic posttraumatic headache

These codes are new and available for use beginning October 1, 2010

780.33	Posttraumatic seizures Note that this code is not to be used for posttraumatic epilepsy, where the appropriate code from category 345.xx should be used
799.50	Unspecified signs and symptoms involving cognition
799.51	Attention or concentration deficit
799.52	Cognitive communication deficit
799.53	Visuospatial deficit
799.54	Psychomotor deficit
799.55	Frontal lobe and executive function deficit Note that the code 310.0 is to be used if the manifestation is due to *brain damage*
799.59	Other signs and symptoms involving cognition

The 799-series codes (different from those mentioned above) allow providers to code emotional/behavioral symptoms without using mental health diagnosis codes. These codes do not replace mental health diagnosis codes. Providers should use these codes when they observe the symptoms but a mental health diagnosis is not established.

While these codes are intended to be used for TBI symptoms, they are not limited to TBI.

799.21: nervousness
799.22: irritability
799.23: impulsiveness
799.24: emotional lability
799.25: demoralization and apathy
799.29: other signs and symptoms involving emotional state

Other manifestations, such as paresis, speech and language disturbances, and sleep disorders, may be found in the *ICD-9-CM* index and are too numerous to list here.

Late Effects of Traumatic Brain Injury

Anytime after the acute phase, manifestations of TBI would be considered "late effects." The first-listed code becomes the manifestation (late effect), and the second code is a "late effect code" appropriate to the injury as listed below:

905.0	Late effect of fracture of skull and facial bones Late effect injury classifiable to 800–804
907.0	Late effect of intracranial injury without mention of skull fracture Late effect of injury classifiable to 850–854

Screening for Traumatic Brain Injury

Especially in the military setting, patients may be screened for possible TBI. The code to be used in this situation is

V80.01	Screening for traumatic brain injury

The military currently uses this code to denote screening for TBI regardless of the outcome of the screening (concussion or no concussion).

Personal History of Traumatic Brain Injury Related to the Global War on Terrorism

This series of codes was developed for the military to assist in tracking TBI, particularly those sustained in relation to the Global War on Terrorism (GWOT). The military requires this code with all TBI documentation. Since it is broken down by relation to GWOT and severity level it provides more significant detail for surveillance purposes. It may be of value in some cases to add the information to a list of diagnoses that a patient has a history of TBI, and instances may occur when no "late effect" is present; this information needs to be captured. In that case, use the code

V15.52_0	Personal History of traumatic brain injury (TBI) not otherwise specified
V15.52_1	Personal History of TBI, Global War on Terrorism (GWOT) Related, *Unknown* Severity Level
V15.52_2	Personal History of TBI, GWOT Related, *Mild*
V15.52_3	Personal History of TBI, GWOT Related, *Moderate*
V15.52_4	Personal History of TBI, GWOT Related, *Severe*
V15.52_5	Personal History of TBI, GWOT Related, *Penetrating* Intracranial Wound, No Level of Severity Assigned
V15.52_6	Personal History of TBI *not* GWOT Related, *Unknown* Level of Severity
V15.52_7	Personal History of TBI *not* GWOT Related, *Mild*
V15.52_8	Personal History of TBI *not* GWOT Related, *Moderate*
V15.52_9	Personal History of TBI *not* GWOT Related, *Severe*
V15.52_A	Personal History of TBI *not* GWOT Related, *Penetrating* Intracranial Wound, No Level of Severity Assigned
V15.52_B	Personal History of TBI, *Unknown* if GWOT Related, *Unknown* Severity Level
V15.52_C	Personal History of TBI, *Unknown* if GWOT Related, *Mild*
V15.52_D	Personal History of TBI, *Unknown* if GWOT Related, *Moderate*
V15.52_E	Personal History of TBI, *Unknown* if GWOT Related, *Severe*
V15.52_F	Personal History of TBI, *Unknown* if GWOT Related, *Penetrating* Intracranial Wound, No Level of Severity Assigned

These codes may not be a first-listed diagnosis.

Coding TBI in the Military Population

The military has unique needs related to coding for TBI. The military has significant instances of

TBI in both combat and the daily life associated with preparing for combat. As a result the military has placed great emphasis on capturing information through ICD-9 coding. In addition to the typical TBI codes used in the civilian sector, the military has created a series of TBI history codes that connect a patient to injury related to the Global War on Terrorism (GWOT). The military also encourages use of the External Injury Codes (E-codes) as appropriate. In particular the E979.2 (Terrorism Involving Other Explosions/Fragments), code is used to document TBI related to Improvised Explosive Devices (IEDs). The military also uses Deployment Status Codes to help determine if injury was related to combat and where care took place. Specifically V70.5_5 (During Deployment Encounter) and V70.5_6 (Post-deployment Encounter) can provide data on where the care of a combat-related injured service member took place. The military relies on the V80.01 (Screening for TBI) to capture screenings regardless of the resulting diagnosis. This code is key to the military surveillance picture because it provides data on how many exposures to potentially concussive events each service member has in relation to the number of diagnosed concussions. When used in combination these codes, both military specific and others, help provide military leaders with a unique blend of data on the current medical status as well as operational impact of TBI in the combat environment.

Quick Guide to Coding in the Military Population

The encounters must be broken down to initial visit and follow-up. At the initial visit, the first code used will be the primary diagnostic code (i.e., 8xx Series code). This is followed by the history of concussion code (V15.52_x). The third position is for any relevant symptom codes. The fourth position is the deployment status code followed by the screening code or the E-code. The TBI screening code can be at the end of the list. On any follow-up visits the first code will be the symptom code. However, the history of TBI code (V15.52_x) will be second. The deployment status code and late effect codes would be next. You do not recode the TBI diagnostic code, E-code or screening code at follow-up visits.

	Code TYPE	Details	Code at initial evaluation	Code for follow-up visit
1.	TBI diagnostic code	• 850.0 concussion without LOC • 850.1 concussion with brief LOC • 850.11 concussion with LOC ≤ 30 min	YES (Code 1st)	NO
2.	Personal history of TBI	• V15.52_1 Injury related to Global War on Terrorism, Unknown • V15.52_2 Injury related to Global War on Terrorism, Mild	YES (Code 2nd)	YES (Code 2nd)
3.	Symptom codes	• Common examples in TBI include: – 784.0 Headache – 388.3 Tinnitus	YES (Code 3rd)	YES (Code 1st)
4.	Late effect code	• 905.0 Late effect of intracranial injury with skull or facial fracture • 907.0 Late effect of intracranial injury w/o skull or facial fracture	NO	YES (Code 3rd)
5.	Deployment status code	• V70.5_5 During deployment encounter	YES (Code 4th)	YES (Code 4th)
6.	TBI screening code	• V80.01 Special Screening for TBI Code	If applicable (Code 5th)	NO
7.	E-code	• E979.2 Terrorism Involving Other Explosions/Fragments	If applicable (Code 6th)	NO

Current Procedural Terminology Coding for Traumatic Brain Injury

Current Procedural Terminology (CPT) coding does not depend on the diagnosis. It depends on the work performed in the service, and more work is needed for more serious presenting problems.

New patients with moderate to severe TBI are usually level 5 consultations CPT 99255 or level 3 admissions CPT 99223 because of the altered mental state and risk of substantial morbidity.

When managing the patient in the intensive care unit, and when the patient is unstable and critically ill, the correct codes are the critical care codes. These codes, CPT 99291 and 99292, use time as the basis for setting level of service instead of bullet points.

New office patients often have concussion, and the level of Evaluation and Management (E/M) service depends on the severity of the presenting problem and risk. For example, a level 3 office new patient visit CPT 99203 would be a high school athlete presenting asymptomatic 4 days after a concussion, requesting permission to return to playing in the football team next week. Symptomatic TBI patients usually require a higher level of service when seen in the office.

Index

J.W. Tsao (ed.), *Traumatic Brain Injury: A Clinician's Guide to Diagnosis, Management, and Rehabilitation*, DOI 10.1007/978-0-387-87887-4, © Springer Science+Business Media, LLC 2012

R

S

MIX
Papier aus verantwortungsvollen Quellen
Paper from responsible sources
FSC® C105338

If you have any concerns about our products,
you can contact us on
ProductSafety@springernature.com

In case Publisher is established outside the EU,
the EU authorized representative is:
Springer Nature Customer Service Center GmbH
Europaplatz 3, 69115 Heidelberg, Germany

Printed by Libri Plureos GmbH
in Hamburg, Germany